NUTRIENT COMPOSITION OF RATIONS FOR SHORT-TERM, HIGH-INTENSITY COMBAT OPERATIONS

Committee on Optimization of Nutrient Composition of Military Rations for Short-Term, High-Stress Situations

Committee on Military Nutrition Research

Food and Nutrition Board

INSTITUTE OF MEDICINE
OF THE NATIONAL ACADEMIES

THE NATIONAL ACADEMIES PRESS
Washington, D.C.
www.nap.edu

THE NATIONAL ACADEMIES PRESS • 500 Fifth Street, N.W. • Washington, DC 20001

NOTICE: The project that is the subject of this report was approved by the Governing Board of the National Research Council, whose members are drawn from the councils of the National Academy of Sciences, the National Academy of Engineering, and the Institute of Medicine. The members of the committee responsible for the report were chosen for their special competences and with regard for appropriate balance.

This study was supported by the United States Army (award number DAMD17-99-1-9478 with the National Academy of Sciences). Any opinions, findings, conclusions, or recommendations expressed in this publication are those of the authors and do not necessarily reflect the views of the sponsoring agency that provided support for the project.

International Standard Book Number: 0-309-09461-3 (Book)
International Standard Book Number: 0-309-54982-5 (PDF)

Additional copies of this report are available from the National Academies Press, 500 Fifth Street, N.W., Lockbox 285, Washington, DC 20055; (800) 624-6242 or (202) 334-3313 (in the Washington metropolitan area); Internet, http://www.nap.edu.

For more information about the Institute of Medicine, visit the IOM home page at: **www.iom.edu.**

The serpent has been a symbol of long life, healing, and knowledge among almost all cultures and religions since the beginning of recorded history. The serpent adopted as a logotype by the Institute of Medicine is a relief carving from ancient Greece, now held by the Staatliche Museen in Berlin.

"Knowing is not enough; we must apply.
Willing is not enough; we must do."
—Goethe

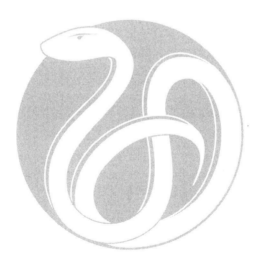

INSTITUTE OF MEDICINE
OF THE NATIONAL ACADEMIES

Advising the Nation. Improving Health.

THE NATIONAL ACADEMIES
Advisers to the Nation on Science, Engineering, and Medicine

The **National Academy of Sciences** is a private, nonprofit, self-perpetuating society of distinguished scholars engaged in scientific and engineering research, dedicated to the furtherance of science and technology and to their use for the general welfare. Upon the authority of the charter granted to it by the Congress in 1863, the Academy has a mandate that requires it to advise the federal government on scientific and technical matters. Dr. Ralph J. Cicerone is president of the National Academy of Sciences.

The **National Academy of Engineering** was established in 1964, under the charter of the National Academy of Sciences, as a parallel organization of outstanding engineers. It is autonomous in its administration and in the selection of its members, sharing with the National Academy of Sciences the responsibility for advising the federal government. The National Academy of Engineering also sponsors engineering programs aimed at meeting national needs, encourages education and research, and recognizes the superior achievements of engineers. Dr. Wm. A. Wulf is president of the National Academy of Engineering.

The **Institute of Medicine** was established in 1970 by the National Academy of Sciences to secure the services of eminent members of appropriate professions in the examination of policy matters pertaining to the health of the public. The Institute acts under the responsibility given to the National Academy of Sciences by its congressional charter to be an adviser to the federal government and, upon its own initiative, to identify issues of medical care, research, and education. Dr. Harvey V. Fineberg is president of the Institute of Medicine.

The **National Research Council** was organized by the National Academy of Sciences in 1916 to associate the broad community of science and technology with the Academy's purposes of furthering knowledge and advising the federal government. Functioning in accordance with general policies determined by the Academy, the Council has become the principal operating agency of both the National Academy of Sciences and the National Academy of Engineering in providing services to the government, the public, and the scientific and engineering communities. The Council is administered jointly by both Academies and the Institute of Medicine. Dr. Ralph J. Cicerone and Dr. Wm. A. Wulf are chair and vice chair, respectively, of the National Research Council.

www.national-academies.org

COMMITTEE ON OPTIMIZATION OF NUTRIENT COMPOSITION OF MILITARY RATIONS FOR SHORT-TERM, HIGH-STRESS SITUATIONS

JOHN W. ERDMAN (*Chair*), Department of Food Science and Human Nutrition, University of Illinois, Urbana-Champaign

BRUCE R. BISTRIAN, Beth Israel Deaconess Medical Center, Harvard Medical School, Boston, MA

PRISCILLA M. CLARKSON, School of Public Health and Health Sciences, University of Massachusetts, Amherst

JOHANNA T. DWYER, Office of Dietary Supplements, National Institutes of Health, Washington, DC

BARBARA P. KLEIN, Department of Food Science and Human Nutrition, University of Illinois, Urbana-Champaign

HELEN W. LANE, Johnson Space Center, National Aeronautics and Space Administration, Houston, TX

MELINDA M. MANORE, Department of Nutrition, Oregon State University, Corvallis

PATRICK M. O'NEIL, Weight Management Center, Institute of Psychiatry, Medical University of South Carolina, Charleston

ROBERT M. RUSSELL, Human Nutrition Research Center on Aging, Tufts University, Boston, MA

BEVERLY J. TEPPER, Department of Food Sciences, Cook College of Rutgers University, New Brunswick, NJ

KEVIN D. TIPTON, School of Sport and Exercise Sciences, University of Birmingham, Birmingham, England

ALLISON A. YATES, Environ Health Sciences Institute, Arlington, VA

Staff

MARIA P. ORIA, Study Director

JON Q. SANDERS, Senior Program Assistant

LESLIE J. SIM, Research Associate

FOOD AND NUTRITION BOARD

Reviewers

This report has been reviewed in draft form by individuals chosen for their diverse perspectives and technical expertise, in accordance with procedures approved by the National Research Council's Report Review Committee. The purpose of this independent review is to provide candid and critical comments that will assist the institution in making its published report as sound as possible and to ensure that the report meets institutional standards for objectivity, evidence, and responsiveness to the study charge. The review comments and draft manuscript remain confidential to protect the integrity of the deliberative process. We wish to thank the following individuals for their review of this report:

E. Wayne Askew, University of Utah, Salt Lake City

Barry Braun, Energy Metabolism Laboratory, University of Massachusetts, Amherst

William J. Evans, University of Arkansas for Medical Sciences, Little Rock

William C. Franke, Rutgers, State University of New Jersey, New Brunswick

Marc K. Hellerstein, University of California, Berkeley

Janet R. Hunt, USDA-ARS Grand Forks Human Nutrition Research Center, ND

Molly Kretsch, United States Department of Agriculture, Beltsville, MD

Ron J. Maughan, School of Sport and Exercise Science, Loughborough University, UK

Robert Nesheim, Salinas, CA

Michael D. Sitrin, Western New York Veterans Administration Medical Center, Buffalo, NY

Douglas W. Wilmore, Ilauea, HI

Although the reviewers listed above have provided many constructive comments and suggestions, they were not asked to endorse the conclusions or recommendations nor did they see the final draft of the report before its release. The review of this report was overseen by Richard N. Miller, M.D. Appointed by the Institute of Medicine, he was responsible for making certain that an independent examination of this report was carried out in accordance with institutional procedures and that all review comments were carefully considered. Responsibility for the final content of this report rests entirely with the authoring committee and the institution.

Preface

This report, titled *Nutrient Composition of Rations for Short-Term, High-Intensity Combat Operations,* is the product of the work of the Committee on Optimization of Nutrient Composition of Military Rations for Short-Term, High-Stress Situations under the auspices of the Standing Committee on Military Nutrition Research (CMNR). The CMNR was established in 1982 to advise the US Department of Defense on the need for and conduct of nutrition research and related issues. This report was produced in response to a request by the US Army Medical Research and Materiel Command to the Institute of Medicine (IOM) to convene a committee to review and recommend the nutritional composition of rations for short-term, high-stress situations. The specific questions posed to the committee evolved from discussions between the standing CMNR and the Military Nutrition Division of the US Army Research Institute of Environmental Medicine (USARIEM) at Natick, Massachusetts.

A 12-member committee was formed that had expertise on micronutrients, protein, energy balance and sports nutrition, gastroenterology, clinical medicine, food processing and technology, eating behavior and intake regulation, clinical nutrition, dietetics, and psychology. The committee's task was to conduct a study to determine the optimal nutrient content of a new combat ration. The committee first discussed the limitations of the current rations for use during future military deployments and combat operations and the expected impact of combat operations on nutrient status, health, and performance. Operating within specific design constrains, the committee then recommended nutritional composition of a new ration designed for short-term use by soldiers during high-tempo, stressful combat missions. The nutritional composition of this new ration was optimized to best sustain physical and cognitive performance and to prevent possible adverse health consequences, despite limitations imposed by ration design and mission constraints. The committee focused on dehydration, the gastrointestinal gut processes, and the function of the immune system as health issues of highest concern. Also, the committee considered the potential health and performance impact of subsistence on this ration during its intended use in combat operations. Although it was not stated in the questions posed, the committee found that some of the answers to the questions needed further confirmation with research that particularly addresses the unique circumstances of combat missions, that is, a combination of multiple stressors that rarely occurs in nonmilitary operations. Therefore, the committee proposed very specific areas of research that are critical to continue improvement of the assault rations.

Among the chief design constraints of this daily ration are that it must fit within 0.12 cubic feet and weigh 3 lb or less. The ration would be targeted for use by average male soldier of 80 kg body mass, 16 percent fat, relatively fit, age range 18–45 years (probably average < 25 years), with no chronic metabolic disease, but potential incidence of some common food allergies. During combat operations, the expected daily energy expenditure is 4,000–4,500 kcal/per day, achieved through intermittent periods of high energy expenditure (> 50 percent VO_2 max) mixed with longer periods of low-intensity movement sustained for 20 hours per day. Soldiers will rely on this ration for three to seven days followed by one to three days of recovery when they will have access to more nutritionally complete meals (i.e., ad lib food availability served in field kitchen setting). These three- to seven-day missions might be repeated several times for up to a month. To provide context for the recommendations, assumptions of the characteristics of the soldiers' diets and health, the missions, and other issues were formulated that were based on information gathered at open sessions with sponsor representatives and other military personnel.

The committee carried out its work over 15 months and held three meetings. The first meeting of the committee was held in conjunction with a two-day workshop. The workshop was hosted by the USARIEM and the Natick Soldier Center (NSC) in Natick, Massachusetts, August 11–13, 2004. Speakers addressed the issues brought to the committee by the USARIEM. These presentations were the basis for the committee's deliberations and recommendations and are included in this report as individually authored papers in Appendix B. Two additional meetings of the committee were held on October 21–22 and November 18–19, 2004.

Throughout the project, the committee had the privilege of having access to information collected directly in the field where soldiers were deployed to military missions of the type relevant to its task. For example, a survey that was designed to collect information on various aspects of eating behavior was conducted in Afghanistan. This very recent data collection was the basis for the committee's outlining of the assumptions and, consequently, the development of the recommendations. The committee would like to express its most sincere appreciation for the work and professionalism of CPT Chad Koenig, Research Dietitian of the Military Nutrition Division (MND) at USARIEM. He not only incorporated the committee's suggestions into the survey and conducted it, but also summarized the survey data for the committee and presented the conclusions at the November meeting.

The committee expresses its appreciation to Douglas Dauphinee, Research Program Coordinator of the MND at USARIEM, for all the help provided during the preparations stages of the workshop at USARIEM. Special thanks go also to Andrew Young, Chief of the MND and representative from the Department of Defense for this task, for generously giving his time and help and for being available to clarify the task of the committee. Special thanks are extended to Scott Montain, Research Physiologist at MND, USARIEM. His assistance was truly invaluable during the committee's work. He helped delineate the task and provided numerous reports and other data to the committee in a timely manner. In addition, the committee thanks COL Karl Friedl who continues to support the work of the CMNR and was readily available to provide the appropriate contacts needed to gather information for the committee.

On behalf of the committee, I sincerely thank the workshop participants and speakers for addressing topics critical to the completion of the committee's work. Each speaker not only provided an excellent presentation, but was available for multiple interactions during the workshop, prepared a manuscript of the presentation (see Appendix B), and worked with IOM staff throughout the revision process. These presentations were important reference sources for the committee and have been used as scientific basis throughout the report.

The committee expresses its deepest appreciation to other staff members at the Combat Feeding Directorate (CFD), Research, Development and Engineering Command, NSC, who offered their insights about the multiple questions on food development at the CFD: Betty Davis, Team Leader of Performance Enhancement and Food Safety; Matthew Kramer, Research Psychologist at Product Optimization and Evaluation Team; and Patrick Dunne, Senior Advisor at the CFD.

In addition, the military leaders that answered and clarified the committee's concerns on health issues during current deployments deserve the committee's most sincere appreciation. They are Mr. Terry Phelps, Deputy Director of the Special Operations Command Surgeon; LTC Christopher, Division Surgeon of the 82nd Airborne Division; and MAJ Steve Lewis, Social Work Officer of the 82nd Airborne Division. Without their contributions many of the health considerations that drove the recommendations would have eluded the committee. We thank MAJ Lolita Burrell for providing such valuable contacts.

The committee owes a strong debt of gratitude to the Food and Nutrition Board (FNB) staff for their professionalism and effectiveness in ensuring that our committee adhered to its task statement, for providing discipline and experience in helping to assemble the report and effectively respond to reviewers, and for providing background research support and organizing our meetings. In particular, we thank Senior Program Officer Maria Oria, who worked tirelessly on numerous drafts and revisions. Ably assisting Dr. Oria in her efforts were

Senior Program Assistant Jon Sanders and Research Associate Leslie Sim. Finally, the committee is also grateful to the overall guidance and continuous support of Linda Meyers, FNB Director. I also extend my deep gratitude to my fellow committee members, who participated in our discussions in this study in a professional and collegial manner, and who approached its task statement with great seriousness and intellectual curiosity. I appreciated the opportunity to work with these colleagues from several disciplines, several of whom I would never have met in my professional research and administration circles.

John W. Erdman, Jr., Chair

Contents

APPENDIXES

Executive Summary

The success of military operations depends to a large extent on the physical and mental status of the individuals involved. The physical demands of combat combined with the mental stress of long days, even if for short-term periods, take a unique toll on soldiers. Extreme environmental stressors encountered by military personnel during combat add further complexity. During sustained operations (SUSOPS), for example, combat foot soldiers carry loads in excess of 50 kg for three to seven days during missions that often last for about a month under weather conditions that vary from cold, mountainous to humid, tropical climates; rest between missions may be as short as two to three days.

An individual's physiological and nutritional status can markedly affect one's ability to maximize performance in sustained high-stress operations and may compromise mission effectiveness. Appropriate nutrition before and during missions can reduce adverse consequences of physical and mental stress, but optimizing soldiers' nutritional status is a continuous challenge. First, from a practical standpoint, it is not possible to implement a single recommended dietary regime before missions. Second, individuals under stress often have diminished appetites. Soldiers usually burn about 4,500 kcal/day but consume only about 2,400 kcal/day during combat, leaving them in a state called "negative energy balance." Finally, the nature of the ration is only one of many factors that determine eating habits during combat. Many less controllable and unpredictable factors, such as individual preferences and climate, come into play to reduce appetite, as was described in the Institute of Medicine (IOM) report, *Not Eating Enough.*

The consequences of being in negative energy balance while under the strenuous circumstances of SUSOPS range from weight loss to fatigue and mental impairments, such as confusion, depression, and loss of vigilance. The military has devoted great efforts to improve the quality of the food rations with the objectives of providing a palatable ration, encouraging consumption, and ensuring proper nutrition for soldiers. First Strike Rations (FSRs) are being developed in collaborative effort by the Combat Feeding Directorate (CFD), Research, Development, and Engineering Command (RDECOM), Natick Soldier Center (NSC) and the US Army Research Institute of Environmental Medicine (USARIEM) and were conceived as a new strategy to optimize the nutritive value of rations created for foot combat soldiers. FSRs are being developed as lightweight rations that contain all essential nutrients and food components with the idea of sustaining physical performance, postponing fatigue, and minimizing other adverse health consequences experienced while in SUSOPS. With the number of SUSOPS increasing, the optimization of these assault rations has become a high priority. The Department of Defense asked the IOM to appoint a committee to guide the design of the nutritional composition of the ration for SUSOPS. Although the focus of this report is soldiers, the recommendations may be applicable to physically fit nonmilitary personnel under similar conditions of high-stress, intense physical activity, especially those experiencing negative energy balance for the repeated, short periods of time outlined here. This may include firefighters, peacekeepers, and other civilian emergency personnel.

COMMITTEE'S TASK AND APPROACH

Under the auspices of the Standing Committee on Military Nutrition Research, the Committee on Optimization of Nutrient Composition of Military Rations for Short-Term, High-Intensity Situations was appointed to recommend the nutritional composition of a new ration designed for short-term use by soldiers during high-tempo, stressful combat missions. The ration is meant to be used for repetitive, three- to seven-day missions that include recovery periods of about 24–72 hours between missions. The nutritional composition of this new ration should be optimized to best sustain physical and cognitive performance and should prevent possible adverse health consequences, focusing on dehydration, the gastrointestinal gut processes, and the function of immune system as health issues of highest concern. Specifically, the committee was asked to respond to questions about the energy content, about levels and types of specific macronutrients and micronutrients, and about amounts of other bioactive substances that may enhance performance during combat missions.

To address this task, the committee convened a workshop hosted by the USARIEM and the NSC in Natick, Massachusetts, August 11–13, 2004, at which speakers addressed the issues brought to the committee by the USARIEM. These presentations were the basis for the committee's deliberations and recommendations and are included in this report as individually authored papers.

Box ES-1
Assumptions Regarding Assault Missions

Population
- Soldiers deployed to assault missions are male with an average body weight of 80 kg, approximately 16 percent body fat who are relatively fit and within an age range of 18–45 years (average < 25 years).

Prior to Assault Mission
- Soldiers may be using dietary supplements and caffeine.
- Immediately prior to a mission soldiers are well hydrated, not abusing alcohol, but may be using tobacco products.

During Assault Mission
- Soldiers may be on a mission for as many as 24 out of 30 days, with each mission lasting three to seven days.
- There may be as much as 20 hr/day of physical activity, with an average of 4 hr/day of sleep. Total daily energy expenditure will be approximately 4,500 kcal.
- Soldiers are likely to have an average energy intake of 2,400 kcal/day.
- Soldiers are likely to have access to 4–5 L of chlorinated water per day.
- Some soldiers may experience diarrhea, constipation, or kidney stones during the assault mission.
- Soldiers have different electrolyte intakes before a mission than during a mission; thus, during a mission a period of biological adjustment may occur.

Ration
- The daily ration must fit within 0.12 cubic feet and weigh 3 lb or less. It will be approximately 12–17 percent water but varying greatly from one item to the other; most items will be energy dense and intermediate in moisture.
- There will be no liquid foods in the rations, although gels and powders may be provided.
- The food available during recovery periods will provide, at a minimum, the nutritional standards for operational rations.

To provide context for the recommendations, the committee also formulated some basic assumptions about the characteristics of the soldiers' diets and health, the missions, and other issues, compiled through open sessions and available literature (see Box ES-1).

The committee used the Dietary Reference Intakes (DRIs) established by the IOM for active young men as the starting point for nutrient content in formulating the assault ration because these values are the most authoritative, up-to-date standards available. Further adjustments were then made to meet the unique needs of soldiers involved in assault conditions.

ANSWERS TO THE MILITARY'S QUESTIONS

1. Should the energy content of the ration (energy density) be maximized so as to minimize the energy debt, or is there a more optimal "mix" of macronutrients and micronutrients, not necessarily producing maximal energy density?

The committee recommends that the basic ration's energy content be approximately 2,400 kcal/day. While this level does not maximize energy density, this is the average daily energy intake that has frequently been reported for soldiers during training. Choosing this caloric level minimizes the possibility of discarding food items that might result in inadequate intakes of necessary micronutrients; however, in case ration items are discarded, micronutrients should be distributed as evenly as possible throughout the food items in the ration (rather than clustering them in a few items) to prevent significant amounts of individual micronutrients from being discarded. It should also be emphasized that rations should only be used over intermittent short terms (three to seven days) that, together, may last for a total of no more than a month.

To develop the recommendation on the total caloric intake of the ration, the committee considered health risks and benefits and information regarding the actual situation in the field. The data included food preferences, degree of satisfaction, and actual consumption of current rations. Data collected during training exercises of various military groups indicate that under stressful field conditions soldiers consume an average energy intake of 2,400 kcal. This level of intake is not enough to maintain body weight; however, the weight loss is moderate if the period of low energy intake is not sustained. Taking this information into account, the committee concluded that a ration with a caloric content of 2,400 kcal—if designed with adequate macronutrients and micronutrients and eaten entirely and for short periods of time such as three to seven days for up to a month— would not pose any health risks.

In addition to the basic ration, the committee recommends provision of high-carbohydrate supplements for energy (400 kcal) in the form of gels, candy, or powder to add to fluids. These may also contain electrolytes to maintain balance. These supplements could serve individuals whose energy intake or need is higher than the one in the basic ration and could also be used at times during the day when physical activity peaks and more energy is needed. They could also be used by individuals who lose excess electrolytes or at times when the climatic conditions may cause higher electrolyte losses than usual.

Although soldiers would still be in a negative energy balance, little evidence exists to suggest that a periodic hypocaloric diet, if otherwise adequate in protein and other essential nutrients, is likely to be harmful when consumed over brief periods of time, even if some weight loss occurs (< 10 percent of body weight). It is recommended that weight loss be measured after one month of use, and if weight loss is greater than 10 percent for a soldier, he should not be sent on assault missions until weight is regained to within 5 percent of initial weight. Also, the ration should not be substituted for Meals, Ready-to-Eat or food services that provide a more appropriate diet for longer periods.

2. What would be the optimal macronutrient balance between protein, fat, and carbohydrate for such an assault ration to enhance performance during combat missions?

3. What are the types and levels of macronutrients (e.g., complex versus simple carbohydrates, proteins with specific amino acid profiles, type of fat, etc.) that would optimize such an assault ration to enhance performance during combat missions?

Answers to questions two and three will be discussed together. The recommendations regarding distribution, level, and type of macronutrients for the ration were developed by considering the major health risks that might be posed by eating a hypocaloric diet in a combat situation.

The typical energy deficit of 50 percent seen in combat operations leads to a negative nitrogen balance that can result in muscle loss, fatigue, and loss of performance. To minimize these potential consequences, the committee recommends that the protein level of the ration be 100–120 g total protein (based on 1.2–1.5 g/kg of body weight for an 80 kg average male soldier). This level will likely spare muscle protein loss as well as attenuate net nitrogen loss and adequately provide for synthesis of serum proteins while the individual is in a hypocaloric state. In addition, this level of protein will likely maintain the immune and cognitive functions requiring protein or amino acids. The committee recommends that the protein added to the ration be of high biological value. At this time, there is insufficient evidence to believe that the addition of specific amino acids or specific proteins with rapid rates of absorption will be of any additional benefit; more evidence is necessary before making a recommendation in this respect.

The carbohydrate content of the ration is an important energy source and also helps maintain gastrointestinal health. Strong evidence that carbohydrate enhances cognitive function is still lacking; however, numerous data suggest that supplementing the diet with carbohydrate throughout periods of continuous physical exercise and stress not only increases energy intake but also optimizes physical performance. The committee recommends that the carbohydrate in the basic ration be 350 g to optimize physical performance. An additional 100 g of carbohydrate should be available as a supplement. Therefore, the overall recommendation is for 450 g. The committee considers palatability to be the major consideration in designing the food products to ensure ration consumption; thus, the food items and the carbohydrate supplement should provide a variety of flavors. The amount of fructose as a monosaccharide in the ration should be limited to avoid the possibility of osmotic diarrhea. Dietary fiber should be 15–17 g and should include both nonviscous, fermentable fiber (e.g., gums, pectin, β-glucans, soy polysaccharides) and viscous, nonfermentable fiber (e.g., cellulose, lignin, hemicellulose).

The primary reason for adding fat to the ration is to provide a readily digestible food source of high energy density. In addition to the essential fatty acids, fat is required to provide palatability and improve taste so that the ration is fully consumed. Among the macronutrients, protein and carbohydrate in adequate levels were considered the priority; the remainder of the macronutrients (up to the energy level of 2,400 kcal) should be provided as fat. The committee recommends that, after protein and carbohydrate needs are met, the ration should provide 58–67 g of fat (22–25 percent of energy intake) to be distributed across a variety of foods. The ration should provide a balance of dietary fatty acids between monounsaturated, polyunsaturated, and saturated fats, with at least 17 g of linoleic acid and 1.6 g of α-linolenic acid, recognizing essential fatty acid needs as well as the undesirable pro-oxidant properties of large amounts of unsaturated fatty acids. This balance can be determined by food formulation criteria. There is no recognized benefit to modifying fatty acid type in or adding structured lipids to the ration.

4. What are the types and levels of micronutrients such as direct antioxidants (e.g., vitamins C and E, carotenoids), cofactors in antioxidant and other biochemical reactions with high metabolic flux (e.g., B vitamins, zinc, manganese, copper), or other bioactives (e.g., caffeine) that could be added to such rations to enhance performance during combat missions?

Table ES-1 shows the recommended levels of micronutrients and other bioactives. The committee followed a general approach to establish these levels as described here. They were primarily based on DRIs and then modified by the committee after considering data about sweat losses and utilization under high energy expenditure and stress. To provide food developers some flexibility, a range of levels was recommended for most micronutrients. In most cases, the ranges are based on the recommended dietary allowance (RDA) or adequate intake and the 95th percentile of intake of the US population. When the 95th percentile dietary intake was higher than the tolerable upper level (UL), then the UL was used as the upper limit of the recommended range.

Exceptions to this general approach include the following: (1) for thiamin, the committee considered the importance of energy expenditure when setting the recommendations, while for vitamin B_6, negative energy balance and the loss of protein were considered; (2) for vitamin C, the committee added 35 mg to the RDA to account for the needs of smokers; and (3) for vitamin A, the committee

TABLE ES-1 Ration Nutrient Composition Recommended by the Committee

Nutrient or Energy Intake	Recommended Amount	Comments
Energy Intake	2,400 kcal in basic ration	Additional 400 kcal should be supplemented as carbohydrate in form of candy, gels, or powder to add to fluids, or all three.
Macronutrients		
Protein	100–120 g	Protein should be of high biological value. Preferable to add sources of protein with low-sulfur amino acids and low oxalate levels to minimize risk of kidney stone formation.
Carbohydrate	350 g 100 g as a supplement	Additional 100 g should be supplemented as carbohydrate in form of candy, gels, or powder to add to fluids, or all three. Amount of fructose as a monosaccharide should be limited to < 25 g.
Fiber	15–17 g	Naturally occurring or added. A mix of viscous, nonfermentable and nonviscous, fermentable fiber should be in the ration for gastrointestinal tract function.
Fat	22–25% kcal 58–67 g	Fat added to the ration should have a balanced mix of saturated, polyunsaturated, and monounsaturated fatty acids with palatability and stability the prime determinants of the specific mixture. Fat should contain 5–10% linoleic acid and 0.6–1.2% α-linolenic acid.
Vitamins		
Vitamin A	300–900 μg RAE[1]	Could be added as preformed vitamin A or provitamin A carotenoids.
Vitamin C	180–400 mg	Highly labile in processed food. If added to foods, encapsulation should be considered to prevent degradation through interaction with pro-oxidants.
Vitamin D	12.5–15 μg	Estimates of dietary intake are not available. Range based on ensuring serum levels of 25-hydroxy-vitamin D.
Vitamin E (α-tocopherol)	15–20 mg	Should be added to foods since natural foods are mainly sources of γ- rather than α-tocopherol.
Vitamin K	No recommended level	Amount in foods would be adequate provided ration is at least 50% whole foods.[2]

continued

TABLE ES-1 Continued

Nutrient or Energy Intake	Recommended Amount	Comments
Thiamin	1.6–3.4 mg	Dependent on energy use and intake. Amount in foods would be adequate provided ration is at least 50% whole foods.
Riboflavin	2.8–6.5 mg	Dependent on energy use.
Niacin	28–35 mg	Dependent on energy use. The amount added to the ration should not be over 35 mg.
Vitamin B_6	2.7–3.9 mg	Dependent on negative energy balance and loss of lean tissue. If a higher protein level is provided, the amount of vitamin B_6 should be increased proportionally.
Folate	400–560 µg	Fortification may be needed.
Vitamin B_{12}	No recommended level	Amount in foods would be adequate provided ration is at least 50% whole foods.
Biotin	No recommended level	Amount in foods would be adequate provided ration is at least 50% whole foods.
Pantothenic Acid	No recommended level	Amount in foods would be adequate provided ration is at least 50% whole foods.
Choline	No recommended level	Amount in foods would be adequate provided ration is at least 50% whole foods.
Minerals		
Calcium	750–850 mg	Major concern for higher levels is the potential formation of kidney stones.
Chromium	No recommended level	Amount in foods would be adequate provided ration is at least 50% whole foods.
Copper	900–1,600 µg	If added to foods, encapsulation should be considered due to its pro-oxidant activity.
Iodine	150–770 µg	Could be added as iodized salt.
Iron	8–18 mg	If added to foods, encapsulation should be considered due to its pro-oxidant activity. Palatability should determine the amount in ration foods.

TABLE ES-1 Continued

Nutrient or Energy Intake	Recommended Amount	Comments
Magnesium	400–550 mg	No more than 350 mg of magnesium salts should be present to meet the minimum daily amount of magnesium recommended. The rest should come from food sources. Also, if salt needs to be added and taste becomes objectionable, encapsulation should be considered.
Manganese	No recommended level	Amount in foods would be adequate provided ration is at least 50% whole foods.
Molybdenum	No recommended level	Amount in foods would be adequate provided ration is at least 50% whole foods.
Phosphorus	700–2,500 mg	Because inorganic phosphates may cause diarrhea, it is recommended that they are added only up to 700 mg. Intakes above this amount should come from food sources only.
Potassium	Aim to 3.3–4.7 g	Foods naturally high in potassium should be included in ration; if added to foods to achieve recommended levels, taste problems might be encountered.
Selenium	55–230 µg	No clear evidence of effects as an enhancer of immune function or performance.
Sodium	≥3 g up to 12 g as supplement	For individuals who lose salt in excess or when in extremely hot or strenuous situations, sodium could be supplemented up to 12 g total. Part of this amount should be included in the form of candy, gels, or powder to add to fluids. Palatability will limit addition of sodium to these products; therefore, salt tablets should also be provided under medical guidance.
Zinc	11–25 mg	If it needs to be added and taste becomes objectionable, encapsulation should be considered.
Ergogenics Caffeine	100–600 mg	Not more than 600 mg in a single dose. There is no evidence of dehydration at this level.

[1]RAE = retinol activity equivalents.
[2]Whole foods = food items prepared to preserve natural nutritive value.

recommends a minimum of 300 µg retinol activity equivalents to minimize the risk of night blindness.

One factor that would affect the micronutrient requirements is sweat and urine losses. Among factors causing increased sweat volume are exercise intensity and environmental temperature. When there were specific data or estimated amounts for additional micronutrient losses in sweat or urine during intense exercise in the heat (e.g., zinc, copper, sodium), then the amount was added to the recommended upper end level.

The committee recommends the micronutrients be provided in whole foods and that fortification or the use of supplements be limited to the extent possible. In cases such as potassium, however, it was recognized that food alone would not provide enough of a particular nutrient and that some form of supplementation might be needed. In other cases, such as for the trace elements molybdenum, manganese, and chromium, no level is recommended because those minerals are widely distributed in foods and a deficiency is not anticipated during the short period of intake of these rations.

The committee cautions about the potential for oxidation or interactions with other nutrients in the ration. Therefore, in addition microbiological tests, chemical analysis should be performed on the final ration following appropriate shelf-life studies.

Other Bioactive Substances

The committee reviewed the effects of several bioactive substances other than nutrients because of their potential benefits in physical or cognitive performance. Caffeine is the only component for which there are compelling data showing effectiveness for combat soldiers; therefore, only caffeine received the endorsement of the committee.

Some other bioactives (e.g., creatine) are consumed already by soldiers with the goal of increasing physical endurance. For the most part, their effects are not clear. The committee recommends that randomized, blinded trials be undertaken to elucidate the risks, including withdrawal effects, and potential benefits of creatine and other popular bioactives; ideally, these trials should be conducted under conditions that mimic combat situations. The flavonoids are a class of compounds that might provide some benefit as antioxidants against the oxidative stress occurring during intense exercise and mental activities. Until more in vivo studies are conducted, foods such as fruits, vegetables, tea, and chocolate, which contain significant amounts of flavonoids, should be included in rations.

WATER NEEDS

Although the committee was not asked to make recommendations regarding water needs, the close links between diet, hydration status, and physiological function cannot be overlooked. Proper hydration is a major factor in maintaining sustained mental and physical performance. Water needs are governed by sweat volume and metabolic rate as well as nutrient intake—primarily protein and salt intake. In this sense, the nature of the ration will also influence the water needs during combat; that is, protein and salt intake provide most of the excreted osmoles as urea and sodium with accompanying anions and, thus, additional fluid is needed for their excretion. The recommendation for 100–120 g of protein per day will result in 0.2–0.4 L more urine than would occur with 80 g of protein. While the protein recommended might add to the needs of water, the comparatively high level of carbohydrate in the ration compensates for some of those needs through improved protein utilization and limitation in the need to excrete sodium salts.

While the committee did not provide specific recommendations for water, adequate amounts of water must be consumed with this ration to maintain and optimize physiological function and performance. Considering the expected level of stress and sweat volumes, and the nature of the ration, water in excess of 4–5 L/day must be available to ensure optimal performance in combat missions in which energy expenditure is high or carried out in hot and humid environments.

FOOD MATRIX CONSIDERATIONS

Food rations that provide complete nutritional needs for short-term, high-intensity military operations present a unique challenge to the product developer and nutritionist. Although the nutrient composition recommended by the committee (see Table ES-1) will place some constraints on the food forms and matrixes used, with careful planning it should be possible to provide complete nutritional needs in a ration with a restricted size and shelf-life of two to three years. For example, although whole foods should be used to the extent possible, the recommended levels for some nutrients may dictate the use of fortification with labile vitamins such as vitamin C as well as with other nutrients such as folate that are likely to be low in the ration due to the types of foods included. Fortification with labile nutrients presents a unique challenge because of the potential interaction with other compounds and decreased bioavailability. Food developers need to carefully consider the shelf-life of the ration to ensure that levels of these labile micronutrients are neither above (if storage period is shorter than anticipated) nor below (due to interactions with other components) the range of recommended levels. To minimize decreased bioavailability due to interactions, the use of encapsulated forms for some nutrients may be necessary.

Because taste is an important factor when soldiers rate foods and because this ration is meant to be eaten entirely, providing a variety of acceptable, palatable products becomes a primary concern. Electrolytes (sodium and potassium) and other minerals (zinc, calcium, and magnesium) are known to have objectionable tastes to some, possibly at the levels recommended. The use of appropriate chemical forms with better taste or technologies to mask the objectionable taste should be a high priority for food developers.

In addition to palatability, satiety and food form should also be taken into consideration for this ration. A mix of carbohydrate-rich and fat-rich foods is needed to provide a satiating balance in the ration and to avoid overconsumption of the less-satiating foods. Foods that are included in a ration should have variety in flavors and textures and should be easy to consume. They should include familiar items in addition to foods that are already available for athletes, such as carbohydrate gels or powders to add to fluids for carbohydrate and electrolyte supplementation. Packaging is also an important consideration for stability, protection, and for ease of consumption. Overall, the use of existing and familiar products, packaging, and technologies is advised.

FUTURE NEEDS

The ration recommended by the committee was designed with the best available data. The majority of the data, however, were derived from studies in which the environment or the subjects were substantially different from the ones for which this ration is targeted. The committee believes that further work needs to be conducted to confirm that the ration provides optimal performance and maintains health or to have the opportunity of improving the ration by making necessary adjustments.

The committee finds that, where gaps in knowledge exist, additional data in the following areas of investigation should prove particularly beneficial to future development and refinement of an optimal ration: (1) additional knowledge regarding the unique nutrient requirements during combat operations, (2) deeper understanding of food preferences under high-stress situations, (3) additional information on the actual use of the ration in the field, and (4) methods to identify individuals at greater risk of excess electrolyte loss and kidney stone formation.

Some of the questions that will help advance knowledge regarding nutrient requirements during combat operations are: (1) What are effects of hypocaloric, high-carbohydrate, high-protein diets on performance and health? (2) What are the effects of micronutrients (e.g., vitamins C and E, B vitamins, zinc, selenium, iron, and copper), combination of antioxidants, or single amino acids on health and performance? (3) What are the potential benefits and risks of taking bioactives to enhance performance? When conducting such research, the physical and cognitive performance outcome measurements should be relevant and appropriate for those conditions (e.g., shot pattern tightness, complex reaction time, vigilance rather than objective or self-reported measurements of mood states). Furthermore, the committee emphasizes the importance of conducting such studies under conditions that approximate circumstances under combat operations.

The committee finds that the USARIEM and the CFD, RDECOM, NSC should continue to follow the existing systematic approach to ration development for combat missions. The approach should incorporate early in the design process issues of palatability and food preferences of end users. To that effect, the military should consider performing studies to test the performance and acceptability of the ration under the real circumstances of combat and under different environments with attention to actual duration of use of such rations. For a continuous improvement of the ration's acceptability, more studies could be conducted to create strategies for the addition of specific nutrients to foods without compromising palatability. Other critical factors that need studying are stability of the rations over the long shelf-life required, for which nutrient interactions and packaging should be considered.

Because this ration was designed to be used under unique circumstances, the actual use of rations with respect to duration and frequency should be monitored to ensure that they are not used when individuals are in garrison or in other types of extended missions.

1

Introduction

The evolution of warfare strategies and the importance of maintaining the fitness of soldiers in military operations are the major driving forces behind the need to continually improve military rations. Also, the level of stress under military operations may affect food consumption in ways not seen to influence the food preferences of the general population. Because the factors that define the eating behavior of soldiers in these environments are still not well understood, ration designs need to be frequently reviewed and revised to adapt to both the soldiers' needs and the demands of changing warfare scenarios. While an understanding of the reasons behind eating behavior observed in the field may be lacking, military rations, especially for soldiers in combat missions, need to be customized to address soldiers' dietary needs and preferences in order to enhance intake. This report addresses those needs and preferences.

Chapter 1, *Introduction*, describes the committee's task and the current concerns of the military regarding improvement of performance under combat, nutritional makeup of current rations for combat situations, and approaches taken to improve rations.

THE COMMITTEE'S TASK

The Department of Defense, through the US Army Research Institute for Environmental Medicine (USARIEM), asked the Institute of Medicine to appoint an ad hoc committee to conduct a study to determine the optimal nutrient content of a new combat ration. The ad hoc committee was to first review existing rations, their limitations for use during future force military deployments and combat operations, and the expected effects of combat operations on nutrient status, health, and performance. The committee was then asked to recommend, within specific design constraints, the nutritional composition of a new ration designed for short-term use by soldiers during high-performance, stressful combat missions. The nutritional composition of this new ration would be optimized to best sustain physical and cognitive performance and to prevent possible adverse health consequences. This was to be done recognizing that the ration would likely have a hypocaloric energy content relative to daily expenditure in short-term assault situations—a limitation imposed by ration design and mission constraints. The committee was asked to focus on health issues of highest concern: dehydration, the gastrointestinal gut processes, and the function of the immune system. The committee was also directed to keep in mind the potential health and performance effects on the soldiers subsisting on this ration during its intended use in combat operations.

To address this task, the committee convened a workshop hosted by the USARIEM and the Natick Soldier Center (NSC) in Natick, Massachusetts, August 11–13, 2004, in which speakers addressed the issues brought to the committee by the USARIEM. The agenda is included in Appendix A. These presentations were the basis for the committee's deliberations and recommendations and are included in this report as individually authored papers in Appendix B.

Ration Design Requirements

Among the chief design constraints of this daily ration as required by USARIEM are that it must fit within 0.12 cubic feet and weigh 3 lb (1.36 kg) or less. The ration is targeted for use by male soldiers who have an average body weight of 80 kg, approximately 16 percent body fat, are relatively fit, are within an age range of 18–45 years (average < 25 years), and who have no chronic metabolic disease but may be vulnerable to some common food allergies. During combat operations, the expected daily energy expenditure is 4,000–4,500 kcal/ day, achieved through intermittent periods of high-energy expenditure (> 50 percent VO_2max) mixed with longer periods of low-intensity movement and sustained for 20 hours per day. The soldier will rely on this ration during missions that last for three to seven days, followed by one to three days of recovery when they will have access to more nutritionally complete meals (i.e., ad libitum food availability served in a field-kitchen setting). The committee has designed this ration with the assumption that soldiers might be deployed to such missions repetitively for a maximum period of one month.

Specific Questions to Be Addressed

The committee task addressed the following four questions:

1. Should the energy content of the ration (energy density) be maximized so

as to minimize the energy debt, or is there a more optimal mix of macro-nutrients and micronutrients not necessarily producing maximal energy density?

2. What would be the optimal macronutrient balance between protein, fat, and carbohydrate for such an assault ration to enhance performance during combat missions?

3. What are the types and levels of macronutrients (e.g., complex versus simple carbohydrates, proteins with specific amino acid profiles, types of fat, etc.) that would optimize such an assault ration to enhance performance during combat missions?

4. What are the types and levels of micronutrients such as direct antioxidants (e.g., vitamins C and E, carotenoids), cofactors in antioxidant and other biochemical reactions with high metabolic flux (e.g., B vitamins, zinc, manganese, copper), or other bioactives (e.g., caffeine) that could be added to such rations to enhance performance during combat missions?

ORGANIZATION OF THE REPORT

The report is organized into an executive summary, chapters, and appendixes. The chapters include an introductory chapter and those chapters that directly answer the four questions that comprise the task of the committee above. Appendix B is composed of the written presentations of the workshop speakers; however, although they were the basis for the committee's answers to the military's questions, they should not be construed as necessarily representing the views of the committee.

This chapter provides some background information on current knowledge regarding the eating behaviors of soldiers under the physical and mental stress of high-intensity operations. The effects of high-intensity operations on performance as well as relevant ration development strategies are also discussed. Chapter 2 provides responses to the four specific questions posed to the committee. In addition, Chapter 2 provides a list of specific research needs for each nutrient that should be of interest to the military. Chapter 3 describes in detail the committee's approach to establishing the levels and types of nutrients required, such as health considerations that were discussed in depth. It also includes a section on food matrix considerations that are critical for food developers who will design the rations. Chapter 3 concludes with a section on overall priority research needs.

The workshop agenda is presented in Appendix A. Appendix B includes the workshop presentations organized by topic: an introduction to information about combat rations; the role of carbohydrate, protein, and fat as fuel sources in performance and health enhancement or maintenance; the effects of micronutrients in performance and health enhancement or maintenance; approaches to improve the immune function and immune responses; prevention of kidney stones and of impairments of gastrointestinal function; and food development considerations, such as strategies to develop food for individuals under stress and factors that may increase food consumption. Finally, the biographical sketches of the speakers and of the committee members are presented in Appendixes C and D, respectively. Appendix E contains a list of acronyms and Appendix F contains a glossary.

ENERGY EXPENDITURE AND FOOD CONSUMPTION DURING MILITARY OPERATIONS OR TRAINING

Data collected during field training indicate that with high energy expenditures of 4,000 kcal/day or more, soldiers tend to consume an average of 3,000 kcal/day, and even less when they depend on operational rations (i.e., rations designed for a wide variety of operations and settings but consumed for a limited period of time). In addition to the potential cognitive decrements due to a variety of stressors during short-term missions, underconsumption may result in a set of consequences ranging from body protein loss and fatigue to deficits in essential micronutrients that may impair physiological functions and result in performance decrements.

The wide range in total energy expenditures of various military groups and factors that appear to contribute to these differences have been described (Tharion et al., 2005). Studies in the field suggest that the typical energy intake of military personnel (soldiers, sailors, airmen, and marines) under a variety of scenarios and climatic conditions is approximately 2,400 kcal/day, even though energy expenditures of soldiers in combat units range from about 4,000–7,131 kcal/day depending on the level of physical activity and environment. Interestingly, these reports note that measured energy deficits for soldiers, whether they are in training school or in combat, were significant (Tharion et al., 2005).

Whereas this might seem normal for training situations due to restricted diets, the reasons for underconsumption during combat are complex, not well understood, and more difficult to avoid or counter. A Committee on Military Nutrition Research (CMNR) report (IOM, 1995) analyzed these reasons and provided recommendations to ameliorate them, focusing largely on the psychology behind eating behaviors during military activities. If the ration is designed to maintain health and performance, consumption of the entire ration (compared to selectively discarding food items) has the advantage of minimizing nutrient deficits resulting in potential adverse consequences in performance and health. Whether it is possible to do this in a combat situation remains to be determined.

IMPACT OF HIGHLY INTENSE OPERATIONS ON
HEALTH AND PERFORMANCE

Physiological Consequences of Combat Operations

As mentioned in other parts of this report, during combat operations soldiers are often under energy deficit that can affect their health and performance. Several field studies have attempted to resolve the question of the minimum energy intake that will maintain military performance for a defined period of time by measuring either body weight loss or performance levels, or both. During the Ranger I and II studies (Moore et al., 1992; Shippee et al., 1994) soldiers completed an eight-week US Army Ranger training program under hypocaloric states and data on body composition, physical performance, cellular immune function, and medical problems were collected. In the first study, students were provided with a single meal of 1,300 kcal (Moore et al., 1992). In the second study (Shippee et al., 1994), an additional 200 kcal were provided in field exercises, which brought the total daily rations up to 1,570 kcal and 50 g of protein per day (IOM, 1992). During these two studies daily caloric deficits resulted in severe weight loss (> 10 percent), although the group that was provided additional calories and protein experienced less weight loss (12 percent versus 15 percent). Improvements in immune function were also seen with additional calories and protein. Both studies showed, however, that those severe hypocaloric states may result in harmful physical and cognitive effects to military personnel health (Moore et al., 1992; Shippee et al., 1994).

Evidence exists, however, showing that a body weight loss of less than 10 percent has no adverse consequences on health or military performance (Consolazio et al., 1979; Keys et al., 1950; Taylor et al., 1957). When rations that are specifically developed for short missions and that provide 2,000 kcal/day were tested, weight loss was around 3 percent of initial body weight. Although this weight loss does not present a major health concern, some measurements of performance were still impaired (Askew et al., 1986). In contrast, the same ration appeared to present no health concern when used with a carbohydrate supplement (Jones et al., 1990), even though the energy deficit was still high—approximately 2,000 kcal.

The loss of body weight as the main consequence of underfeeding during sustained operations (SUSOPS) results from reductions in both fat and lean body mass. Fat loss is an essential feature of starvation because body fat acts as an energy source when energy expenditure exceeds energy consumption. The reasons for protein loss, however, are not as well understood and such a loss of body protein could have adverse consequences for military performance. One of the first studies to illustrate that starvation causes body protein loss was the Minnesota starvation experiment (Keys et al., 1950). Recently, fat and lean tissue losses of 1.2 and 1.5 kg, respectively, were reported over a 72-hour SUSOPS (Nindl et al., 2002). Similarly, 38 percent of the ~12 kg body weight loss that occurred during Ranger training (due to severe underfeeding) was attributable to nonfat tissue loss (Moore et al., 1992). A recent study conducted on the physiological and psychological effects of eating three different menus during 12 days of military training in a tropical environment (Booth et al., 2003) has been reported. Three groups of Australian Air Field Defense Guards received either freshly prepared foods, one combat ration pack (CRP), or half of a CRP, respectively, containing 3,600 kcal, 3,600 kcal, or 1,800 kcal. The menus were designed to provide a similar percent of energy from macronutrients as a percentage of total energy. There was substantial underconsumption in the CRP group versus the half-CRP group, which resulted in similar weight loss (about 1.7 and 2.6 percent, respectively), protein catabolism, and immune suppression in both of these groups; they also reported greater fatigue than the group eating fresh foods. Despite underconsumption, all groups ate sufficient protein to meet the military daily recommended intake for protein. It should be noted, however, that hypocaloric intakes raise protein requirements for maximal protein-sparing, and, therefore, the standard military daily recommended intake might not be sufficient.

Protein loss is one of the main consequences of combat operations and minimizing the protein loss might well be one strategy to maintain military performance. It has been suggested that this could be accomplished by a soldier storing an appropriate amount of body fat to be used during the mission, preventing severe body fat depletion, maintaining some level of physical activity, and increasing protein intake (see Hoffer, 2004 in Appendix B).

Other consequences of stress and underconsumption during combat likely include impairments in the immune and endocrine systems, dehydration, kidney stone formation, or gastrointestinal disturbances (see Montain, 2004 in Appendix B).

Impact of Combat Operations on Physical Performance

As described by Montain (see Montain, 2004 in Appendix B), performance of simple and well-learned motor tasks (e.g., weapon handling) do not appear to be compromised by sustained operational stress (Haslam, 1982). Endurance time, however, is frequently impaired during aerobic exercise tasks (VanHelder and Radomski, 1989), and there is an increased perception among subjects of the effort needed to perform the same task. Nindl and colleagues (2002) reported a 25 percent lower level of work productivity on a physical persistence task (building a wall for 25 minutes) when soldiers were fed a hypocaloric diet (a diet that contained > 50 percent less kilocalories than the soldiers' energy expenditures) and allowed to sleep for only 1 hr/day over a four-day period as compared to the control. This is consistent with the hypothesis that SUSOPS compromise performance when tasks are prolonged and monotonous. Independent of energy intake (Rognum et al., 1986), operational effectiveness is also affected if sleep is inadequate. The sections below describe studies that show various factors affecting military performance.

Effects of Weight Loss and Energy Intake

Studies with prolonged operations lasting several weeks and associated with substantial losses of lean body mass (Moore et al., 1992; Shippee et al., 1994) have shown reductions in physical performance. The caloric deficit and weight loss associated with SUSOPS scenarios, however, appear to have inconsistent effects on soldier performance (Montain and Young, 2003). One of the difficulties with these studies is that physical performance is measured with a variety of tests that may or may not be reliable or indicative of work productivity. In addition, confounding factors, such as small sample sizes, lead to scores that were improved with time. Generally, earlier studies of short-term duration suggest that several days of underfeeding have limited ill effect on muscle strength and aerobic endurance; however, physical performance also depends on the degree of energy deficit and length of the mission.

Shorter duration studies with minimal lean body mass loss generally showed little or no decrement in muscle strength, power, or fatigability (Bulbulian et al., 1996; Guezennec et al., 1994; VanHelder and Radomski, 1989). In the study described above (Booth et al., 2003), no differences were evident among the three groups in the areas of physical fitness (as tested by chin-ups or sit-ups and running times), daily activity, sleeping quality, or cognitive function, despite a weight loss of approximately 3 percent reported in the groups on the CRP diets. The authors concluded that a 3 percent weight loss after 12 days was unlikely to be detrimental to military performance, and the loss of protein was not considered significant.

The lack of performance decrements with short-term operations, however, is not universal (Legg and Patton, 1987). A SUSOPS scenario lasting less than one week resulted in reduced maximal aerobic power and endurance (Guezennec et al., 1994), as have sleep-deprivation studies (Van HElder and Raomski, 1989).

Earlier studies suggested that if mineral supplements were included in the ration, health and performance may be maintained over a short period of time (10 days) (Consolazio et al., 1967a, b). In this case, however, performance was measured as handgrip strength, which might not be a good measurement of military performance. No differences, either in time to complete an assault course or in prone marksmanship performance, were reported when cadet soldiers were provided 1,500 or 8,000 kcal/day during a five-day scenario (Rognum et al., 1986). In another study, an 8 percent reduction in maximal aerobic power was noted when soldiers were restricted to 1,800 kcal/day, but no reductions were apparent when soldiers were fed 3,200 or 4,200 kcal/day (Guezennec et al., 1994). Similarly, reductions in shot group tightness on a marksmanship task were reported after sustained road marching during which soldiers were fed

250 g/day of carbohydrate, but no change was noted when soldiers consumed a daily diet with 400 or 550 g of carbohydrate (Tharion and Moore, 1993). Military performance, measured by aerobic performance, psychomotor and vigilance tasks, and military performance test scores, were no different for subjects on a hypocaloric diet (2,400 kcal/day) versus those on eucaloric diets for 7 to 10 days while energy expenditures were 3,800 kcal/day (Rai et al., 1983).

Most of these studies, however, were not conducted under the stressful circumstances of actual combat, which might alter the results. As has been noted by others (Montain and Young, 2003), despite confounding factors, the data available suggest that moderate levels of weight loss have limited ill effects on the ability of the soldier to perform tests of accuracy and coordination, anaerobic power, and endurance.

Effects of Eating Schedule and Nutrient Intake

Time of ingestion and content of the previous meal may be an explanation for the divergent results described above regarding the effects of varying energy intake on performance. A study found a relationship in that an increase in energy (or carbohydrate) intake sustains uphill run time over three days of physically demanding field training (Montain et al., 1997). Moreover, when provided with the same amounts of carbohydrate and energy, soldiers who best sustained their uphill run time performance had eaten carbohydrate during the four hours preceding the uphill run, while soldiers with the greatest decrement had eaten none of their rations since the previous night's meal. The results of this study suggest that soldiers subsisting on diets at these energy and carbohydrate levels during high-paced operations are receiving nearly the minimum level of energy needed to sustain performance, necessitating good food discipline (i.e., eating the food provided) or acceptable food choices (i.e., eating the carbohydrate-containing foods), or both, to preserve physical performance.

Effects of Sleep Deprivation

According to recent surveys conducted in the field during combat missions, some soldiers sleep an average of 4 hr/day; most of them, however, sleep 5–6 hr/day (personal communication, C. Koenig, USARIEM, November 15, 2004). Current military doctrine requires that units operate around the clock during times of conflict because the success of battlefield operations depends, at least in part, on maintaining the momentum of continuous day–night operations (US Department of the Army, 1997), especially with the technological advances that have enhanced night-fighting capabilities.

A recent CMNR report reviewed the consequences of sleep deprivation on military personnel (IOM, 2004b). It was noted that depriving humans of proper restorative sleep produces attention lapses and slower reaction times, which are associated with poor performance (Krueger, 1991). Sleep-deprived personnel lost approximately 25 percent of their ability to perform useful mental work with each 24-hour period of sleep loss (Belenky et al., 1994). The CMNR report also noted that, by the end of three days without sleep, combat service members may be considered totally ineffective in the operational setting, especially if they are performing complex tasks such as operating computerized command-and-control centers. Although under SUSOPS this is not the usual sleep interval, decreases in cognitive function may still be expected given that assault operations providing little time to sleep can last up to a month.

Over the past several years, the problem of sleep loss and fatigue has escalated due to the increased requirements on military forces caused by reductions in manpower and other resources (IOM, 2004b). The efficiency of combatants in SUSOPS can be significantly compromised by inadequate sleep (Krueger, 1991). Vigilance and attention suffer, reaction time is impaired, mood declines, and some personnel begin to experience perceptual disturbances. Cognitive abilities suffer a 30 percent reduction after only one night without sleep, and a 60 percent reduction after a second sleepless night (Angus and Heslegrave, 1985). In this way, marksmanship can be compromised by sustained operation activities. Significantly impaired marksmanship occurred after 73–74 hr of total sleep deprivation during Navy Seal training (Tharion et al., 1997). Specifically, there was a greater distance from the center of mass (by 20 percent) as well as increased dispersion of shot groups, both indicative of reduced marksmanship. These adverse findings occurred despite a 50 percent slower sighting time. In contrast, no negative results were observed during nine days of SUSOPS (which allowed two days of no sleep and four hours of sleep for the seven remaining days) on shot group clustering when troops fired in the prone supported position (Haslam, 1982). The ability to acquire and accurately hit a randomly appearing target, however, declined progressively during the first two days of the study and was 10 percent below baseline performance (only 5 hits versus 6 of 9 hits) after nine days. SUSOPS duration may be a factor. Despite soldiers' rating of the marksmanship task as more difficult to perform after 48 and 72 hours of SUSOPS, in another study there was no reduction in the number of randomly appearing targets hit during the test (Johnson et al., 2001). When task durations extend beyond 15 to 20 minutes, performance deteriorations from fatigue become far more pronounced than when the task durations are shorter (Caldwell and Ramspott, 1998; Wilkinson, 1969; Wilkinson et al., 1966).

Although not all types of performance are affected to the same degree by sleep loss, the fatigue from prolonged duty periods clearly jeopardizes unit readiness in the operational context. This is especially the case for tasks that are lengthy, devoid of performance feedback, or boring.

DEVELOPMENT OF RATIONS FOR MILITARY OPERATIONS

Improvement of Rations Throughout Time

Since the Civil War, and especially after the end of World War II, the US military has devoted a great deal of effort to develop and improve the existing rations for soldiers both in combat and in garrison. The military recognized that, rather than simply providing a nutritionally balanced diet, rations needed to be targeted to the specific situation in which military personnel operate. The environment (i.e., geographical location and climate) was recognized as an important factor that influenced ration development; changes in warfare tactics have also resulted in new dietary needs and consumption habits. For example, nutrient requirements for extended operations in temperate climates might not be the same as those for short-term extreme conditions during which sweating might be severe and physical activity strenuous. In 1947 (US Department of the Army, 1947), the military had recognized the importance of maintaining personnel performance as well as the need to provide acceptable foods to adequately maintain their stability and nutritional needs.

Throughout the ensuing years, many types of rations have been and continue to be developed to provide for the nutritional needs of soldiers in specific situations. As components of the Department of Defense, (1) Combat Feeding Directorate (CFD), Research, Development and Engineering Command, NSC, and (2) the Operational Ration Business Unit of the Defense Supply Center, Philadelphia's Directorate of Subsistence, collaborate to develop, test, evaluate, procure, and support all military rations. In developing the rations, food technologists at the CFD collaborate with nutritionists and physiologists at USARIEM, which has the responsibility of setting the nutrient composition of the rations in compliance with nutrition standards established by the Surgeon General of the US Army (US Departments of Army, Navy, and Air Force, 2001). The nutritional standards for rations have evolved as knowledge about human nutrient requirements has expanded. The Military Dietary Reference Intakes (MDRIs) are quantitative reference values for nutrient intakes to be used for planning and assessing diets for the healthy military population.

Operational and restricted rations are designed for military personnel in a wide variety of operations and settings to be used during limited periods of time. "Operational" rations are designed to be nutritionally adequate, whereas "restricted" rations are incomplete and used for shorter periods of time. See Table 1-1 for a comparison of nutrient reference values and energy levels for military rations and for the general population (Dietary Reference Intakes or DRIs). MDRIs are mostly based on the DRIs, with some modifications that consider the special needs of military personnel.

Increasing the food intake of soldiers during times of high energy expenditure has been a constant challenge for those responsible for developing military

TABLE 1-1 Military Recommended Intakes for Men in Garrison Feeding, Operational and Restricted Rations Compared to Recommended Intakes for the General Population, Men 19–30 Years of Age

Nutrient or Energy	RDA, AI, or AMDR (per day)	Military Daily Recommended Intake	Operational Ration Daily Minimum Intake	Restricted Ration Daily Minimum Intake
Energy Intake (kcal)	3,600	3,250	3,600	1,500
Protein (for an 80 kg male) (g) (% of kcal)	64 (10–30%)	91 (10–15%)	91 (10–15%)	50 (10–15%)
Fat (% of kcal)	25–35%	≤ 35%	≤ 35%	≤ 35%
PUFA (% kcal)				
n-3 as α-linolenic	0.6–1.2 %	NS	NS	NS
n-6 as linoleic acid	5–10 %	NS	NS	NS
Carbohydrate (g) (% of kcal)	130 (40–65%)	NS	494	200
Vitamin A (μg)	900 RAE	1,000 RE	1,000 RE	500 RE
Vitamin C (mg)	90	90	90	45
Vitamin D (μg)	5	5	5	3
Vitamin E (mg)	15	15	15	8
Vitamin K (μg)	120	80	80	40
Thiamin (mg)	1.2	1.2	1.2	0.6
Riboflavin (mg)	1.3	1.3	1.3	0.7
Niacin (mg NE)	16	16	16	8
Vitamin B_6 (mg)	1.3	1.3	1.3	0.7
Folate (μg DFE)	400	400	400	200
Vitamin B_{12} (μg)	2.4	2.4	2.4	1.2
Biotin (μg)	30	NS	NS	NS
Pantothenic Acid (mg)	5	NS	NS	NS
Choline (mg)	550	NS	NS	NS
Calcium (mg)	1,000	1,000	1,000	500
Chromium (μg)	35	NS	NS	NS
Copper (μg)	900	NS	NS	NS
Fluoride (mg)	4	4	4	2
Iodine (μg)	150	150	150	75
Iron (mg)	8	10	15	8
Magnesium (mg)	400	420	420	210
Manganese (mg)	2.3	NS	NS	NS
Molybdenum (μg)	45	NS	NS	NS
Phosphorus (mg)	700	700	700	350
Potassium (mg)	4,700	3,200	3,200	2,000
Selenium (μg)	55	55	55	28
Sodium (mg)	1,500; ≤ 2,300	5,000; (4,550–5,525)	5,000–7,000	2,500–3,500
Zinc (mg)	11	15	15	8

NOTE: AI = adequate intake; AMDR = acceptable macronutrient distribution ranges; DFE = dietary folate equivalents; NE = niacin equivalents; NS = not specified; PUFA = polyunsaturated fatty acids; RAE = retinol activity equivalents; RE = retinol equivalents; RDA = recommended dietary allowance. SOURCE: IOM, 2004a; US Departments of Army, Navy, and Air Force, 2001.

rations. As mentioned in other parts of this report, palatability is a critical factor that greatly determines energy intake by soldiers. To adapt the ration items to the wants and needs of the soldier, an important aspect of ration development is the information gathered from surveys in the field regarding soldiers' food preferences, their acceptance of rations, and their resultant behavior. For example, Meals, Ready-to-Eat (MREs), which are rations to sustain soldiers for no more than 10 days and in the absence of food service, have been improved since their introduction in 1993 as a result of survey findings. The MREs' menus have increased from 12 to 24 varieties and now include four vegetarian meals and 150 new items.

One of the surveys (unpublished data) was conducted with soldiers stationed at Ft. Drum, New York, during a 10-day field training exercise in 1996; the study tested the acceptability of a new MRE developed as a result of prior studies that concluded preferences for larger serving sizes and more variety in menus. This study revealed that an increased number of fruits and snacks were favored and that a decrease in total calories would be desirable.

Another study with the 28th Combat Support Hospital personnel assessed a test ration in comparison to that year's version of the MRE during energy expenditures averaging 4,000 kcal/day for 11 days (Baker-Fulco et al., 2002). The test ration contained new items and more carbohydrate and less fat than the control MRE. Subjects increased energy intake as intended but changes in protein intake were marginal with the test ration. For both rations, underconsumption resulted in most subjects not meeting the military recommended intakes for a number of nutrients. This study showed that manipulation of the food items and of the distribution of macronutrients in the ration could reduce energy deficits in military personnel. Studies such as these are critical to determine the food preferences and the eating behavior of soldiers, such as which items are discarded or eaten more frequently, in specific situations. Improvements in the MRE and research efforts in food technology have been described in an earlier CMNR report (IOM, 1995).

Current Efforts to Improve Rations

Although MREs are envisioned as rations to sustain soldiers in the absence of food service facilities of field kitchens (as in the case of SUSOPS), MREs are designed for use for periods of no more than 10 days, at which time field kitchens or other facilities are to be made available. As the number of SUSOPS has increased in recent years, the need to reevaluate existing ration designs and develop a new lightweight ration specifically to meet the metabolic needs of soldiers during SUSOPS (e.g., three- to seven-day operations) is a high priority. MREs are not suitable for these operations because of the weight they add to the already heavy loads that soldiers carry when no resupply is planned. When MREs were provided for SUSOPS, anecdotal evidence revealed that, in an attempt to lighten the loads, soldiers selectively discarded food items; this practice has become a widespread problem and may result in unbalanced diets that could possibly jeopardize a soldier's health or performance or both during an assault operation.

With these issues in mind, new assault ration prototypes have been under development by USARIEM and the NSC. The current concept is a lightweight ration to be eaten "on the go" that, unlike the MREs, requires no preparation. Items in the current prototype ration include fruit bars, dried fruit, meat pockets, a dairy bar, and beef jerky. The acceptability of these prototype food items has been tested in the laboratory and in garrison situations, and the results to date are promising (personal communication, A. Young, USARIEM, August 11, 2004). Although it is appropriate to initially conduct such tests, testing under the unique circumstances of a combat situation is a critical step to confirm acceptability and revisit the ration design if poorly accepted. Currently, these rations are being tested in the field, and results from those tests, as well as the recommendations in this report, are expected to help military food developers and nutritionists optimize the utility of the assault ration.

REFERENCES

Angus RG, Heslegrave RJ. 1985. Effects of sleep loss on sustained cognitive performance during a command and control simulation. *Behav Res Method Instrum Comp* 17(1):55–67.

Askew EW, Claybaugh JR, Cucinell SA, Young AJ, Szeto EG. 1986. *Nutrient Intakes and Work Performance of Soldiers During Seven Days of Exercise at 7,200 Ft Altitude Consuming the Meal, Ready-to-Eat Ration.* Technical Report T3-87. Fort Detrick, MD: US Army Medical Research and Development Command.

Baker-Fulco CJ, Kramer FM, Lesher LL, Merrill E, Johnson J, DeLany J. 2002. *Dietary Intakes of Female and Male Combat Support Hospital Personnel Subsisting on Meal-Focused or Standard Versions of the Meal, Ready-to-Eat.* Technical Report T-01/23. Natick, MA: US Army Research Institute of Environmental Medicine.

Belenky G, Penetar DM, Thorne D, Popp K, Leu J, Thomas M, Sing H, Balkin T, Wesensten N, Redmond D. 1994. The effects of sleep deprivation on performance during continuous combat operations. In: Marriott BM, ed. *Food Components to Enhance Performance.* Washington, DC: National Academy Press. Pp. 127–135.

Booth CK, Coad RA, Forbes-Ewan CH, Thomson GF, Niro PJ. 2003. The physiological and psychological effects of combat ration feeding during a 12-day training exercise in the tropics. *Mil Med* 168(1):63–70.

Bulbulian R, Heaney JH, Leake CN, Sucec AA, Sjoholm NT. 1996. The effect of sleep deprivation and exercise load on isokinetic leg strength and endurance. *Eur J Appl Physiol Occup Physiol* 73(3–4):273–277.

Caldwell JA, Ramspott S. 1998. Effects of task duration on sensitivity to sleep deprivation using the multi-attribute task battery. *Behav Res Method Instru Comput* 30(4):651–660.

Consolazio CF, Johnson HL, Nelson RA, Dowdy R, Krzywicki HJ, Daws TA, Lowry LK, Waring PP, Calhoun WK, Schwenneker BW, Canham JE. 1979. *The Relationship of Diet to the Performance of the Combat Soldier. Minimal Calorie Intake during Combat Patrols in a Hot Humid Environment (Panama).* Technical Report 76. San Francisco, CA: Letterman Army Institute of Research.

Consolazio CF, Matoush LO, Johnson HL, Nelson RA, Krzywicki HJ. 1967a. Metabolic aspects of acute starvation in normal humans (10 days). *Am J Clin Nutr* 20(7):672–683.

Consolazio CF, Nelson RA, Johnson HL, Matoush LO, Krzywicki HJ, Isaac GJ. 1967b. Metabolic aspects of acute starvation in normal humans: Performance and cardiovascular evaluation. *Am J Clin Nutr* 20(7):684–693.

Guezennec CY, Satabin P, Legrand H, Bigard AX. 1994. Physical performance and metabolic changes induced by combined prolonged exercise and different energy intakes in humans. *Eur J Appl Physiol Occup Physiol* 68(6):525–530.

Haslam DR. 1982. Sleep loss, recovery sleep, and military performance. *Ergonomics* 25(2):163–178.

Hoffer LJ. 2004 (August 9). *Optimum Protein Intake in Hypocaloric States.* Paper presented at the Institute of Medicine Workshop on the Optimization of Nutrient Composition of Military Rations for Short-Term, High-Stress Situations, Natick, MA. Institute of Medicine Committee on Optimization of Nutrient Composition of Military Rations for Short-Term, High-Stress Situations.

IOM (Institute of Medicine). 1992. *A Nutritional Assessment of US Army Ranger Training Class 11/ 91.* Washington, DC: Institute of Medicine.

IOM. 1995. *Not Eating Enough.* Washington, DC: National Academy Press.

IOM. 2004a. *Dietary Reference Intakes Tables—The Complete Set.* [Online]. Available: http://www.iom.cdu/Object.File/Master/21/372/0.pdf [accessed February 24, 2005].

IOM. 2004b. *Monitoring Metabolic Status. Predicting Decrements in Physiological and Cognitive Performance.* Washington, DC: The National Academies Press.

Johnson RF, Merullo DJ, Montain SJ, Castellani JW. 2001. Marksmanship during simulated sustained operations. *Proceedings of the Human Factors and Ergonomics Society. 45th Annual Meeting, 2001.* 45:1382–1385.

Jones TE, Hoyt RW, Baker CJ, Hintlian CB, Walczak PS, Kluter RA, Shaw CP, Schilling D, Askew EW. 1990. *Voluntary Consumption of a Liquid Carbohydrate Supplement by Special Operations Forces During a High Altitude Cold Weather Field Training Exercise.* Technical Report T20-90. Natick, MA: US Army.

Keys A, Brozek J, Henschel A, Mickelsen O, Taylor HL. 1950. *The Biology of Human Starvation.* Minneapolis, MN: The University of Minnesota Press.

Krueger GP. 1991. Sustained military performance in continuous operations: Combatant fatigue, rest and sleep needs. In: Gal R, Mangelsdorff AD, eds. *Handbook of Military Psychology.* New York: John Wiley & Sons. Pp. 255–277.

Legg SJ, Patton JF. 1987. Effects of sustained manual work and partial sleep deprivation on muscular strength and endurance. *Eur J Appl Physiol Occup Physiol* 56(1):64–68.

Montain SJ. 2004 (August 9). *Physiological Demands of Combat Operations.* Paper presented at the Institute of Medicine Workshop on the Optimization of Nutrient Composition of Military Rations for Short-Term, High-Stress Situations, Natick, MA. Institute of Medicine Committee on Optimization of Nutrient Composition of Military Rations for Short-Term, High-Stress Situations.

Montain SJ, Young AJ. 2003. Diet and physical performance. *Appetite* 40(3):255–267.

Montain SJ, Shippee RL, Tharion WJ. 1997. Carbohydrate-electrolyte solution effects on physical performance of military tasks. *Aviat Space Environ Med* 68(5):384–391.

Moore RJ, Friedl KE, Kramer TR, Martinez-Lopez LE, Hoyt RW, Tulley RE, DeLany JP, Askew EW, Vogel JA. 1992. *Changes in Soldier Nutritional Status & Immune Function During the Ranger Training Course.* Technical Report T13-92. Natick, MA: US Army Medical Research and Development Command.

Nindl BC, Leone CD, Tharion WJ, Johnson RF, Castellani JW, Patton JF, Montain SJ. 2002. Physical performance responses during 72 h of military operational stress. *Med Sci Sports Exerc* 34(11):1814–1822.

Rai RM, Sridharan K, Swamy YV, Mukherjee AK, Radhakrishnan U, Kumaria MML, Grover SK, Bhardwaj SK, Upadhyay TN, Patil SKB, Sampatkumar T, Rao YBM, Pillai PBS, Arora BS, Phool HS. 1983. *Effect of Repeated Strenuous Exercise Under Low Energy Intake on Physical Performance.* AFMRC Report 874/77. Delhi Cantt, India: Defence Institute of Physiology and Allied Sciences.

Rognum TO, Vartdal F, Rodahl K, Opstad PK, Knudsen-Baas O, Kindt E, Withey WR. 1986. Physical and mental performance of soldiers on high- and low-energy diets during prolonged heavy exercise combined with sleep deprivation. *Ergonomics* 29(7):859–867.

Shippee R, Friedl K, Kramer T, Mays M, Popp K, Askew E, Fairbrother B, Hoyt R, Vogel J, Marchitelli L, Frykman P, Martinez-Lopez L, Bernton E, Kramer M, Tulley R, Rood J, Delany J, Jezior D, Arsenault J. 1994. *Nutritional and Immunological Assessment of Ranger Students With Increased Caloric Intake.* Technical Report T95-5. Fort Detrick, MD: US Army Medical Research and Materiel Command.

Taylor HL, Ruskirk ER, Brozek J, Anderson JT, Grande F. 1957. Performance capacity and effects of caloric restriction with hard physical work on young men. *J Appl Physiol* 10(3):421–429.

Tharion WJ, Moore RJ. 1993. *Effects of Carbohydrate Intake and Load Bearing Exercise on Rifle Marksmanship Performance.* Technical Report T5-93. Natick, MA: US Army Research Institute of Environmental Medicine.

Tharion WJ, Lieberman HR, Montain SJ, Young AJ, Baker-Fulco CJ, Delany JP, Hoyt RW. 2005. Energy requirements of military personnel. *Appetite* 44(1):47–65.

Tharion WJ, Shukitt-Hale B, Coffey B, Desai M, Strowman SR, Tulley R, Lieberman HR. 1997. *The Use of Caffeine to Enhance Cognitive Performance, Reaction Time, Vigilance, Rifle Marksmanship and Mood States in Sleep-Deprived Navy SEAL (BUD/ S) Trainees.* Technical Report T98-4. Natick, MA: US Army Research Institute of Environmental Medicine.

US Department of the Army. 1947. *Nutrition.* AR 40-250. Washington, DC: Department of the Army.

US Department of the Army. 1997. *Army Aviation Operations.* FM-100. Feburary 21. Washington, DC: Department of the Army.

US Departments of Army, Navy, and Air Force. 2001. *Nutrition Standards and Education.* AR 40-25/BUMEDINST 10110.6/AFI 44-141. Washington, DC: US Department of Defense Headquarters.

VanHelder T, Radomski MW. 1989. Sleep deprivation and the effect on exercise performance. *Sports Med* 7(4):235–247.

Wilkinson R. 1969. Some factors influencing the effect of environmental stressors upon performance. *Psychol Bull* 72(4):260–272.

Wilkinson RT, Edwards RS, Haines E. 1966. Performance following a night of reduced sleep. *Psychon Sci* 5(12):471–472.

2

Answers to the Military's Questions

This chapter presents the committee's conclusions and recommendations regarding the specific questions posed by the military on the optimal nutrient composition of the assault ration. Chapter 3 provides additional comments and suggestions related to food ration development because the success of the ration is ultimately associated with its acceptability by the soldiers in the field.

The need for specific nutrients is influenced by the health status and specific scenario and environmental conditions in which soldiers are deployed. To provide context for the recommendations, assumptions of the characteristics of the soldiers' diets and health, the missions, and other issues were formulated. These assumptions were compiled throughout the deliberations of the committee, open sessions with sponsor representatives and other military personnel, information from a field survey conducted in Afghanistan, and available literature. As a result, a worst-case scenario was constructed so that the recommended assault ration would diminish, to the extent possible, significant losses of body fat and protein, which, if allowed to occur, might prevent soldiers completing an assault mission from being redeployed to a subsequent mission in the immediate future.

Finally, where the committee identified gaps in the information available, research needs to establish nutrient requirements and to unravel food technology challenges are provided. This chapter presents the assumptions, along with the committee's conclusions and recommendations, and research needs specific for each nutrient.

ASSUMPTIONS

The assault ration recommended in this report is designed for healthy male soldiers with an average body weight of 80 kg, approximately 16 percent body fat who are relatively fit and within an age range of 18–45 years (average < 25 years) while on military assault missions. As evident in Table 1-1, the ration recommended does not meet the military recommended nutrient intakes for garrison in AR 40-25 (US Departments of Army, Navy, and Air Force, 2001) nor does it meet the recommended nutrient intakes for civilians (IOM, 1997a, 1998, 2000, 2001b, 2002a, 2004). For very active male soldiers in the field, daily energy intakes rarely are over 3,000 kcal (IOM, 1995) and unpublished data suggest they average 2,400 kcal (see Montain, 2004 in Appendix B), which in the event of energy expenditures of 4,500 kcal are significantly hypocaloric. Prolonged and continuous use of this hypocaloric ration as the sole source of sustenance at such high energy expenditures will lead to substantial weight loss. The committee emphasizes that this ration is meant to be used for repetitive three- to seven-day missions that last for a maximum total period of one month and that include recovery periods of 24 to 72 hours between missions. With the expected energy expenditures of 4,500 kcal/day during the missions, it is possible that some soldiers might lose as much as 10 percent body weight before the end of the month, even with refeeding between missions; this degree of weight loss could result in adverse, but mild performance decrements. However, there is not likely to be any serious consequences for health. Therefore, it is recommended that weight loss be measured after one month of use, and if weight loss is higher than 10 percent for a soldier, he should not be sent on assault missions until weight is regained to within 5 percent of initial weight.

Scenarios Before and After Deployment on Assault Missions

The committee assumes that, before being deployed on a mission, soldiers may be living in one of three general scenarios:

1. A base in the United States or a foreign country in which food is relatively abundant and consumed on an ad libitum, uncontrolled basis. Soldiers have ready access to beverages, often including alcohol, and dietary supplements.
2. A more highly controlled environment in a military theatre of operations. In such an environment, food consumption is ad libitum from either field kitchens or conventional foods in a garrison situation. There is a variable but generally more limited availability of other substances including food and dietary supplements.
3. A recovery site where soldiers are in the process of rehabilitation from a prior assault mission. Food choice is even more limited, with fewer menu

items available, and provided ad libitum but in a more controlled environment than in the field kitchen. Nevertheless, the amount of food and calories available are more abundant than while deployed on an assault mission.

The probability of soldiers deploying from any of these scenarios will no doubt vary, depending on the theatre of operations for the assault mission.

Diets Prior to Assault Mission

Food Consumption

It is unclear what foods and beverages soldiers would be likely to consume before an assault mission. Existing literature and soldier interviews indicate that their food usually comes from a field kitchen. The soldiers may be eating Meals, Ready-to-Eat (MREs) or hot meals with bread and dessert served in a portable cafeteria line, but without fresh fruits or vegetables. Food in the pre-deployment setting is generally provided ad libitum. The committee assumes that the soldiers' diet prior to the assault mission is ad libitum from a field kitchen without fresh fruits or vegetables.

Alcohol Consumption

Although military policy strictly prohibits alcohol consumption in the field operations, some alcoholic beverages are probably available in the local environment in many theatres of military operations. Some soldiers may have consumed alcohol in the days immediately before the mission. The likelihood of this happening depends on whether soldiers are deployed to the mission from a controlled environment or not (see scenarios above). Available information suggests that excessive alcohol consumption is unlikely to be a major problem among those being deployed on assault missions in the field. The committee assumes that soldiers may consume alcohol before the assault mission, but this is unlikely to be a major problem.

Use of Dietary Supplements and Other Substances

Dietary supplements, caffeine, and other substances such as tobacco may be available locally from several sources, as well as from shipments from home. As a result, effects of these on nutrient requirements as well as withdrawal symptoms may be relevant. The committee assumes that a soldier may use supplements and caffeine before the assault mission and withdrawal symptoms may interfere with performance. The general use of tobacco products is also assumed.

Diets Immediately Before Assault Mission

Existing reports suggest that immediately (i.e., a day or hours) before the assault mission, soldiers are well hydrated. Indeed, because soldiers know that fluids are likely to be limited during the mission, with only four to five liters of water available, they may attempt to overhydrate themselves for a few hours before the mission. While a soldier could eat in excess or use protein-rich supplements in the period immediately prior to deployment on an assault mission, in general it has been reported that soldiers pay little attention to nutritional considerations during this time. It has also been reported that approximately 40 percent of the soldiers increase energy intake (primarily as carbohydrate) prior to deployment. Alcohol is strictly prohibited, although some alcohol may be available from the local environment; alcohol use was not reported as a problem. It is estimated that 20–30 percent of the soldiers smoke and as many as 60 percent chew or dip tobacco. The committee assumes that immediately prior to a mission soldiers are well hydrated, often use tobacco products, and do not abuse alcohol.

Scenario During Assault Mission

Duration of Mission

The worst-case scenario is depicted as three- to seven-day missions that will be repeated several times with little rehabilitation in between missions, leading to increased physiological stress. Based on experiences in Afghanistan, in a 30-day period soldiers might be in assault operations as many as 24 days. The committee assumes that a soldier is in an assault mission 24 out of 30 days, with each mission lasting three to seven days.

Physical Activity and Energy Expenditure

The energy expenditure of soldiers while on an assault mission is reported to be approximately 4,500 kcal/day due to intermittent periods of high energy expenditure (> 50 percent VO_2max) and periods of low-intensity, sustained movement. According to the experiences in Afghanistan, during a mission many soldiers sleep about five to six hours per day; the average sleep time, however, was four hours. The committee assumes that a soldier is physically active for a total of 20 hours per day, gets four hours per day of sleep, and expends about 4,500 kcal/day.

Consumption of Ration Food Items

Observational data from testing First Strike Rations (FSRs), a lightweight ration prototype being developed for assault missions by the US Department of

Defense Combat Feeding Directorate in Natick, Massachusetts, showed little wastage at approximately 2,400 kcal when used in military training. Some reports, however, suggest that with other higher-calorie rations, soldiers trade and selectively discard items (stripping) according to individual preferences. It appears that there is less stripping of the FSR than was the case in Desert Storm using MREs in the early 1990s (personal communication, S. Montain, US Army Research Institute of Environmental Medicine [USARIEM], August 9, 2004). When stripping of rations does occur, the carbohydrate-rich (e.g., candies) and protein-rich (or those entrees that are perceived as high in protein) meal items are the ones most frequently preserved. Items stripped depend on the environment; some items are favored in hot climates and others in cold climates. Relevant to these discussions is the fact that during Ranger Training in which one MRE per day plus a bread item (1,600 kcal/day) was provided, the rangers did not discard but rather ate 100 percent of the ration; however, their daily energy expenditure averaged 4,000 kcal and the period of training in the field was twice as long (56 days) as the time being considered in this report (Shippee et al., 1994). Other observations indicate that during recent Iraq missions troops discarded food items from MREs to carry more ammunition and then became hungry. It is not known what or how much was thrown away.

The committee assumes that, if palatable, when provided with an assault ration of 2,400 kcal or less per day, soldiers expending 4,500 kcal per day will consume virtually 100 percent of the ration.

Accessibility to Water

It is assumed that soldiers have four to five liters of chlorinated water (i.e., 2-5 ppm chlorine) available during the mission. Water will be resupplied or obtained from other sources during the mission.

Health Issues

Little specific information is available on prevalence of diarrhea during recent assault missions in Afghanistan. Cases of diarrhea were reported as being a problem when soldiers ate local foods. Very few of the cases of diarrhea resulted in dehydration so severe that personnel had to be evacuated from the theatre of operation, although many more cases were probably treated medically in the field. Constipation in the field appears not to be of concern, according to interviews and information available to the committee. There is little information on the prevalence of kidney stones in the field, but it was mentioned as a concern in anecdotal reports. Some cases of kidney stones, though, were thought to be not the result of the rations consumed but of some preexisting condition previous to deployment (personal communication, C. Koenig, USARIEM, November 19, 2004). It is assumed that cases of diarrhea and kidney stones occur during missions and are an important consideration when making recommendations on nutritional composition of assault rations.

Environmental Conditions

The climatic conditions and geographical sites in which combat can take place vary from hot, dry deserts to cold, high-altitude mountain terrains. Deployment to these varying environments can affect the nutrient requirements of soldiers due to differences in fluid intake as well as in sweat and excretory losses of nutrients. Even more unknown are the effects of these varied environments on food preferences, acceptability, and eating behavior. Although there was no attempt to consider all the possible environmental conditions, two environmental temperatures (20 and 30°C) were assumed in cases in which losses of a particular nutrient through sweat could be significant. In line with the committee's philosophy of assuming the worst-case scenario, when sweat losses of minerals are significant (i.e., could lead to adverse health effects), an extra amount of the nutrient was included to cover the losses endured by soldiers engaged in significant energy expenditure (4,500 kcal) in warm temperatures.

Physiological Compensation for Changes in Electrolyte Intake

Electrolyte, especially sodium, intake in garrison and on mission may be very different. Adaptation to a lower level of intake is fairly rapid as reequilibrium of serum levels occurs quickly (e.g., within a few days for potassium and sodium; Luft et al., 1979; Ruppert et al., 1994). It is assumed that soldiers have different electrolyte intakes before a mission than during a mission but that the period of biological adjustment to these changes will be relatively short and thus of little consequence.

Assault Ration

Size and Weight Limits

The daily assault ration for sustained operations could be distributed in various components but must fit in 0.12 cubic feet (e.g., a 6-inch cube) and weigh no more than 3 lb (1.36 kg). Packaging material constitutes 0.181 kg of the 1.36 kg. It is assumed that the ration is on average approximately 12–17 percent water, varying greatly from one item to the other; most items are energy dense, intermediate moisture food products with negligible packaging material weight.

Form of Food

In addition to food products of intermediate moisture, gels or powders high in carbohydrate and/or electrolytes that can be added to water and candy are possible food forms that can be used in an assault ration. The committee assumed that there will be no liquid foods in the rations, and that gels, powders, or candy are alternate forms of food.

Micronutrients

Electrolytes may be supplemented as candy, gels, or powders to be added to fluid. It is assumed that all other required micronutrients, however, are provided within the food items making up the basic ration.

Food Consumption During Recovery After Deployment on Assault Missions

It is difficult to determine whether soldiers consciously attempt to gain weight during recovery or rehabilitation after missions. Anecdotal information indicates that after an assault mission and during recovery, soldiers generally eat to appetite if food is readily available, and most do not attempt to gain or lose weight. A complete reversal of the deficits incurred during the assault mission may not occur during the 1–3-day recovery period of time. For example, a report from recent operations in Afghanistan suggests that personnel are re-deployed on repeated assault missions with little time for recovery between missions. Thus, soldiers would rarely have adequate time to build up bodily stores for the next assault exercise. The committee assumes that food consumption after return from an assault mission will not allow for complete rehabilitation. However, it is also assumed that the food available during recovery will provide at a minimum the nutritional standards for operational rations as delineated in AR 40-25 (US Departments of Army, Navy, and Air Force, 2001).

QUESTION A

Should the energy content of the ration (energy density) be maximized so as to minimize the energy debt, or is there a more optimal mix of macro-nutrients and micronutrients, not necessarily producing maximal energy density?

RECOMMENDATION: The basic ration's energy content should be approximately 2,400 kcal/day. While this level does not maximize energy density, this is the average daily energy intake that has frequently been reported for soldiers during training. Choosing this caloric level minimizes the possibility of discarding food items that might result in inadequate intakes of necessary micronutrients; however, in case ration items are discarded, micronutrients should be distributed as evenly as possible throughout the food items in the ration (rather than clustering them in a few items) to prevent significant amounts of individual micronutrients from

being discarded. It should also be emphasized that rations should only be used over intermittent short terms (three to seven days) that, together, may last for a total of no more than a month.

Options for the Energy Content of the Ration

The committee discussed options that provide different macronutrient profiles and caloric content to meet the needs of soldiers on assault missions. Given the weight and size constraints of the ration (0.12 cubic feet, 1.36 kg) and unique circumstances encountered in the assault scenario, three options that represent the spectrum of possibilities were developed, and the most feasible option based on review of expected benefits and drawbacks was identified.

The first option was to design a ration that would provide enough energy (i.e., 4,500 kcal) to meet the expected needs during the mission. The advantage of such a ration, if it were eaten completely, would be that soldiers would maintain energy equilibrium and avoid the adverse consequences of a periodic hypocaloric diet. The major disadvantage of this first option would be that when food items are discarded, as is often the case when higher-calorie rations are provided, nutrients would be discarded as well, potentially resulting in inadequate intakes of essential nutrients. Therfore, a major challenge with this scenario is to design a ration of sufficient palatability so that it is eaten in its entirety. When soldiers in the field do not consume all of their ration items when they are provided with enough MREs to meet their energy needs (personal communication, C. Koenig, USARIEM, November 19, 2004), then the risk of soldiers discarding foods containing rich sources of essential nutrients and increased risk for nutrient deficiency cannot be dismissed. Although it might be possible to design a ration in which nutrients are equally distributed among items, the acceptability of such a ration would be low compared to a ration that included foods that offer variety and familiarity (see Chapter 3, *Food Matrix Considerations*). Given the routine practice of stripping based on food preferences, providing a ration with a variety of highly acceptable products that ensures 100 percent consumption is more important than providing a ration with a high caloric value that may result in important components being discarded.

A second option was to design a ration that would provide the usual energy needs of soldiers when not on assault operations; such energy needs are assumed to be approximately 3,500 kcal/day. The major advantage of this second option is that it would create a comparatively small energy deficit when energy expenditure is at the level of 4,500 kcal/day. However, this option design presents the same challenges as the one above, namely to design a ration that is fully eaten when the caloric content is higher than what they would normally eat. Given the challenge of designing a highly acceptable ration that is fully eaten by soldiers under stress in an assault operation, and due to concerns about selective discarding of some items in the ration, this is also not a viable design.

The third energy level option would provide as a basic ration 2,400 kcal/day, with a supplemental source of energy. Observations in the field indicate that during training and with 3,600 kcal (3 MREs), a soldier's voluntary energy intake is approximately 2,400 kcal/day, even when the energy expenditure is high (>7,000 kcal for marines at high altitudes and cold temperatures or ~ 6,000 kcal for Army rangers in warm temperatures) (see Montain, 2004 in Appendix B); therefore, 2,400 kcal/day represents an energy level at which virtually all of the ration should be consumed (personal communication, A. Young, USARIEM, August 9, 2004). The ration would include 100 to 120 g of protein, 350 g of carbohydrate, and the remainder as fat (approximately 22–25 percent) (see questions B and C and Box 2-1) for a total of 2,400 kcal, as well as the micronutrient recommendations which follow (see questions D and E).

BOX 2-1
General Design of the Recommended Assault Ration

Basic Ration:

Protein	100–120 g (400–480 kcal; 17–20% kcal)
Carbohydrate	350 g (1,400 kcal; 58% kcal)
Fat	58–67 g (520–600 kcal; 22–25% kcal)
Water	105 g (assuming an average of 17% moisture)
Total weight (kcal)	613–642 g (2,400 kcal)

Carbohydrate (and Electrolyte) Supplement:

Carbohydrate	100 g (400 kcal)
Water	17 g (assuming an average of 17% moisture)
Sodium	up to 12 g (based on palatability)
Potassium	up to 3.3–4.7 g (based on palatability)
Total Weight (kcal)	117 g (400 kcal)

Salt Tablets (Available Through Medical Personnel):

Sodium	up to 12 g
Potassium	up to 4.7 g
Total Weight	16.7 g

Packaging:	181 g
Total Weight	**0.95 kg**
Total Energy Content	**2,800 kcal**

NOTE: This ration is intended for use over three- to seven-day missions for up to a month. Prolonged and continuous use of these rations as a sole source of sustenance may lead to substantial weight loss. Constraints: weight of 3 lb (1.36 kg) and volume of 0.12 cubic feet.

To provide an energy level closer to the level of energy expended, 400 additional kcal should be supplemented to the basic ration, increasing the total energy content of the ration to 2,800 kcal/day. This can be accomplished with the addition of supplements in individual, small packages with a total amount of up to 100 g (400 kcal) of carbohydrate in four forms: as a powder to be dissolved in a liquid, as a gel, as candy, or as some combination of these depending on the delivery system. Although soldiers would still be in a negative energy balance, little evidence exists to suggest that a periodic hypocaloric diet, if otherwise adequate in protein and other essential nutrients as specified in the following sections, is likely to be harmful when consumed over brief periods of time (repetitive three to seven days, up to a month), even if some weight loss occurs (< 10 percent of body weight). However, with the expected energy expenditures of 4,500 kcal/day during the missions, it is possible that some soldiers might lose as much as 10 percent body weight before the end of the month, even with refeeding between missions; this degree of weight loss could result in adverse, but mild, performance decrements. However, this level of weight loss is not likely to be of any serious consequences for health. Therefore, it is recommended that weight loss be measured after one month of use, and if weight loss is higher than 10 percent for a soldier, he should not be sent on assault missions until weight is regained to within 5 percent of initial weight.

Rationale for Energy Content

Energy expenditures of soldiers during combat assault missions have been reported to be high (about 4,500 kcal/day). The committee based its recommendation for energy level on the premise that, to maintain health and performance, it is critical that soldiers have adequate nutrient intakes and that, based on experience, in this type of military operations voluntary daily energy intakes approximates 2,400 kcal.

While it is possible to construct a ration with up to 4,500 kcal within the constraints of weight and size, given the research reviewed and anecdotal information, soldiers would most likely selectively discard unwanted items ("cherry pick") and, in this way, would likely consume less of essential nutrients. A strategy to avoid nutrient inadequacies due to stripping would be to design a ration with nutrients equally distributed among items. While this might appear ideal and highly desirable from the nutritional standpoint, it is unlikely that a ration can be designed that, in addition to having nutrients equally distributed, is also palatable and acceptable, two key requirements to enhancing intake. Typically, nutrients in palatable, commercially available products are not equally distributed. To maximize acceptability and encourage consumption, the ration should contain a variety of foods that are similar to those commercially available rather than relying on the "bar" type of product fortified to contain the recommended levels of all nutrients. Moreover, given the fact that water needs increase with caloric intake, a lower calorie ration may be advantageous. Providing a ration with a variety of highly acceptable products that ensure 100 percent consumption is more important than providing a ration with a high caloric value that may result in important components being discarded.

Given the weight and volume restrictions and considerations described above, a 2,400 kcal basic ration is the most nutritionally appropriate choice among the three options discussed above (i.e., energy content of 4,500, 3,600, and 2,400 kcal). Recent experience with prototype FSRs at approximately similar levels of energy content (approximately 2,400 kcal) indicates that selective discarding of menu items in the rations was not widely practiced (personal communication, A. Young, USARIEM, August 9, 2004). A ration of 2,400 kcal, although hypocaloric, will be above the basal level necessary for covering resting metabolism in all individuals in the military. Since the caloric deficit is not likely to be sustained for more than three to seven days at a time during the assault mission, the concern about the potential inadequate intake of important nutrients when stripping a higher caloric ration outweighs the concern about the effects of multiple hypocaloric periods.

In addition to the enery content of the basic ration of 2,400 kcal, an additional 100 g (400 kcal) of carbohydrate would be a readily available source of carbohydrate. This supplemental energy source could be consumed on a periodic basis in bolus doses to keep energy (and electrolytes) at more satisfactory levels or as a supplement of energy for individuals with even greater caloric expenditure. Also, such energy-dense snacks appear to be particularly popular among the troops (personal communication, C. Koenig, USARIEM, November 19, 2004).

Even with such a low-caloric ration, specific items containing concentrated sources of a particular nutrient may be selectively discarded, leading to an increased risk of nutrient deficits. This is particularly true for items other than high-carbohydrate foods. Therefore, to further ensure the maximum consumption of all essential nutrients in the ration, the micronutrients and macronutrients should be distributed as evenly as possible; this should be accomplished without compromising acceptability across menu items in the ration.

Research Needs Related to Energy Content

- Test the acceptability of the prototype assault ration under field conditions and determine the actual amounts eaten. The extent of discarding ration items under combat conditions needs to be evaluated in field surveys, and the findings must be taken into account in ration development and refinement.

QUESTIONS B AND C

What would be the optimal macronutrient balance between protein, fat, and carbohydrate for such an assault ration to enhance performance during combat missions?

What are the types and levels of macronutrients (e.g., complex versus simple carbohydrates, proteins with specific amino acid profiles, type of fat, etc.) that would optimize such an assault ration to enhance performance during combat missions?

Protein

RECOMMENDATION: The protein level of the ration should be 100–120 g total protein (based on 1.2–1.5 g/kg of body weight for an 80 kg average male soldier). This level will likely spare muscle protein loss as well as attenuate net nitrogen loss and adequately provide for synthesis of serum proteins while the individual is in a hypocaloric state. In addition, this level of protein will likely maintain the immune and cognitive functions requiring protein or amino acids.

The committee recommends that the protein added to the ration be of high biological value. At this time, there is insufficient evidence to believe that the addition of specific amino acids or specific proteins with rapid rates of absorption would be of any additional benefit; more evidence is necessary before making a recommendation in this respect.

Background

The multiple stressors (e.g., sleep deprivation, increased energy expenditure, hypocaloric diet) during short-term combat missions may result in decrements of mental and physical function that would compromise military success and may even jeopardize lives. Optimizing the ration's protein and carbohydrate levels may be particularly important for muscle performance and cognitive function. The Recommended Dietary Allowance (RDA) for dietary protein set by the Institute of Medicine (IOM) of 0.8 g/kg of body weight per day (IOM, 2002a) and the safe amount of dietary protein to maintain body weight and nitrogen balance set for healthy persons in international dietary standards of 0.75 g/kg of body weight per day (FAO/WHO/UNU, 1985) do not necessarily apply to individuals under stress. The combination of physical and psychological stressors during combat missions presents a complex and unique situation. Nutritional needs and impact on performance in such situations have yet to be examined. Therefore, until more data become available, the committee concluded, it is prudent to include liberal amounts of protein high in biological value to avoid possible short-falls.

Limited energy intake (approximately, 2,400 kcal/day) combined with high levels of physical activity results in energy deficits of about 50 percent for a three- to seven-day assault mission and can result in muscle loss and impairments in performance. Muscle loss during simulated sustained operations has not been clearly demonstrated (Montain and Young, 2003; Nindl et al., 2002), but this is possibly due to the poor sensitivity of the methodology used to estimate losses. Other evidence, however, suggests that such energy deficits will result in muscle loss.

Many classical studies have demonstrated the importance of energy balance for body nitrogen balance (Butterfield and Calloway, 1984; Todd et al., 1984). Nitrogen balance could clearly not be maintained over the long term when energy intake was 15 percent less than expenditure, and nitrogen balance was shown to be better maintained when energy balance was positive or at least zero (Todd et al., 1984). Presumably, a major source of this nitrogen loss would be from the body's predominant and readily accessible source of nitrogen, muscle protein. Energy restriction over longer time periods results in loss of lean mass during very low-calorie dieting (Layman et al., 2003); however, the metabolic mechanisms remain to be delineated. Animal studies also showed similar findings (Anthony et al., 2000). These perturbations in muscle metabolism due to energy deficits may occur very rapidly, as evidenced by the immediate signs of muscle catabolism stimulated by a 20 percent energy intake reduction in a study that included males and females (Tipton et al., 2003). Taken together, these findings suggest that soldiers participating in missions during which energy intake is half of the energy output would be losing nitrogen; most nitrogen would be from muscle protein, although some might also come from the gastrointestinal or other internal organs.

In addition to the effects due to a hypocaloric diet, the loss of muscle protein may also be exacerbated by the intensity of the physical activity. Evidence from studies on very strenuous physical activity and muscle metabolism in rats (Anthony et al., 1999) suggests that, rather than increasing protein utilization, the physical activity involved in prolonged military missions may be detrimental to muscle protein metabolism. Although sports experts advise athletes to consume approximately 1.5 g protein per kg every day (ACSM/ADA/DA, 2000), which is nearly twice the RDA (IOM, 2002a), insufficient evidence was found to conclude that high-level physical activity alone increases the normal protein requirement. More recent reviews have come to the same conclusion (Fielding and Parkington, 2002; Tipton and Wolfe, 2004).

It thus appears that the energy deficit combined with the stressful situation found in combat alters muscle protein metabolism during missions of this type.

Rationale for the Level of Protein

Although there is a great deal of controversy over the protein requirements for athletes and active individuals, it is a reasonable and conservative hypothesis that increased protein intake would be advantageous in a situation in which the substantial energy deficit is exacerbated by high levels of physical activity (see Hoffer, 2004 in Appendix B).

Lean Tissue and Nitrogen Balance. Under eucaloric conditions, the RDA for protein (0.8 g/kg/day) (IOM, 2002a) will maintain lean tissue and normal values of its usual physiologic and laboratory markers—lean tissue maintenance and nitrogen balance—but this amount of protein might not be adequate when energy is restricted. As mentioned above, improvements in protein metabolism may be produced by increasing the protein intake. A recent study demonstrated that a greater proportion of weight lost during energy restriction came from fat rather than lean mass when protein intake was increased (Layman et al., 2003). Although this study was conducted on obese individuals, most of whom were female, in weight loss situations and they did not involve exercise, it may be inferred from the data that under mild energy deficits a higher level of protein in a diet is protein sparing.

The level of protein intake that will be necessary to assure nitrogen balance depends on the severity of the energy deficit but it will be somewhat greater than the RDA of 0.8g/kg/day (IOM, 2002a). At severe energy deficits of less than 50 percent of total energy expenditure, an intake of about 1.5 g/kg of body weight will maximize protein sparing effects (Hoffer et al., 1984). This study showed that moderately obese females on a diet to lose weight for periods of up to 4 weeks with caloric intakes of about 600–800 kcal and twice the energy expenditures achieved nitrogen equilibrium at 1.5 g/kg ideal body weight but not at 0.8g/kg protein (under eucaloric conditions). It has also been shown that in severely burned patients there is no further protein sparing when 1.4 g protein/kg versus 2.3 g protein/kg are provided (Patterson et al., 1997). Increases in energy expenditure through physical activity do not markedly alter protein requirements; thus, despite a likely energy deficit of 50 percent under combat mission conditions, protein intakes of somewhat less than 1.5 g/kg body weight/day would probably be sufficient for optimal sparing of lean tissue. Parenthetically, at this level of 1.5 g protein/kg body weight/day, this is also the maximal level of protein sparing found during severe catabolic illness and during repletion of malnourished subjects (Bistrian and Babineau, 1998; Wolfe et al., 1983). Thus, a recommendation of 1.2–1.5 g protein/kg body weight/day (i.e., 100–120 g total protein daily for an average body size of 80 kg) for the assault ration would be the committee's best estimate to attenuate net nitrogen and lean body mass loss at the recommended energy level. This amount is in fact the intake by the average American (although, in percentage, is greater than the average intake). Although it can be argued that a high protein level will increase energy expenditures due to protein thermogenesis, based on a regression analysis by Westerterp (2004), the difference in thermogenesis for a diet with 0.8 or 1.5 g/kg of protein is estimated to be about 40 kcal, a rather small difference compared to the overall energy expenditures.

Synthesis of Serum Proteins. Over the expected short-term duration of assault missions, achievement of nitrogen balance may not be a sufficient criterion to establish the desirable protein level for the ration. Another criterion to be considered is the proper functioning of antioxidant systems. The stress response, whether due to intense physical activity or systemic inflammatory response leading to oxidative stress, may impair the amino acid and protein component of the antioxidant systems (Jackson et al., 2004). The glutathione redox cycle is one such antioxidant system and one of the most important body defense systems against metabolic stress. Glutathione is a tripeptide composed of the amino acids cysteine, glutamate, and glycine. Cysteine is the rate-limiting amino acid for glutathione synthesis (Lu, 1998). It has been postulated that feeding diets marginal in protein may affect glutathione synthesis given its need for a constant amino acid supply to produce the peptide (Jackson et al., 2004). The existence of an adaptation period to lower protein diets in experimental studies is well known. For example, when switching from a usual protein intake of 1.13 g/kg/day to the lower intake of 0.75 g/kg/day, nitrogen balance was negative for the first few days and reestablished after 10 days (Gibson et al., 2002). Other studies have found similar results (Pacy et al., 1994); nitrogen balance is restored by reducing whole-body protein turnover and net protein catabolism, which maintains the endogenous rate of indispensable amino acid synthesis (Gibson et al., 2002). However, although the plasma levels of albumin, HDL apolipoprotein A1, retinol-binding protein, transthyretin, haptoglobulin, and fibrinogen are maintained, the synthetic rates of nutrient transport proteins are not (Afolabi et al., 2004). In their latest study in which on days 3 and 10 the usual protein intake was decreased, erythrocyte glutathione concentrations and synthetic rates decreased by day 3 and recovered by day 10, but erythrocyte concentrations of the constituent amino acids of glutathione were still elevated at day 10, suggesting that functional changes occurred that were related to this lower level of protein intake (Jackson et al., 2004).

Although not studied in this experimental model, amino acid availability would also be an important factor in optimizing immune function (Moldawer et al., 1978). Prior to going into combat missions, trained soldiers will likely have a protein intake greater than the 1.13 g/kg used in these studies. They then will undergo metabolic or physical stress that will exacerbate the need for essential amino acids to mount an optimal stress response. This greater need constitutes an additional reason to provide a higher protein level than the RDA.

In summary, it is likely that neither nitrogen balance nor synthesis of serum proteins will be maintained with the RDA level of protein intake when consuming a hypocaloric diet under a highly stressful scenario. A high protein intake not only will spare muscle protein but also will contribute to energy needs. Although some of the findings are ambiguous, a higher protein level may also help improve immune function (Booth et al., 2003; Keenan et al., 1982) and cognitive function (Dye et al., 2000; Fischer et al., 2002; Holt et al., 1999; IOM, 1995; Keys et al., 1950).

Food Quality. Maintaining nitrogen balance and serum protein synthesis are, by themselves, valid reasons from a physiological standpoint to recommend a high protein level for this ration. Equally important is the need to enhance the sensory properties of food items to optimize acceptability. Food items with higher amounts of protein may in fact encourage higher consumption since a ration composed of foods that are naturally high in protein, such as meats, poultry, and nuts, introduces a variety of flavors and textures that have been shown to enhance food intake (Sorensen et al., 2003).

In conclusion, both from a physiological and food quality standpoint, a higher-protein ration is superior. There is little reason to believe that a hypocaloric diet, if otherwise adequate in protein as justified above and in other essential nutrients, presents any potential for harm when consumed over multiple brief periods of time (repetitive three- to seven-day periods for up to a month) even if some weight loss occurs. However, with the expected energy expenditures of 4,500 kcal/day during the missions, it is possible that some soldiers might lose as much as 10 percent body weight before the end of the month, even with refeeding between missions; this degree of weight loss could result in adverse, but mild, performance decrements. However, this level of weight loss is not likely to be of any serious consequences for health. Therefore, it is recommended that weight loss be measured after one month of use, and if weight loss is higher than 10 percent for a soldier, he should not be sent on assault missions until weight is regained to within 5 percent of initial weight.

Rationale for the Source of Protein

Evidence from acute metabolic studies in fasting subjects suggests that increased muscle protein synthesis and net muscle protein synthesis result from provision only of indispensable amino acids. That is, dispensable amino acids are unnecessary to stimulate muscle protein accretion (Borsheim et al., 2002; Tipton and Wolfe, 2001; Tipton et al., 1999, 2003). Furthermore, acute metabolic studies of fasting subjects showed that, following resistance exercise, 6 g of indispensable amino acids resulted in amino acid uptake that was more than double that of 20 g of whole proteins (Borsheim et al., 2002; Tipton et al., 2004). Another recent study showed that indispensable amino acids, when combined with exercise, ameliorated the amino acid release from muscle in response to a 20 percent energy deficit (Tipton et al., 2003). Although the addition of amino acids might benefit performance, however, the use of amino acids as a source of protein might not present additional benefits over and above the high-protein ration recommended by the committee.

The committee considered the addition of some specific amino acids, such as branched amino acids, glutamine, or arginine, because their consumption might result in physiological effects of interest. For example, glutamine has been promoted as an immune-enhancing nutrient, particularly when catabolic stress is present as in trauma or infection; however, most of this benefit has been shown with glutamine delivered by parenteral routes (Novak et al., 2002) so that high serum glutamine levels could be achieved. Since the gastrointestinal tract metabolizes glutamine, it is difficult to achieve sufficient oral intake of glutamine to alter serum levels. Therefore, most clinical trials of oral glutamine have not been effective. Furthermore, glutamine is quite unstable and has a short shelf-life. Arginine has also been promoted for its immune-enhancing properties. It has some ability to improve hospital outcome in postsurgical patients, but only when provided with other putative immune-enhancing nutrients (Beale et al., 1999; Heyland et al., 2001; Heys et al., 1999). When provided alone, arginine has not been beneficial (Luiking et al., 2005) except in incidences of sepsis in critically ill patients. In addition, postsurgical patients are clinically much more susceptible to infection than are soldiers. Thus, inclusion of arginine as an amino acid supplement to the ration is not a high priority at this time.

Finally, the branched-chain amino acids isoleucine, leucine, and valine have been purported to improve skeletal muscle metabolism. The committee, however, concluded that at levels greater than those in 1.2 g/kg/day of high-biological-value protein, which contains 15–20 percent branched-chain amino acids, there is little likelihood that further provision of branched chain amino acids would be effective.

When whole proteins are added to food items, the biological value of the protein is an important consideration. Whole protein of high biological value is recommended for the ration. Examples include soy, casein, whey, and egg. Protein sources need to be relatively low in sulfur amino acids to maintain elevated urinary pH, because this decreases risk of stone formation. Although soy protein would be a good option as a protein source because it is low in sulfur amino acids, its relatively high level of oxalate could also increase the risk of stone formation (Massey et al., 2002). Net protein synthesis might also be influenced by the speed with which protein is absorbed (slow- versus fast-absorption protein) (Dangin et al., 2003). The committee concluded that, at the high level of protein intake recommended and with the high energy deficit, the rate of absorption from the small intestine will not significantly affect protein deposition.

Research Needs

- Investigate the effects of the higher protein level recommended compared to maintenance protein intakes under high energy expenditure situations resulting in hypocaloric conditions and stress on muscle loss, physical and cognitive performance, and immune function. Muscle loss should be assessed by state-of-the-art techniques such as dual energy X-ray absorptiometry or whole-body nitrogen measurement. Physical performance should be assessed by measurement of maximal oxidative capacity, endurance, and strength. Immune function should be measured by both in vitro and in vivo methods.

- Continue research efforts on the potential to improve physical and cognitive performance and immune function by supplementing diets with indispensable amino acids compared to supplementing with whole protein.
- Conduct further research on the potential benefits of adding specific amino acids in addition to protein when subjects are consuming a hypocaloric diet under the environmental conditions and high-stress situations of combat missions. There is suggestive evidence obtained under significantly different conditions that warrants continuing research, specifically with arginine for immune enhancement and wound healing, and glutamine for intestinal function and immune function.
- Investigate the influence of individual variability on the effect of high-protein diets on performance in hypocaloric states.
- Study body composition and physical activity as factors that influence protein sparing and prevention of muscle loss.

Carbohydrate

RECOMMENDATION: The carbohydrate in the basic ration should be 350 g to optimize physical performance. An additional 100 g of carbohydrate should be available as a supplement. Therefore, the overall recommendation is for 450 g.

The committee considers palatability to be the major consideration in designing the food products to ensure ration consumption; thus, the food items and the carbohydrate supplement should provide a variety of flavors. The amount of fructose as a monosaccharide should be less than 25 g to avoid the possibility of osmotic diarrhea. Dietary fiber should be 15–17 g and should include both nonviscous, fermentable fiber (e.g., gums, pectin, β-glucans, soy polysaccharides) and viscous, nonfermentable fiber (e.g., cellulose, lignin, hemicellulose).

Background

Carbohydrate as an Energy Source. Carbohydrate is the major energy source for skeletal muscle and the brain. After ingestion, carbohydrate is digested into monosaccharides in the small intestine, absorbed, transported in the blood to the liver by way of the hepatic portal system, and then either removed by the liver or released into the circulation (Williams, 2005). Monosaccharides can be stored as glycogen in the liver or muscle or be used as immediate fuel by muscle and brain cells. Muscle glycogen is metabolized anaerobically through glycolysis in the cytoplasm, where glucose is converted to lactic acid units with the formation of small amounts of adenosine triphosphate (ATP), and aerobically, through glycolysis in the cytoplasm and the tricarboxylic acid cycle-electron transport system in the mitochondria, resulting in the production of substantially more ATP (Powers and Howley, 1997; Wilmore and Costill, 1999).

In skeletal muscle, anaerobic glycolysis can produce a limited supply of ATP at a rapid rate compared with aerobic glycolysis, which can produce a greater amount of ATP, but at a slower rate (Powers and Howley, 1997; Williams, 2005, p. 91; Wilmore and Costill, 1999). Hence, short-term, high-intensity exercise, in which ATP is needed rapidly, relies predominantly on anaerobic glycolysis, while longer endurance activity relies predominantly on aerobic glycolysis. Glucose (or carbohydrate) ingested during exercise enters directly into these muscle metabolic pathways rather than being stored as muscle glycogen (Williams, 2005). Thus, carbohydrate is a versatile, important energy source in muscle for a wide array of physical activities.

Glucose is also the obligatory energy substrate for the brain (Rosenthal et al., 2001). Because glycogen levels in the brain are low compared to liver and muscle, a constant supply of glucose from the blood is necessary. Blood glucose is tightly regulated by hormonal control (insulin and glucagon) to maintain levels in a narrow range for optimal usage by brain cells. It has been proposed that high cognitive demand may activate specific brain areas and deplete glucose in that area, resulting in cognitive dysfunction (Rosenthal et al., 2001). Functional magnetic resonance imaging has been used to show that the brain oxygenation state is altered by hypoglycemia (Rosenthal et al., 2001). Whether increased cognitive demands during physical activity alter brain glucose needs is unknown.

Carbohydrate for Physical Performance. In the muscle, stored carbohydrate (glycogen) can be used for both anaerobic (short-term, high-intensity) and aerobic (endurance) activity (Powers and Howley, 1997; Williams, 2005; Wilmore and Costill, 1999). During rest, carbohydrate supplies about 15–20 percent of the muscle's energy need, while during moderate intensity exercise, carbohydrate use increases to over 50 percent and becomes greater as the intensity of exercise is increased (Williams, 2005). Muscle can also draw glucose from the circulation and from the liver to augment energy production. Carbohydrate is more efficient than fat as a fuel, and the rate of supply of ATP for muscle contraction is faster than that of fat. Therefore, maintaining muscle glycogen and blood glucose levels is important for optimal physical performance.

Muscle glycogen levels are directly related to the amount of carbohydrate in the diet. On high-carbohydrate diets (80 percent of total energy), more muscle glycogen is stored compared to a normal carbohydrate diet (55 percent of total energy) (Bergstrom et al., 1967). Early studies found that endurance performance (time to exhaustion) (Ahlborg et al., 1967; Bergstrom et al., 1967) or ability to maintain optimal running pace (Karlsson and Saltin, 1971) was directly related to the initial muscle glycogen level in the exercising muscle.

Athletes ingesting a low-carbohydrate diet (40 percent of total calories) were not able to maintain muscle glycogen levels compared with athletes who ingested a high-carbohydrate diet (70 percent of total calories) (Costill and Miller, 1980).

Diets low in carbohydrate and low muscle glycogen levels were associated with suboptimal performance (Costill and Miller, 1980; Costill et al., 1988). The consumption of either normal or amplified food rations (increased calories and the proportion of carbohydrate) showed no difference in the effect on muscle glycogen level during 4.5 days of field exercises, although in both cases muscle glycogen was severely depleted (Jacobs et al., 1983). These data suggest that extra carbohydrate is used immediately for energy production in muscle, rather than being stored as muscle glycogen. Sufficient carbohydrate is important for maintaining optimal performance during sustained military operations (see Tipton, 2004 in Appendix B).

Carbohydrate Supplementation to Optimize Performance. Because those engaged in strenuous physical activity require an increased amount of carbohydrate to optimize performance, carbohydrate is often supplemented, especially in the form of beverages that also serve to maintain hydration. As reviewed by Coyle (2004 in Appendix B), carbohydrate ingestion has been shown to benefit performance of moderate- to high-intensity continuous or intermittent exercise lasting more than one hour. Convertino et al. (1996) recommended that carbohydrate be ingested at a rate of 30–60 g/hour to maintain carbohydrate oxidation and delay fatigue. Friedl and Hoyt (1997) reviewed the history of military nutrition research in the past century and concluded that one way to deal with the reduced energy intake ($\leq 3,000$ kcal/day) during field training when energy expenditure could be 4,000 kcal/day or higher was to provide soldiers with a carbohydrate-electrolyte beverage supplement. Typical carbohydrate intake of soldiers in the field is about 300 g/day (Friedl and Hoyt, 1997), which would fall short of the 464–608 g/day or more that may be needed as cited in the next section, Rationale for the Level of Carbohydrate. Therefore, some means to supplement carbohydrate in the diet would appear critical for optimizing performance of soldiers in the field.

Although most research studies examined the effect of supplemental carbohydrate on sport or exercise performance (Coyle, 2004 in Appendix B), research has demonstrated that carbohydrate will also improve performance on military tasks. Tharion and Moore (1993) randomly assigned 15 male soldiers to a 250, 400, or 550 g carbohydrate diet (with total caloric content and protein constant) for a four-day period. These subjects performed a marching exercise on a treadmill for up to 4 hours at the rate of 3.5 mph while carrying a 45 kg backpack. Accuracy and speed for a rifle shooting test were assessed before and after the exercise. A significant deterioration in shooting performance occurred after the exercise when the 250 g carbohydrate diet was followed, but there was no significant decrement in performance for the 400 or 550 g carbohydrate diet.

To evaluate the effect of supplemented carbohydrate on total food intake and activity, the voluntary energy and carbohydrate intake of Marines who were randomly assigned to either a carbohydrate-beverage supplement or a noncaloric placebo beverage during an 11-day field training exercise was estimated, along with energy expenditure (Tharion et al., 2004). Both groups received a similar total amount of carbohydrate in the food ration. Energy expenditure was assessed by doubly labeled water techniques. Exercises included bouts of repetitive lifting of a 45 kg weight, running, calisthenics, and routine manual work. The total carbohydrate ingested by the carbohydrate-supplemented group averaged 470 g (293 g in the ration, 177 g supplemented), and the corresponding values for the placebo group were 317 g (310 g and 7 g, respectively). Total energy intake of the carbohydrate-supplemented and the placebo groups was 3,120 kcal (13.1 MJ) and 2,670 kcal (11.2 MJ), respectively. Total energy expenditure was 4,380 kcal (18.4 MJ) and 3,840 kcal (16.1 MJ) for the carbohydrate-supplemented and the placebo group, respectively, with no significant difference between groups. The carbohydrate-supplemented group consumed an additional 153 g of carbohydrate and 450 kcal (1.9 MJ)/day of energy. Thus, providing a carbohydrate beverage may reduce energy and carbohydrate deficits that commonly occur during field training (Tharion et al., 2004). It should be noted that this increase in carbohydrate intake was concomitant with a slight decrease in protein intake (105 g protein intake in the placebo group versus 93 g in the experimental group). Although such a slight decrease might not result in adverse effects, the committee cautions that protein intake should remain at the recommended level and should not be compromised when a carbohydrate supplement is provided to increase energy intake.

In another study of military subjects, 27 infantry soldiers were fed diets containing approximately 2,600 kcal/day during three days of field training in hot humid conditions (30°C, 60 percent relative humidity) (Montain et al., 1997). The soldiers were randomly assigned to groups receiving a carbohydrate-electrolyte, placebo, or water beverage. The carbohydrate-electrolyte beverage provided an additional 1,000 kcal/day. The groups ingested on average a total of 462, 175, and 217 g/day of carbohydrate, respectively, while fluid intake was not different among the groups. Soldiers drinking the carbohydrate-electrolyte beverage were more likely to maintain their performance during the uphill run and the marksmanship performance.

Environmental factors also affect the amount of carbohydrate needed. Montain and Young (2003) summarized a study of Askew et al. (1987) who showed that soldiers who ingested carbohydrate-electrolyte drinks compared to a placebo during four days at an altitude of 4,100 m consumed 250 additional grams of carbohydrate and covered more distance during a two-hour run than the placebo group. In hot environments, greater muscle glycogen use during exercise in the heat (41°C) than in cold conditions (9°C) has been demonstrated in a number of studies (Febbraio et al., 1996, Fink et al., 1975). Although two studies have reported that supplemental carbohydrate during exercise in the heat did not improve performance (Febbraio, 2001; Febbraio et al., 1996), the addition of 204 g of carbohydrate in water was found to be more effective in maintaining cycling performance over two hours than water or carbohydrate alone (Fritzsche et al., 2000). These last results suggest that carbohydrate supplementation during endurance performance in the heat, when dehydration is not a factor, benefits performance by increasing blood glucose uptake and oxidation. Thus, supplemental carbohydrate in a fluid should provide a valuable energy source in field situations that require continuous physical activity.

Carbohydrate for Cognitive Performance. Nutrient influences on psychological and behavioral functions have been reviewed (Dye and Blundell, 2002) and the results of trials exploring nutrient effects on commonly assessed aspects of cognitive performance summarized. Cognitive performance functions include reaction time (simple and complex), vigilance/attention, information processing, memory, reasoning, and psychomotor performance. Nutritional interventions that increase blood glucose appear to improve reaction times in a few studies, while carbohydrate-rich foods may impair reaction times under some circumstances in other studies. Still others find either no effect or improvement (Dye and Blundell, 2002). Similarly, various studies of vigilance and attention found that high-carbohydrate meals, compared to low-carbohydrate meals, led to performances that were better, worse, or no different. Memory is improved when glucose is given, but carbohydrate in other forms has had more variable effects (Dye and Blundell, 2002).

These generally inconclusive results are not surprising given that the studies typically involved very brief (often, one meal) nutritional interventions usually of unstressed adults in sedentary conditions, in addition to varying the methodologies and nutritional manipulations. Importantly, "It is also clear that cognitive performance is normally well protected by a regulatory process that maintains a stable output" (Dye and Blundell, 2002).

Studies of the effects of nutritional interventions on cognitive performance in more challenging settings of high-energy output and physical or psychological stress are therefore more germane to the uses of the assault ration. Such studies offer situations that are more analogous to the demands of assault missions in that they may draw on the participants' resources to the point at which cognitive decrements might ordinarily be observed.

Other reviews have pointed out that, although performance benefits from supplemental carbohydrate can often be ascribed to effects on metabolism, other factors may also play a role (Coyle, 2004; Kaplan, 2004 in Appendix B). In this regard, several studies have reported the benefits of supplemental carbohydrate feeding when fatigue is not due to a lack of aerobic or anaerobic carbohydrate energy. The exercise tasks used in these studies are general stop-and-go, high-intensity exercise (Coyle, 2004). Performance benefits in this case may be due to preventing a decline in cognitive function. For example, in one study subjects ingested either a carbohydrate-electrolyte beverage or placebo before and during a shuttle-running protocol (Welsh et al., 2002). The carbohydrate-electrolyte beverages (overall ~127.5 g supplemented carbohydrate) enhanced performance, and there was a self-reported reduction of perceived fatigue (assessed by Profile of Mood States [POMS] and improved motor skill performance). In a randomized cross-over design, a high-carbohydrate (8.5 g/kg body weight/day) diet was compared to normal carbohydrate diet (5.4 g/kg body weight/day) over the course of 11 days, including seven days of intense physical training (Achten et al., 2004). The high-carbohydrate diet resulted in better maintenance of running performance and global mood state (assessed by the POMS test). Both groups, however, were on fairly high-carbohydrate diets (e.g., for an 80 kg person approximately 432 g and 680 g, respectively).

Using a within-subjects design, changes in reaction times after 100-minute runs were assessed in well-trained athletes, but gender was not specified (Collardeau et al., 2001). The reaction time trials consisted of (1) simple reaction time, where subjects were instructed to lift their thumb off a button in response to a stimulus, and (2) choice reaction time, where subjects were instructed to move a handle in one of four directions as indicated by an arrow on a computer screen. The time to respond to the stimulus was the criterion measured. Subjects received 8 ml/kg body weight of a solution prior to the session followed by a 2 ml/kg body weight every 15 minutes. The solution contained either 5.5 percent carbohydrate (glucose, fructose, maltodextrins) or placebo, with equal electrolyte content. While no effect of supplementation was observed on simple reaction time, the carbohydrate solution (but not the placebo solution) was associated with a significant improvement in complex reaction time immediately after the exercise session, as well as a smaller increase in ratings of perceived exertion over the session.

In another study, 143 young healthy male soldiers were randomly assigned to one of three groups who were given the following supplemented beverage: 6 percent carbohydrate (2.1 g/kg), 12 percent carbohydrate (4.2 g/kg), or placebo beverage. Over the 10-hour study, subjects performed a 19.3 km road march and two 4.8 km runs interspersed with rest and other activities (Lieberman et al., 2002). Vigilance as measured by reaction to an auditory signal improved in a dose-related manner with the percentage of carbohydrate. The negative components of mood (confusion, lack of vigor) as assessed by the standardized POMS test were reduced with the additional carbohydrate. Although carbohydrate supplementation appeared to enhance cognitive performance in individuals engaged in sustained, intense physical activity (Lieberman, 2003), it should be noted that no eucaloric control was used. Thus, increased energy intake may have produced the improvements in vigilance and mood.

It is important to note that the POMS test was designed to measure changes in mood states occurring over a period of a week or more (Lorr et al., 2003) and that it was originally designed to measure mood states among psychiatric patients. Since then, it has been used to measure mood changes in other populations (including sport psychology studies of athletes and studies of medical patients). POMS has not been validated to assess psychologically healthy individuals or to assess changes within shorter time frames (e.g., pre- and postexercise bouts). In addition, the POMS test assesses self-rated emotional states rather than objectively measured neurocognitive performance. While both are psychological domains, they typically are treated separately and there is usually little reason to assume that findings in one domain apply to the other.

Rationale for the Level of Carbohydrate

Carbohydrate Needs for Intense Physical Activity. The new Acceptable Macronutrient Distribution Range (AMDR) of the Dietary Reference Intakes (DRIs) (IOM, 2002a) states that normal, healthy adults should get 45–65 percent of their calories from carbohydrates. The amount of carbohydrate that others have recommended for athletes is 60–70 percent of total energy intake (Anonymous, 1991). It has been suggested, however, that the daily recovery amount of carbohydrate for athletes be expressed in grams per kilogram body weight, and the amount recommended should depend on the level of training (Burke et al., 2004). Using this approach, recommendations for recovery from moderate-duration, low-intensity training are 5–7 g/kg body weight/day, moderate to heavy endurance training 7–12 g/kg body weight/day, and extreme exercise (defined as > 4 hr/day) 10–12 g/kg body weight/day (Burke et al., 2004). For an 80 kg man, the amount of carbohydrate for recovery from moderate to heavy endurance training would be 560 to 960 g. Reviews of diet surveys of nonendurance and endurance male athletes showed daily carbohydrate intakes of 5.8 and 7.6 g/kg body weight/ day respectively, which, for an 80 kg male athlete would range from 464 to 608 g (Burke et al., 2004). Given the weight and volume constraints of the ration and needs for other nutrients, the committee recommends including 350 g/day of carbohydrate in the basic ration. This level, however, will not be sufficient to meet the needs of soldiers in high-intensity military operations. In addition to the 350 g in the basic ration, the committee recommends including an extra 100 g of carbohydrate as supplements in the form of gels, candy, or powder to be added to beverage. In this way, the total recommended amount of carbohydrate is 450 g. This amount is the minimal amount of carbohydrate needed to meet the needs of soldiers experiencing intense physical activity.

Carbohydrate Needs for Cognitive Function. Although some studies described above have found that carbohydrate may improve vigilance and reaction time, improvements in other cognitive domains associated with carbohydrate consumption have not been found. Hence, there is a lack of conclusive results on the effect of carbohydrate on cognitive performance. Also, most studies have relied on subjective methodologies that have not been validated for the scenarios of concern. The committee recommends that researchers seeking to determine the effects of carbohydrate on cognitive function develop and use tests that fall within the domain of neurocognitive functioning (e.g., attention, vigilance, short-term memory, reaction time, problem-solving ability) rather than the emotional domain (e.g., depression, anxiety, anger). In summary, although some studies have found that carbohydrate may improve vigilance and reaction time, there is no conclusive evidence to recommend specific levels of carbohydrate to enhance cognitive function.

Rationale for Type of Carbohydrate

The type of carbohydrate in the food ration menu items should be a mixture of complex and simple carbohydrates so that the food is palatable (not too sweet). Fructose as a monosaccharide should be limited due to the association between dietary fructose and diarrhea (Skoog and Bharucha, 2004). Some studies have found that dietary glucose increases the absorption of fructose, so the recommended use of a mixture of carbohydrates should limit the malabsorption of fructose (Skoog and Bharucha, 2004; Truswell et al., 1988). Because reports that consumption of 25 g of fructose as a monosaccharide for three consecutive days caused malabsorption symptoms in healthy adults (Born et al., 1994), the amount of fructose as a monosaccharide should be less than 25 g.

The supplemental carbohydrate should be available in easily digestible forms, such as powder to mix in with water (to a 4–8 percent solution) (Coyle and Montain, 1992), in carbohydrate gels, or in candy. A study by Murray and colleagues in which gastric emptying of exercising subjects was measured after drinking water or carbohydrate beverages suggests that gastric emptying significantly decreases after the 8 percent carbohydrate beverage; this decrease was not observed with either water or 4 or 6 percent carbohydrate beverages. The authors concluded that such a delay is not optimal for fluid replacement (Murray et al., 1999). Therefore, the concentration (and possibly type of carbohydrate) should be an important consideration when developing a carbohydrate beverage. As mentioned in the section above, supplemental carbohydrate delivered in fluid form should provide the most benefit to performance compared to carbohydrate alone (Fritzsche et al., 2000).

Rationale for Amount and Type of Dietary Fiber

The adequate intake (AI) for dietary fiber is based on 14 g dietary fiber/1,000 kcal, a level that has been shown to decrease risk of cardiovascular disease by virtue of its presence in foodstuffs in the gut (IOM, 2002a). Although the consumption of high amounts of total dietary fiber is desirable to reduce the risks of chronic diseases, in the case of short-term missions, avoiding diarrhea and constipation and decreasing stool weight are of greater concern to the military. Therefore, it is recommended that the range of dietary fiber in the assault ration be based on a minimum amount to avoid constipation to the extent possible and on estimates of the intake of young men in the US population. It is assumed that these amounts should prevent diarrhea and constipation. The estimated median intake and the 95th percentile intake from the Continuing Survey of Food Intake for Individuals in 1994–1996 (CSFII, 1998) in the United States for men 19–30 years old is 17.4 and 32.3 g/day of total dietary fiber, respectively (IOM, 2002a). When adjusted for the lower energy intake of the soldiers (approximately 2,400 kcal) compared to the normal population (median and 95th percentile intake of 2,718 and 4,374 kcal, respectively [IOM, 2002a]), the median intake and the 95th percentile would be approximately 15 and 17 g/day, respectively.

The type of fiber is also important. Both viscous and nonviscous fiber typically found in foods of plant and vegetable origin are important (IOM, 2002a). The available literature suggests that the viscous (liquid-like but thick and resistant to flow), nonfermentable fiber can alter blood glucose and cholesterol concentrations and optimize laxation; nonviscous, fermentable fiber can also impart beneficial effects, such as act as immunomodulators. Beta-glucan might be included as an example of a nonviscous, fermentable fiber. Beta-glucan has been evaluated as an immunostimulant and can be fermented into short-chain fatty acids in the large bowel, which improves intestinal function (i.e., acts as prebiotics) (Brown and Gordon, 2003; Frank et al., 2004). In addition, β-glucan may decrease blood cholesterol levels, and, therefore, the risk of coronary heart disease. The Food and Drug Administration recently recognized these benefits by approving the health claim that β-glucan may reduce the risk of coronary heart disease (Food Labeling. Specific Requirements for Health Claims. 21 C.F.R. §101, 2002).

Based on the median and 95th percentile intake adjusted for energy intake, the committee recommends including total dietary fiber in the range of 15–17 g/day. The committee concluded that a mixture rather than a single source of fiber might be better tolerated physiologically and may help prevent constipation. Therefore, the committee recommends that the amount provided include nonviscous, fermentable fiber (e.g., gums, pectin, β-glucans, soy polysaccharides) as well as viscous, nonfermentable fiber (e.g., cellulose, lignin, hemicellulose).

Research Needs

- Investigate the type of carbohydrate (disaccharides versus starches) that best enhances physical and cognitive performance.
- Determine whether specific fiber types will reduce the incidence of diarrhea.
- Determine the carbohydrate "dosing/delivery" schedule (e.g., continuous versus bolus) that will contribute to best improving physical and cognitive performance.
- Confirm the effects of carbohydrate on performance and cognition under conditions analogous to the high-stress situations of military operations.

Fat

RECOMMENDATION: After protein and carbohydrate needs are met, the ration should provide 58–67 g fat (22–25 percent of energy intake) to be

distributed across a variety of foods. The ration should provide a balance of dietary fatty acids between monounsaturated, polyunsaturated, and saturated fats, with at least 17 g linoleic acid and 1.6 g α-linolenic acid, recognizing essential fatty acid needs as well as the undesirable pro-oxidant properties of large amounts of unsaturated fatty acids. This balance can be determined by food formulation criteria. There is no recognized benefit to modifying fatty acid type in the ration or to adding structured lipids.

Background

The primary reason for fat in the ration is to provide a readily digestible, palatable, energy-dense source of calories to help soldiers perform physically and cognitively demanding military operations. Since appetite may be depressed under conditions of high-intensity physical activity and stress, maximal consumption of the ration is a primary goal. Fat provides a highly palatable source of calories that can be expected to promote ration intake. Among energy sources, fat has been shown to be less satiating (Gerstein et al., 2004; Mattes, 2004 in Appendix B), which should increase consumption under field conditions. In addition, recent studies indicated that greater satiety results from consumption of foods higher in protein and carbohydrate than fat (see also Chapter 3). While the desire to increase ration consumption as much as possible would support the addition of a higher level of fat, increasing the fat content would result in a decrease in the amount of carbohydrate or protein in the ration. The committee believes that, although increasing consumption is desirable, satiety is only one of the many factors that influence consumption, and the available data do not yet provide an unequivocal answer. A better understanding of the influence of nutrient composition on satiety is needed before considering it as the basis for nutrient level recommendations.

Other roles of fat must be considered as well. The ration must also satisfy essential fatty acid needs. In addition, dietary fat is frequently the vehicle for intake and absorption of fat-soluble vitamins. It can be assumed, however, that healthy young men will have adequate fat-soluble vitamin stores and that, as depot fat is utilized to meet energy needs, such fat will be the main source of fat-soluble vitamins. Thus, this role of dietary fat is not of consequence, although some supplementation with fat-soluble vitamins beyond what is naturally present in the food items may be required.

Rationale for Level of Fat

Fat as a Fuel Source. Several factors were taken into consideration in setting the fat level. First, the levels of macronutrients recommended are meant to optimize protein and carbohydrate intake. The rationale for setting the levels of protein and carbohydrate in the ration are described in detail earlier in this chapter.

Briefly, they are based on the facts that the physical demands of high-intensity military operations require a high contribution of protein to preserve lean mass, and that a high contribution of carbohydrate will maintain vigilance and physical performance. The committee concludes that, after protein and carbohydrate needs are met, fat should be used to maximize palatability and energy density.

Maintaining carbohydrate availability to muscle is critical for sustained, intense, physical activity. Numerous studies show that carbohydrate benefits performance. For example, Coyle and colleagues (1986) demonstrated that feeding carbohydrate during prolonged strenuous exercise results in high enough carbohydrate oxidation to delay fatigue. Hawley and colleagues showed improved performance capacity with high-carbohydrate diets (Hawley et al., 1997). Whether the improvement in performance occurs because the intake of carbohydrate spares muscle glycogen or because blood glucose levels are maintained is still not clear. Conversely, fat feeding induces a higher rate of fat oxidation and a rapid repletion of muscle triacylglycerol stores (Hawley, 2000). Carbohydrate, however, is more efficient than fat as a fuel and carbohydrate's rate of supply of ATP for muscle contraction is faster than that of fat. Among the macronutrients used as fuel, fat offers the advantage of providing the highest amount of calories per gram; that is fat, provides 9 kcal/g of energy compared with 4 kcal/g for protein and carbohydrate. A recent theory suggests that high-fat feeding (≥ 65 percent energy) provides an alternate fuel source, which might help to preserve muscle glycogen or slow its rate of use (Burke and Hawley, 2002; Helge, 2000). Accordingly, there might be some advantage to manipulating the diet to modify the pattern of fuel utilization to preserve or enhance performance. Currently, however, evidence in support of this theory is not convincing. A recent review of the literature concluded that fat adaptation over one to three days was not sufficient to elicit the purported metabolic shift in favor of fat utilization (Burke and Hawley, 2002). Likewise, fat adaptation over a longer period (more than seven days) did not provide performance benefits, and in some cases led to performance decrements. Switching from fat adaptation to high-carbohydrate intake did result in higher rates of fat oxidation and concomitant muscle glycogen sparing; however, this strategy did not benefit physical performance (Helge, 2000; see Helge, 2004 in Appendix B).

Two studies compared the effects of high-fat versus high-carbohydrate feeding on cognitive outcomes during endurance training. In both studies, subjects were able to complete the training, but those on high-fat feeding experienced higher perceived exertion and reported that they required more mental effort to complete the task than those on high-carbohydrate feeding (Marsh and Murlin, 1928; Stepto et al., 2002).

During military operations, high energy expenditure is likely to occur in the context of an energy deficit. None of the studies cited above considered the dual burdens of intense physical work and energy deficit on physical performance. This situation is somewhat unique to the military, and few research studies have investigated this interaction; however, one study in men who traversed the Greenland icecap on cross-country skis pulling sleds is instructive (Helge et al., 2003). The men were in energy deficit of approximately 1,000–1,500 kcal/day and consumed 30–40 percent energy as fat and 50–60 percent energy as carbohydrate. This macronutrient mix was sufficient for the men to complete their task.

Another study with distance runners varied the amount of dietary fat (17 percent, 31 percent, or 44 percent energy as fat) to maximize energy and nutrient intakes. Energy intakes were lower than energy expenditure under all feeding conditions, over approximately 30 days. However, energy intakes were higher on the medium- and high-fat diets, and subjects reported being less hungry on them. While on the 31 percent fat diet, male runners consumed 2,900 kcal/day, and intakes of essential fatty acids and vitamins were adequate (Horvath et al., 2000). For the purposes of energy delivery, it seems desirable to provide 30–40 percent of the energy in the ration as fat. Increasing the fat beyond this level does not appear to improve physical or cognitive performance. In addition, a period of 14–21 days is needed to metabolically adapt to a high-fat diet, which is beyond the period of intermittent use for this ration (Phinney et al., 1983). Given the energy recommendation of 2,400 kcal/day as well as protein and carbohydrate needs for health and performance, a ration providing 22–25 percent energy as fat appeared to be a reasonable level of intake. This level of total fat will likely provide acceptable palatability while serving as an important source of energy. In support of this level, the energy density of the average man's food is 1.91 kcal/g (Ledikwe et al., 2005) which is similar to the recommended ration's energy density of 2.03 kcal/g (1,360 g [total weight]–181 g [packaging] = 1,179 g; 2,400 kcal/1,179 g = 2.03 kcal/g).

Fat and Palatability. An ongoing concern for the military is that soldiers do not eat enough during field operations (IOM, 1995), particularly during high-intensity combat situations (Popper et al., 1989). Intense physical activity and stress are known to reduce food intake in trained athletes (King et al., 1997); however, the combined effects of highly intense physical activity, acute stress, and energy deficit on appetite mechanisms are poorly understood. Again, this combination of factors is rarely encountered outside the military context and has been seldom studied. Since both hunger and the motivation to eat may be compromised in soldiers during high-intensity field operations, it seems prudent to maximize the palatability of the ration to the extent possible.

It is well known that taste is a primary determinant of food choices (Glanz et al., 1998). Energy-dense foods such as fats are generally preferred over low-energy foods and seem to enhance overall food intake (Drewnowski, 1997). Nevertheless, there is considerable individual variation in the preferred level of fat in specific foods and for the diet as a whole (Cooling and Blundell, 2001; Mela and Sacchetti, 1991). The biological and personal factors that contribute to these differences are not well understood and need further study.

For the purposes of this report, typical intakes could be considered as an index of acceptable levels of fat in the diet. The mean estimated fat intake of young adult men in the general population is 33 percent (IOM, 2002a). Also, evidence from population studies suggests that diets providing less than 30 percent energy as fat can be well tolerated, particularly by highly motivated individuals. In the Women's Health Initiative, participants in the intervention group adhered to a diet providing approximately 25–27 percent energy as fat for five years (Women's Health Initiative Study Group, 2004). The FSRs, which are under development by the USARIEM, provide approximately 27 percent energy as fat. The military reports that FSRs are almost completely consumed in limited field tests (personal communication, C. Koenig, USARIEM, November 19, 2004). Whether the FSR provides the preferred level of fat for elite war fighters is unknown and should be ascertained in future studies. Nevertheless, based on previous experience, it is reasonable to assume that a ration providing 22–25 percent energy as fat will be relatively well accepted by soldiers in the field. Every effort should be made to optimize fat content and palatability of the ration design.

Rationale for Type of Fat

The polyunsaturated fatty acids (PUFA) omega-6 (n-6) and omega-3 (n-3) are essential in the human diet. The ration should contain, at a minimum, the recommended amounts of linoleic and α-linolenic acid to satisfy essential fatty acid needs. The effects of fatty acid type, including n-3 and n-6 fatty acids, on physical and cognitive performance, immune function, and gene expression. There is some evidence that feeding n-3 fatty acids improves endurance performance in rats (Ayre and Hulbert, 1996) and increases aerobic capacity and intracellular fatty acid transport in skeletal muscle (Clavel et al., 2002); however, the evidence for these effects in humans is extremely limited (Lukaski et al., 2001). Other evidence suggests that n-3 fatty acids, especially in combination with protein supplements, increase muscle mass and protect against muscle wasting in cancer patients (Barber et al., 1999; Fearon et al., 2003). Although these findings are provocative, they have little application to the military context at this time.

Recommended intakes of PUFA for the assault ration are thus set at the AI for men ages 19–30 years and should be at least 17 g/day of n-6 PUFA (as linoleic acid) and 1.6 g/day of n-3 PUFA (as α-linolenic acid) (IOM, 2002a). In addition, the committee believes the ration should provide for the potential health benefits of PUFA related to cardiovascular disease without unduly increasing potential pro-oxidant activity (IOM, 2002a). To that end, the committee recommends that the AMDR for these fatty acids (5–10 percent of energy from linoleic acid and 0.6–1.2 percent of energy from n-3 fatty acids [as α-linolenic acid; IOM, 2002a]) be taken into consideration in formulating food products for the ration.

The effects of structured lipids (including medium-chain triglycerides and conjugated linoleic acid) on exercise performance were also considered. Studies reviewed by Jandacek (IOM, 1994) and more recent data (Vistisen et al., 2003) found no improvement in performance with structured lipids. The committee concluded that there is insufficient evidence at this time supporting a benefit of these lipids on performance. The committee recommends that the ration contain a balance mix of saturated, polyunsaturated, and monounsaturated fatty acids, with palatability and stability the prime determinants of the specific mixture.

Research Needs

- Study the combined effects of intense physical activity, acute stress, and energy deficit on hunger and appetite.
- Explore the potential role of n-3 and n-6 fatty acids in immune and brain function.
- Investigate the biological and personal factors that influence food preferences and diet palatability.
- Develop a systematic approach to optimizing ration palatability, which would incorporate the wants and needs of end-users, early in the design process.

QUESTION D

What are the types and levels of micronutrients such as direct antioxidants (e.g., vitamin C and E, carotenoids), cofactors in antioxidant and other biochemical reactions with high metabolic flux (e.g., B vitamins, zinc, manganese, copper), or other bioactives (e.g., caffeine) that could be added to such rations to enhance performance during combat missions?

Vitamin A

RECOMMENDATION: The assault ration should contain at least 300 μg retinol activity equivalents (RAE)/day and no more than 900 μg RAE/day based on prevention of night blindness and the current RDA.

Background

Vitamin A is essential for vision, growth, cellular differentiation, integrity of epithelial cells, and the reproductive and immune systems. The RDA is set at 900 μg RAE/day for men (IOM, 2001b) based on the amount required to maintain a body pool in well-nourished subjects with liver reserves of 20 μg RAE/g (estimated four months of body storage) (Haskell et al., 1997; IOM, 2001b). The

Tolerable Upper Level (UL) for men was established at 3,000 µg of preformed vitamin A per day based on risk of liver abnormalities (IOM, 2001b).

In National Health and Nutrition Examination Survey (NHANES) III, the median and the 95th percentile dietary intake of vitamin A for 19- to 30-year-old men in the United States was 744 and 1,487 µg RAE/day, respectively (IOM, 2001b). There is no evidence of vitamin A inadequacy among the adult US population. An early symptom of actual deficiency is night blindness; that is, the inability to adapt to night vision due to impaired regeneration of rhodopsin. Although vitamin A deficiency is not a public health problem in the United States, it is a continuous concern in developing countries, and when diets are inadequate, supplementation reduces the risk of mortality of children and infants.

Rationale for Levels of Vitamin A

As much as 90 percent of vitamin A total body stores is in the liver (Olson, 1987), and liver stores of vitamin A are high in the US population. Using radio-isotopic methods, researchers have estimated the retention of consumed vitamin A to be 50 percent (Bausch and Rietz, 1977; Sauberlich et al., 1974). There is little or no evidence of vitamin A inadequacy among the adult US population (IOM, 2001b).

An adequate level of vitamin A is critical for successful performance of certain tasks in the military. For example, optimal night vision is a consideration that may determine vitamin A requirements for the combat ration. Although there is a clear association between vitamin A deficiency and night blindness, the high liver stores exhibited by the US population would ensure an adequate supply of vitamin A to peripheral tissues. Moreover, there are no known reports of night blindness among the troops. Nevertheless, to err on the conservative side, the committee recommends a level of vitamin A that would prevent night blindness. Studies on adaptation to darkness in developing countries or clinical research studies (Batchelder and Ebbs, 1943; Blanchard and Harper, 1940; Hume and Krebs, 1949; Sauberlich et al., 1974) indicate that 300 µg RAE is the median intake in adults to prevent night blindness (i.e., the Estimated Average Requirement [EAR] because an RDA for night blindness prevention could not be calculated due to the high variability in the data) (IOM, 2001b). This level, 300 µg RAE, should be considered the minimum amount in the short-term assault rations. The committee recommends an upper limit of 900 µg RAE/day. This level represents the RDA for men, which is estimated to provide four months of liver stores of vitamin A for 97–98 percent of the population (IOM, 2001b). There are no toxicity concerns at these levels.

Food Form

The sources of vitamin A could be included as preformed vitamin A or provitamin A carotenoids. All of these forms could be found naturally in foods (e.g., animal-derived foods, fruits, vegetables, and cereals); food could also be fortified to achieve a level of vitamin A within the recommended range.

Vitamin C

RECOMMENDATION: The assault rations should include a vitamin C level of 180–400 mg. This level considers the current RDA for US males 19–30 years old, 90 mg/day, plus 35 mg/day to account for the higher vitamin C requirements of smokers; to establish the lower limit of the range (180 mg), another 50 percent was added due to the potential degradation of vitamin C over the shelf-life of the ration. The upper level is the 95th percentile dietary intake of vitamin C. To minimize its interaction with pro-oxidants in the ration and further degradation, encapsulation of vitamin C should be considered. If shelf-life of the ration is such that degradation would not occur, then a lower amount (< 400 mg) should be considered as the upper end of the range.

Background

The biological function of vitamin C comes from its ability to donate reducing equivalents to reactions, including reduction of reactive oxygen that damages cells. Vitamin C is the electron donor for eight enzymes involved in collagen hydroxylation, carnitine biosynthesis, and hormone and amino acid biosynthesis. Vitamin C deficiency is characterized by impairments in connective tissue, specifically impairment of collagen synthesis. Vitamin C has also been shown to affect components of the immune response (IOM, 2000). The RDA for vitamin C was based on maintaining near-maximal neutrophil concentrations with minimal urinary loss at 90 mg for men. The median intake and the 95th percentile intake of US males ages 19–30 is 127 mg and 400 mg, respectively. The UL is set at 2 g/day based on a criterion of gastrointestinal disturbance (IOM, 2000).

Rationale for Levels of Vitamin C

Vitamin C as Antioxidant. Although the properties of vitamin C as an antioxidant suggest that a high level of vitamin C intake might prevent oxidative damage and muscle injury associated with high-intensity exercise, recent studies have indicated that supplementing the diet with vitamin C at doses of 200 and 1,000 mg does not affect markers of muscle damage, soreness, or interleukin (IL)-6 after eccentric exercise (Thompson et al., 2001, 2004). In addition, contrary to the antioxidant theory, other studies suggest that high-dose vitamin C supplementation could result in pro-oxidant adverse effects (Childs et al., 2001).

Vitamin C could exert an antioxidant effect by serving as an electron donor to oxidized vitamin E that is created (in reaction to oxidative stress) during exercise (Evans, 2000). The combination of vitamin C (500 mg) and vitamin E (up to 1,200 international units [IU]), however, shows mixed effects on signs and symptoms of muscle damage (e.g., muscle soreness and swelling were not affected, whereas maximal voluntary isometric contraction force and eccentric contractile torque and work were affected by the supplementation) (Shafat et al., 2004). The potential benefits of antioxidant supplementation were investigated in a study that provided ultramarathon runners with vitamins E (300 mg) and C (1,000 mg) for six weeks. The supplemented group was protected from lipid oxidation as evidenced by the lower level of F2-isoprostanes; however, there was no marked effect on inflammatory markers, muscle damage markers. or DNA damage markers (Mastaloudis et al., 2004a, b). For a more detailed explanation of these studies, the reader is referred to Traber and Mastaloudis (2004) in Appendix B. Similar findings were reported by Dawson et al. (2002). Animal studies show that intake of vitamin E alone after stress was more effective in lowering lipid peroxidation than other treatments, including vitamin C supplementation. In addition, an IOM committee (IOM, 1999) concluded in a letter report that there is little evidence to support the idea that supplementation with vitamin C beyond the military nutrient reference value (90 mg/day) would protect against short-term acute oxidative stress. The committee concurs with this conclusion and finds that, although future studies may prove that under certain circumstances supplementation with vitamin C or vitamin E or both might prove beneficial, at this time there is no consistent evidence that either of the vitamins alone or in combination enhances performance or health. Since the time of publication of that letter report, there has been no evidence to the contrary.

Vitamin C and Immune Function. The effectiveness of vitamin C against the common cold is also a matter of controversy. To date, supplementation with vitamin C has not been unequivocally shown to reduce the incidence or severity of the common cold (Hemila, 1994, 1997; Hemila et al., 2002; Takkouche et al., 2002)—except perhaps in those with low vitamin C intakes (e.g., males in the United Kingdom) (Hemila, 1997). Furthermore, significant effects on other aspects of the immune function have not been proven (IOM, 2000).

Vitamin C and Tobacco Consumption. One factor that the committee considered to be important in determining the level of vitamin C in the ration was the fact that most soldiers are, or become, tobacco users while being deployed. According to two studies using radiolabeled tracer ascorbic acid in healthy male smokers and nonsmokers, the metabolic turnover of the vitamin C was about 35 mg/day greater in smokers than in nonsmokers (Kallner et al., 1979, 1981). Considering the high percentage of smokers among US soldiers, the committee decided to factor in an additional 35 mg/day for the recommended level of vitamin C.

Food Form

Due to issues involving the lack of stability of vitamin C, an additional 50 percent over the desired intake level would need to be added to the food (IOM, 1997b), resulting in approximately 180 mg/day (125 + 60) in the ration. The 95th percentile intake for adult men in the United States is 400 mg/day. The committee believes that this amount will not increase the risk of stone formation since a review of the evidence for an RDA concluded that levels below 1,000 mg/day are considered safe based on risk stone formation (Levine et al., 1996). The committee recommends that food developers aim at including 180 mg but no more than 400 mg of vitamin C in the ration. If shelf-life of the ration is such that degradation would not occur, then a lower amount (< 400 mg) should be considered as the upper end of the range to avoid potential for increased stone formation.

Dried fruits that naturally contain vitamin C could be included in the ration; ration foods can also be fortified with vitamin C. If fortification is considered, vitamin C may be coated with various substances, such as ethyl cellulose, cyclodextrins, or lipids, to prevent contact with iron, copper, or nickel. As explained in Chapter 3, encapsulation of vitamin C slows its degradation under high heat and moisture conditions and protects it from oxidation by metals.

Research Needs

- Investigate the potential synergistic effects of a mixture of antioxidants on physical performance and immune function in a randomized trial.
- Conduct studies on the effects of vitamin C supplementation with high dietary levels of the vitamin, rather than pharmacological levels. Before conducting such studies, valid markers of antioxidant activity that will permit comparison of studies across laboratories are needed.
- Explore the use of vitamin C supplementation to prevent colds in young people.
- Determine the stability of vitamin C in the food under extreme environmental conditions during shelf-life of rations.
- Investigate the effects of smokeless tobacco use on vitamin C.

Vitamin D

RECOMMENDATION: The assault ration should contain 12.5–15 µg of vitamin D based on the amount of vitamin D needed to maintain a serum level of 70 nmol /L of 25(OH)D and on the amount shown to maintain serum 25(OH)D levels in military personnel assigned to submarine duty over a three-month period.

Background

Vitamin D is essential in that it maintains normal serum levels of calcium and phosphorus. Other roles of vitamin D, such as in immune disorders and cancer, are still not clear, although there is enough evidence from studies with animal models to suggest important functions (Deluca and Cantorna, 2001; Griffin et al., 2003; van Etten et al., 2002). The endogenous synthesis of pre-vitamin D from 7-dehydrocholesterol by the action of ultraviolet B (UVB) light on skin is a major contributor to the pool of vitamin D in the human body. People with dark skin, however, have high melanin levels that block UVB light; thus, they tend to be at risk of vitamin D deficiency due to a decrease in the amount of UVB light that is available for cutaneous vitamin D synthesis. In addition, the number of sunlight hours also affects the amount of endogenous synthesis. Therefore, latitude and season are factors that should be considered when determining the amount needed in the assault ration.

Unlike most other nutrients, estimates of dietary intake are not available from NHANES or the CSFII. Estimates of average vitamin D intakes for men 19–30 years old based on modeling of food and supplement intake from two nutrition surveys (NHANES III from food and supplements; CFSII from food only) have been made, and are 8 and 4.8 μg/day, respectively (Moore et al., 2004). Due to the numerous factors that affect vitamin D status, in 1997 the AI for adults was derived by increasing the amount shown to maintain adequate levels of serum 25(OH)D (> 30 nmol/L) in women during winter in Nebraska, 3.3 to 3.4 μg/day, to a total of 5 μg to cover the needs of adults 19–50 years regardless of exposure to sunlight. The UL of 50 μg/day was based on vitamin D intakes resulting in hypercalcemia (IOM, 1997a).

Rationale for Levels of Vitamin D

Using assumptions required to estimate vitamin D intakes (Moore et al., 2004), intakes of men 19–30 years old appear to approach the AI level of 5 μg/day. It is possible, however, that some soldiers may enter missions with low levels of serum 25(OH)D. Although liver storage could be expected to ensure sufficient amounts of vitamin D during short-term assault missions, recent epidemiological studies showed prominent vitamin D deficiency (defined as serum 25 (OH)D levels less than 37.5 nmol/L) in US adolescents, especially among African Americans (37 percent compared to 6 percent and 22 percent for white and Hispanic adolescents, respectively) (Gordon et al., 2004). Higher frequencies of insufficiency in the African-American population (Calvo and Whiting, 2003) and lower serum concentrations of 25(OH)D in the Mexican-American population (Reasner et al., 1990) as compared with the white population, are of concern. Because the level of sunlight will vary with the particular environment of military missions (e.g., desert versus mountainous environments), it is appropriate to assume the conservative scenario that most vitamin D will be derived from the diet.

In addition to concerns about vitamin D status for some subpopulations within the military, based on new studies experts are now questioning whether the cutoff for the accepted criterion of adequacy, serum concentration of 25(OII)D, should be higher (e.g., > 80 nmol/L) (Holick, 2004) than that used in 1997 (> 30 nmol/L) when the current AI was established (IOM, 1997a). This criterion of adequacy was based on estimates of intake and the related 25(OH)D serum levels of women in Nebraska (> 30 nmol/L), where sunlight is more limited. The question, however, remains whether this level indicates optimal health. A recent intervention study reported that during winter an oral intake level of 12.4 µg/day was required to sustain serum 25(OH)D levels at or above an average of 70 nmol/L (Heaney et al., 2003). Others have recommended that indicators of chronic disease, rather than levels 25(OH)D, might provide a better basis to establish the AI (Specker, 2005). The possible need for amounts in excess of the AI, along with reports of apparent vitamin D deficiency in adolescents and young men, suggests that the level of vitamin D for the assault ration be set at 12.5 µg/day, a level that should maintain serum vitamin D levels at 70 nmol/L without depending on sunlight exposure or body liver stores to contribute to available vitamin D. In support of this, a study with submariners showed that a dietary intake of 15 µg of vitamin D could generally maintain serum concentrations of 25(OH)D for three months. Using the conservative assumption that sunlight exposure during missions may be lacking, to prevent depletion of body stores and to remediate possible previous inadequate intakes, particularly in African-American soldiers, the committee recommends that the ration contain from 12.5 to 15 µg of vitamin D. The lower level of the range is based on possible benefits to optimal health and is based on the amount of vitamin D needed to maintain a level of 70 nmol/L of 25(OH)D in serum over time, while the upper end of the range is based on an amount shown to maintain serum 25(OH)D levels in military personnel assigned to submarine duty over a three-month period (15 µg). The committee recommends that, as the new data indicating the need for reviewing the AI and the UL are further evaluated, the military consider revising the range in light of such deliberations.

Food Form

Very few foods are good sources of vitamin D. Most vitamin D in the diet comes from fortified foods, with the exception of small amounts in animal products. Cereals and milk products are typically fortified with vitamin D in the United States, whereas in other countries, margarine and other staples are fortified. It is envisioned that food items in the ration will need to be fortified with vitamin D.

Research Needs

- Evaluate the effect of clothing on vitamin D status parameters in soldiers while in field operations.
- Evaluate vitamin D status of soldiers in the field in different environments, particularly after deployments in cold weather, at high latitudes, and at high altitudes where sunlight will be limited.
- Examine ethnic differences in vitamin D status in these military environments.

Vitamin E

RECOMMENDATION: The ration should contain a level in the range of 15–20 mg of α-tocopherol, based on the RDA to prevent erythrocyte lysis and on dietary intake levels. If necessary, this form can be added into the food products because natural foods are limited in this form of tocopherol.

Background

The main role of vitamin E (by definition, α-tocopherol; IOM, 2000) is as an antioxidant that prevents the propagation of free radical formation, a process that may be related to many of the chronic diseases of aging, such as cardiovascular disease, cancer, and diabetes. Overt signs of vitamin E deficiency occur very rarely in humans and have not been reported as a result of low dietary intakes, except when combined with moderate to severe malnutrition. Individuals who have overt signs of deficiency of vitamin E, due to a genetic abnormality in vitamin E transport or to fat malabsorption, develop scaly skin and eventually neurological symptoms. The RDA for vitamin E is set at 15 mg for men 19–50 years of age. This requirement was based on maintaining plasma tocopherol concentration at a level that limited hemolysis in red blood cells due to peroxide exposure to less than 12 percent. According to NHANES III serum data, this amount would ensure that at least 95 percent of the population is protected against vitamin E deficiency. The median and the 95th percentile dietary intake of α-tocopherol are 9 and 19 mg/day, respectively, for men 19–30 years of age (NHANES III; IOM, 2000). The UL of vitamin E was established at 1,000 mg based on hemorrhagic effects.

Rationale for Levels of Vitamin E

Vitamin E as Antioxidant. High levels of physical activity create oxidative damage, and, as with vitamin C, vitamin E requirements might differ for individuals under physical stress. Although dietary vitamin E appears to have a protective role against oxidative stress, the studies conducted until now have not clearly shown a benefit either in reducing muscle injury due to exercise or in improving performance (Sacheck and Blumberg, 2001). The effect of vitamin E on exercise-induced changes in creatine kinase (CK), oxidative damage to lipids, and markers for DNA damage is uncertain. One study showed that supplementing 800 IU/day of vitamin E for 60 days actually promoted lipid peroxidation and inflammatory markers after a triathlon, as evidenced by an increase in plasma F_2-isoprostanes and IL-6; however, there was no effect on performance (Nieman et al., 2004).

The existing data on the effects of vitamin E as an antioxidant and enhancer of performance often come from studies that used pharmacologic doses of the vitamin. An added difficulty comes from appropriately choosing antioxidant indicators of oxidative stress and muscle damage. For example, Cannon et al. (1990) questioned whether an increase of CK after exercise reflects undesirable muscle damage. Their research comparing young and old subjects (Cannon et al., 1990) suggests that the increase in CK might be due to the need to clear damaged proteins with an increase in muscle protein turnover (Cannon et al., 1991). There are studies that show that supplementation with vitamin C and E together (compared to vitamin C or E alone) is more effective in protecting from oxidative stress due to regeneration of vitamin E by vitamin C. For more details, the reader is referred to the section on vitamin C above.

Vitamin E and Immune Function. Vitamin E has been investigated as a potentiator of immune function. At levels from 60–800 mg/day for 4–8 months, vitamin E was shown to increase immune status markers in the elderly; no adverse effects were reported (Meydani et al., 1997, 1998). Studies have also specifically looked at the effect of vitamin E on the incidence of common colds. A recent study found that supplementing the diet with 220 mg/day during one year lowered the incidence of common colds in elderly nursing home residents (Meydani et al., 2004). Another study, however, reported no beneficial effect of supplementing the diet of noninstitutionalized elderly individuals with the same amount (Graat et al., 2002). Unfortunately, most studies have been conducted with the elder population, and data on effects of vitamin E supplementation on the immune system of young adults are scarce.

The committee concludes that there is no clear evidence that providing high, pharmacologic levels (> 60 mg) of vitamin E in the ration is efficacious whether to improve performance or to enhance the immune function. Therefore, the level recommended is based on the RDA for this age group and dietary intake validated by chemical analysis of duplicate samples. The committee does not consider using the UL for the general population (1,000 mg/day) (IOM, 2000) as reasonable due to reports on the risk of hemorrhage, increased prothrombin time, and interruption of blood coagulation (Booth et al., 2004). A recent meta-analysis (Miller et al., 2005) suggests that such high amounts of vitamin E may be associated with other adverse events, including increased death rate. Therefore, rather than using the UL, the committee based the upper limit of the recommendation on chemically measured dietary intakes. It is recognized that, although the RDA was set at 15 mg/day, dietary intakes are likely underestimated. For example, in Holland, chemical testing showed that conventional menus contained 20.9 mg of α-tocopherol (van het Hof et al., 1999). The committee concluded that these data justify setting a range of 15–20 mg/day of vitamin E for combat rations. There are concerns also with the use of aspirin, or other drugs with anticoagulant properties, in combination with vitamin E due to the potential additive, adverse effects on coagulation.

A recent study showed that plasma α-tocopherol disappearance was faster in smokers compared to nonsmokers and that these rates correlated with plasma ascorbic acid concentration in smokers but not in nonsmokers. The authors concluded that smokers have an increased requirement for α-tocopherol (Bruno et al., 2005). At this time, however, it is premature to recommend the addition of a specific amount of α-tocopherol due to smoking.

Food Form

Since many common food sources are generally low in α-tocopherol, it is expected that the committee recommendation will not be met by the foods in the ration. Because only the α-tocopherol form of vitamin E can be transported by transfer proteins in the liver, and other forms (β-, γ-, and δ-tocopherols and the tocotrienols) will be excreted, foods should be fortified with vitamin E as α-tocopherol. Other forms (β-, γ-, and, δ-tocopherols and the tocotrienols) will be present as natural components of food in the ration.

Research Needs

- Investigate the potential synergistic effects of a mixture of antioxidants in a randomized trial on physical performance and immune function. Before conducting such studies, valid markers of antioxidant activity that will permit comparison of studies across laboratories are needed.
- Conduct studies on the effects of vitamin E supplementation on physical performance and immune function using more physiologic levels of the vitamin (15–60 mg), rather than pharmacologic levels.
- Explore the use of supplementation of vitamin E to prevent colds in young people.
- Determine if smokers need supplemental levels of vitamin E.
- Study the use of aspirin by individuals consuming a diet high in vitamin E, since the action of both may affect coagulation.
- Further study adverse events associated with vitamin E.

Vitamin K

RECOMMENDATION: The committee assumes that enough vitamin K would occur naturally in the ration foods; therefore, additional vitamin K is not necessary.

Background

Vitamin K acts as a cofactor during the synthesis of blood coagulation enzymes. The median and 95th percentile dietary intake for men 19–30 years old are 101.1 and 181.3 µg/day, respectively (NHANES III; IOM, 2001b). The AI is based on dietary intake data for healthy individuals and was established at 120 µg/day for adult men. There have been no adverse events reported, so no UL was established (IOM, 2001b).

Rationale for Levels of Vitamin K

Turnover from lipid fraction is rapid and hepatic reserves deplete rapidly if the intake of vitamin K is restricted (Usui et al., 1990). The committee believes that for the short terms of the combat mission, however, it is not essential to add vitamin K to the ration because it is stored in the liver and is naturally present in foods. In addition, vitamin K deficiency is rare.

Thiamin

RECOMMENDATION: Assuming an energy content of 2,400 kcal in the assault ration and an average energy expenditure of 4,500 kcal/day, the assault ration should contain a level of 1.6–3.4 mg of thiamin.

Background

Thiamin is essential in the metabolism of carbohydrate and branched-chain amino acids. Thiamin is a coenzyme that affects the cardiovascular, muscular, nervous, and gastrointestinal system (Tanphaichitr, 1999). The RDA for men ages 19–30 years is set at 1.2 mg/day thiamin (IOM, 1998). The 95th percentile intake of thiamin is 3.4 mg/day for men between the ages of 19–30 years (IOM, 1998). Thiamin deficiency signs and symptoms include anorexia, weight loss, mental dysfunction, muscle weakness, and cardiovascular effects. A UL was not set because there have been no sufficient data on adverse effects associated with thiamin consumption.

Rationale for the Levels of Thiamin

Thiamin is required for the metabolism of carbohydrate (conversion of pyruvate to acetyl CoA), branched-chain amino acids, and fat (tricarboxylic acid [TCA] cycle enzymes). There are no metabolic feeding studies examining the amount of thiamin required to maintain good status in active individuals. The EAR for thiamin is based on the need for 0.3 mg thiamin/1,000 kcal (IOM, 1998), assuming individuals were in energy balance. Rather than basing the amount in the assault ration on its caloric level, given the restriction in energy intake of soldiers, a recommendation for thiamin based on energy expenditure is a reasonable approach. Assuming a 4,500 kcal/day energy expenditure, a minimum recommended daily intake of 1.6 mg of thiamin/day would be calculated, based on increasing the EAR of 0.3 mg/day/1,000 kcal by 20 percent for twice the assumed CV of requirements for thiamin of 10 percent (0.3 mg/day/1,000 kcal × 4.5 × 120 percent = 1.6 mg/day needed) (IOM, 1998). In addition, based on NHANES III data, the 95th percentile intake of thiamin is 3.4 mg/day for men between the ages of 19 and 30 (IOM, 1998). Using these numbers, the committee concluded that 1.6–3.4 mg/day of thiamin, which is above the current RDA for men (1.3 mg/day), would cover the thiamin needs of the soldiers. There are no reports available of adverse effects from consumption of excess thiamin by ingestion of food or supplements (IOM, 1998). Thiamin can be either naturally occurring in food or added to the food.

Riboflavin

RECOMMENDATION: Assuming an energy content of 2,400 kcal in the assault ration and an average energy expenditure of 4,500 kcal/day, the assault ration should contain a level of 2.8–6.5 mg of riboflavin.

Background

Riboflavin is an essential nutrient due to its function as a coenzyme in numerous redox reactions. Riboflavin is involved in numerous metabolic pathways and in energy production. Signs and symptoms of deficiency include sore throat, hyperemia and edema of the pharyngeal and oral mucosal membranes, cheilosis, angular stomatitis, among others (McCormick, 1999). The RDA in healthy males of ages 19–30 years is 1.3 mg/day riboflavin (IOM, 1998). The 95th percentile intake of riboflavin is 6.5 mg/day for men between the ages of 19 and 30 (IOM, 1998). A UL has not been set because there is insufficient data on adverse effects associated with riboflavin consumption.

Rationale for Levels of Riboflavin

Riboflavin is important for physical activity because it is involved in carbohydrate, protein, and fat metabolism, and in the conversion of vitamin B_6 and folate to their active forms (IOM, 1998; Manore, 2000). Data from Belko et al. (1985) provided information about riboflavin needs under conditions of low energy intake and exercise. This study used the same level of energy restriction experienced by the soldiers (approximately 50 percent of energy needs). Thus, their estimate based on energy intake was used for the calculation of riboflavin needs. This differs from the approach used in developing the EAR (and thus, the RDA) (IOM, 2000) in which estimates were based on requirements at normal activity levels where a relationship to energy intake was not demonstrated. Using the recommendations in Belko et al. (1985) and an energy intake of 2,400 kcal/day, soldiers on assault missions would need approximately 2.78 mg of riboflavin to maintain good nutritional status (1.16 mg riboflavin $\times$ 2.4 = 2.78 mg). In addition, according to NHANES III data, the 95th percentile intake of riboflavin is 6.5 mg/day for men between the ages of 19 and 30 (IOM, 1998). Using these numbers, the committee agreed that 2.8–6.5 mg/day of riboflavin would cover the need of the soldiers. This range is above the current RDA for riboflavin (1.3 mg) for men 19–30 years old. There are no adverse effects associated with riboflavin consumption from food or supplements (IOM, 1998). Riboflavin can be either naturally occurring in food or added to the food.

Niacin

RECOMMENDATION: Assuming an energy content of 2,400 kcal in the daily ration and an average energy expenditure of 4,500 kcal/day, the assault ration should contain a level of 28–35 mg of niacin equivalents (NE).

Background

Niacin is an essential precursor of nucleotides that are key components of redox reactions, ATP synthetic pathways, and adenosine diphosphate ribose transfer reactions. The RDA for men ages 19–30 years is set at 16 mg/day of NE (IOM, 1998). The 95th percentile intake of niacin for men between the ages of 19 and 30 years is 45 mg/day (NHANES III; IOM, 1998). Deficiency manifests itself as pellagra with signs and symptoms like rash, diarrhea, or constipation associated with changes in digestive tract as well as neurological symptoms such as fatigue and loss of memory. Due to flushing that has been seen in studies of subjects given an excess of the vitamin, the UL is set at 35 mg/day of NE from forms added to foods or as supplements only.

Rationale for Levels of Niacin

Niacin (NAD and NADP) is required for the metabolism of carbohydrate (glycolysis and electron transport) and fat (β-oxidation of fats) and for protein synthesis. No metabolic feeding studies examined the amount of niacin required to maintain good status in active individuals. In addition, no studies have examined the impact of dieting and exercise on niacin status. The EAR for niacin was determined to be 4.8 NE/1,000 kcal, assuming that individuals were in energy balance (IOM, 1998). Because the energy intake of soldiers is low during missions, basing the recommendation for niacin on energy expenditure instead of intake would be a reasonable approach. Assuming a 4,500 kcal/day energy expenditure, a minimum recommended daily intake of 28 mg of niacin/day would result, based on increasing the EAR of 4.8 mg/day/1,000 kcal by 30 percent for twice the assumed CV of requirements for thiamin of 15 percent (4.8 mg/day/ 1,000 kcal × 4.5 × 130 percent = 28.1 mg/day needed) (IOM, 1998). Since the UL of niacin (35 mg/day) is below the NHANES III 95th percentile intake of niacin for men 19–30 years old (45 mg/day) (IOM, 1998), the committee recommends a range of 28–35 mg/day of niacin. This recommended range is above the RDA (16 mg/day) and below the UL for this age range (35 mg/day). Thus, it should ensure adequate amounts and minimal risk of adverse effects. If adequate amounts of niacin are provided, endogenous synthesis of niacin from tryptophan will be minimized. The niacin can be either naturally occurring or added to the food. A minimum of 28 mg should be present in the ration, and not more than 35 mg be added to foods.

Vitamin B$_6$

RECOMMENDATION: Based on an estimated body protein loss of approximately 52 g/day due to the soldiers' negative energy balance and a minimum protein intake of 100 g/day, the assault ration should contain a level of 2.7–3.9 mg/day of vitamin B$_6$; if a higher protein level is provided, this amount should be increased proportionally.

Background

Vitamin B$_6$ is an essential coenzyme for metabolism of amino acids, glycogen, and sphingoid bases. It is essential for immune and nervous system function and affects gluconeogenesis, niacin formation, red cell metabolism, and steroid function. Classical signs and symptoms of deficiency of vitamin B$_6$ include stomatitis, cheilosis, glossitis, irritability, depression, and confusion (Leklem, 1999). The RDA set for healthy normal men 19–30 years is 1.3 mg/day of vitamin B$_6$ (IOM, 1998). The 95th percentile intake of vitamin B$_6$ is 3.91 mg/day for men between the ages of 19 and 30 (NHANES III; IOM, 1998). The UL, based on the risk of developing sensory neuropathy, is 100 mg/day of vitamin B_6 (IOM, 1998).

Rationale for Levels of Vitamin B_6

Vitamin B_6 is required for the metabolism of carbohydrate (gluconeogenesis and glycogen breakdown) and protein (transamination reactions). Thus, vitamin B_6 is important in helping to provide energy to exercising muscles (Manore, 2000). Based on the recent metabolic feeding data by Huang et al. (1998) and Hansen et al. (2001), in order to maintain adequate vitamin B_6 status, 0.019–0.020 mg B_6/g protein was required in sedentary young women who were weight stable and consuming 70–85 g protein/day. The committee assumes that the soldiers will be consuming 2,400 kcal/day while expending 4,500 kcal/day. Under these conditions, the soldier is exercising vigorously and losing weight. Using data collected on male soldiers consuming 1,600 kcal/day and expending 4,500 kcal/day, Nindl et al. (2002) found a loss of 1.5 kg fat-free mass (FFM) in three days. In order to calculate the amount of body protein lost in the Nindl et al. study (2002), the committee assumed that 50 percent of this FFM weight was water loss. Assuming a nitrogen-to-lean tissue ratio of 30:1 and a 6.25 factor to convert nitrogen to protein, there would be a protein loss of 156 g in 3 days or 52 g/day in this study. In applying these data to the combat assault situation posed here, the committee assumed about 33 percent less protein was lost (100 g or 33 g/day), since intake of energy (2,400 kcal/day) and protein (100 g/day) would be higher. Thus, protein metabolism would include components of both dietary protein (100 g) and protein lost from the body (33 g) for a total of 133 g protein. Using a requirement of 0.020 mg B_6/g protein (Hansen et al., 2001), 2.7 mg/day of B_6 of would be needed to metabolize 133 g of protein. In NHANES III data, the 95th percentile intake of vitamin B_6 is 3.91 mg/day for men between the ages of 19 and 30 (IOM, 1998). Using the calculations above and the 95th percentile intake of vitamin B_6, providing 2.7–3.9 mg/day B_6 would cover the needs of the soldiers. This range falls above the current RDA for vitamin B_6 (1.3 mg/day) and below the UL for vitamin B_6 (100 mg/day). Vitamin B_6 can be either naturally occurring in food or added to the food.

Research Needs

• Determine the requirements of niacin, riboflavin, thiamine, and vitamin B_6 when individuals are consuming a hypocaloric diet under the environmental conditions and high-stress situations of combat missions (e.g., intense physical activity, high energy expenditure, reduced caloric intake, and hot and humid conditions).

Folate

RECOMMENDATION: The assault ration should contain 400–560 μg of folate (either as food folate or folate added to foods), based on the current RDA for folate and the 95th percentile intake for folate.

Background

Folate is essential in single-carbon transfers in the metabolism of nucleic and amino acids. The RDA for healthy men 19–30 years of age is 400 μg/day of dietary folate equivalents (DFEs) (IOM, 1998). The 95th percentile intake of folate is 564 μg/day for men between the ages of 19 and 30 (NHANES; IOM, 1998). The UL for folate is 1,000 μg/day from fortified food or supplements (IOM,1998).

Rationale for Levels of Folate

Folate is involved in a number of metabolic processes associated with physical activity. Folate is important for red blood cell (RBC) formation and, thus, for the transport of oxygen to the working muscle. Folate is also involved in the synthesis of pyrimidine and purine nucleotides, protein synthesis, and normal cell growth.

As reviewed by the IOM (1998), naturally existing folate from food is only 50 percent bioavailable. Folate added to foods fortified with folic acid has much higher bioavailability, about 85 percent (i.e., a bioavailability ratio of 1.7). When a mixture of folic acid plus food folate is consumed, as in the assault ration, dietary folate equivalents are estimated as follows:

$$\mu g \text{ of DFEs provided} = \mu g \text{ of food folate} + (1.7 \times \mu g \text{ of folic acid})$$

This formula can also be used to calculate the EAR. No metabolic feeding studies have examined the amount of folate required to maintain good status in active individuals. In general, studies examining dietary intakes of active males report that mean intakes of folate are adequate (Manore and Thompson, 2000). These adequate intakes can be attributed to the relatively high-energy intakes of these individuals. Poor folate status has been associated with depression in healthy subjects between the ages of 15 and 39 (Morris et al., 2003) and poor cognitive function (Calvaresi and Bryan, 2001) but data are mixed (Malouf et al., 2003). NHANES III data, which were collected before folate fortification, indicate that the median and 95th percentile intake of folate from foods is 277 and 564 μg/day for men between the ages of 19 and 30, respectively (IOM, 1998). Based on the RDA and the 95th percentile intake, providing 400–564 μg/day of folate to soldiers would cover their folate needs.

Food Form

Folate occurs naturally in food or can be added to the food. The formula described above should be used to derive the dietary folate equivalents from food, which takes into consideration the availability of both the food folate and the added folic acid.

Vitamin B_{12}

RECOMMENDATION: The committee assumes that enough vitamin B_{12} would occur naturally in the ration, if some of the protein is of animal source and, therefore, that additional vitamin B_{12} is not necessary.

Background and Rationale

Vitamin B_{12} is necessary for RBC formation, normal cell growth, and proper folate metabolism. The RDA for men between the ages of 19 and 30 is 2.4 µg/day vitamin B_{12} (IOM, 1998). There is no UL for vitamin B_{12} (IOM, 1998). In normal, healthy men vitamin B_{12} stores have been estimated as sufficient for 2 years (IOM, 1998); the risk of depletion over a few days is low. Thus, there is no compelling reason to add B_{12} to the ration to supplement what would occur naturally in food.

Biotin

RECOMMENDATION: The committee assumes that enough biotin would occur naturally in the ration foods; therefore, additional biotin is not necessary.

Background and Rationale

Biotin is required for a number of metabolic functions related to physical activity. It is required for the metabolism of carbohydrate (gluconeogenesis), amino acid (leucine degradation), and fat (TCA cycle), and for fat synthesis. No metabolic feeding studies have examined the amount of biotin required to maintain good status in active individuals. In addition, no studies have examined the impact of dieting and exercise on biotin status. There is no UL for biotin. Currently, the AI for biotin is 30 µg/day for men (IOM, 1998).

Pantothenic Acid (CoA)

RECOMMENDATION: The committee assumes that enough pantothenic acid would occur naturally in the ration foods; therefore, additional pantothenic acid is not necessary.

Background and Rationale

Pantothenic acid (CoA) is required for the metabolism of carbohydrate (gluconeogenesis and glycolysis), fat (β-oxidation, TCA cycle), and protein. No metabolic feeding studies have examined the amount of pantothenic acid required to maintain good status in active individuals. In addition, no studies have examined the impact of dieting and exercise on pantothenic acid status. There is no UL for pantothenic acid. Currently, the AI for pantothenic acid is 5 mg/day for men (IOM, 1998).

Choline

RECOMMENDATION: The committee assumes that enough choline would occur naturally in the ration foods; therefore, additional choline is not necessary.

Background and Rationale

Choline accelerates the synthesis and release of acetylcholine, an important neurotransmitter involved in memory storage, muscle storage and muscle control; its deficiency is marked by changes in liver enzymes. The AI for choline is 550 mg/day for men between the ages of 19 and 30. The UL for choline is 3.5 g/day for adults 19 years of age or older, based on fishy body odor and hypotension (IOM, 1998).

Calcium

RECOMMENDATION: The assault ration should contain 750–850 mg of calcium. This range is based on a factorial approach to estimating calcium requirements and potential sweat losses during prolonged exercise, also taking into account concerns about renal stone formation.

Background

The AI for men 19–30 years of age is 1,000 mg/day based on balance studies to determine intakes at which there are gains in bone mineral content. The UL for adults was established at 2,500 mg/day based on the risk of nephrolithiasis (formation of renal stones) (IOM, 1997a).

Intestinal absorption of calcium is enhanced at low levels of calcium intake (approximately 300 mg) due to an active transport process in the proximal small intestine, resulting in an increased fractional absorption of calcium (Ireland and Fordtran, 1973). Absorption of additional calcium from higher intakes occurs via passive cell-mediated diffusion not requiring the action of 1,25-dihydroxyvitamin D_3 (calcitriol).

Calcium requirements in the field are based on a number of factors that affect its absorption as well as its excretion via urine and sweat. Sweat losses may be appreciable given the expected level of energy expenditure and possible environmental heat. In addition, renal stone formation has been reported in troops deployed to the Middle East (personal communication, C. Koenig, USARIEM, November 19, 2004). Therefore, the major concerns considered in deriving the recommended range for calcium in the assault ration are sweat losses and the prevention of renal stone formation.

Rationale for Levels of Calcium

Effect of Energy Expenditure on Calcium Absorption and Excretion. Some evidence is available that indicates the fractional rates of calcium absorption are slightly higher in response to aerobic exercise in endurance trained athletes than in the untrained (Zittermann et al., 2002). In spite of this increase, however, markers of bone collagen formation were decreased in that study. Other studies have shown a slight but significant increase in 24-hour renal calcium excretion in trained young men compared to matched untrained control subjects (Zittermann et al., 2000) who also had higher calcium absorption rates as well as plasma calcitriol levels. Thus, it appears that endurance exercise at levels less than that expected in the soldier during active assault periods may result in both increased calcium absorption and increased urinary calcium excretion and decreased bone formation. These studies did not evaluate the extent of increased losses of calcium via sweat due to the high energy level expended.

Effect of Calcium Lost via Sweat. Calcium concentration of sweat in soldiers has been measured (Armstrong et al., 1992). Sweat calcium concentration declines as the volume of sweat increases. Intermittent exercise over 6 hours at 30°C resulted in a lower concentration of calcium in sweat with higher volumes of sweat, decreasing from 250 mg/L at a sweat rate of 0.37 L/hour to 70 mg/L at a rate of 0.62 L/hour (Armstrong et al., 1992).

Methodological problems may, in part, be responsible for differences in estimated calcium losses via sweat in the few available studies (Consolazio et al., 1966; Shirreffs and Maughan, 1997). Additionally, urinary calcium excretion in response to changes in sweat volume declines (Armstrong et al., 1992; Bullen et al., 1999). Unfortunately, compensatory changes in calcium absorption have not been estimated. For soldiers who are assumed to be sweating due to heavy prolonged exercise in hot, humid climates, it is important to ensure adequate calcium intakes to replace these potential calcium losses.

Effect of Sodium Intake. High sodium chloride intake has been shown to result in increased urinary excretion of calcium in hypertensive individuals (Kurtz et al., 1987). Quantitatively, 100 mmol (2,300 mg) of sodium as sodium chloride increased urinary calcium excretion by 1 mmol (40 mg) in postmenopausal women (Nordin and Polley, 1987). While this appears to occur at moderate and high calcium intakes, it is not evident at lower calcium intakes (less than 300 mg/day), possibly due to modulation by parathyroid hormone (Dawson-Hughes et al., 1996).

Based on the results of Nordin and Polley (1987), the potential increased loss (i.e., 80–240 mg/day) due to the high sodium content of the diet (4–12 g) will not be considered in setting the minimum amount of calcium for the assault ration for the following reasons:

- increased urinary losses will be balanced to some extent by increased fractional absorption of calcium due to the higher level of physical activity expected (see above); and
- there is concern about the increased risk of hypercalciuria and renal stones when fluid restriction is combined with a comparatively high amount of dietary calcium, such as the daily median dietary intake for calcium for young men in the United States (954 mg; IOM, 1997a). Although it might appear to be sensible and without adverse consequences to provide this level when the recommended daily level of sodium (AI = 1,000 mg; IOM, 1997a) is also close to the median intake of sodium, under conditions of fluid restriction the potential for adverse effects cannot be overlooked.

Effect of Dietary Protein Level. Although increased dietary protein intake increases calcium excretion (Linkswiler et al., 1981; Margen et al., 1974; Walker and Linkswiler, 1972), this effect of protein is due in part to the content of sulfur amino acids and it was demonstrated at protein intake levels higher than the range recommended for the assault ration (100–120 g/day). Also, more recent research suggests that the calciuretic effect of protein is partly explained by increased calcium absorption, and that calciuretic effects are considerably modified by long-term adaptation (Dawson-Hughes et al., 2004; Kerstetter et al., 2005). Thus, this potential effect will not be considered further in establishing a range for the assault ration.

Effect of Calcium Intake on Fat Oxidation. Recent studies evaluating the effect of consumption of dairy products and weight loss have implicated calcium in enhancing whole-body fat oxidation (Davies et al., 2000, Melanson et al., 2003; Zemel et al., 2000) while other studies have not (Jacobsen et al., 2005) except only for fecal fat excretion. This is an area of recent interest and little has been well established; however, given the concern with maintaining body weight to the extent possible while in combat missions, the potential adverse effects of higher calcium intakes on body weight should continue to be investigated. At the same time there is also evidence that losses in bone mass are attenuated on hypocaloric diets when calcium intakes are relatively high (Ricci et al., 1998); these effects should also be evaluated.

Effect of Lower Levels of Calcium Intake on Calcium Balance. A recommended daily dietary intake level of approximately 800 mg/day should result in both passive as well as active absorption, assuming that vitamin D included in the food packet of the ration is provided in the same food items and is at or above 5 µg per day (IOM, 1997a).

Effect of Calcium Intake on Stone Formation. High intakes of calcium along with possibly lower than normal urinary volumes due to water scarcity may result in hypercalciuria and consequently renal stone formation. Based on observations in military field hospitals in Iraq and Afghanistan (personal communication, C. Koenig, USARIEM, November 19, 2004), a comparatively high incidence of renal stone formation (urolithiasis) has been noted in soldiers in these theaters of operation, possibly due to lower fluid consumption concomitant with significant losses of sweat due to high environmental temperatures and a high level of physical activity.

Renal stone formation is due to crystallization of calcium oxalate, calcium phosphate, or both (Tiselius, 1997). Urine supersaturated with these components enhances crystal formation and growth. The most important determinants of supersaturation in forming calcium oxalate crystals are the presence of high amounts of oxalate, calcium, citrate, and magnesium, and for calcium phosphate crystals, urinary pH, high amounts of calcium, phosphate, and citrate. Citrate inhibits growth of both types of renal stones, while magnesium inhibits growth of calcium phosphate stones (Tiselius, 1997). Increasing urine volume to greater than 2 L has been shown to halve stone recurrence following first idiopathic calcium stone episodes (Borghi et al., 1996).

Renal oxalate stone formation is also enhanced with higher intakes of oxalate, particularly in individuals who are intestinal hyperabsorbers of oxalate (Siener et al., 2003). Endogenous synthesis of oxalate, while a factor, is not the significant component contributing to calcium oxalate stone formation. There is controversy regarding the contribution of both dietary oxalate and dietary ascorbic acid to urinary oxalate (Holmes, 2000; Williams and Wandzilak, 1989). A study by Baker and colleagues (1966) which showed about 40 percent of the urinary oxalate is from ascorbate breakdown has been criticized because there is question about the pH to which urine samples were exposed prior to analysis for oxalate when estimates of breakdown rates from ascorbate to oxalate were made (Holmes, 2000). Hepatic synthesis is estimated to be 10–20 mg/day, with estimates of urinary oxalate derived from the diet via intestinal absorption varying from 10–20 percent (de O G Mendonca et al., 2003) to 67 percent (Holmes et al., 1995). Recent studies have shown that lower calcium diets (400 mg compared to 1,000 or 1,200 mg per day) lead to increased oxalate absorption, probably due to the decreased amount of unabsorbable calcium-oxalate complexes formed, thus allowing more free oxalate to be absorbed and subsequently excreted, thereby contributing to oxalate stone formation (Borghi et al., 2002; Holmes et al., 2001).

Determination of Estimated Needs. The committee's concern about stone formation stems from the soldiers' high volumes of sweat and possibly curtailed fluid intake. Therefore, risk of stone formation is a major factor in determining the recommended range for calcium. The expected loss of calcium due to significant sweat production is also a major factor. While the AI of 1,000 mg for this age group (IOM, 1997a) is at a level which, in normal situations, does not lead to hypercalciuria, given the environmental temperatures in the field and the energy expenditure expected, a lower level of calcium intake than the AI is recommended. Although exercise involving weight-bearing activity itself will result in less bone loss, the level of calcium should be as high as possible to prevent bone resorption, given that the ration may be consumed for a total of up to 24 days in a 30-day period. The level should be above 400 mg/day to minimize oxalate absorption and below 1,200 mg/day to minimize the risk of stone formation. Intake between these two levels (e.g., 800 mg/day) should provide for oxalate binding in the gut as well as diminishing bone loss resulting from hypercalciuria brought on by the potential level of dehydration expected in this environment. A range of 750–850 mg of calcium is thus recommended. This level assumes a sweat loss of 6.5 L/day in acclimatized individuals expending approximately 4,500 kcal/day under temperatures of approximately 20°C (IOM, 2004). In hotter environments (e.g., 30°C), sweat loss is assumed to be 10.5 L/day on average (IOM, 2004).

While additional sweat losses of calcium with higher ambient temperatures may result, no further increase in the calcium content of the ration is recommended. In all likelihood, the total fluid intake may not increase equivalently, resulting in increased urinary concentration and enhancing the risk of stone formation. Under these conditions, the additional sweat will have lower concentrations of calcium, and less additional calcium will be lost. It is also assumed that, due to the increased level of physical activity and any additional body demand for calcium, fractional absorption of calcium will increase to cover some of the additional sweat losses.

In summary, the level of 750–850 mg/day of calcium is recommended. This level will minimize hypercalciuria while allowing for both active and passive absorption. It also will enhance gut formation of unabsorbable calcium-oxalate complexes in asymptomatic individuals considered oxalate hyperabsorbers.

Food Form

Most of the calcium in foods comes from dairy products. The ration will likely have cheese spreads but not in quantities enough to meet the level of calcium recommended. In addition, cereals and fruits have some calcium. In order to achieve the amount of calcium recommended in the ration (750–850 mg), ration items, such as cereals will have to be fortified with calcium; such fortified products are already commercially available and therefore acceptability is not anticipated to be an issue.

Research Needs

- While enhancements to encourage fluid intake need to be sought, additional research is needed on the relationships between calcium, magnesium, and phosphorus on the maintenance of bone mineral density in hot environments resulting in significant sweating. This should include determining the appropriate levels of intake to maintain bone mineral density while diminishing hypercalciuria to the extent possible.

Chromium

RECOMMENDATION: The committee assumes that enough chromium would occur naturally in the ration foods; therefore, additional chromium is not necessary.

Background

Chromium is essential because it promotes the action of insulin so that the body can utilize fats, carbohydrates, and protein. Chromium is a potentiator of insulin activity (Mertz, 1969, 1993; Mertz et al., 1961). It is hypothesized to function by complexing with a low-molecular-weight chromium-binding substance that binds and activates the insulin receptor of insulin-dependant cells.

The AI for chromium is based on estimated mean intakes and is 35 µg/day (IOM, 2001b). No UL was established due to few known serious adverse effects. Also, evidence of deficiency in humans is limited to individuals on prolonged total parenteral nutrition therapy. In these cases, individuals affected developed weight loss and peripheral neuropathy that was reversed upon chromium administration.

Rationale for Levels of Chromium

The committee does not consider it necessary to provide supplemental chromium in the ration in spite of its possible role in potentiating the effects of insulin. It is assumed that, because of the wide distribution of chromium in foods (Anderson et al., 1992), food items in the ration will have enough chromium to meet the needs of soldiers. Given the lack of reports indicating deficiencies in individuals in the population, concerns about inadequate intake while consuming food based diets are minimal, especially for the short terms of combat missions. Additionally, there is no conclusive evidence that chromium supplementation enhances performance (Clarkson, 1997; Lukaski, 2001).

Research Needs

- Determine whether supplementation with chromium affects physical performance for individuals on a hypocaloric diet under the environmental conditions of combat missions.

Copper

RECOMMENDATION: The assault ration should contain copper at a level in the range of 900–1,600 µg/day based on the RDA and potential sweat losses.

Background

Copper is a component of many metalloenzymes that act as oxidases, such as amine oxidases, ferroxidases, and superoxidase dismutase. Due to the ubiquity of copper, its deficiency affects many physiological functions: outcomes of deficiency include connective tissue defects, anemia, and immune and cardiac dysfunction. Copper deficiency in humans is rare but has been seen in premature infants and in patients receiving parenteral nutrition (IOM, 2001b). Even in the absence of signs and symptoms of deficiency, various immune system parameters may be altered (Percival, 1998) if copper status is deficient. Copper toxicity, which can also occur, results in increased lipid peroxidation and DNA damage.

The RDA is based on a factorial method and is set at 900 µg/day for men. The factorial method takes into account the amount needed in the diet to replace obligatory losses (i.e., losses from sweat, hair, nails). The UL level for men is 10 mg/day and is based on a level that presents no toxicity to the liver (IOM, 2001b). Susceptibility to copper toxicity depends on numerous factors, including the efficiency of absorption and expression of copper transport and storage proteins (Bremner, 1998). The median intake and the 95th percentile of intake of men 19–30 years old in the US is estimated to be 1,630 and 2,650 µg/day, respectively (NHANES III; IOM, 2001b).

Rationale for Levels of Copper

There is no consistent evidence of deficient copper status in the US population. Also, there is no strong evidence that inadequate copper intake leads to in any chronic disease (Jacob et al., 1981). Although copper status could affect energy metabolism based on its presence in key enzymes involved, there is no scientific literature supporting a benefit from supplementing copper on either cognition or physical performance.

Some evidence indicates that excess copper may have a pro-oxidant effect through catalyzing the formation of hydroxyl groups (Bremner, 1998). A recent study explored the effects of a high copper diet, in which supplements of 7.0 mg/day (compared to 1.6 mg/day) were given. After almost five months of a high-copper diet, subjects had a lower concentrations of neutrophils (as a percentage of total white blood cells) and a lower concentration of IL-2 receptor; in addition, their antibody titer after influenza immunization decreased (Turnlund et al., 2004).

A study by the military reported that under hot conditions, sweat, skin and hair copper losses may increase several fold from the average basal amount of 250 µg/day to up to 1,600 µg/7 hour at 37.8°C (Consolazio et al., 1964). It is not known, however, whether such high increased losses are sustained.

Given the concern about possible pro-oxidant effects of large amounts of added copper, it is not recommended to raise the level of copper in the assault ration above the level to replace the high obligatory losses. As mentioned above, there are reports of higher copper losses in the heat (up to 1,600 µg/7 hr at 37.8°C). The committee concludes that these losses need to be considered and recommends an upper limit of 1,600 µg/day in the ration. Levels above this might result in interferences with the bioavailability of other nutrients (see Food Form section below).

Food Form

The committee assumes that copper will occur naturally in food items of the assault ration. Copper is a pro-oxidant and catalyzes unsaturated fat and oil oxidation, as well as ascorbic acid oxidation; it could also interfere with bio-availability of other minerals, such as zinc, although this has not been proven in humans at the levels recommended here (Lonnerdal, 2000). Furthermore, this would occur most likely only if fortification is needed, an unlikely event since copper would be naturally present in food in sufficient amounts.

Research Needs

- Measure copper sweat losses in studies which simulate the environment encountered by soldiers in similar types of operations (e.g., intense physical activity, high energy expenditure, reduced caloric intake, in hot and humid conditions) in order to evaluate the additional requirements for copper.

Iodine

RECOMMENDATION: The assault ration should contain 150–770 µg of iodine. This range is based on the RDA and the 95th percentile intake from food sources.

Background

Iodine is essential for the diet because it is a component of thyroid hormones and therefore involved in many key biochemical reactions critical to life. Most iodine deficiency disorders affect growth and development due to insufficient thyroid hormones. The most severe disorders affect the developing brain. The RDA is set at 150 µg/day for men 19–50 years of age. It was estimated from thyroidal radio-iodine accumulation in turnover studies. The UL was established at 1,100 µg/day based on elevated concentrations of thyroid stimulating hormone. The median dietary intake and the 95th percentile dietary intake are 240–300 and 920 µg/day (from food sources [770 µg] and supplements [150 µg]), respectively, for men 19–30 years old (US Food and Drug Administration, Total Diet Study; IOM, 2001b).

Rationale for Levels of Iodine

The committee considers that it is important to ensure an adequate intake of iodine to minimize the risk of goiter and other impairments of the thyroid function, particularly if the ration is used repeatedly. Excess intake iodine would not create concerns because of the mechanisms that permit the thyroid to adapt to increases in iodine (Aurengo et al., 2002). A range of 150–770 mg iodine/day is recommended based on the RDA and 95th percentile of iodine intake of US adult men.

Food Form

The most feasible way to introduce iodine in the ration will be in the form of iodized salt. It is recommended that iodized salt contains 20–40 mg of iodine per kg of salt (IOM, 2002b). When all the salt in the ration is iodized, about 250 µg of iodine will be provided per 1,000 kilocalories, which is within the range recommended here.

Iron

RECOMMENDATION: The assault ration should contain iron in the range of 8–18 mg per day. The lower level of the range is based on the RDA; the higher level of the range is based on increasing the RDA to account for the potential losses of iron in sweat during high energy expenditures and for a potential lower bioavailability from the ration foods. Since iron deficiency is rare in men, if there are palatability or stability problems, the level could be closer to the 8 mg level, the RDA for men.

Background

Iron functions in oxygen transport and energy utilization as a cofactor for a number of enzymes involved in energy metabolism. The RDA for men, 8 mg/day, is based on estimated basal requirements of body losses (i.e., an average of 0.9–1.0 mg/day, based on studies using radiolabeled iron [Green et al., 1968]) and an estimated bioavailability from foods of 18 percent. Basal losses include fecal losses, urinary losses, and losses due to normal skin and miscellaneous losses. The UL for adults is 45 mg/day based on the risk of gastrointestinal distress. The median dietary intake is 17.9 mg and the 95th percentile is 31.1 mg/day for men 19–30 years old (NHANES III; IOM, 2001b). Clinical effects of deficiency include impaired physical and cognitive performance.

The estimate of bioavailability (18 percent) is based on an assumption that 10 percent of the iron in the daily diet will come from heme iron, 25 percent of which is absorbed (Hallberg and Rossander-Hulten, 1991), and 90 percent will come from non-heme iron sources, of which approximately 17 percent is absorbed (Cook et al., 1991). In the absence of heme iron, estimates of bioavailability drop to 10 percent (IOM, 2001b). As iron stores rise, there is a decrease in the percent of dietary iron that is absorbed, thus decreasing the availability of dietary iron.

Rationale for Levels of Iron

Iron Status and Physical Performance. The impact of adequate iron and iron supplements on maintenance and possibly enhancement of physical performance was evaluated during sports training and in endurance athletes (Newhouse and Clement, 1988). Most studies of iron were with female athletes, many of whom had evidence of iron depletion or anemia or both (see Lukaski and Penland, 2004 in Appendix B). Hematological parameters such as hematocrit, hemoglobin, and serum iron were decreased in response to intense exercise maintained over time. This phenomenon is known as "sports anemia" (Aguilo et al., 2004).

Based on review of over 20 years of research on iron and athletic performance and health, Beard and Tobin (2000) concluded that reductions in hemoglobin concentration and tissue iron content can be detrimental to exercise performance, and that iron status is negatively altered in many populations of chronically exercising individuals. Decreased hematocrit and hemoglobin impair the delivery of oxygen to the tissues and lead to a reduced VO_2max. Supplementation of individuals with iron to a normal hematocrit improves VO_2max (Beard and Tobin, 2000) and, hence, exercise capacity and performance (Woodson, 1984).

Deficits of the nonheme iron that is associated with enzyme systems (e.g., electron transport) can also result in significant detrimental effects on athletic performance (Beard and Tobin, 2000), while constituting only 1 percent of total body iron. Iron-depleted, nonanemic women engaged in aerobic training were studied for six weeks with or without iron supplementation (Brownlie et al., 2002, 2004; Hinton et al., 2000). Improvements in measures of endurance capacity with training were lower in those with tissue iron deficiency and provision of supplementary iron reversed this decrease. A subsequent placebo-controlled study from the same laboratory in similar iron-depleted, nonanemic women found that iron supplementation improved indices of progressive muscle fatigue resistance (Brutsaert et al., 2003). Note that these were untrained women, which may not be analogous to what might be expected among men in assault operations.

A study of Australian soldiers consuming combat rations during operations in Australia (Booth et al., 2003) found serum ferritin levels declining by 13 percent over 12 days in a field exercise in tropical conditions while consuming an estimated 2,850 kcal/day (Booth et al., 2003). Ferritin levels in those soldiers receiving only one-half the combat ration pack (estimated to consume about 1,600 kcal) dropped by 17 percent over the 12-day operation. However, in this paper, no conclusion was made about the consequences of the alteration in ferritin status on health or performance. It is unknown whether soldiers involved in assault operations who expend significant energy (approximately 4,500 kcal/day) may present altered iron status.

Iron Status and Mental Performance. The association of iron deficiency anemia with impaired mental performance has been noted for many years, particularly in infants and young children (IOM, 2001b). Of interest to developing the assault ration are data on the use of iron supplementation to improve attention and short-term memory in adolescent girls who were iron deficient but not anemic (Bruner et al., 1996). Accuracy and attention-, memory-, and learning-reaction times were directly related to higher ferritin and transferrin saturation in young women while, in other studies, markers of cortical activation were directly related to serum iron and ferritin levels (see Lukaski and Penland, 2004 in Appendix B). Given the reported increased feelings of fatigue, loss of vigor, and confusion as well as decreased serum ferritin levels and dehydration when consuming restricted rations (Booth et al., 2003), maintaining adequate iron status is probably an important component of preserving brain function and mental performance.

Iron Status and Immune Function. Exercise affects iron requirements and metabolism (Gleeson et al., 2004). Reallocation of available circulating and body iron stores occurs due to significant physical activity and resulting high energy expenditure and iron sweat losses may result in impaired immune function.

Maintaining optimal resistance to infection is a complex process that involves many nutrients, including iron. Some studies have shown that infection by specific pathogenic organisms (e.g., *Plasmodium falciparum*, which causes malaria) that require iron to replicate may be less frequent in individuals who appear to be iron deficient (Nyakeriga et al., 2004). In addition, other studies suggest that continued use of oral or parenteral iron or the presence of excess stored iron as a result of hemochromatosis may be associated with enhanced susceptibility to infections (Gleeson et al., 2004; Keusch, 1999), perhaps due to release of free iron radicals that facilitate bacterial growth or an increase in the formation of destructive hydroxyl radicals (Shephard and Shek, 1998).

In individuals who are mildly iron deficient and are treated with oral iron, such as may be the case in those engaged in assault operations, data to demonstrate an adverse effect on infection rate or severity is scarce (Keusch, 1999).

Iron Losses Through Sweat. Studies have been conducted to estimate the amount of potential losses of iron due to sweating in hot environments and as a result of exercise. Sweat loss of whole-body iron has been estimated to be 0.09 $mg/m^2/hour$ in men during 60 minutes of exercise on a cycle ergometer at 50 percent VO_2max in a hot environment ($35°C$). The concentration decreased with time during the exercise (within the first 30 minutes of exercise) and was less than that seen with sweat during heat without exercise, which also produced less sweat (Waller and Haymes, 1996).

In a subsequent study, the iron content of sweat in recreational cyclists who exercised for 120 minutes at 50 percent VO_2max in a temperate environment ($23°C$) was estimated (DeRuisseau et al., 2002). Sweating rates (volume/time) increased during the first hour, and then remained constant during the second hour. Sweat iron concentration was significantly lower during the second hour. Sweat iron concentrations during the second hour were approximately 0.10 mg/L at a rate of about 0.43 $L/m^2/hour$ while sweat concentrations during the first hour were approximately 0.17 mg/L at the same rate as the second; the average iron lost for the two-hour study period in the male subjects was about 0.23 mg.

These studies alone show that during combat missions sweat losses may be appreciable due to high rates of energy expenditure (generating internal body heat) and high humidity and climatic temperatures in which the activity is conducted. Losses are difficult to estimate, as they vary considerably due to the following factors: (1) environmental conditions; (2) method of sweat collection; (3) whether sweat losses include dermal losses; (4) the level of acclimation to a given environmental condition, and (5) the body size of the individual. While estimates vary significantly, loss of iron in sweat does not appear related to dietary intake (Vellar, 1968). The sweating rate (volume/time) is greater at higher temperatures, but sweat iron concentration (mg/volume) has been shown to be lower when higher volumes are produced (Waller and Haymes, 1996). The available data are too varied to adequately determine the differences between estimates in temperate versus hot environments. Therefore, taking into account only the estimated values from studies conducted in hot climates or with exercise, where the final measurement (cell-free, if available) was taken after a period of sweating, and using the lowest value if using two methods or doing a series of measurements, the estimate of the average iron content in sweat is 0.156 mg/L (Brune et al., 1986; Cohn and Emmett, 1978; Consolazio et al., 1964; DeRuisseau et al., 2002; Jacob et al., 1981; Vellar, 1968; Waller and Haymes, 1996).

Iron Losses Through Urine. In athletes, especially runners, hemoglobin and myoglobin often appear in urine (Jones and Newhouse, 1997; Weaver and Rajaram, 1992). This is thought to result from repeated foot contact with the ground where RBCs are crushed, a process termed foot-strike hemolysis. Other studies have found an increase in the loss of hemoglobin in urine or feces of endurance runners, perhaps indicating irritation and bleeding in the gastrointestinal tract (Horn and Feller, 2003).

Bioavailability. The absorption rate of iron from a typical US diet with a mix of animal and vegetable protein was estimated to be 18 percent when establishing the RDA (IOM, 2001b). If the assault ration is formulated primarily with cereal based food ingredients, it may contain more inhibitors of iron absorption, such as polyphenols in tea and coffee (Disler et al., 1975), calcium (Hallberg et al., 1991), and phytate in legumes, rice, and grains (Brune et al., 1992; Cook et al., 1997). Therefore, 10 to 18 percent bioavailability should be used when calculating the levels of iron in the assault ration depending on the source of foods in the ration. This range is in line with the 1988 Food and Agriculture Organization (FAO)/World Health Organization (WHO) recommendation that "constrained vegetarian diets" were judged to be 10 percent bioavailable (FAO/WHO, 1988) and with the value estimated for bioavailability (18 percent) if more animal foods (containing heme iron) are included in the ration (IOM, 2001b).

Determination of Estimated Needs. The RDA for men at the 97.5 percentile of estimated requirements is 8.49 mg /day (IOM, 2001b), assuming an absorption rate of 18 percent. When adjusted for a bioavailability of 10 percent, minimum daily dietary iron needed in the assault ration increases to approximately 15 mg/day.

It has been recommended that, in order to conservatively cover the increased iron losses associated with exercise and endurance training among athletes, the estimated EAR should be increased by 30 percent (IOM, 2001b). This would increase the amount required from 15 mg/day to a level at or above 20 mg /day. With significant sweating due to heavy work, high relative humidity, and high environmental temperature, iron losses of the soldier will substantially increase in field operations. If calculated by considering a loss of 6.5 L (IOM, 2004, see Figure 2-1) in temperate climates (20°C) at energy expenditures of 4,500 kcal/ day, an additional 1.0 mg/day would be lost (6.5 L × 0.156 mg/L). With a rate of absorption of approximately 10 percent, this would mean that an additional 10 mg/day of dietary iron would be needed, for a total of 25 mg /day, more than two-thirds the estimated amount of 15 mg needed to meet basal losses when consuming foods with lower bioavailable iron.

Following the same approach, at 30°C the estimated volume of water lost is approximately 10.5 L/day (IOM, 2004, and Figure 2-1), which at 0.156 mg/L and a 10 percent rate of absorption, would require an additional 16.4 mg of iron each day above the 15 mg/day for basal losses (i.e., 31 g/day).

Other factors such as increased iron needs (Cook et al., 1974), the presence of ascorbic acid (see vitamin C recommendation), which has been shown to

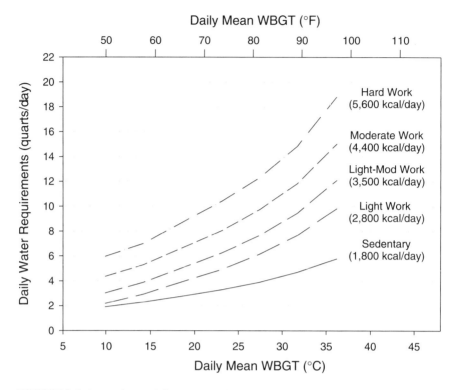

FIGURE 2-1 Approximate daily water requirements as a function of climatic temperature (wet bulb globe temperature, WBGT) and total energy expenditure (kcal).
SOURCE: Sawka and Montain (2001), *International Life Sciences Institute*, used with permission.

increase absorption of nonheme iron (Allen and Ahluwalia, 1997), and the reduction of phytate and tannins to the extent possible should improve the amount absorbed. Calcium has been shown to decrease absorption as well (Hallberg et al., 1991), so it would be advantageous to limit the amount of calcium contained in individual ration components that have higher iron content.

Recommending that the assault ration should contain such a high level of iron (25 or 31 g/day) might put some individuals in the military at risk of iron accumulation; namely those who carry the genetic disorder for hemochromatosis. Of special concern are those who have not been diagnosed as being homozygous at risk of iron accumulation (occult hemochromatosis). Other factors in support of a lower level of iron are that bioavailability might be closer to 18 percent, depending on the protein sources used in the ration, and that iron deficiency is rare in men. Thus, the recommendation for the assault ration is kept to 8–18 mg iron /day. The lower level of 8 mg is based on the RDA with the expectation that the rate of absorption will increase as the body's demand increases and that bioavailability from foods may be more than 10 percent. In situations of strenuous exercise, the higher amount of 18 mg will provide an additional 3 mg to cover the additional needs due to sweat and energy expenditure above that estimated to meet basal losses in 97.5 percent of young men, assuming a rate of absorption of 10 percent. This level of 18 mg is also the estimated median intake of men in the 19–30 age group from NHANES III (IOM, 2001b). A higher level, such as the 95th percentile of intake (31 mg/day), was not chosen due to the concerns of occult hemochromatosis and potential for interactions with other nutrients if iron fortification is needed.

In summary, since iron deficiency in men is rare, the recommended range chosen is based on current RDA, potential losses in sweat, and potential lower bioavailability from foods.

Food Form

There are possible shelf stability issues inherent in providing 18 mg iron (the majority of which is derived from supplemental sources) in the assault ration (Hurrell, 2002a, b; see also Chapter 3). Depending on which food items in the ration contain iron, it is possible that flavor may also be adversely affected (see Chapter 3). Since the primary concern in formulating this ration is to provide highly palatable food to increase energy intake to the extent possible, the level of iron could be reduced as needed to the minimum of 8 mg/day. As noted above, the committee concludes that US men have generally enough iron storages and iron deficiency would be rare and, therefore, low levels of iron intake for brief periods will have no appreciable effect on iron stores and no adverse physiologic effects.

Research Needs

- Measure iron fecal, sweat, and urine losses in studies which simulate the environment encountered by soldiers in similar types of operations (e.g., intense physical activity, high energy expenditure, reduced caloric intake, in hot and humid conditions) in order to evaluate the additional require-ments for iron.

Magnesium

RECOMMENDATION: The assault ration should contain magnesium in the range of 400–550 mg/day. This range covers the current RDA based on magnesium balance and the 95th percentile of intake of adult men.

Background

Magnesium is the second most abundant intracellular cation and functions in muscle metabolism and bone (50–60 percent of the magnesium in the body is found in bone). Magnesium is a required cofactor for hundreds of enzyme systems (Wacker and Parisi, 1968), including energy generation via the Mg-ATP complex or directly as an enzyme activator (Garfinkel and Garfinkel, 1985). In magnesium depletion, intracellular calcium increases, affecting skeletal and smooth muscle contraction.

The 95th percentile of intake is 553 mg for men 19–30 years old. The RDA for men 19–30 years old is 400 mg. The UL was established at 350 mg for magnesium from supplements, because supplements are the only known sources of adverse effects; no adverse effect is known from ingesting magnesium from food (IOM, 1997a).

Rationale for Levels of Magnesium

Magnesium and Physical Performance. Reviews of magnesium nutrition and performance have suggested that magnesium supplementation may not enhance performance although more research may be warranted (Clarkson and Haymes, 1995; McDonald and Keen, 1988). During chronic endurance exercise, however, plasma or serum magnesium concentrations fall, as does urinary magnesium (Buchman et al., 1998). This might suggest a need for additional magnesium in the diet of those who exercise regularly and strenuously. In contrast, provision of magnesium supplements were shown neither to enhance performance in a study of marathon runners (Terblanche et al., 1992), nor to increase serum or muscle magnesium levels or improve endurance performance in athletes who received 500 mg of magnesium for three weeks (Weller et al., 1998).

Other studies have found various effects on physical performance. During submaximal exercise, decreased oxygen uptake was noted when physically active men were supplemented with magnesium (270 mg/day for 4 weeks), but there was no increase in run-time to exhaustion (Brilla and Gunter, 1995). During a progressive rowing test, men receiving 360 mg of magnesium daily for 4 weeks had reduced serum lactate concentrations and oxygen uptake (Golf et al., 1993). In another study in which physically active men were evaluated, magnesium supplementation at a level of 250 mg/day for 7 weeks [total intake of 500mg/day (diet + supplementation)] increased muscle strength and power in a strength-training regimen; however, the placebo group had an average lower magnesium intake than the recommended level (Brilla and Haley, 1992). Thus, the weight of the data suggests that magnesium supplementation over recommended levels of intake has little to no effect on exercise performance.

Magnesium and Mental Performance. One study evaluated the effect of decreased magnesium levels (not necessarily due to magnesium depletion) on mental performance. Electroencephalograms of male and female athletes with low serum magnesium levels showed decreased alpha activity compared to those with normal serum magnesium levels (Delorme et al., 1992). Other studies have not been described in the literature.

Magnesium and Immune Function. A few recent studies have evaluated the role of magnesium status on immune function in athletes (Konig et al., 1998; Mooren et al., 2003; Shephard and Shek, 1998). Magnesium in vitro mediates cell immune function (Mooren et al., 2003) via its effect on granulocyte function; however, supplementing students for two months with 365 mg/day of magnesium in a placebo-controlled study did not change blood, intracellular, or extracellular free, ionized, or total magnesium concentrations, nor did it register the alterations in immune cell function typically seen with exhaustive exercise, perhaps because the students were not considered deficient in magnesium (Mooren et al., 2003). While potentially applicable to the soldier in special operations, given the information currently available, providing additional magnesium above predicted requirements would not be of benefit.

Effect of High Levels of Dietary Magnesium. Increasing dietary magnesium intake has been shown to decrease calcium phosphate renal stone growth in individuals with previous calcium phosphate stones (Tiselius, 1997). A high-protein, low-carbohydrate diet also resulted in decreased magnesium intake, and consequently lower magnesium excretion (Reddy et al., 2002). Provision of 252 mg of magnesium as a potassium-magnesium citrate supplement (which provided 1,640 mg of potassium and 4 g of citrate total per day as well) to patients who had at least two previous episodes of calcium oxalate stones markedly reduced the risk of recurrent stone formation (Ettinger et al., 1997). No data were provided on their intake of dietary magnesium from food, nor on the extent to which the potassium and citrate provided could have contributed to the decreased rate.

Bolus doses have been demonstrated to produce diarrhea (Bashir et al., 1993) when given as a magnesium salt. Because diarrhea was reported in the study to a greater extent in patients receiving the potassium-magnesium-citrate supplement compared to the placebo (Ettinger et al., 1997), caution is warranted in using magnesium salts to enhance the magnesium content of the ration.

In summary, providing magnesium at a level equivalent to or greater than the RDA (400 mg for 19- to 30-year-old men; IOM, 1997a) should provide higher levels of intake than generally consumed (median intake 328 mg/day for 19 to 30 year-old men; 1994 CSFII; IOM, 1997a). This level of intake should have a positive influence on decreasing formation of calcium phosphate stones. Possible benefits to increasing intake above this level are not well established.

Due to adverse reactions (e.g., diarrhea) to magnesium in mineral supplements, and given the concerns about the potential for taste disturbances, it is recommended that the higher end of the range in the ration be no greater than the 95th percentile of intake of 553 mg, if it must be supplemented to ration foods as a salt (IOM, 1997a). A ration containing magnesium at levels above 553 mg would not be of concern if no magnesium fortificant was required in the product formulation. Magnesium fortification should only be used if the lower level of 400 mg cannot be met with food sources. In this case, the supplemented amount would be at levels substantially below 350 mg, the UL for magnesium supplements.

Food Form

It is assumed that most of the magnesium in the assault ration would occur naturally in foods and food ingredients. Significant experience in the use of magnesium salts resulting in a bitter and sour taste (Lawless et al., 2003) and the potential for gastrointestinal distress at higher levels limits the advisability of adding magnesium salts to the assault ration in substantial quantities. Although it is possible, however, for magnesium salts to partially replace sodium salts in breads without deterioration in the sensory properties of the food product (Salovaara, 1982), if the added magnesium salts to achieve the recommended lower level of the range (400 mg) result in taste problems, encapsulation could be considered.

Research Needs

- Study the effect of higher levels of magnesium on enhancing both physical and cognitive performance in studies which simulate the environment encountered by soldiers in similar types of operations (e.g., intense physical activity, high energy expenditure, reduced caloric intake, in hot and humid conditions).
- Study the role of magnesium in maintaining and enhancing immune function and response under the same conditions as above.

Manganese

RECOMMENDATION: The committee assumes that enough manganese would occur naturally in the ration foods; therefore, additional manganese is not necessary.

Background and Rationale

Manganese is a component with various proteins, including metalloenzymes (e.g., arginase, glutamine synthetase, and manganese superoxide dismutase) and other manganese-activated enzymes; it participates in formation of bone and in amino acid, cholesterol, and carbohydrate metabolism. An AI was set at 2.3 mg/day for men 19 years and older based on median intakes (US Food and Drug Administration Total Diet Study; IOM, 2001b). The UL was established at 11 mg/day based on the risk of neurotoxicity (IOM 2001b).

The committee believes that, under the assumed conditions of short-term intake, additional manganese is not necessary and that food items in the ration will have enough manganese to avoid deficiencies. In addition, clinical signs and symptoms of deficiency have not been clearly associated with poor dietary intakes (IOM, 2001b).

Molybdenum

RECOMMENDATION: The committee assumes that enough molybdenum would occur naturally in the ration foods; therefore, additional molybdenum is not necessary.

Background and Rationale

Molybdenum is a cofactor for various enzymes mostly involved with catabolism of sulfur amino acids and heterocyclic compounds such as purines and pyridines. Its essentiality derives from the discovery of a genetic disease in which sulfite oxidase is not synthesized; that is, molybdenum is only essential when this genetic disease is present. The RDA is 45 μg/day based on balance studies. A UL was set at 2,000 μg/day (IOM, 2001b).

The committee believes that, under the assumed conditions of short-term intake, additional molybdenum is not necessary and that food items in the ration will have enough molybdenum for deficiencies not to occur. In addition, no deficiencies have been observed in healthy people and no symptoms of deficiency have been achieved in animals even when the activity of molybdoenzymes was greatly suppressed.

Phosphorus

RECOMMENDATION: The assault ration should contain 700–2,500 mg/day of phosphorus. This range is based on the RDA and 95th percentile of intake for adult men to maintain serum inorganic phosphate levels while taking into account concerns about renal stone formation observed at high levels of intake. Ration formulation at levels above 700 mg should be from food ingredients, not from the addition of phosphate salts, due to concern about diarrhea.

Background

Phosphorus, most commonly as phosphate, is found broadly in all animal and plant tissues. Most of it (85 percent) in adults is in bone. Dietary and bone phosphorus is initially found in blood and extracellular fluid. Inorganic phosphorus is then either excreted in urine or made into structural or high-energy phosphate.

Phosphorus stores and transfers energy, activates proteins, and maintains pH through its buffering capacity. The 95th percentile of intake for 19- to 30-year-old individuals in the United States is nearly 2,500 mg (CSFII; IOM, 1997a). The RDA is 700 mg for men 19–50 years of age, using serum inorganic phosphorus as the functional indicator. Hypophosphatemia occurs as a result of inadequate intake and is expressed as anorexia, muscle weakness, increased susceptibility to infection, bone pain, and mental impairment. The UL of 4.0 g was established based on normal inorganic phosphorus in the serum because dietary hyperphosphatemia has not been reported.

Adults fed mixed diets absorb about 60–65 percent of the phosphorus in foods (Heaney and Recker, 1982; Wilkinson, 1976). Phytate phosphorus in unleavened bread and cereal is poorly absorbed (IOM, 1997a).

Rationale for Levels of Phosphorus

The effects of inadequate dietary phosphorus have been studied in individuals who experience periods of significant energy expenditure. Oral or parenteral refeeding of individuals following significant energy depletion due to heavy endurance exercise, without adequate attention to supplying phosphorus, can precipitate extreme, even fatal, hypophosphatemia (Bushe, 1986; Dale et al., 1986). Thus, it is important to ensure that phosphorus is present in most of the individual items making up the ration. While phosphorus is found both in bone and soft tissue, little evidence is available to suggest that additional requirements due to high rates of energy expenditure or high levels of physical activity demand higher intakes. Estimates of phosphorus content of sweat indicate negligible amounts (less than 2.6 mg/L) of phosphorus (Consolazio et al., 1963; Nishimuta et al., 2004).

Calcium phosphate and calcium oxalate stone formation can be a concern when fluid intake is suboptimal (Borghi et al., 1996). It appears that the recommended intake for soldiers engaging in multiple assault operations should be the same as that for other individuals; thus, a level at or above the RDA should be sufficient. It is expected that the phosphorus level of the ration may well be above the RDA due to its presence in most foods and food ingredients.

While intakes above the 95th percentile of intake (2,500 mg, IOM, 1997a) in individuals consuming high-energy diets (more than 6,000 kcal/day) have not caused harmful effects, high levels of dietary phosphorus (above 3,500 mg) can result in serum inorganic phosphate levels above normal (> 1.4 mmol/L) (IOM, 1997a). Such high levels act to reduce urinary calcium loss, renal synthesis of 1,25 dihydroxyvitamin D, and serum-ionized calcium, all of which can increase serum parathyroid hormone levels (Portale et al., 1989), which increases calcium released from bone and phosphorus urine loss. If prolonged, elevated phosphorus levels can result in ectopic calcification of kidney and soft tissue (Janigan et al., 1997; Wood et al., 1988). The inorganic phosphate levels, however, must be high enough to prevent increased bone resorption, but not so high as to increase the formation of calcium phosphate renal stones. Therefore, the range proposed, 700–2,500 mg/day, will be adequate to meet needs but not so high as to increase renal stone formation.

Food Form

Inorganic phosphates are used as cathartics and result in diarrhea in amounts above 1 g of phosphorus/dose (Grimm et al., 2001; Whybro et al., 1998). Based on this concern, it is recommended that phosphate salts be used in the assault ration only to attain the level of 700 mg, but not to increase the daily intake above 2,500 mg. Intakes from 700 mg to 2,500 mg should come from foods and food ingredients only.

Research Needs

- Given the role of phosphorus as both a nutrient required for normal intracellular function and as well as a structural component of bone formation, studies are needed to evaluate changes (if any) in the ability of soldiers to perform physical and mental function tests under varying levels of phosphorus intake.

Potassium

RECOMMENDATION: Food developers should aim for a level of potassium in the ration of 3.3–4.7 g based on 50th percentile dietary intake and the AI for adult men.

Background

Potassium is the major intracellular cation in the body and is needed for cellular function. Potassium deficiency results in cardiac arrhythmias, muscle weakness, and glucose intolerance. The AI of 4.7 g/day for adult men was established based on effects on reduction of blood pressure and renal stone formation. The reduction of both blood pressure and renal stone formation seen with high potassium intakes appears to be related to a decrease in the sodium-to-potassium ratio. However, although there is a clear relationship between sodium and potassium, there is not enough evidence to establish requirements on the basis of this dependency. The median intake and 95th percentile for US men 19–30 years old is 3.3 and 4.3 g/day, respectively (NHANES III; IOM, 2004).

Rationale for Levels of Potassium

Potassium Losses Through Sweat. Mild potassium depletion can occur under military operations if potassium intake is not adequate. Malhotra et al. (1981) showed that male soldiers working in winter-cold conditions developed negative potassium balance at intakes of 1.76–2.15 g/day. Balance was achieved at 3.32 g/day. A review by Knochel (1993) predicted negative potassium balance in soldiers engaged in prolonged training in hot weather. They reported sweat levels around 0.3 to 0.4 g/L. Assuming that these extreme conditions and work loads produce 10.5 L of sweat (Figure 2-1), the potassium sweat losses potentially could be 3–4 g/day. In addition, aldosterone secretion increases with exercise to promote sodium retention; the sodium retention could enhance potassium losses (Sacks et al., 2001), although most studies show no difference in total body potassium under these conditions (Knochel, 1993). Finally, soldiers may experience some muscle loss due to extensive exercise and hypocaloric diets (see Friedl, 1997; Hoffer, 2004 in Appendix B). This muscle loss will release muscle potassium that may be available for metabolic functions or may be lost in the urine.

Potassium and Renal Stones. The role of potassium in preventing renal stones formation is relevant when establishing levels of potassium due to the high protein level recommended in the assault ration (100–120 g/day), even though the primary protein source may not be of animal origin. Metabolic acidosis due to protein metabolism produces increased bone resorption leading to hypercalciuria. The combination of metabolic acidosis (Arnett, 2003; Frassetto et al., 1998) and dehydration increases the risk of renal stone formation. The addition of dietary potassium, however, may ameliorate this risk. Intake of dietary potassium at the AI of 4.7 g/day (IOM, 2004) in relation to the recommended intake of 100–120 g/day of protein may decrease endogenous noncarbonic acid production (Frassetto et al., 1998; Zwart et al., 2004) and reduce the risk of renal stone formation.

Potassium-to-Sodium Ratios. Although the relationship is not clear, there is an association between sodium-to-potassium ratio and urinary excretions of both cations, salt sensitivity, and blood pressure responses to dietary electrolyte intake. The IOM report (2004) does not make a specific recommendation on the potassium-to-sodium ratio, although using the AI for potassium and sodium, the ratio is calculated to be over 3 (4.7/1.5). Based on the committee's recommendations, the ration's ratio of potassium to sodium (see sodium section) is calculated to be about 1.5 (4.7/3). This ratio is above what the US population consumes, which is less than 1; for many individuals it is less than 0.5. The committee concluded that, given the importance of palatability, the risk on stone formation, the loss of sodium through sweat, and the need to maintain body levels of sodium and potassium, a potassium-to-sodium ratio of 1.5 is reasonable.

In summary, recognizing that this might be a challenge for the development of the assault ration, the committee recommends aiming for 3.3–4.7 g/day of potassium in the ration; this range is based on the median intake for the US population (3.3 g/day), an attainable level, and the AI (4.7 g/day). The AI of 4.7g/day is based on long-term health consequences, including protection from hypertension and bone loss. There is no rationale for increasing potassium intake above the AI value because potassium sweat losses are as low as 0.090–0.626 g/L (IOM, 2004). The importance of adequate potassium intake for cardiac and muscle function (IOM, 2004) and to reduce the risk of renal stone formation (Curhan et al., 1993) supports the recommended AI level. Hypokalemia (serum potassium level below 136 mmol/L) may cause cardiac arrhythmias, muscle weakness, hypercalciuria, and glucose intolerance (IOM, 2004), all of which are dangerous in combat conditions. Potassium balance is affected by level of dietary potassium and sodium as well as other dietary factors such as fiber. In addition to the benefits of maintaining an adequate potassium status, the committee finds that, with the high dietary sodium levels recommended, potassium levels must be equally high.

Food Form

The difficulty in recommending high levels of potassium relates to maintaining palatability. The US diet can provide the AI level from foods depending on consumption of green leafy vegetables, fruits, root vegetables and legumes— all foods not normally part of a combat ration. Furthermore, according to NHANES III data, the US diet intake ranges from 2.9 to 3.3 g/day (IOM, 2004). It appears that providing 4.7 g/2,400 kcal in the assault ration may be difficult. The committee's recommendation is to include foods with naturally high potassium levels in the ingredients (e.g., banana chips or spinach products that have 150 mg/oz, or nuts such as almonds), or to fortifiy foods with forms of potassium such as citrate, rather than chloride, to maintain palatability.

Another strategy to provide more potassium would be to include it as part of supplements in the form of powder to add to fluids, gels, or candy. Whether potassium is added to the basic ration foods or to supplements, however, the flavor of potassium chloride is difficult to mask; therefore, the committee believes it would be advantageous to develop palatable products that increase potassium intakes.

Research Needs

- Identify new ways to increase potassium levels in the food and still maintain palatability.

Selenium

RECOMMENDATION: The ration should include at least 55 µg selenium but not more than 230 µg. This is based on the current RDA and 95th percentile of dietary intake for adult men.

Background

Selenium functions through its association with selenoproteins. Glutathione peroxidases and iodothyronine deiodinases are selenium-dependent enzymes whose action might affect physical performance; in addition, the stressful situations under consideration might affect their level of activity. Numerous studies have demonstrated the increase in reactive oxygen species and oxidative stress developed in muscle after intense exercise; this increase might result in muscle damage and fatigue and can be attenuated by a properly developed antioxidant defense system. Glutathione peroxidases are critical enzymes in that they participate in one of the most essential antioxidant systems in the body by catalyzing the decomposition of oxygen-reactive species that form during exercise. In this regard, the supplementation of diets with selenium has been considered as a way to ensure the proper functioning of glutathione peroxidases. Selenium also forms complexes with iodothyronine deiodinases, which regulate thyroid hormone metabolism.

The EAR was based on two intervention studies and was established at 45 µg/day for men 19–30 years old, with the RDA established at 55 µg/day for this same group. The median intake was 154 µg/day for males 19–30 years old and the 95th percentile of dietary intake is 230 µg/day (NHANES III, IOM, 2000). The UL for adults was based on the appearance of signs of seleniosis and was established at 400 µg/day (IOM, 2000). When selenium deficiency occurs in association with other deficiencies or stresses, it can lead to biochemical changes that predispose soldiers to illness. On its own, however, selenium deficiency does not appear to be a real concern.

Rationale for Levels of Selenium

As with other micronutrients, the need to recommend a different selenium level from the established RDA for assault rations depends upon possible increased selenium needs for the soldiers due to stress, immune function, and level of physical activity. There are data that show the effect of selenium on immune function (Broome et al., 2004; Ravaglia et al., 2000), activity of anti-oxidant glutathione peroxidase during exercise (Clarkson and Thompson, 2000; Sen and Packer, 2000), and energy needs related to thyroid function (Arthur et al., 1993; Bianco et al., 2002; Vanderpas et al., 1993). Selenium is involved in both antioxidant metabolism through glutathione peroxidases and thyroid function; thus, any change in oxidation status that includes exercise and stress and energy metabolism with includes thyroid function would be impacted by deficiency in selenium. For healthy individuals under combat conditions, however, there is no clear evidence to support raising the requirement of selenium.

Research Needs

- Investigate the effects on performance of supplementation with selenium for periods of high-energy expenditure and physical and mental stress comparable to those encountered by soldiers in assault missions.

Sodium

RECOMMENDATION: The assault ration should contain 3 or more grams of sodium, the specific amount depending on palatability and acceptability of the ration. In addition, to ensure that the needs of individuals who lose salt in excess or who are in extremely hot or strenuous situations are met, additional sodium up to 12 g should be available as a supplement and in salt tablets. Food developers should aim at including sodium and other electrolytes as a supplement in the form of candy, gels, or powder to be mixed with fluid; however, because palatability will limit the amount of additional sodium that can be added to these products, sodium should also be available in the form of tablets to be provided by medical personnel or under medical guidance when needed.

Background

Sodium is the main cation in the extracellular fluid and is required to maintain plasma volume. Sodium also maintains the potential of the membrane, playing an important role in active transportation of molecules through the membrane. A low level of sodium or hyponatremia affects blood lipids, insulin resistance, and cardiovascular disease. It often is not associated with low dietary intake but rather with excessive losses (e.g., during exercise) or consumption of hypotonic fluids. The AI value of 1.5 g/day (65 mmoles/day) for men 19–50 years old (IOM, 2004) is based on the replacement of daily obligatory losses of sodium of up to 0.18 g/day calculated by adding urinary losses (0.005–0.035 g/day), stool losses (0.01–0.125 g/day), and nominal sweat (0.025 g/day) (see Shirreffs, 2004 in Appendix B). Other considerations in setting the AI were the evidence supporting that 1.5 g/day would minimize potential adverse effects on blood lipid concentrations and insulin resistance and the fact that this intake would also be met with a typical Western diet. In addition, that level would cover sodium losses by unacclimatized individuals. The UL is 2.3 g/day and considers the risk of high blood pressure (IOM, 2004).

Rationale for Levels of Sodium

Sodium Losses Through Sweat. As part of the electrolyte regulatory system, urinary sodium losses increase with increases in dietary sodium intakes. In addition, urinary sodium and sweat sodium concentrations decrease when individuals become dehydrated, causing a decrease in plasma volume. Conn (1949) showed sodium balance in healthy persons sweating 5–9 L/day with an intake of sodium 0.76 g/day (33.2 mmoles/day) to 1.28 g/day (55 mmoles/day). As mentioned above, the AI value for sodium (1.5 g/day) accounts for sweat losses for unacclimatized individuals in addition to achieving balance in relatively sedentary individuals.

There also is a large variability in sodium losses between individuals due in part to variations in adaptation to heat and exercise capabilities. Thus, the committee's recommendation is based on the assumption that soldiers doing moderate work (4,400 kcal/day) could lose up to 10.5 L water in sweat each day (see Figure 2-1), with ranges of sweat sodium concentrations between 0.12 and 4.2 g/L depending on the sodium intakes, subject characteristics, ambient conditions, and length and type of activities (Armstrong et al., 1985; Consolazio et al., 1963; Costill et al., 1976b; Dill et al., 1976). Calculations that included the maximum potential sodium losses from sweat could lead to high sodium losses, such as 10–12 g/day. Costill et al. (1976a) reported increases in aldosterone secretion and decreases in urinary sodium losses with 60 min of 60 percent VO_2max and 30°C; thus, the body compensates for the elevated sweat sodium losses.

The recommended value of 3 or more grams per day was increased from the AI (1.5 g/day) to allow for the increased sodium losses that occur with elevated energy expenditure and ambient temperatures. Allsopp et al. (1998) showed that acclimated individuals at ambient temperature of 40°C and dietary sodium intakes of 4 g/day for 8 days had sweat losses of 1.8 g/day. Taking this approach and assuming that the AI level includes 0.1 g sweat losses, then the value for sodium need would be 3.2 g/day (1.8 + 1.4 = 3.2). A second approach is to assume heavy exercise, approximately 4,400 kcal/day under two different ambient temperatures. If the temperature is high (30°C), then the total sweat losses will increase to about 10.5 L water/day (IOM, 2004, or Figure 2-1). With the sweat sodium concentrations varying from 0.23 g/L (Allan and Wilson, 1971, no dietary information, 40°C, 60 min of exercise) to 1.4 g/L (Inoue et al., 1999, no dietary information, at 43°C, 90 min of exercise), sweat sodium losses can be 2.3 g to 14 g/day. Using the lower level of 0.23 g/L, assuming 10.5 L of sweat, the calculated value for sodium needs is 3.7 g/day ([0.23 * 10] + 1.4 [AI – 0.1]) = 3.7). If the temperature is low (20°C), then the sweat losses will be less—about 6.5 L/water per day (IOM, 2004 or Figure 2-1)—but the concentration of sodium in the sweat will likely be more. For example, if 1.4 g/L were used, then as much as 9.1 g/day could be lost. Consolazio and co-workers (1963) showed a range of sodium sweat losses from 1.6–11.0 g/day when working at 37.7°C for 7.5 hr.

Given the large variations in energy level, ambient conditions, and individual acclimatization to ambient conditions (Conn, 1949), the recommendation is to provide ≥3 g/day of sodium, with additional sodium up to a total of 12 g provided through supplementation. Palatability will be a factor that limits the amount in the ration. Based on intake data for the US healthy population, it is not envisioned that an amount significantly higher than 3 g would be acceptable (see Food Form below).

When sodium intake does not meet losses, aldosterone secretion increases to conserve sodium by reducing urinary sodium levels (Costill et al., 1976a). Given the body's natural conservation, combined with decreases in sweat sodium concentration in acclimatized subjects in most work and heat conditions, a level of approximately 3 g/day of sodium is adequate.

Other Sodium Losses. For nonacclimatized soldiers or for those who lose excessive salt, extra salt may be needed. In addition, when average daily temperatures increase above 30°C/day and work load exceeds 2,800 kcal/day, sweat losses may exceed dietary intakes (Figure 2-1). Therefore, for these cases, extra sodium should be available (up to 12 g). The committee recommends that this be provided through a supplement, either to be added to their water supply or in candy or gel preparations. Palatability will limit the amount of sodium that can be added to these products and, therefore, sodium should also be available in the form of tablets to be provided by medical personnel or under medical guidance when needed.

In addition to fluid loss through sweat, more fluid may be lost due to diarrhea. For these cases, dry powder preparations that could be mixed with water should be available during combat or upon return to the base.

Sodium and Renal Stones. The committee had concerns about renal stones because soldiers could easily become dehydrated, and renal stones have occurred among troops (personal communication, C. Koenig, USARIEM, November 19, 2004). It is generally assumed that urinary calcium excretion reflects urinary sodium especially at urinary sodium levels above 2 g/day (Devine et al., 1995; Goulding and Lim, 1983; Massey and Whiting, 1996). Dawson-Hughes et al. (1996) showed that healthy men and women over age 65 had positive correlations of sodium and calcium excretion when calcium intake was over 1,000 mg/day with a normal sodium intake. Space flight data demonstrate a similar relationship (Whitson et al., 1997). The calcium recommendation for this ration is 750–850 mg/day, a level that should not promote renal stones with the sodium intakes of 4 g/day.

Food Form. The committee evaluated the feasibility of providing 3 or more grams of sodium per 2,400 kcal without compromising palatability. Intake data from NHANES III for 1988–1998 estimate that males 19–50 years of age consume 1.9–8.2 g/day of sodium (IOM, 2004) at energy intakes of 1,223–4,703 kcal (IOM, 2002a). These data suggest that males in this group would find 3 g/2,400 kcal acceptable. Acceptability of sodium levels in foods has been well studied; studies on salt levels with highest acceptability in specific foods have been conducted (Norton and Noble, 1991). Some people prefer high-salt diets when exercising (Leshem et al., 1999). The available data support the recommendation that ≥3 g/day of sodium would not only be acceptable but necessary for palatability for individuals who may have some decreases in appetite due to stress and exercise (Beauchamp et al., 1991).

Due to the impact of dehydration on performance after heavy activity, individuals should be encouraged to take extra sodium (see Shirreffs, 2004 in Appendix B). To ensure that the needs of individuals who lose salt in excess or who are in extremely hot or strenuous situations are met, additional sodium up to 12 g should be available as a supplement and in salt tablets. For the supplemental sodium, carbohydrate gels—some of them already commercially available—are easy to consume and carry and provide a feasible form to add sodium. Due to palatability issues, however, the amount of sodium in these products is only about 1 percent. Commercially available beverage supplements contain between 2.8 and 4.5 g of sodium per liter of water. With good rehydration procedures, this concentration of sodium in water would easily replace sodium sweat losses (Maughan and Shirreffs, 1997). To the extent possible, this supplemental amount (up to 12 g) should be included in the form of candy, gels, or powder to be mixed with fluid. However, because palatability will limit addition of sodium to these products, salt tablets should also be available and provided by medical personnel or under medical guidance when needed.

In summary, the AI for adult men (1.5 g/day) accounted for sodium sweat losses for unacclimatized individuals, but this level is not appropriate for individuals who are highly active, are exposed to prolonged heat, or who lose sodium in excess. The committee's sodium recommendation is based on estimates of sodium losses due to heavy exercise in potentially extreme temperatures, the interaction of high sodium and protein intakes with calcium losses in an environment prone to dehydration (Giannini et al., 1999; Whitson et al., 1997), and the importance of palatable food. Although this recommendation (≥3 g/day) is higher than the UL (2.3 g/day), the committee does not anticipate any adverse health effects on high blood pressure because the UL was established considering chronic intakes and not for short periods envisioned for the consumption of the assault ration; in any case, palatability issues will limit the amount of sodium in the ration and the tablet supplements should only be provided under medical guidance to individuals that lose excess salt or in extremely hot or strenuous situations.

Research Needs

- Evaluate the additional requirements for sodium and measure fecal, sweat, and urine losses in studies which simulate the environment encountered by soldiers in similar types of operations (e.g., exercise, high energy expenditure and reduced caloric intake, in high humidity and temperature).

Zinc

RECOMMENDATION: The assault ration should contain a level in the range of 11–25 mg of zinc. This range is based on the RDA for adult men, established with a factorial approach, and potential sweat losses during intense physical activity.

Background

Zinc participates in many physiological functions with catalytic, structural, immunologic, and regulatory roles that are essential for life. More than 100 enzymes depend on it for activity, and it is due to its properties as an electron acceptor that zinc becomes an essential element for enzymatic activity. Zinc-containing enzymes participate in macronutrient metabolism. Its importance in the proper functioning of the immune system derives in part from its structural role in the binding of tyrosine kinase to T-cell receptors. Because zinc has multiple roles, deficiency presents multiple signs and symptoms. Some of the clinical effects seen in zinc deficiencies are depressed growth, immune dysfunction, diarrhea, altered cognition, and altered appetite.

The RDA is set at 11 mg/day for adult men and was based on a factorial approach in which the principal indicator was the minimal quantity of absorbed zinc adequate to replace endogenous losses. The UL was set at 40 mg/day based on evidence of no adverse effects noted at this level (i.e., no suppression of immune response, no decrease in high-density lipoprotein cholesterol, and no reduced copper status). The median intake and 95th percentile intake in healthy US men age 19–30 years is 14.8 and 23.9 mg/day, respectively (IOM, 2001b).

Rationale for Levels of Zinc

Zinc Losses Through Sweat. Intense exercise is considered to affect zinc status. One of the factors affecting plasma levels is zinc loss either through urine or sweat. Urinary losses of zinc have been documented to rise from 0.4–0.7 mg/day during a 34-day training exercise in military field conditions (Miyamura et al., 1987). When sweat losses were studied over 16 days in the heat and after submaximal exercise, zinc losses ranged from 13.7 mg/day (first 4 days) to 2.2 mg/day (day 5 to day 12) with declining losses during acclimatization (Consolazio et al., 1964). Whereas one might have expected a rise in plasma zinc due to muscle damage or turnover, these losses were accompanied by small declines in serum zinc. Tipton et al. (1993) found that when sweat rates were included in the calculations, the rate of zinc loss was the same under hot (35°C) and neutral (25°C) conditions. Zinc losses in sweat might reach significant amounts and should be considered when recommending a level for the ration. The committee recommends a range of 11–25 mg in the ration. The lower limit of the range is based on the RDA for adult men; the upper limit is based on the addition of potential sweat losses during intense physical activity (14 mg) for a total of 25 mg.

Zinc and the Immune System. The beneficial effect of zinc as a modulator of the immune system and, particularly, in the prevention of upper respiratory infections is promising (Bhaskaram, 2002), but research findings have not reached clear, definite conclusions. Studies with the elderly population have shown either no effect of supplementation with zinc (Bogden et al., 1988), a mix of beneficial and adverse effects (Bogden et al., 1990), or beneficial effects only when mixed with other micronutrients (Bogden, 2004). There is conflicting evidence on whether zinc supplements shorten duration of colds; however, there is no evidence that supports the idea that zinc supplements prevent upper respiratory infections (Eby et al., 1984; Farr et al., 1987; Jackson et al., 2000; Prasad et al., 2000; Turner and Cetnarowski, 2000). Several immune function parameters decline with zinc deficiency, but zinc supplements at either 15 or 100 mg/day suppressed delayed-type skin hypersensitivity (an indicator of immune system function) in subjects > 60 years (Bogden et al., 1990). Similar findings on the impairment of the immune function were observed by Chandra (1984) when healthy adults were given 300 mg of zinc for 6 weeks. Unfortunately, there are no data on the effects of 15 mg/day on immunity in young healthy adults.

Zinc is one of the essential minerals that, due to its involvement as a cofactor with up to 100 enzymes, has been considered a dietary supplement for athletes. A review of the published literature, however, reveals that there is no strong evidence that zinc supplements in normally nourished individuals have an effect on immunity or physical and cognitive performance (Lukaski, 2004). A balance study conducted with obese men for over 40 days found that restricted-calorie diets (400 kcal) resulted in an increase in serum zinc, and also an increase in urine and fecal zinc; but zinc balance was not negative until 30–40 days (Lowy et al., 1986). The relevance of this study for the highly fit individuals who consume combat rations is not known.

Other Considerations. The committee is concerned that accurately assessing zinc status in stress conditions might not be feasible due to shifts between compartments (via cytokines) and the high variability in sweat and urine losses. Zinc intakes can be quite low even under normal dietary conditions and deficits resulting in health and performance effects could possibly develop. Meetings with the USARIEM representatives revealed that soldiers probably consume insufficient amounts of zinc during military operations, and that they could become mildly zinc deficient under stress. Due to these uncertainties (i.e., variable sweat losses, difficulties in assessing zinc status, marginal zinc status of many soldiers), the committee is taking a conservative approach, recommending zinc in the range of 11–25 mg. The higher end is meant to account for potential sweat losses of about 14 mg/day. It is unlikely that this amount (25 mg) will have any adverse effects on the immune system of young healthy adults. Although several studies reported gastrointestinal adverse effects at higher doses of zinc (> 100 mg/day) when ingested as zinc lozenges (Al-Gurairi et al., 2002; Garland and Hagmeyer, 1998), side effects at the level recommended here (25 mg/day) are not anticipated. The committee has concerns, however, that a higher limit of 40 mg/day, which is the UL for adults, might result in interactions with other minerals and undesirable anorexic effects or some gastrointestinal tract intolerance. Although supplementing with high amounts of iron (in the range of 34–400 mg) might interfere with zinc absorption (Kordas and Stoltzfus, 2004; Solomons and Jacob, 1981; Troost et al., 2003), with the amounts of iron recommended here (8–18 mg/day) there should be no such interference.

Questions regarding the bioavailability of zinc from the ration foods remained unanswered (see *Food Form* below).

Food Form

Zinc will be naturally present in ration foods such as cereals and red meats but may also need to be added to foods. Due to palatability issues, fortification with zinc should be done in foods, in which off-flavors can be masked, rather than in gels, candy, or powder forms. In addition to palatability issues, food developers should consider that the range of zinc recommended might affect appetite, a concern for soldiers in combat operations who already undereat.

As mentioned above, the bioavailability of zinc from the ration foods, whether zinc is naturally occurring or added, is not known. Estimates of absorption of zinc from foods differ depending on the data used (total diet data compared to single meal data) and on the nature of the diet considered. For example, the estimated absorption of zinc used in establishing the EAR (and, thus, the RDA) was 41 percent (IOM, 2001b) when data from studies conducted with male subjects were considered in a single diet category; in comparison, the International Zinc Nutrition Consultative Group (IZiNCG, 2004) estimated 26 and 18 percent absorption when calculated as a function of the diet type (i.e., mixed or cereal-based diet, respectively) and with data from studies conducted with both male and female subjects. When zinc doses up to 12 mg were given as a supplement to male and female subjects, average intestinal absorption was 55 percent (Payton et al., 1982). Another study in which subjects were given a total level of zinc of approximately 15 mg/day reported an average absorption of 64 percent (August et al., 1989). Thus, while there is substantial variability in estimates of zinc bioavailability and the bioavailability of recommended 14 mg added to the RDA is not known, it is likely to be in the same range of 45 to 65 percent.

Research Needs

- Determine the effects of supplemental levels of zinc on suppressing appetite for those in a stressful situation and under the hypocaloric rations in the field.

- Determine the effects of zinc on flavor and palatability of rations and identify ways to mask objectionable flavors.
- Measure fecal, sweat, and urine losses in studies which simulate the environment encountered by soldiers in similar types of operations (e.g., exercise, high energy expenditure and reduced caloric intake, in high humidity and temperature) in order to evaluate the additional requirements for zinc.

Other Bioactives and Dietary Supplements

General Background

In recent years there has been increased interest among athletes in augmenting traditional diets to optimize physical and mental performance. Earlier approaches of adding more protein or "carbo-loading" are still practiced by athletes. In addition, there has been increased use of herbals and bioactive components of foods; these include a variety of substances ranging from essential and nonessential amino acids, metabolites, energy enhancers, "muscle builders," and stimulants such as caffeine. Frontline soldiers wishing to gain a performance edge may well seek out and use such nontraditional food components, stimulants, and herbals. The key question is whether any of these compounds enhance performance with relatively few adverse effects at levels of use. Of importance to developing a ration for short-term, high-energy assault operations is whether any of these compounds should be provided in the ration to enhance performance.

A number of classes of compounds might be considered performance enhancers that could fall into the broad category of "other bioactive food components." Supradietary levels of traditional nutrients such as tyrosine, tryptophan, or carotenoids can be considered to function as bioactives. Megadose levels of vitamin E or C would be in this category because these levels are consumed for pharmacological effects. These nutrients are discussed in earlier sections of this chapter. Supplements of biological metabolites like creatine, L-carnitine, or coenzyme Q_{10} are also part of this category. In addition, thousands of plant polyphenols such as the flavonoids make up a huge category of compounds that in some situations have antioxidant and perhaps other properties. Stimulants such as caffeine have been shown to maintain cognitive performance. Finally, herbals such as ginkgo, ginseng, and tea and berry extracts contain potentially bioactive compounds and are reported in some studies to maintain or enhance performance.

Costello and Chrousos (2004 in Appendix B) evaluated the potential performance-enhancing effects of a number of bioactive food and dietary supplements. Among the materials reviewed were the neurotransmitter precursors tyrosine and L-tryptophan, the potential energy enhancers L-carnitine and coenzyme Q_{10}, and several herbals reported to increase energy or cognitive function. They did not find compelling evidence that any of these compounds enhanced performance. Except for creatine, few studies have been carried out in a randomized and blinded manner. Enough evidence warrants continued investigation of some of the components reviewed. As Costello and Chrousos suggest, a number of issues need to be considered in the design of future studies, including overtly controlling for coping status of subjects because those coping poorly under stress may respond better to the supplemented bioactive component than those who are coping well. The researchers also suggest future studies to identify food matrixes that can serve as delivery vehicles for bioactive substances. The committee discussed a variety of bioactive compounds or extracts (e.g., carnitine, creatine, *Ginkgo biloba* extract, glutamine) and concluded that, with the exception of caffeine, inclusion in the assault ration is not appropriate at this time. The following paragraphs highlight the committee's conclusions and recommendations on selected bioactive compounds that enhance performance (e.g., caffeine) and others that show promise but need further study as performance enhancers (e.g., creatine) or promising antioxidants (e.g., flavonoids).

Caffeine: Recommendation and Rationale

RECOMMENDATION: The committee supports the recommendations of past IOM committees regarding caffeine use for the military. Rations for combat missions should be supplemented with caffeine at levels of 100–600 mg, with no more than 600 mg in a single dose.

The effect of caffeine as a restorative compound when subjects are sleep deprived and as a performance enhancer for athletes or soldiers in sustained military operations is well documented (IOM, 2001a; Kalmar and Cafarelli, 2004; Magkos and Kavouras, 2004; Penetar et al., 1994). The Committee on Military Nutrition Research (CMNR) has been asked to evaluate the use of nutrients for performance enhancement in previous requests from the US Army Medical Research and Material Command. In 1994, the report *Food Components to Enhance Performance* (IOM, 1994) recommended that the military conduct research on the mechanisms of caffeine's effects on cognitive performance, on the feasibility of including caffeine in a different food vehicle in the ration, and on the optimized levels of caffeine that could help develop maximum performance for both caffeine-habituated individuals and casual caffeine users. That committee concluded that caffeine is a safe ingredient at levels necessary to maintain alertness and to overcome the cognitive function detriment resulting from sleep deprivation. For those used to caffeine, levels of 300–600 mg/70 kg person were recommended for alertness.

In 1998, as a result of new research on caffeine completed by the military and the need to make management decisions about its use, the military asked the CMNR to confirm its previous recommendations on caffeine use, and to provide recommendations on health risks of readily available caffeine. The committee was also charged with recommending safe levels for efficacy, better alternatives to caffeine, feasible vehicles to deliver caffeine, as well as recommendations on whether including it with other compounds would increase its effectiveness.

That committee concluded in the report *Caffeine for the Sustainment of Mental Task Performance* that caffeine in doses of 100–600 mg may be used to maintain cognitive performance, especially when an individual is sleep deprived or when fast reactions and acute vigilance may be needed (IOM, 2001a). A level of 200–600 mg was found to enhance physical endurance. Those amounts might be best provided in increments of 100 mg every 3–4 hours, and a single dose should not exceed 600 mg regardless of the habituation level. A recent review indicated that at those moderate doses the diuretic effect of caffeine is minimal (Maughan and Griffin, 2003). Another literature review to assess potential effects of caffeine during exercise suggested that athletes will not incur detrimental fluid-electrolyte imbalances or dehydration if they consume caffeine beverages in moderation (Armstrong, 2002). The committee also concluded that there were no current alternatives to caffeine for enhancing physical and cognitive performance when soldiers are sleep deprived, but that research should be conducted on the synergistic effects of using a combination of carbohydrate and caffeine. Chewing gums and food bars were suggested as the best delivery methods for caffeine (IOM, 2001a).

Caffeine is currently consumed by many Americans on a daily basis to maintain cognitive function. Soldiers also consume this stimulant regularly and would suffer withdrawal symptoms if caffeine were not available during the assault phases of operations. Provision of caffeine supplements in rations with the appropriate user advice is recommended, especially for those soldiers who will have minimal opportunities for sleep.

More recent published literature supports the recommendations of the IOM committee. The effects of caffeine ingestion on target detection and rifle marksmanship following a military exercise were investigated. When two doses were provided at 5 and 2.5 mg/kg of body weight prior to and following the exercise, respectively, target detection and engagement speed was improved. More complex tasks, such as friend-foe discrimination and shooting performance, were unaffected by this caffeine supplementation regime (Gillingham et al., 2004). Similar findings were reported by Tikuisis et al. (2004) when supplementing caffeine to sleep-deprived subjects. At the end of a 22-hour period without sleep, subjects who consumed a single dose of 400, 100, and 100 mg of caffeine at different times prior to the task showed improvement in target detection (a measure of cognitive function) versus decrements reported by the subjects who did not use caffeine. Caffeine, however, was not effective in restoring decrements in shooting accuracy and precision (a measure of psychomotor function) that occur with sleep deprivation.

Caffeine has also been studied in connection with improving physical performance. One study showed that physical performance as measured by rating of perceived exertion, time to complete a task, and time to exhaustion was also improved with a single dose of 400 mg and with two 100 mg doses of caffeine at intervals of a few hours during 24 hours of wakefulness (McLellan et al., 2004). Improvements in physical performance with caffeine were also reported with high-intensity cycling studies (Doherty et al., 2004).

Research Needs

- Determine the optimal levels of caffeine supplementation in hot and cold climates and at high altitude.
- Conduct further research on the optimal delivery methods of caffeine in rations.

Muscle Mass Enhancement Bioactives—Creatine and Other Bioactives

Dietary supplements are frequently used by athletes in an attempt to increase muscle mass or lean body mass (Clarkson and Rawson, 1999). Among the supplements used for this purpose have been the hormone dehydroepiandrosterone, β-methyl-hydroxy-β-methybutryrate), amino acid and protein supplements, elements (e.g., chromium and boron) as well as creatine. Reviews of such practices have concluded that "overall, it appears that there is little scientific documentation that most nutritional supplements will increase muscle mass as purported…" (Clarkson and Rawson, 1999, p. 324). The authors called for further research to document efficacy of supplements, possible mechanisms of action, and long-term safety. They did note that there was some evidence for the effectiveness of creatine in increasing muscle mass from a review of more than 15 studies.

Reports from observers in field operations (personal communication, C. Koenig, USARIEM, November 19, 2004) indicate widespread use of dietary supplements by soldiers. Given the lack of demonstration of efficacy and the potential for abuse of such substances, concern is warranted.

RECOMMENDATION: The committee notes the reports of substantial current use of the supplement creatine by troops. The potential efficacy of creatine on muscle performance during combat situations appears to be very limited. The committee is concerned about the metabolic effects of long-term use of this supplement, as well as the potential impact of withdrawal effects due to a sudden consumption decrease of creatine as troops begin assault operations. Both of these issues require attention.

Creatine continues to be a popular oral supplement among soldiers who are interested in enhancing muscle mass and athletic performance. The committee was informed by a team of military medical officers (personal communication, F. Christopher, S. Lewis, T. Phelps, US Army, October 22, 2004) that many combat troops currently consume creatine supplements. Thus, the efficacy and safety of this supplement is of special interest to the committee.

In 2000, the American College of Sports Medicine (Terjung et al., 2000) issued a consensus statement on the physiological and health effects of oral creatine supplementation. That panel noted that creatine supplementation can increase muscle phosphocreatine content in some individuals, leads to weight gain within a few days of supplementation, likely due to water retention, and is associated with an enhanced accrual of strength in strength-training programs. Performance enhancements, however, are small and are found only under specific exercise conditions. The group concluded that "the apparent high expectations for performance enhancement, evident by the extensive use of creatine supplementation, are inordinate" (Terjung et al., 2000, p. 706). A recent review of the creatine literature identified roughly 300 studies that have been carried out to evaluate the effects of creatine on exercise performance and concluded that it appears that creatine allows some athletes, perhaps due to their genetic makeup, to train with higher work loads; thus, it promotes strength gain in a resistance training program (Rawson and Clarkson, 2003). Creatine appears to improve performance in repeated, high-intensity exercises each lasting less than 30 seconds (e.g., sprinting activities) (Rawson and Clarkson, 2003).

Research Need

- Pursue randomized, well-controlled trials to elucidate the risks (e.g., withdrawal effects) and potential benefits (e.g., cognitive performance) of taking selected bioactives that are often consumed in the field, such as creatine; these trials should be conducted under conditions that mimic combat situations.

Food-Based, Mixed Antioxidants: Recommendation and Rationale

RECOMMENDATION: Food items should be designed to contain whole pieces or purees of fruit and other foods high in flavonoids and other polyphenols in order to enhance acceptability of rations and increase the quantity of naturally occurring antioxidants.

Antioxidant defense systems protect the human organism from tissue injury that occurs during chronic or acute exercise. Antioxidant nutrients such as vitamins C and E, the carotenoids, and selenium have received a great deal of scientific interest regarding their abilities to enhance a body's ability to cope with excess oxidative stress brought on by exercise. These nutrients and food components are also under study for their abilities to enhance or maintain cognitive functions. The committee's conclusions regarding those nutrients are found earlier in this chapter under each nutrient discussion.

Many foods of plant origin, especially foods derived from fruits, whole grains, and vegetables, contain a host of other less well characterized compounds that may function as cellular antioxidants and have the potential to aid in enhancing performance or decreasing the time of recovery after acute energy expenditure. Moreover, some of these other food components may act in synergy with other antioxidant defense systems to enhance performance. Antioxidant defense mechanisms in the body include a variety of enzymes such as catalase, superoxide dismutase, and glutathione peroxidase as well as nonenzymatic counterparts including vitamins C and E, carotenoids, and glutathione (Nijveldt et al., 2001).

One class of antioxidant compounds from plant-based foods is the polyphenols. Several hundred polyphenols have been isolated from edible plants. While they are primarily secondary metabolites of plants and serve in defense mechanisms in those plants, they have structural elements that suggest that they may play a role in prevention of oxidative stress in mammals (Manach et al., 2004).

Flavonoids, a subclass of the polyphenols with about 4,000 compounds, have received extensive research attention. Flavonoids occur naturally in fruits, vegetables, and beverages such as tea and wine (Nijveldt et al., 2001). There are a number of favorable in vitro investigations on the impact of various flavonoids on biomarkers of disease or symptoms such as cardiovascular events, inflammation, antitumor activity, and thrombosis. While outcomes of these studies need to be verified in vivo and in clinical trials and thus are less relevant to the combat soldier during assault missions, the general antioxidant effect of these compounds may be important to overall performance.

More relevant to the combat soldier during assault missions is the maintenance of an antioxidant defense system that optimizes the body's ability to cope with oxidative stress during periods of high physical and mental activity. The antioxidant defense systems should protect the body systems from excess production of reactive oxygen and nitrogen species. While it is not known whether the plant polyphenol substances specifically can enhance performance or decrease recovery time, it has been hypothesized that flavonoids may have additive effects with the endogenous reactive species' scavenging mechanisms (Liu, 2004). Various flavonoids, at least in vitro, have been shown to directly scavenge free radicals and to interact in antioxidant enzyme systems (Nijveldt et al., 2001). Much more work is needed in the context of assault operations to determine the synergy of these compounds with endogenous enzyme protection systems and with known dietary antioxidants.

Flavonoids are found in high concentrations in foods like fruits, vegetables, tea, and chocolate. It is important for the components of rations to have both good taste and optimal nutritional value. Both goals can be achieved by using food matrixes that contain some of these food sources. For example, dried fruit or fruit pastes (e.g., blueberry, grape, and cranberry) can be used in food items such as fruit roll-ups, cookies, purees, or gels. These fruit items contain significant levels of flavonoids as well as carotenoids and potentially vitamin C if processing conditions are mild. Concentrated fruit can also be fortified with vitamins C and E. Chocolate items have always been widely accepted by soldiers and have concentrated sources of flavonoids and other polyphenols. Coffee, and to a lesser extent tea, are also consumed by soldiers and, thus, provide flavonoids as well. There is no compelling reason to provide supplements or pills of concentrated flavonoids at this time. There are ample opportunities to include foods and beverages high in polyphenols for both acceptability and possibly for health reasons.

Research Needs

- Determine whether the addition of foods, food extracts, and beverages that are all high in antioxidant polyphenols enhances the acceptability of the rations.
- Determine whether the addition of foods, food extracts, and beverages that are high in antioxidant polyphenols would reduce the effects of oxidative stress under similar combat conditions, either along or through synergy with endogenous enzyme protection systems and known dietary antioxidants.

WATER REQUIREMENTS

Although the committee was not charged with making recommendations regarding water needs, the close links between diet, hydration status, and physiological function cannot be overlooked. Proper hydration is a major factor in maintaining sustained mental and physical performance. Information provided to the committee indicates that 4–5 L of water per day is made available during a combat mission. Part of these water needs is used to replace fluid losses due to the intense exercise. For example, assuming 4,400 kcal of energy expenditure, it can be estimated that sweat volumes could be as high as 6.5 and 10.5 L at 20 and 30°C, respectively.

In addition to sweat losses and metabolic rate, water needs are governed by nutrient intake, primarily protein and salt intake. Protein and sodium provide most of the excreted osmoles as urea and sodium and accompanying anions. The recommendation of 100–120 g of protein per day, while reasonable from a nutritional standpoint, will induce a higher water excretion via the kidneys to handle the increased solute load due to the production of approximately 16–19 g of urea nitrogen, 2–5 g more than with a 80 g protein intake. This additional increment of urea would require about 0.2 L more of urine, assuming a urinary concentration of 800 mOsm or as much as 0.4 L assuming a more conservative urine concentration of 400 mOsm. Maximal urinary concentration is approximately 1,200 mOsm. When such estimates are experimentally determined, subjects are usually in nitrogen balance, that is, urinary excretion of nitrogen equals nitrogen intake. Gamble (1947) found that 50–100 g of carbohydrate per day was more beneficial than protein to reduce renal water excretion and enhance hydration in fasting individuals. Other studies have shown that 100 g of carbohydrate reduce the deficit of body water by preventing ketosis (thus, decreasing ketones contribution to the osmolar excretion requirements) as well as reducing required urine volume due to the antinatriuretic effect of insulin stimulated by the dietary glucose. In the present situation, the provision of some energy and ample carbohydrate improves protein utilization over that in a fasting and severely hypocaloric state, resulting in a decreased production of urea from accelerated tissue protein breakdown. While the protein recommended by the committee (100–120 g) will add to the need for water, the high level of carbohydrate in the ration (450 g) should compensate for some of this need through improved protein utilization and limitation of renal excretion of sodium and its anions. Thus, the recommended carbohydrate in the ration constitutes an advantage in this regard.

While the committee did not provide specific recommendations for water, adequate amounts of water must be consumed with this ration to maintain and optimize physiological function and performance. Considering the expected level of stress and sweat volumes and the nature of the ration, water in excess of the 4–5 L/day must be available to ensure optimal performance in combat missions in which energy expenditure is high or carried out in hot and humid environments.

REFERENCES

Achten J, Halson SL, Moseley L, Rayson MP, Casey A, Jeukendrup AE. 2004. Higher dietary carbohydrate content during intensified running training results in better maintenance of performance and mood state. *J Appl Physiol* 96(4):1331–1340.

ACSM/ADA/DA (American College of Sports Medicine/American Dietetic Association/Dietitians of Canada). 2000. Joint postition statement. Nutrition and athletic performance. *Med Sci Sports Exerc* 32(12):2130–2145.

Afolabi PR, Jahoor F, Gibson NR, Jackson AA. 2004. Response of hepatic proteins to the lowering of habitual dietary protein to the recommended safe level of intake. *Am J Physiol Endocrinol Metab* 287(2):E327–E330.

Aguilo A, Tauler P, Fuentespina E, Villa G, Cordova A, Tur JA, Pons A. 2004. Antioxidant diet supplementation influences blood iron status in endurance athletes. *Int J Sport Nutr Exerc Metab* 14(2):147–160.

Ahlborg B, Bergstrom J, Ekelund LG, Hultman E. 1967. Muscle glycogen and muscle electrolytes during prolonged physical exercise. *Acta Physiol Scand* 70(2):129–142.

Al-Gurairi FT, Al-Waiz M, Sharquie KE. 2002. Oral zinc sulphate in the treatment of recalcitrant viral warts: Randomized placebo-controlled clinical trial. *Br J Dermatol* 146(3):423–431.

Allan JR, Wilson CG. 1971. Influence of acclimatization on sweat sodium concentration. *J Appl Physiol* 30(5):708–712.

Allen LH, Ahluwalia N. 1997. *Improving Iron Status through Diet. The Application of Knowledge Concerning Dietary Iron Bioavailability in Human Populations.* OMNI Technical Papers, No. 8. Arlington, VA: John Snow International.

Allsopp AJ, Sutherland R, Wood P, Wootton SA. 1998. The effect of sodium balance on sweat sodium secretion and plasma aldosterone concentration. *Eur J Appl Physiol* 78(6):516–521.

Anderson RA, Bryden NA, Polansky MM. 1992. Dietary chromium intake. Freely chosen diets, institutional diet, and individual foods. *Biol Trace Elem Res* 32:117–121.

Anonymous. 1991. Foods, nutrition, and sports performance. Final consensus statement. *J Sports Sci* 9:iii.

Anthony JC, Anthony TG, Layman DK. 1999. Leucine supplementation enhances skeletal muscle recovery in rats following exercise. *J Nutr* 129(6):1102–1106.

Anthony JC, Anthony TG, Kimball SR, Vary TC, Jefferson LS. 2000. Orally administered leucine stimulates protein synthesis in skeletal muscle of postabsorptive rats in association with increased eIF4F formation. *J Nutr* 130(2):139–145.

Armstrong LE. 2002. Caffeine, body fluid-electrolyte balance, and exercise performance. *Int J Sport Nutr Exerc Metab* 12(2):189–206.

Armstrong LE, Hubbard RW, Szlyk PC, Matthew WT, Sils IV. 1985. Voluntary dehydration and electrolyte losses during prolonged exercise in the heat. *Aviat Space Environ Med* 56(8):765–770.

Armstrong LE, Szlyk PC, De Luca JP, Sils IV, Hubbard RW. 1992. Fluid-electrolyte losses in uniforms during prolonged exercise at 30 degrees C. *Aviat Space Environ Med* 63(5):351–355.

Arnett T. 2003. Regulation of bone cell function by acid-base balance. *Proc Nutr Soc* 62(2):511–520.

Arthur JR, Nicol F, Beckett GJ. 1993. Selenium deficiency, thyroid hormone metabolism, and thyroid hormone deiodinases. *Am J Clin Nutr* 57(2 Suppl):236S–239S.

Askew EW, Claybaugh GM, Hashiro GM, Stokes WS, Sato A, Cucinell SA. 1987. *Mauna Kea III: Metabolic Effects of Dietary Carbohydrate Supplementation During Exercise at 4,100 m Altitude.* Technical Report No. T12-87. Fort Detrick, MD: US Army Medical Research and Development Command.

August D, Janghorbani M, Young VR. 1989. Determination of zinc and copper absorption at three dietary Zn-Cu ratios by using stable isotope methods in young adult and elderly subjects. *Am J Clin Nutr* 50(6):1457–1463.

Aurengo A, Leenhardt L, Aurengo H. 2002. Adaptation of thyroid function to excess iodine. *Presse Med* 31(35):1658–1663.

Ayre KJ, Hulbert AJ. 1996. Effects of changes in dietary fatty acids on isolated skeletal muscle functions in rats. *J Appl Physiol* 80(2):464–471.

Baker EM, Saari JC, Tolbert BM. 1966. Ascorbic acid metabolism in man. *Am J Clin Nutr* 19(6):371–378.

Barber MD, Ross JA, Preston T, Shenkin A, Fearon KC. 1999. Fish oil-enriched nutritional supplement attenuates progression of the acute-phase response in weight-losing patients with advanced pancreatic cancer. *J Nutr* 129(6):1120–1125.

Bashir Y, Sneddon JF, Staunton HA, Haywood GA, Simpson IA, McKenna WJ, Camm AJ. 1993. Effects of long-term oral magnesium chloride replacement in congestive heart failure secondary to coronary artery disease. *Am J Cardiol* 72(15):1156–1162.

Batchelder EL, Ebbs JC. 1943. Some observations of dark adaptation in mand and their bearing on the problem of human requirement for vitamin A. *Rhode Island Agricultural Experiment Station Bulletin.* No. 645:295–302.

Bausch J, Rietz P. 1977. Method for the assessment of vitamin A liver stores. *Acta Vitaminol Enzymol* 31(1–5):99–112.

Beale RJ, Bryg DJ, Bihari DJ. 1999. Immunonutrition in the critically ill: A systematic review of clinical outcome. *Crit Care Med* 27(12):2799–2805.

Beard J, Tobin B. 2000. Iron status and exercise. *Am J Clin Nutr* 72(2 Suppl):594S–597S.

Beauchamp GK, Bertino M, Engelman K. 1991. Human salt appetite. In: Friedman ME, Tordoff MG, Kare MR, eds. *Chemical Senses.* Vol. 4. New York: Marcel Dekker. Pp. 85–107.

Belko AZ, Meredith MP, Kalkwarf HJ, Obarzanek E, Weinberg S, Roach R, McKeon G, Roe DA. 1985. Effects of exercise on riboflavin requirements: Biological validation in weight reducing women. *Am J Clin Nutr* 41(2):270–277.

Bergstrom J, Hermansen L, Hultman E, Saltin B. 1967. Diet, muscle glycogen and physical performance. *Acta Physiol Scand* 71(2):140–150.

Bhaskaram P. 2002. Micronutrient malnutrition, infection, and immunity: An overview. *Nutr Rev* 60(5 Pt 2):S40–S45.

Bianco AC, Salvatore D, Gereben B, Berry MJ, Larsen PR. 2002. Biochemistry, cellular and molecular biology, and physiological roles of the iodothyronine selenodeiodinases. *Endocr Rev* 23(1):38–89.

Bistrian BR, Babineau T. 1998. Optimal protein intake in critical illness? *Crit Care Med* 26(9):1476–1477.

Blanchard EL, Harper HA. 1940. Measurement of vitamin A status of young adults by the dark adaptation technic. *Arch Int Med* 66:661–669.

Bogden JD. 2004. Influence of zinc on immunity in the elderly. *J Nutr Health Aging* 8(1):48–54.

Bogden JD, Oleske JM, Lavenhar MA, Munves EM, Kemp FW, Bruening KS, Holding KJ, Denny TN, Guarino MA, Holland BK. 1990. Effects of one year of supplementation with zinc and other micronutrients on cellular immunity in the elderly. *J Am Coll Nutr* 9(3):214–225.

Bogden JD, Oleske JM, Lavenhar MA, Munves EM, Kemp FW, Bruening KS, Holding KJ, Denny TN, Guarino MA, Krieger LM. 1988. Zinc and immunocompetence in elderly people: Effects of zinc supplementation for 3 months. *Am J Clin Nutr* 48(3):655–663.

Booth CK, Coad RA, Forbes-Ewan CH, Thomson GF, Niro PJ. 2003. The physiological and psychological effects of combat ration feeding during a 12-day training exercise in the tropics. *Mil Med* 168(1):63–70.

Booth SL, Golly I, Sacheck JM, Roubenoff R, Dallal GE, Hamada K, Blumberg JB. 2004. Effect of vitamin E supplementation on vitamin K status in adults with normal coagulation status. *Am J Clin Nutr* 80(1):143–148.

Borghi L, Meschi T, Amato F, Briganti A, Novarini A, Giannini A. 1996. Urinary volume, water and recurrences in idiopathic calcium nephrolithiasis: A 5-year randomized prospective study. *J Urol* 155(3):839–843.

Borghi L, Schianchi T, Meschi T, Guerra A, Allegri F, Maggiore U, Novarini A. 2002. Comparison of two diets for the prevention of recurrent stones in idiopathic hypercalciuria. *N Engl J Med* 346(2):77–84.

Born P, Zech J, Stark M, Classen M, Lorenz R. 1994. Carbohydrate substitutes: Comparative study of intestinal absorption of fructose, sorbitol and xylitol. *Med Klin (Munich)* 89(11):575–578.

Borsheim E, Tipton KD, Wolf SE, Wolfe RR. 2002. Essential amino acids and muscle protein recovery from resistance exercise. *Am J Physiol Endocrinol Metab* 283(4):E648–E657.

Bremner I. 1998. Manifestations of copper excess. *Am J Clin Nutr* 67(5 Suppl):1069S–1073S.

Brilla LR, Gunter KB. 1995. Effect of magnesium supplementation on exercise time to exhaustion. *Med Exerc Nutr Health* 4:230–233.

Brilla LR, Haley TF. 1992. Effect of magnesium supplementation on strength training in humans. *J Am Coll Nutr* 11(3):326–329.

Broome CS, McArdle F, Kyle JAM, Andrews F, Lowe NM, Hart CA, Arthur JR, Jackson MJ. 2004. An increase in selenium intake improves immune function and poliovirus handling in adults with marginal selenium status. *Am J Clin Nutr* 80(1):154–162.

Brown GD, Gordon S. 2003. Fungal beta-glucans and mammalian immunity. *Immunity* 19(3):311–315.

Brownlie T 4th, Utermohlen V, Hinton PS, Giordano C, Haas JD. 2002. Marginal iron deficiency without anemia impairs aerobic adaptation among previously untrained women. *Am J Clin Nutr* 75(4):734–742.

Brownlie T 4th, Utermohlen V, Hinton PS, Haas JD. 2004. Tissue iron deficiency without anemia impairs adaptation in endurance capacity after aerobic training in previously untrained women. *Am J Clin Nutr* 79(3):437–443.

Brune M, Magnusson B, Persson H, Hallberg L. 1986. Iron losses in sweat. *Am J Clin Nutr* 43(3):438–443.

Brune M, Rossander-Hulten L, Hallberg L, Gleerup A, Sandberg AS. 1992. Iron absorption from bread in humans: Inhibiting effects of cereal fiber, phytate and inositol phosphates with different numbers of phosphate groups. *J Nutr* 122(3):442–449.

Bruner AB, Joffe A, Duggan AK, Casella JF, Brandt J. 1996. Randomised study of cognitive effects of iron supplementation in non-anaemic iron-deficient adolescent girls. *Lancet* 348(9033):992–996.

Bruno RS, Ramakrishnan R, Montine TJ, Bray TM, Traber MG. 2005. α-Tocopherol disappearance is faster in cigarette smokers and is inversely related to their ascorbic acid status. *Am J Clin Nutr* 81(1):95–103.

Brutsaert TD, Hernandez-Cordero S, Rivera J, Viola T, Hughes G, Haas JD. 2003. Iron supplementation improves progressive fatigue resistance during dynamic knee extensor exercise in iron-depleted, nonanemic women. *Am J Clin Nutr* 77(2):441–448.

Buchman AL, Keen C, Commisso J, Killip D, Ou CN, Rognerud CL, Dennis K, Dunn JK. 1998. The effect of a marathon run on plasma and urine mineral and metal concentrations. *J Am Coll Nutr* 17(2):124–127.

Bullen DB, O'Toole ML, Johnson KC. 1999. Calcium losses resulting from an acute bout of moderate-intensity exercise. *Int J Sport Nutr* 9(3):275–284.

Burke LM, Hawley JA. 2002. Effects of short-term fat adaptation on metabolism and performance of prolonged exercise. *Med Sci Sports Exerc* 34(9):1492–1498.

Burke LM, Kiens B, Ivy JL. 2004. Carbohydrates and fat for training and recovery. *J Sports Sci* 22(1):15–30.

Bushe CJ. 1986. Profound hypophosphataemia in patients collapsing after a "fun run". *Br Med J* 292(6524):898–899.

Butterfield GE, Calloway DH. 1984. Physical activity improves protein utilization in young men. *Br J Nutr* 51(2):171–184.

Calvaresi E, Bryan J. 2001. B vitamins, cognition, and aging: A review. *J Gerontol B Psychol Sci Soc Sci* 56(6):P327–P339.

Calvo MS, Whiting SJ. 2003. Prevalence of vitamin D insufficiency in Canada and the United States: Importance to health status and efficacy of current food fortification and dietary supplement use. *Nutr Rev* 61(3):107–113.

Cannon JG, Meydani SN, Fielding RA, Fiatarone MA, Meydani M, Farhangmehr M, Orencole SF, Blumberg JB, Evans WJ. 1991. Acute phase response in exercise. II. Associations between vitamin E, cytokines, and muscle proteolysis. *Am J Physiol* 260(6 Pt 2):R1235–R1240.

Cannon JG, Orencole SF, Fielding RA, Meydani M, Meydani SN, Fiatarone MA, Blumberg JB, Evans WJ. 1990. Acute phase response in exercise: Interaction of age and vitamin E on neutrophils and muscle enzyme release. *Am J Physiol* 259(6 Pt 2):R1214–R1219.

Chandra RK. 1984. Excessive intake of zinc impairs immune responses. *J Am Med Assoc* 252(11):1443–1446.

Childs A, Jacobs C, Kaminski T, Halliwell B, Leeuwenburgh C. 2001. Supplementation with vitamin C and N-acetyl-cysteine increases oxidative stress in humans after an acute muscle injury induced by eccentric exercise. *Free Radic Biol Med* 31(6):745–753.

Clarkson PM. 1997. Effects of exercise on chromium levels. Is supplementation required? *Sports Med* 23(6):341–349.

Clarkson PM, Haymes EM. 1995. Exercise and mineral status of athletes: Calcium, magnesium, phosphorus, and iron. *Med Sci Sports Exerc* 27(6):831–843.

Clarkson PM, Rawson ES. 1999. Nutritional supplements to increase muscle mass. *Crit Rev Food Sci Nutr* 39(4):317–328.

Clarkson PM, Thompson HS. 2000. Antioxidants: What role do they play in physical activity and health? *Am J Clin Nutr* 72(2 Suppl):637S–646S.

Clavel S, Farout L, Briand M, Briand Y, Jouanel P. 2002. Effect of endurance training and/or fish oil supplemented diet on cytoplasmic fatty acid binding protein in rat skeletal muscles and heart. *Eur J Appl Physiol* 87(3):193–201.

Cohn JR, Emmett EA. 1978. The excretion of trace metals in human sweat. *Ann Clin Lab Sci* 8(4):270–275.

Collardeau M, Brisswalter J, Vercruyssen F, Audiffren M, Goubault C. 2001. Single and choice reaction time during prolonged exercise in trained subjects: Influence of carbohydrate availability. *Eur J Appl Physiol* 86(2):150–156.

Conn JW. 1949. The mechanism of acclimatization to heat. *Adv Int Med* 3:373–393.

Consolazio CF, Matoush LO, Nelson RA, Harding RS, Canham JE. 1963. Excretion of sodium, potassium, magnesium and iron in human sweat and the relation of each to balance and requirements. *J Nutr* 79:407–415.

Consolazio CF, Matoush LO, Nelson RA, Isaac GJ, Canham JE. 1966. Comparisons of nitrogen, calcium and iodine excretion in arm and total body sweat. *Am J Clin Nutr* 18(6):443–448.

Consolazio CF, Nelson RA, Matoush LO, Hughes RC, Urone P. 1964. *The Trace Mineral Losses in Sweat*. Report No. 284. Denver, CO: US Army Medical Research and Nutrition Laboratory.

Convertino VA, Armstrong LE, Coyle EF, Mack GW, Sawka MN, Senay LC, Sherman WM. 1996. American College of Sports Medicine Position Stand on exercise and fluid replacement. *Med Sci Sports Exerc* 28(1):i–vii.

Cook JD, Dassenko SA, Lynch SR. 1991. Assessment of the role of nonheme-iron availability in iron balance. *Am J Clin Nutr* 54(4):717–722.

Cook JD, Lipschitz DA, Miles LE, Finch CA. 1974. Serum ferritin as a measure of iron stores in normal subjects. *Am J Clin Nutr* 27(7):681–687.

Cook JD, Reddy MB, Burri J, Juillerat MA, Hurrell RF. 1997. The influence of different cereal grains on iron absorption from infant cereal foods. *Am J Clin Nutr* 65(4):964–969.

Cooling J, Blundell JE. 2001. High-fat and low-fat phenotypes: Habitual eating of high- and low-fat foods not related to taste preference for fat. *Eur J Clin Nutr* 55(11):1016–1021.

Costello RB, Chrousos GP. 2004 (August 10). *Other Bioactive Food Components and Dietary Supplements*. Paper presented at the Institute of Medicine Workshop on Optimization of Nutrient Composition of Military Rations for Short-Term, High-Stress Situations, Natick, MA. Institute of Medicine Committee on Optimization of Nutrient Composition of Military Rations for Short-Term, High-Stress Situations.

Costill DL, Miller JM. 1980. Nutrition for endurance sport: Carbohydrate and fluid balance. *Int J Sports Med* 1(1):2–14.

Costill DL, Branam G, Fink W, Nelson R. 1976a. Exercise induced sodium conservation: Changes in plasma renin and aldosterone. *Med Sci Sports* 8(4):209–213.

Costill DL, Cote R, Fink W. 1976b. Muscle water and electrolytes following varied levels of dehydration in man. *J Appl Physiol* 40(1):6–11.

Costill DL, Flynn MG, Kirwan JP, Houmard JA, Mitchell JB, Thomas R, Park SH. 1988. Effects of repeated days of intensified training on muscle glycogen and swimming performance. *Med Sci Sports Exerc* 20(3):249–254.

Coyle EF. 2004 (August 9). *Carbohydrate Ingestion Prior To and During Intense Activity*. Paper presented at the Institute of Medicine Workshop on Optimization of Nutrient Composition of Military Rations for Short-Term, High-Stress Situations, Natick, MA. Institute of Medicine Committee on Optimization of Nutrient Composition of Military Rations for Short-Term, High-Stress Situations.

Coyle EF, Montain SJ. 1992. Benefits of fluid replacement with carbohydrate during exercise. *Med Sci Sports Exerc* 24(9 Suppl):S324–S330.

Coyle EF, Coggan AR, Hemmert MK, Ivy JL. 1986. Muscle glycogen utilization during prolonged strenuous exercise when fed carbohydrate. *J Appl Physiol* 61(1):165–172.

Curhan GC, Willett WC, Rimm EB, Stampfer MJ. 1993. A prospective study of dietary calcium and other nutrients and the risk of symptomatic kidney stones. *N Engl J Med* 328(12):833–838.

Dale G, Fleetwood JA, Inkster JS, Sainsbury JR. 1986. Profound hypophosphataemia in patients collapsing after a "fun run". *Br Med J (Clin Res Ed)* 292(6518):447–448.

Dangin M, Guillet C, Garcia-Rodenas C, Gachon P, Bouteloup-Demange C, Reiffers-Magnani K, Fauquant J, Ballevre O, Beaufrere B. 2003. The rate of protein digestion affects protein gain differently during aging in humans. *J Physiol* 549(Pt 2):635–644.

Davies KM, Heaney RP, Recker RR, Lappe JM, Barger-Lux MJ, Ratterty K, Hinders S. 2000. Calcium intake and body weight. *J Clin Endocrinol Metab* 85(12):4635–4638.

Dawson B, Henry GJ, Goodman C, Gillam I, Beilby JR, Ching S, Fabian V, Dasig D, Morling P, Kakulus BA. 2002. Effect of Vitamin C and E supplementation on biochemical and ultra-structural indices of muscle damage after a 21 km run. *Int J Sports Med* 23(1):10–15.

Dawson-Hughes B, Fowler SE, Dalsky G, Gallagher C. 1996. Sodium excretion influences calcium homeostasis in elderly men and women. *J Nutr* 126(9):2107–2112.

Dawson-Hughes B, Harris SS, Rasmussen H, Song L, Dallal GE. 2004. Effect of dietary protein supplements on calcium excretion in healthy older men and women. *J Clin Endocrinol Metab* 89(3):1169–1173.

de O G Mendonca C, Martini LA, Baxmann AC, Nishiura JL, Cuppari L, Sigulem DM, Heilberg IP. 2003. Effects of an oxalate load on urinary oxalate excretion in calcium stone formers. *J Ren Nutr* 13(1):39–46.

Delorme O, Bourdin H, Viel JF, Rigaud ML, Kantelip JP. 1992. Spectral analysis of electro-encephalography data in athletes with low erythrocyte magnesium. *Magnes Res* 5(4):261–264.

Deluca HF, Cantorna MT. 2001. Vitamin D: Its role and uses in immunology. *FASEB J* 15(14):2579–2585.

DeRuisseau KC, Cheuvront SN, Haymes EM, Sharp RG. 2002. Sweat iron and zinc losses during prolonged exercise. *Int J Sport Nutr Exerc Metab* 12(4):428–437.

Devine A, Criddle RA, Dick IM, Kerr DA, Prince RL. 1995. A longitudinal study of the effect of sodium and calcium intakes on regional bone density in postmenopausal women. *Am J Clin Nutr* 62(4):740–745.

Dill DB, Soholt LF, Oddershede IB. 1976. Physiological adjustments of young mean to five-hour desert walks. *J Appl Physiol* 40(2):236–242.

Disler PB, Lynch SR, Charlton RW, Torrance JD, Bothwell TH, Walker RB, Mayet F. 1975. The effect of tea on iron absorption. *Gut* 16(3):193–200.

Doherty M, Smith P, Hughes M, Davison R. 2004. Caffeine lowers perceptual response and increases power output during high-intensity cycling. *J Sports Sci* 22(7):637–643.

Drewnowski A. 1997. Taste preferences and food intake. *Annu Rev Nutr* 17:237–253.

Dye L, Blundell J. 2002. Functional foods: Psychological and behavioral functions. *Br J Nutr* 88(Suppl 2):S187–S211.

Dye L, Lluch A, Blundell JE. 2000. Macronutrients and mental performance. *Nutrition* 16(10):1021–1034.

Eby GA, Davis DR, Halcomb WW. 1984. Reduction in duration of common colds by zinc gluconate lozenges in a double-blind study. *Antimicrob Agents Chemother* 25(1):20–24.

Ettinger B, Pak CY, Citron JT, Thomas C, Adams-Huet B, Vangessel A. 1997. Potassium-magnesium citrate is an effective prophylaxis against recurrent calcium oxalate nephrolithiasis. *J Urol* 158(6):2069–2073.

Evans WJ. 2000. Vitamin E, vitamin C, and exercise. *Am J Clin Nutr* 72(2 Suppl):647S–652S.

FAO/WHO (Food and Agriculture Organization/World Health Organization). 1988. *Requirements of Vitamin A, Iron, Folate, and Vitamin B_{12}*. FAO Food Nutrition Series No. 23. Rome: FAO. Pp. 33–50.

FAO/WHO/UNU (Food and Agriculture Organization/World Health Organization/United Nations University). 1985. *Energy and Protein Requirements*. Technical Report Series 724. Geneva: World Health Organization.

Farr BM, Conner EM, Betts RF, Oleske J, Minnefor A, Gwaltney JM Jr. 1987. Two randomized controlled trials of zinc gluconate lozenge therapy of experimentally induced rhinovirus colds. *Antimicrob Agents Chemother* 31(8):1183–1187.

Fearon KC, Von Meyenfeldt MF, Moses AG, Van Geenen R, Roy A, Gouma DJ, Giacosa A, Van Gossum A, Bauer J, Barber MD, Aaronson NK, Voss AC, Tisdale MJ. 2003. Effect of a protein and energy dense N-3 fatty acid enriched oral supplement on loss of weight and lean tissue in cancer cachexia: A randomised double blind trial. *Gut* 52(10):1479–1486.

Febbraio MA. 2001. Alterations in energy metabolism during exercise and heat stress. *Sports Med* 31(1):47–59.

Febbraio MA, Murton P, Selig SE, Clark SA, Lambert DL, Angus DJ, Carey MF. 1996. Effect of CHO ingestion on exercise metabolism and performance in different ambient temperatures. *Med Sci Sports Exerc* 28(11):1380–1387.

Fielding RA, Parkington J. 2002. What are the dietary protein requirements of physically active individuals? New evidence on the effects of exercise on protein utilization during post-exercise recovery. *Nutr Clin Care* 5(4):191–196.

Fink WJ, Costill DL, Van Handel PJ. 1975. Leg muscle metabolism during exercise in the heat and cold. *Eur J Appl Physiol Occup Physiol* 34(3):183–190.

Fischer K, Colombani PC, Langhans W, Wenk C. 2002. Carbohydrate to protein ratio in food and cognitive performance in the morning. *Physiol Behav* 75(3):411–423.

Frank J, Sundberg B, Kamal-Eldin A, Vessby B, Aman P. 2004. Yeast-leavened oat breads with high or low molecular weight beta-glucan do not differ in their effects on blood concentrations of lipids, insulin, or glucose in humans. *J Nutr* 134(6):1384–1388.

Frassetto LA, Todd KM, Morris RC Jr, Sebastian A. 1998. Estimation of net endogenous noncarbonic acid production in humans from diet potassium and protein contents. *Am J Clin Nutr* 68(3):576–583.

Friedl KE. 1997. Variability of fat and lean tissue loss during physical exertion with energy deficit. In: Kinney JM, Tucker HN, eds. *Physiology, Stress, and Malnutrition: Functional Correlates, Nutritional Intervention.* Philadelphia: Lippincott-Raven. Pp. 431–450.

Friedl KE, Hoyt RW. 1997. Development and biomedical testing of military operational rations. *Annu Rev Nutr* 17:51–75.

Fritzsche RG, Switzer TW, Hodgkinson BJ, Lee SH, Martin JC, Coyle EF. 2000. Water and carbohydrate ingestion during prolonged exercise increase maximal neuromuscular power. *J Appl Physiol* 88(2):730–737.

Gamble JL. 1947. Physiological information gained from studies on the life raft ration. In: The Harvey Society of New York, eds. *The Harvey Lectures.* Lancaster, PA: The Sciences Press Printing Co. Pp. 247–273.

Garfinkel L, Garfinkel D. 1985. Magnesium regulation of the glycolytic pathway and the enzymes involved. *Magnesium* 4(2–3):60–72.

Garland ML, Hagmeyer KO. 1998. The role of zinc lozenges in treatment of the common cold. *Ann Pharmacother* 32(1):63–69.

Gerstein DE, Woodward-Lopez G, Evans AE, Kelsey K, Drewnowski A. 2004. Clarifying concepts about macronutrients' effects on satiation and satiety. *J Am Diet Assoc* 104(7):1151–1153.

Giannini S, Nobile M, Sartori L, Dalle Carbonare L, Ciuffreda M, Corro P, D'Angelo A, Calo L, Crepaldi G. 1999. Acute effects of moderate dietary protein restriction in patients with idiopathic hypercalciuria and calcium nephrolithiasis. *Am J Clin Nutr* 69(2):267–271.

Gibson NR, Jahoor F, Ware L, Jackson AA. 2002. Endogenous glycine and tyrosine production is maintained in adults consuming a marginal-protein diet. *Am J Clin Nutr* 75(3):511–518.

Gillingham RL, Keefe AA, Tikuisis P. 2004. Acute caffeine intake before and after fatiguing exercise improves target shooting engagement time. *Aviat Space Environ Med* 75(10):865–871.

Glanz K, Basil M, Maibach E, Goldberg J, Snyder D. 1998. Why Americans eat what they do: Taste, nutrition, cost, convenience, and weight control concerns as influences on food consumption. *J Am Diet Assoc* 98(10):1118–1126.

Gleeson M, Nieman DC, Pedersen BK. 2004. Exercise, nutrition and immune function. *J Sports Sci* 22(1):115–125.

Golf SW, Bohmer D, Nowacki PE. 1993. Is magnesium a limiting factor in competitive exercise? A summary of relevant scientific data. In: Golf S, Dralle D, Vecchiet L, eds. *Magnesium 1993.* London: John Libbey & Co. Pp. 209–219.

Gordon CM, DePeter KC, Feldman HA, Grace E, Emans SJ. 2004. Prevalence of vitamin D deficiency among healthy adolescents. *Arch Pediatr Adolesc Med* 158(6):531–537.

Goulding A, Lim PE. 1983. Effects of varying dietary salt intake on the fasting urinary excretion of sodium, calcium and hydroxyproline in young women. *N Z Med J* 96:853–854.

Graat JM, Schouten EG, Kok FJ. 2002. Effect of daily vitamin E and multivitamin-mineral supplementation on acute respiratory tract infections in elderly persons: A randomized controlled trial. *J Am Med Assoc* 288(6):715–721.

Green R, Charlton R, Seftel H, Bothwell T, Mayet F, Adams B, Finch C, Layrisse M. 1968. Body iron excretion in man. A collaborative study. *Am J Med* 45:336–353.

Griffin MD, Xing N, Kumar R. 2003. Vitamin D and its analogs as regulators of immune activation and antigen presentation. *Annu Rev Nutr* 23:117–145.

Grimm M, Muller A, Hein G, Funfstuck R, Jahreis G. 2001. High phosphorus intake only slightly affects serum minerals, urinary pyridinium crosslinks and renal function in young women. *Eur J Clin Nutr* 55(3):153–161.

Hallberg L, Rossander-Hulten L. 1991. Iron requirements in menstruating women. *Am J Clin Nutr* 54(6):1047–1058.

Hallberg L, Brune M, Erlandsson M, Sandberg AS, Rossander-Hulten L. 1991. Calcium: Effect of different amounts on nonheme- and heme-iron absorption in humans. *Am J Clin Nutr* 53(1):112–119.

Hansen CM, Shultz TD, Kwak HK, Memon HS, Leklem JE. 2001. Assessment of vitamin B-6 status in young women consuming a controlled diet containing four levels of vitamin B-6 provides an estimated average requirement and recommended dietary allowance. *J Nutr* 131(6):1777–1786.

Haskell MJ, Handelman GJ, Peerson JM, Jones AD, Rabbi MA, Awal MA, Wahed MA, Mahalanabis D, Brown KH. 1997. Assessment of vitamin A status by the deuterated-retinol-dilution technique and comparison with hepatic vitamin A concentration in Bangladeshi surgical patients. *Am J Clin Nutr* 66(1):67–74.

Hawley J. 2000. Nutritional strategies to enhance fat oxidation during aerobic exercise. In: Burke L, Deakin V, eds. *Clinical Sports Nutrition.* 2nd ed. Roseville, Australia: McGraw Hill Australia. Pp. 428–454.

Hawley JA, Schabort EJ, Noakes TD, Dennis SC. 1997. Carbohydrate-loading and exercise performance. An update. *Sports Med* 24(2):73–81.

Heaney RP, Recker RR. 1982. Effects of nitrogen, phosphorus, and caffeine on calcium balance in women. *J Lab Clin Med* 99(1):46–55.

Heaney RP, Davies KM, Chen TC, Holick MF, Barger-Lux MJ. 2003. Human serum 25-hydroxycholecalciferol response to extended oral dosing with cholecalciferol. *Am J Clin Nutr* 77(1):204–210.

Helge JW. 2000. Adaptation to a fat-rich diet. Effects on endurance performance in humans. *Sports Med* 30(5):347–357.

Helge JW. 2004 (August 9). *Optimization of Macronutrient Composition for Carbohydrate and Fat Intake: What is the Optimal Balance.* Paper presented at the Institute of Medicine Workshop on Optimization of Nutrient Composition of Military Rations for Short-Term, High-Stress Situations, Natick, MA. Institute of Medicine Committee on Optimization of Nutrient Composition of Military Rations for Short-Term, High-Stress Situations.

Helge JW, Lundby C, Christensen DL, Langfort J, Messonnier L, Zacho M, Andersen JL, Saltin B. 2003. Skiing across Greenland icecap: Divergent effects on limb muscle adaptations and substrate oxidation. *J Exp Biol* 206(Pt 6):1075–1083.

Hemila H. 1994. Does vitamin C alleviate the symptoms of the common cold? A review of current evidence. *Scand J Infect Dis* 26(1):1–6.

Hemila H. 1997. Vitamin C intake and susceptibility to the common cold. *Br J Nutr* 77(1):59–72.

Hemila H, Kaprio J, Albanes D, Heinonen OP, Virtamo J. 2002. Vitamin C, vitamin E, and beta-carotene in relation to common cold incidence in male smokers. *Epidemiology* 13(1):32–37.

Heyland DK, Novak F, Drover JW, Jain M, Su X, Suchner U. 2001. Should immunonutrition become routine in critically ill patients? A systematic review of the evidence. *J Am Med Assoc* 286(8):944–953.

Heys SD, Walker LG, Smith I, Eremin O. 1999. Enteral nutritional supplementation with key nutrients in patients with critical illness and cancer: A meta-analysis of randomized controlled clinical trials. *Ann Surg* 229(4):467–477.

Hinton PS, Giordano C, Brownlie T, Haas JD. 2000. Iron supplementation improves endurance after training in iron-depleted, nonanemic women. *J Appl Physiol* 88(3):1103–1111.

Hoffer LJ. 2004 (August 9). *Optimum Protein Intake in Hypocaloric States.* Paper presented at the Institute of Medicine Workshop on Optimization of Nutrient Composition of Military Rations for Short-Term, High-Stress Situations, Natick, MA. Institute of Medicine Committee on Optimization of Nutrient Composition of Military Rations for Short-Term, High-Stress Situations.

Hoffer LJ, Bistrian BR, Young VR, Blackburn GL, Matthews DE. 1984. Metabolic effects of very low calorie weight reduction diets. *J Clin Invest* 73(3):750–758.

Holick MF. 2004. Vitamin D: Importance in the prevention of cancers, type 1 diabetes, heart disease, and osteoporosis. *Am J Clin Nutr* 79(3):362–371.

Holmes RP. 2000. Oxalate synthesis in humans: Assumptions, problems, and unresolved issues. *Mol Urol* 4(4):329–332.

Holmes RP, Goodman HO, Assimos DG. 1995. Dietary oxalate and its intestinal absorption. *Scanning Microsc* 9(4):1109–1120.

Holmes RP, Goodman HO, Assimos DG. 2001. Contribution of dietary oxalate to urinary oxalate excretion. *Kidney Int* 59(1):270–276.

Holt SH, Delargy HJ, Lawton CL, Blundell JE. 1999. The effects of high-carbohydrate vs high-fat breakfasts on feelings of fullness and alertness, and subsequent food intake. *Int J Food Sci Nutr* 50(1):13–28.

Horn S, Feller ER. 2003. Gastrointestinal (GI) bleeding in endurance runners. *AMAA J* 16(1):5–6, 11.

Horvath PJ, Eagen CK, Ryer-Calvin SD, Pendergast DR. 2000. The effects of varying dietary fat on the nutrient intake in male and female runners. *J Am Coll Nutr* 19(1):42–51.

Huang YC, Chen W, Evans MA, Mitchell ME, Shultz TD. 1998. Vitamin B-6 requirement and status assessment of young women fed a high-protein diet with various levels of vitamin B-6. *Am J Clin Nutr* 67(2):208–220.

Hume EM, Krebs HA. 1949. *Vitamin A Requirement of Human Adults. An Experimental Study of Vitamin A Deprivation in Man.* Medical Research Council Special Report Series No. 264. London: His Majesty's Stationaery Office.

Hurrell RF. 2002a. Fortification: Overcoming technical and practical barriers. *J Nutr* 132(4 Suppl):806S–812S.

Hurrell R. 2002b. How to ensure adequate iron absorption from iron-fortified food. *Nutr Rev* 60(7 Pt 2):S7–S15.

Inoue Y, Havenith G, Kenney WL, Loomis JL, Buskirk ER. 1999. Exercise- and methylcholine-induced sweating responses in older and younger men: Effect of heat acclimation and aerobic fitness. *Int J Biometeorol* 42(4):210–216.

IOM (Institute of Medicine). 1994. *Food Components to Enhance Performance.* Washington, DC: National Academy Press.

IOM. 1995. *Not Eating Enough.* Washington, DC: National Academy Press. Pp. 285–302.

IOM. 1997a. *Dietary Reference Intakes. Calcium, Phosphorus, Magnesium, Vitamin D, and Fluoride.* Washington, DC: National Academy Press.

IOM. 1997b. *Vitamin C Fortification of Food Aid Commodities.* Washington, DC: National Academy Press.

IOM. 1998. *Dietary Reference Intakes. Thiamin, Riboflavin, Niacin, Vitamin B_6, Folate, Vitamin B_{12}, Pantothenic Acid, Biotin, and Choline.* Washington, DC: National Academy Press.

IOM. 1999. *Letter Report to the Office of the Surgeon General United States Army on Antioxidants and Oxidative Stress in Military Personnel.* Washington, DC: Institute of Medicine.

IOM. 2000. *Dietary Reference Intakes for Vitamin C, Vitamin E, Selenium, and Carotenoids.* Washington, DC: National Academy Press.

IOM. 2001a. *Caffeine for the Sustainment of Mental Task Performance. Formulations for Military Operations.* Washington, DC: National Academy Press.

IOM. 2001b. *Dietary Reference Intakes. Vitamin A, Vitamin K, Arsenic, Boron, Chromium, Copper, Iodine, Iron, Manganese, Molybdenum, Nickel, Silicon, Vanadium, and Zinc.* Washington, DC: National Academy Press.

IOM. 2002a. *Dietary Reference Intakes. Energy, Carbohydrate, Fiber, Fat, Fatty Acids, Cholesterol, Protein, and Amino Acids.* Washington, DC: The National Academies Press.

IOM. 2002b. *High-Energy, Nutrient-Dense Emergency Relief Food Product.* Washington, DC: National Academy Press.

IOM. 2004. *Dietary Reference Intakes. Water, Potassium, Sodium, Chloride, and Sulfate.* Washington, DC: The National Academies Press.

Ireland P, Fordtran JS. 1973. Effect of dietary calcium and age on jejunal calcium absorption in humans studied by intestinal perfusion. *J Clin Invest* 52(11):2672–2681.

IZiNCG (International Zinc Nutritional Consulative Group). 2004. Assessment of the risk of zinc deficiency in populations and options for its control. Hotz C, Brown KH, eds. *Food Nutr Bull* 25(1 Suppl 1):S91–S204.

Jackson AA, Gibson NR, Lu Y, Jahoor F. 2004. Synthesis of erythrocyte glutathione in healthy adults consuming the safe amount of dietary protein. *Am J Clin Nutr* 80(1):101–107.

Jackson JL, Lesho E, Peterson C. 2000. Zinc and the common cold: A meta-analysis revisited. *J Nutr* 130(5S Suppl):1512S–1515S.

Jacob RA, Sandstead HH, Munoz JM, Klevay LM, Milne DB. 1981. Whole body surface loss of trace metals in normal males. *Am J Clin Nutr* 34(7):1379–1383.

Jacobs I, Anderberg A, Schele R, Lithell H. 1983. Muscle glycogen in soldiers on different diets during military field maneuvers. *Aviat Space Environ Med* 54(10):898–900.

Jacobsen R, Lorenzen JK, Toubro S, Krog-Mikkelsen I, Astrup A. 2005. Effect of short-term high dietary calcium intake on 24-h energy expenditure, fat oxidation, and fecal fat excretion. *Int J Obes Relat Metab Disord* 29(3):292–301.

Janigan DT, Perey B, Marrie TJ, Chiasson PM, Hirsch D. 1997. Skin necrosis: An unusual complication of hyperphosphatemia during total parenteral nutrition therapy. *J Parenter Enteral Nutr* 21(1):50–52.

Jones GR, Newhouse I. 1997. Sport-related hematuria: A review. *Clin J Sport Med* 7(2):119–125.

Kallner A, Hartmann D, Hornig D. 1979. Steady-state turnover and body pool of ascorbic acid in man. *Am J Clin Nutr* 32(3):530–539.

Kallner AB, Hartmann D, Hornig DH. 1981. On the requirements of ascorbic acid in man: Steady-state turnover and body pool in smokers. *Am J Clin Nutr* 34(7):1347–1355.

Kalmar JM, Cafarelli E. 2004. Caffeine: A valuable tool to study central fatigue in humans? *Exerc Sport Sci Rev* 32(4):143–147.

Kaplan RJ. 2004 (August 9). *Macronutrient Composition of Military Rations for Cognitive Performance in Short-Term, High-Stress Situations.* Paper presented at the Institute of Medicine Workshop on Optimization of Nutrient Composition of Military Rations for Short-Term, High-Stress Situations, Natick, MA. Institute of Medicine Committee on Optimization of Nutrient Composition of Military Rations for Short-Term, High-Stress Situations.

Karlsson J, Saltin B. 1971. Diet, muscle glycogen, and endurance performance. *J Appl Physiol* 31(2):203–206.

Keenan RA, Moldawer LL, Yang RD, Kawamura I, Blackburn GL, Bistrian BR. 1982. An altered response by peripheral leukocytes to synthesize or release leukocyte endogenous mediator in critically ill, protein-malnourished patients. *J Lab Clin Med* 100(6):844–857.

Kerstetter JE, O'Brien KO, Caseria DM, Wall DE, Insogna KL. 2005. The impact of dietary protein on calcium absorption and kinetic measures of bone turnover in women. *J Clin Endocrinol Metab* 90(1):26–31.

Keusch GT. 1999. Iron metabolism, microbial virulence, and host defenses. In: Institute of Medicine. *Military Strategies for Sustainment of Nutrition and Immune Function in the Field.* Washington, DC: The National Academy Press. Pp. 317–336.

Keys A, Brozek J, Henschel A, Mickelsen O, Taylor HL. 1950. *The Biology of Human Starvation.* Minneapolis, MN: The University of Minnesota Press. Vol. II.

King NA, Tremblay A, Blundell JE. 1997. Effects of exercise on appetite control: Implications for energy balance. *Med Sci Sports Exerc* 29(8):1076–1089.

Knochel JP. 1993. Potassium deficiency as the result of training in hot weather. In: Institute of Medicine. *Fluid Replacement and Heat Stress.* Washington, DC: National Academy Press. Pp. 117–126.

Konig D, Weinstock C, Keul J, Northoff H, Berg A. 1998. Zinc, iron, and magnesium status in athletes—influence on the regulation of exercise-induced stress and immune function. *Exerc Immunol Rev* 4:2–21.

Kordas K, Stoltzfus RJ. 2004. New evidence of iron and zinc interplay at the enterocyte and neural tissues. *J Nutr* 134(6):1295–1298.

Kurtz TW, Al-Bander HA, Morris RC Jr. 1987. "Salt-sensitive" essential hypertension in men. Is the sodium ion alone important? *N Engl J Med* 317(17):1043–1048.

Lawless HT, Rapacki F, Horne J, Hayes A. 2003. The taste of calcium and magnesium salts and anionic modifications. *Food Qual Pref* 14(4):319–325.

Layman DK, Boileau RA, Erickson DJ, Painter JE, Shiue H, Sather C, Christou DD. 2003. A reduced ratio of dietary carbohydrate to protein improves body composition and blood lipid profiles during weight loss in adult women. *J Nutr* 133(2):411–417.

Ledikwe JH, Blanck HM, Khan LK, Serdula MK, Seymour JD, Tohill BC, Rolls BJ. 2005. Dietary energy density determined by eight calculation methods in a nationally representative United States population. *J Nutr* 135(2):273–278.

Leklem JE. 1999. Vitamin B_6. In: Shils ME, Olson JA, Shike M, Ross AC, eds. *Modern Nutrition in Health and Disease.* 9th ed. Baltimore, MD: Williams and Wilkins. Pp. 413–421.

Leshem M, Abutbul A, Eilon R. 1999. Exercise increases the preference for salt in humans. *Appetite* 32(2):251–260.

Levine M, Conry-Cantilena C, Wang Y, Welch RW, Washko PW, Dhariwal KR, Park JB, Lazarev A, Graumlich JF, King J, Cantilena LR. 1996. Vitamin C pharmacokinetics in healthy volunteers: Evidence for a recommended dietary allowance. *Proc Natl Acad Sci USA* 93(8):3704–3709.

Lieberman HR. 2003. Nutrition, brain function and cognitive performance. *Appetite* 40(3):245–254.

Lieberman HR, Falco CM, Slade SS. 2002. Carbohydrate administration during a day of sustained aerobic activity improves vigilance, as assessed by a novel ambulatory monitoring device, and mood. *Am J Clin Nutr* 76(1):120–127.

Linkswiler HM, Zemel MB, Hegsted M, Schuette S. 1981. Protein-induced hypercalciuria. *Fed Proc* 40(9):2429–2433.

Liu RH. 2004. Potential synergy of phytochemicals in cancer prevention: Mechanism of action. *J Nutr* 134(12 Suppl):3479S–3485S.

Lonnerdal B. 2000. Dietary factors influencing zinc absorption. *J Nutr* 130(5S Suppl):1378S–1383S.

Lorr M, McNair DM, Heuchert JW. 2003. Profile of Mood States (POMS). [Online]. Multi-Health Systems, Inc. Available: https://www.mhs.com/ecom/product.asp?Cou=USA&AppGrpID= BEM&RptGrpID=POM&SubAppGrpID=BHE&node= [accessed December 13, 2004].

Lowy SL, Fisler JS, Drenick EJ, Hunt IF, Swendseid ME. 1986. Zinc and copper nutriture in obese men receiving very low calorie diets of soy or collagen protein. *Am J Clin Nutr* 43(2):272–287.

Lu SC. 1998. Regulation of hepatic glutathione synthesis. *Semin Liver Dis* 18(4):331–343.

Luft FC, Rankin LI, Bloch R, Weyman AE, Willis LR, Murray RH, Grim CE, Weinberger MH. 1979. Cardiovascular and humoral responses to extremes of sodium intake in normal black and white men. *Circulation* 60(3):697–706.

Luiking YC, Poeze M, Ramsay G, Deutz NE. 2005. The role of arginine in infection and sepsis. *J Parenter Enteral Nutr* 29(1 Suppl):S70–S74.

Lukaski HC. 2001. Magnesium, zinc, and chromium nutrition and athletic performance. *Can J Appl Physiol* 26 (Suppl):S13–S22.

Lukaski HC. 2004. Vitamin and mineral status: Effects on physical performance. *Nutrition* 20(7–8):632–644.

Lukaski HC, Penland JG. 2004 (August 9). *Zinc, Magnesium, Copper, Iron, Selenium, and Calcium in Assault Rations: Roles in Promotion of Physical and Mental Performance.* Paper presented at the Institute of Medicine Workshop on Optimization of Nutrient Composition of Military Rations for Short-Term, High-Stress Situations, Natick, MA. Institute of Medicine Committee on Optimization of Nutrient Composition of Military Rations for Short-Term, High-Stress Situations.

Lukaski HC, Bolonchuk WW, Klevay LM, Milne DB, Sandstead HH. 2001. Interactions among dietary fat, mineral status, and performance of endurance athletes: A case study. *Int J Sport Nutr Exerc Metab* 11(2):186–198.

Magkos F, Kavouras SA. 2004. Caffeine and ephedrine: Physiological, metabolic and performance-enhancing effects. *Sports Med* 34(13):871–889.

Malhotra MS, Sridharan K, Venkataswamy Y, Rai RM, Pichan G, Radhakrishnan U, Grover SK. 1981. Effect of restricted potassium intake on its excretion and on physiological responses during heat stress. *Eur J Appl Physiol* 47(2):169–179.

Malouf M, Grimley EJ, Areosa SA. 2003. Folic acid with or without vitamin B_{12} for cognition and dementia. *Cochrane Database Syst Rev* (4):CD004514.

Manach C, Scalbert A, Morand C, Remesy C, Jimenez L. 2004. Polyphenols: Food sources and bioavailability. *Am J Clin Nutr* 79(5):727–747.

Manore MM. 2000. Effect of physical activity on thiamine, riboflavin, and vitamin B-6 Requirements. *Am J Clin Nutr* 72(2 Suppl):598S–606S.

Manore M, Thompson J. 2000. *Sport Nutrition for Health and Performance.* Champaign, IL: Human Kinetics.

Margen S, Chu JY, Kaufmann NA, Calloway DH. 1974. Studies in calcium metabolism. I. The calciuretic effect of dietary protein. *Am J Clin Nutr* 27(6):584–589.

Marsh E, Murlin JR. 1928. Muscular efficiency on high carbohydrate and high fat diets. *J Nutr* 1:105–137.

Massey LK, Whiting SJ. 1996. Dietary salt, urinary calcium, and bone loss. *J Bone Miner Res* 11(6):731–736.

Massey LK, Grentz LM, Horner HT, Palmer RG. 2002. Soybean and soyfood consumption increase oxalate excretion. *Top Clin Nutr* 17:49–59.

Mastaloudis A, Morrow JD, Hopkins DW, Devaraj S, Traber MG. 2004a. Antioxidant supplementation prevents exercise-induced lipid peroxidation, but not inflammation, in ultramarathon runners. *Free Rad Biol Med* 36(10):1329-1341.

Mastaloudis A, Yu TW, O'Donnell RP, Frei B, Dashwood RH, Traber MG. 2004b. Endurance exercise results in DNA damage as detected by the comet assay. *Free Rad Biol Med* 36(8):966–975.

Mattes RD. 2004 (August 11). *Food Intake Regulation: Liquid versus Solid.* Paper presented at the Institute of Medicine Workshop on Optimization of Nutrient Composition of Military Rations for Short-Term, High-Stress Situations, Natick, MA. Institute of Medicine Committee on Optimization of Nutrient Composition of Military Rations for Short-Term, High-Stress Situations.

Maughan RJ, Griffin J. 2003. Caffeine ingestion and fluid balance: A review. *J Hum Nutr Dietetics* 16(6):411–420.

Maughan RJ, Shirreffs SM. 1997. Recovery from prolonged exercise: Restoration of water and electrolyte balance. *J Sports Sci* 15(3):297–303.

McCormick DB. 1999. Riboflavin. In: Shils ME, Olson JA, Shike M, Ross AC, eds. *Modern Nutrition in Health and Disease.* 9th ed. Baltimore, MD: Williams and Wilkins. Pp. 391–399.

McDonald R, Keen CL. 1988. Iron, zinc and magnesium nutrition and athletic performance. *Sports Med* 5(3):171–184.

McLellan TM, Bell DG, Kamimori GH. 2004. Caffeine improves physical performance during 24 h of active wakefulness. *Aviat Space Environ Med* 75(8):666–672.

Mela DJ, Sacchetti DA. 1991. Sensory preferences for fats: Relationships with diet and body composition. *Am J Clin Nutr* 53(4):908–915.

Melanson EL, Sharp TA, Schneider J, Donahoo WT, Grunwald GK, Hill JO. 2003. Relation between calcium intake and fat oxidation in adult humans. *Int J Obes Relat Metab Disord* 27(2):196–203.

Mertz W. 1969. Chromium occurrence and function in biological systems. *Physiol Rev* 49(2):163–239.

Mertz W. 1993. Chromium in human nutrition: A review. *J Nutr* 123(4):626–633.

Mertz W, Roginski EE, Schwarz K. 1961. Effect of trivalent chromium complexes on glucose uptake by epididymal fat tissue of rats. *J Biol Chem* 236(2):318–322.

Meydani SN, Leka LS, Fine BC, Dallal GE, Keusch GT, Singh MF, Hamer DH. 2004. Vitamin E and respiratory tract infections in elderly nursing home residents: A randomized controlled trial. *J Am Med Assoc* 292(7):828–836.

Meydani SN, Meydani M, Blumberg JB, Leka LS, Pedrosa M, Diamond R, Schaefer EJ. 1998. Assessment of the safety of supplementation with different amounts of vitamin E in healthy older adults. *Am J Clin Nutr* 68(2):311–318.

Meydani SN, Meydani M, Blumberg JB, Leka LS, Siber G, Loszewski R, Thompson C, Pedrosa MC, Diamond RD, Stollar BD. 1997. Vitamin E supplementation and in vivo immune response in healthy elderly subjects. A randomized controlled trial. *J Am Med Assoc* 277(17):1380–1386.

Miller ER 3rd, Pastor-Barriuso R, Dalal D, Riemersma RA, Appel LJ, Guallar E. 2005. Meta-analysis: High-dosage vitamin E supplementation may increase all-cause mortality. *Ann Intern Med* 142(1):37–46.

Miyamura JB, McNutt SW, Lichton IJ, Wenkam NS. 1987. Altered zinc status of soldiers under field conditions. *J Am Diet Assoc* 87(5):595–597.

Moldawer LL, Trerice MS, Flatt JP, Bistrian BR, Blackburn GL. 1978. A protein sparing model in the rat during hypocaloric feeding: Factors determining preservation of visceral protein function. *J Surg Res* 25(5):424–432.

Montain SJ. 2004 (August 9). *Physiological Demands of Combat Operations.* Paper presented at the Institute of Medicine Workshop on Optimization of Nutrient Composition of Military Rations for Short-Term, High-Stress Situations, Natick, MA. Institute of Medicine Committee on Optimization of Nutrient Composition of Military Rations for Short-Term, High-Stress Situations.

Montain SJ, Young AJ. 2003. Diet and physical performance. *Appetite* 40(3):255–267.

Montain SJ, Shippee RL, Tharion WJ. 1997. Carbohydrate-electrolyte solution effects on physical performance of military tasks. *Aviat Space Environ Med* 68(5):384–391.

Moore C, Murphy MM, Keast DR, Holick MF. 2004. Vitamin D intake in the United States. *J Am Diet Assoc* 104(6):980–983.

Mooren FC, Golf SW, Volker K. 2003. Effect of magnesium on granulocyte function and on the exercise induced inflammatory response. *Magnes Res* 16(1):49–58.

Morris MS, Fava M, Jacques PF, Selhub J, Rosenberg IH. 2003. Depression and folate status in the US Population. *Psychother Psychosom* 72(2):80–87.

Murray R, Bartoli W, Stofan J, Horn M, Eddy D. 1999. A comparison of the gastric emptying characteristics of selected sports drinks. *Int J Sport Nutr* 9(3):263–274.

Newhouse IJ, Clement DB. 1988. Iron status in athletes. An update. *Sports Med* 5(6):337–352.

Nieman DC, Henson DA, McAnulty SR, McAnulty LS, Morrow JD, Ahmed A, Heward CB. 2004. Vitamin E and immunity after the Kona Triathlon World Championship. *Med Sci Sports Exerc* 36(8):1328–1335.

Nijveldt RJ, van Nood E, van Hoorn DE, Boelens PG, van Norren K, van Leeuwen PA. 2001. Flavonoids: A review of probable mechanisms of action and potential applications. *Am J Clin Nutr* 74(4):418–425.

Nindl BC, Leone CD, Tharion WJ, Johnson RF, Castellani JW, Patton JF, Montain SJ. 2002. Physical performance responses during 72 h of military operational stress. *Med Sci Sports Exerc* 34(11):1814–1822.

Nishimuta M, Kodama N, Morikuni E, Yoshioka YH, Takeyama H, Yamada H, Kitajima H, Suzuki K. 2004. Balances of calcium, magnesium and phosphorus in Japanese young adults. *J Nutr Sci Vitaminol (Tokyo)* 50(1):19–25.

Nordin BE, Polley KJ. 1987. Metabolic consequences of the menopause. A cross-sectional, longitudinal, and intervention study on 557 normal postmenopausal women. *Calcif Tissue Int* 41 (Suppl 1):S1–S59.

Norton VP, Noble JM. 1991. Acceptance of quantity recipes with zero added salt by a military population. *J Am Diet Assoc* 91(3):312–315.

Novak F, Heyland DK, Avenell A, Drover JW, Su X. 2002. Glutamine supplementation in serious illness: A systematic review of the evidence. *Crit Care Med* 30(9):2022–2029.

Nyakeriga AM, Troye-Blomberg M, Dorfman JR, Alexander ND, Back R, Kortok M, Chemtai AK, Marsh K, Williams TN. 2004. Iron deficiency and malaria among children living on the coast of Kenya. *J Infect Dis* 190(3):439–447.

Olson JA. 1987. Recommended dietary intakes (RDI) of vitamin A in humans. *Am J Clin Nutr* 45(4):704–716.

Pacy PJ, Price GM, Halliday D, Quevedo MR, Millward DJ. 1994. Nitrogen homeostasis in man: The diurnal responses of protein synthesis and degradation and amino acid oxidation to diets with increasing protein intakes. *Clin Sci* 86(1):103–118.

Patterson BW, Nguyen T, Pierre E, Herndon DN, Wolfe RR. 1997. Urea and protein metabolism in burned children: Effect of dietary protein intake. *Metabolism* 46(5):573–578.

Payton KB, Flanagan PR, Stinson EA, Chodirker DP, Chamberlain MJ, Valberg LS. 1982. Technique for determination of human zinc absorption from measurement of radioactivity in a fecal sample of the body. *Gastroenterology* 83(6):1264–1270.

Penetar DM, McCann U, Thorne D, Schelling A, Galinski C, Sing H, Thomas M, Belenky G. 1994. Effects of caffeine on cognitive performance, mood, and alertness in sleep-deprived humans. In: *Food Components to Enhance Performance*. Washington, DC: National Academy Press.

Percival SS. 1998. Copper and immunity. *Am J Clin Nutr* 67(5 Suppl):1064S–1068S.

Phinney SD, Bistrian BR, Wolfe RR, Blackburn GL. 1983. The human metabolic response to chronic ketosis without caloric restriction: Physical and biochemical adaptation. *Metabolism* 32(8):757–768.

Popper R, Smits G, Meiselman HL, Hirsch E. 1989. Eating in combat: A survey of US Marines. *Mil Med* 154(12):619–623.

Portale AA, Halloran BP, Morris RC Jr. 1989. Physiologic regulation of the serum concentration of 1,25-dihydroxyvitamin D by phosphorus in normal men. *J Clin Invest* 83(5):1494–1499.

Powers SK, Howley ET. 1997. *Exercise Physiology. Theory and Application to Fitness and Performance.* 3rd ed. Boston, MA: McGraw-Hill.

Prasad AS, Fitzgerald JT, Bao B, Beck FW, Chandrasekar PH. 2000. Duration of symptoms and plasma cytokine levels in patients with the common cold treated with zinc acetate. A randomized, double-blind, placebo-controlled trial. *Ann Intern Med* 133(4):245–252.

Ravaglia G, Forti P, Maioli F, Bastagli L, Facchini A, Mariani E, Savarino L, Sassi S, Cucinotta D, Lenaz G. 2000. Effect of micronutrient status on natural killer cell immune function in healthy free-living subjects aged >/=90 y. *Am J Clin Nutr* 71(2):590–598.

Rawson ES, Clarkson PM. 2003. Scientifically debatable: Is creatine worth its weight? *Gatorade Sports Science Institute: Sports Science Exchange #91* 16(4):1–6.

Reasner CA 2nd, Dunn JF, Fetchick DA, Liel Y, Hollis BW, Epstein S, Shary J, Mundy GR, Bell NH. 1990. Alteration of vitamin D metabolism in Mexican-Americans. *J Bone Miner Res* 5(1):13–17.

Reddy ST, Wang CY, Sakhaee K, Brinkley L, Pak CY. 2002. Effect of low-carbohydrate high-protein diets on acid-base balance, stone-forming propensity, and calcium metabolism. *Am J Kidney Dis* 40(2):265–274.

Ricci TA, Chowdhury HA, Heymsfield SB, Stahl T, Pierson RN Jr, Shapses SA. 1998. Calcium supplementation suppresses bone turnover during weight reduction in postmenopausal women. *J Bone Miner Res* 13(6):1045–1050.

Rosenthal JM, Amiel SA, Yaguez L, Bullmore E, Hopkins D, Evans M, Pernet A, Reid H, Giampietro V, Andrew CM, Suckling J, Simmons A, Williams SC. 2001. The effect of acute hypoglycemia on brain function and activation: A functional magnetic resonance imaging study. *Diabetes* 50(7):1618–1626.

Ruppert M, Overlack A, Kolloch R, Kraft K, Lennarz M, Stumpe KO. 1994. Effects of severe and moderate salt restriction on serum lipids in nonobese normotensive adults. *Am J Med Sci* 307(Suppl 1):S87–S90.

Sacheck JM, Blumberg JB. 2001. Role of vitamin E and oxidative stress in exercise. *Nutrition* 17(10):809–814.

Sacks FM, Svetkey LP, Vollmer WM, Appel LJ, Bray GA, Harsha D, Obarzanek E, Conlin PR, Miller ER 3rd, Simons-Morton DG, Karanja N, Lin PH. 2001. Effects on blood pressure of reduced dietary sodium and the Dietary Approaches to Stop Hypertension (DASH) diet. DASH-Sodium Collaborative Research Group. *N Engl J Med* 344(1):3–10.

Salovaara H. 1982. Sensory limitations to replacement of sodium with potassium and magnesium in bread. *Cereal Chem* 59(5):427–430.

Sauberlich HE, Hodges RE, Wallace DL, Kolder H, Canham JE, Hood J, Raica N Jr, Lowry LK. 1974. Vitamin A metabolism and requirements in the human studied with the use of labeled retinol. *Vitam Horm* 32:251–275.

Sawka MN, Montain SJ. 2001. Fluid and electrolyte balance: Effects on thermoregulation and exercise in the heat. In: Bowman BA, Russell RM, eds. *Present Knowledge in Nutrition.* 8th ed. Washington, DC: ILSI Press. Pp. 115–124.

Sen CK, Packer L. 2000. Thiol homeostasis and supplements in physical exercise. *Am J Clin Nutr* 72(2 Suppl):653S–669S.

Shafat A, Butler P, Jensen RL, Donnelly AE. 2004. Effects of dietary supplementation with vitamins C and E on muscle function during and after eccentric contractions in humans. *Eur J Appl Physiol* 93(1–2):196–202.

Shephard RJ, Shek PN. 1998. Immunological hazards from nutritional imbalance in athletes. *Exerc Immunol Rev* 4:22–48.

Shippee R, Friedl K, Kramer T, Mays M, Popp K, Askew E, Fairbrother B, Hoyt R, Vogel J, Marchitelli L, Frykman P, Martinez-Lopez L, Bernton E, Kramer M, Tulley R, Rood J, Delany J, Jezior D, Arsenault J. 1994. *Nutritional and Immunological Assessment of Ranger Students with Increased Caloric Intake.* Technical Report No. T95-5. Fort Detrick, MD: US Army Medical Research and Materiel Command.

Shirreffs S. 2004 (August 10) *Optimization of Nutrient Composition of Military Rations for Short-Term, High-Stress Situations: Sodium, Potassium and Other Electrolytes.* Paper presented at the Institute of Medicine Workshop on Optimization of Nutrient Composition of Military Rations for Short-Term, High-Stress Situations, Natick, MA. Institute of Medicine Committee on Optimization of Nutrient Composition of Military Rations for Short-Term, High-Stress Situations.

Shirreffs SM, Maughan RJ. 1997. Whole body sweat collection in humans: An improved method with preliminary data on electrolyte content. *J Appl Physiol* 82(1):336–341.

Siener R, Ebert D, Nicolay C, Hesse A. 2003. Dietary risk factors for hyperoxaluria in calcium oxalate stone formers. *Kidney Int* 63(3):1037–1043.

Skoog SM, Bharucha AE. 2004. Dietary fructose and gastrointestinal symptoms: A review. *Am J Gastroenterol* 99(10):2046–2050.

Solomons NW, Jacob RA. 1981. Studies on the bioavailability of zinc in humans: Effects of heme and nonheme iron on the absorption of zinc. *Am J Clin Nutr* 34(4):475–482.

Sorensen LB, Moller P, Flint A, Martens M, Raben A. 2003. Effect of sensory perception of foods on appetite and food intake: A review of studies on humans. *Int J Obes Relat Metab Disord* 27(10):1152–1166.

Specker B. 2005 (December 8). *Vitamin D Requirements.* Presented at the Institute of Medicine Symposium on Dietary Reference Intakes: Framing the Next Generation, Washington, DC: Food and Nutrition Board.

Stepto NK, Carey AL, Staudacher HM, Cummings NK, Burke LM, Hawley JA. 2002. Effect of short-term fat adaptation on high-intensity training. *Med Sci Sports Exerc* 34(3):449–455.

Takkouche B, Regueira-Mendez C, Garcia-Closas R, Figueiras A, Gestal-Otero JJ. 2002. Intake of vitamin C and zinc and risk of common cold: A cohort study. *Epidemiology* 13(1):38–44.

Tanphaichitr V. 1999. Thiamin. In: Shils ME, Olson JA, Shike M, Ross AC, eds. *Modern Nutrition in Health and Disease.* 9th ed. Baltimore, MD: Williams and Wilkins. Pp. 381–389.

Terblanche S, Noakes TD, Dennis SC, Marais D, Eckert M. 1992. Failure of magnesium supplementation to influence marathon running performance or recovery in magnesium-replete subjects. *Int J Sport Nutr* 2(2):154–164.

Terjung RL, Clarkson P, Eichner ER, Greenhaff PL, Hespel PJ, Israel RG, Kraemer WJ, Meyer RA, Spriet LL, Tarnopolsky MA, Wagenmakers AJ, Williams MH. 2000. American College of Sports Medicine roundtable. The physiological and health effects of oral creatine supplementation. *Med Sci Sports Exerc* 32(3):706–717.

Tharion WJ, Moore RJ. 1993. *Effects of Carbohydrate Intake and Load Bearing Exercise on Rifle Marksmanship Performance.* Technical Report No. T5-93. Natick, MA: US Army Medical Research and Development Command.

Tharion WJ, Hoyt RW, Cline AD, DeLany JP, Lieberman HR. 2004. Energy expenditure and water turnover assessed by doubly labeled water during manual work in a dry and warm environment. *J Human-Environ Syst* 7(1):11–17.

Thompson D, Bailey DM, Hill J, Hurst T, Powell JR, Williams C. 2004. Prolonged vitamin C supplementation and recovery from eccentric exercise. *Eur J Appl Physiol* 92(1–2):133–138.

Thompson D, Williams C, Kingsley M, Nicholas CW, Lakomy HK, McArdle F, Jackson MJ. 2001. Muscle soreness and damage parameters after prolonged intermittent shuttle-running following acute vitamin C supplementation. *Int J Sports Med* 22(1):68–75.

Tikuisis P, Keefe AA, McLellan TM, Kamimori G. 2004. Caffeine restores engagement speed but not shooting precision following 22 h of active wakefulness. *Aviat Space Environ Med* 75(9):771–776.

Tipton KD. 2004 (August 9). *Carbohydrate/Protein Balance for Muscle Performance.* Paper presented at the Institute of Medicine Workshop on Optimization of Nutrient Composition of Military Rations for Short-Term, High-Stress Situations, Natick, MA. Institute of Medicine Committee on Optimization of Nutrient Composition of Military Rations for Short-Term, High-Stress Situations.

Tipton KD, Wolfe RR. 2001. Exercise, protein metabolism, and muscle growth. *Int J Sport Nutr Exerc Metab* 11(1):109-132.

Tipton KD, Wolfe RR. 2004. Protein and amino acids for athletes. *J Sports Sci* 22(1):65–79.

Tipton KD, Borsheim E, Wolf SE, Sanford AP, Wolfe RR. 2003. Acute response of net muscle protein balance reflects 24-h balance after exercise and amino acid ingestion. *Am J Physiol Endocrinol Metabol* 284(1):E76–E89.

Tipton KD, Elliott TA, Cree MG, Wolf SE, Sanford AP, Wolfe RR. 2004. Ingestion of casein and whey proteins result in muscle anabolism after resistance exercise. *Med Sci Sports Exerc* 36(12):2073–2081.

Tipton KD, Ferrando AA, Phillips SM, Doyle D Jr, Wolfe RR. 1999. Postexercise net protein synthesis in human muscle from orally administered amino acids. *Am J Physiol* 276(4 Pt 1):E628–E634.

Tipton K, Green NR, Haymes EM, Waller M. 1993. Zinc loss in sweat of athletes exercising in hot and neutral temperatures. *Int J Sport Nutr* 3(3):261–271.

Tiselius HG. 1997. Risk formulas in calcium oxalate urolithiasis. *World J Urol* 15(3):176–185.

Todd KS, Butterfield GE, Calloway DH. 1984. Nitrogen balance in men with adequate and deficient energy intake at three levels of work. *J Nutr* 114(11):2107–2118.

Traber MG, Mastaloudis A. 2004 (August 9). *Vitamin C and E in the Prevention of Oxidative Stress, Inflammatory and Fatigue from Exhaust Exercise.* Paper presented at the Institute of Medicine Workshop on Optimization of Nutrient Composition of Military Rations for Short-Term, High-Stress Situations, Natick, MA. Institute of Medicine Committee on Optimization of Nutrient Composition of Military Rations for Short-Term, High-Stress Situations.

Troost FJ, Brummer RJ, Dainty JR, Hoogewerff JA, Bull VJ, Saris WH. 2003. Iron supplements inhibit zinc but not copper absorption in vivo in ileostomy subjects. *Am J Clin Nutr* 78(5):1018–1023.

Truswell AS, Seach JM, Thorburn AW. 1988. Incomplete absorption of pure fructose in healthy subjects and the facilitating effect of glucose. *Am J Clin Nutr* 48(6):1424–1430.

Turner RB, Cetnarowski WE. 2000. Effect of treatment with zinc gluconate or zinc acetate on experimental and natural colds. *Clin Infect Dis* 31(5):1202–1208.

Turnlund JR, Jacob RA, Keen CL, Strain JJ, Kelley DS, Domek JM, Keyes WR, Ensunsa JL, Lykkesfeldt J, Coulter J. 2004. Long-term high copper intake: Effects on indexes of copper status, antioxidant status, and immune function in young men. *Am J Clin Nutr* 79(6):1037–1044.

US Departments of Army, Navy, and Air Force. 2001. *Nutrition Standards and Education.* AR 40-25/BUMEDINST 10110.6/AFI 44-141. Washington, DC: US Department of Defense Headquarters.

Usui Y, Tanimura H, Nishimura N, Kobayashi N, Okanoue T, Ozawa K. 1990. Vitamin K concentrations in the plasma and liver of surgical patients. *Am J Clin Nutr* 51(5):846–852.

van Etten E, Decallonne B, Mathieu C. 2002. 1,25-dihydroxycholecalciferol: Endocrinology meets the immune system. *Proc Nutr Soc* 61(3):375–380.

van het Hof KH, Brouwer IA, West CE, Haddeman E, Steegers-Theunissen RP, van Dusseldorp M, Weststrate JA, Eskes TK, Hautvast JG. 1999. Bioavailability of lutein from vegetables is 5 times higher than that of beta-carotene. *Am J Clin Nutr* 70(2):261–268.

Vanderpas JB, Contempre B, Duale NL, Deckx H, Bebe N, Longombe AO, Thilly CH, Diplock AT, Dumont JE. 1993. Selenium deficiency mitigates hypothyroxinemia in iodine-deficient subjects. *Am J Clin Nutr* 57(2 Suppl):271S–275S.

Vellar OD. 1968. Studies on sweat losses of nutrients. II. The influence of an oral iron load on the iron content of whole body cell-free sweat. *Scand J Clin Lab Invest* 21(4):344–346.

Vistisen B, Nybo L, Xu X, Hoy CE, Kiens B. 2003. Minor amounts of plasma medium-chain fatty acids and no improved time trial performance after consuming lipids. *J Appl Physiol* 95(6):2434–2443.

Wacker WE, Parisi AF. 1968. Magnesium metabolism. *N Engl J Med* 278(12):658–663.

Walker RM, Linkswiler HM. 1972. Calcium retention in the adult human male as affected by protein intake. *J Nutr* 102(10):1297–1302.

Waller MF, Haymes EM. 1996. The effects of heat and exercise on sweat iron loss. *Med Sci Sports Exerc* 28(2):197–203.

Weaver CM, Rajaram S. 1992. Exercise and iron status. *J Nutr* 122(3 Suppl):782–787.

Weller E, Bachert P, Meinck HM, Friedmann B, Bartsch P, Mairbaurl H. 1998. Lack of effect of oral Mg-supplementation on Mg in serum, blood cells, and calf muscle. *Med Sci Sports Exerc* 30(11):1584–1591.

Welsh RS, Davis JM, Burke JR, Williams HG. 2002. Carbohydrates and physical/mental performance during intermittent exercise to fatigue. *Med Sci Sports Exerc* 34(4):723–731.

Westerterp KR. 2004. Diet induced thermogenesis. *Nutr Metab (Lond)* 1(1):5–9.

Whitson PA, Pietrzyk RA, Pak CY. 1997. Renal stone risk assessment during Space Shuttle flights. *J Urol* 158(6):2305–2310.

Whybro A, Jagger H, Barker M, Eastell R. 1998. Phosphate supplementation in young men: Lack of effect on calcium homeostasis and bone turnover. *Eur J Clin Nutr* 52(1):29–33.

Wilkinson R. 1976. Absorption of calcium, phosphorus, and magnesium. In: Nordin BEC, ed. *Calcium, Phosphate, and Magnesium Metabolism. Clinical Physiology and Diagnostic Procedures.* New York: Churchill Livingstone. Pp. 36–112.

Williams HE, Wandzilak TR. 1989. Oxalate synthesis, transport and the hyperoxaluric syndromes. *J Urol* 141(3 Pt 2):742–749.

Williams MH. 2005. *Nutrition for Health, Fitness, and Sport.* 7th ed. Boston, MA: McGraw-Hill.

Wilmore JH, Costill DL. 1999. *Physiology of Sport and Exercise.* 2nd ed. Champaign, IL: Human Kinetics. Pp. 115–154.

Wolfe RR, Goodenough RD, Burke JF, Wolfe MH. 1983. Response of protein and urea kinetics in burn patients to different levels of protein intake. *Ann Surg* 197(2):163–171.

Women's Health Initiative Study Group. 2004. Dietary adherence in the Women's Health Initiative Dietary Modification Trial. *J Am Diet Assoc* 104(4):654–658.

Wood RJ, Sitrin MD, Rosenberg IH. 1988. Effect of phosphorus on endogenous calcium losses during total parenteral nutrition. *Am J Clin Nutr* 48(3):632–636.

Woodson RD. 1984. Hemoglobin concentration and exercise capacity. *Am Rev Respir Dis* 129(2 Pt 2):S72–S75.

Zemel MB, Shi H, Greer B, Dirienzo D, Zemel PC. 2000. Regulation of adiposity by dietary calcium. *FASEB J* 14(9):1132–1138.

Zittermann A, Sabatschus O, Jantzen S, Platen P, Danz A, Dimitriou T, Scheld K, Klein K, Stehle P. 2000. Exercise-trained young men have higher calcium absorption rates and plasma calcitriol levels compared with age-matched sedentary controls. *Calcif Tissue Int* 67(3):215–219.

Zittermann A, Sabatschus O, Jantzen S, Platen P, Danz A, Stehle P. 2002. Evidence for an acute rise of intestinal calcium absorption in response to aerobic exercise. *Eur J Nutr* 41(5):189–196.

Zwart SR, Hargens AR, Smith SM. 2004. The ratio of animal protein intake to potassium intake is a predictor of bone resorption in space flight analogues and in ambulatory subjects. *Am J Clin Nutr* 80(4):1058–1065.

3

General Considerations and
Summary of the Ration Design

This chapter summarizes the general approach followed in designing the nutrient composition of a ration for short-term, high-stress combat missions. The chapter also describes the main health concerns that were taken into consideration when recommending the nutrient composition of the ration. Some of the factors related to the food choices and ration design that might affect the level of consumption and availability of the required nutrients are also discussed. Finally, high-priority areas of research that should provide a basis for the future development of rations are highlighted.

COMMITTEE'S APPROACH TO RATION DESIGN

The committee used the Dietary Reference Intakes (DRIs) established by the Institute of Medicine for active young men (IOM, 2004) as the starting point or benchmark for nutrient content in formulating the assault ration because these values are the most authoritative and up-to-date standards available. Further adjustments were then made to meet the unique needs of soldiers involved in assault conditions. The Military Dietary Reference Intakes (US Departments of Army, Navy, and Air Force, 2001) were not used as the standard values because they have not yet been revised to reflect all of the new DRIs. Although the focus of this report is soldiers during sustained operations, the recommendations (see Table 3-1) may be applicable to physically fit nonmilitary personnel (e.g., firefighters, peacekeepers, and other civilian emergency personnel) under similar conditions of high-stress, intense physical activity, and negative energy balance and for the short periods of time outlined here. The committee emphasizes that this ration is meant to be used for repetitive three- to seven-day missions

TABLE 3-1 Ration Nutrient Composition Recommended by the Committee

Nutrient or Energy Intake	Recommended Amount	Comments
Energy Intake	2,400 kcal in basic ration	Additional 400 kcal should be supplemented as carbohydrate in form of candy, gels, or powder to add to fluids, or all three.
Macronutrients		
Protein	100–120 g	Protein should be of high biological value. Preferable to add sources of protein with low-sulfur amino acids and low oxalate levels to minimize risk of kidney stone formation.
Carbohydrate	350 g 100 g as a supplement	Additional 100 g should be supplemented as carbohydrate in form of candy, gels, or powder to add to fluids, or all three. Amount of fructose as a monosaccharide should be limited to < 25 g.
Fiber	15–17 g	Naturally occurring or added. A mix of viscous, nonfermentable and nonviscous, fermentable fiber should be in the ration for gastrointestinal tract function.
Fat	22–25% kcal 58–67 g	Fat added to the ration should have a balanced mix of saturated, polyunsaturated, and monounsaturated fatty acids with palatability and stability the prime determinants of the specific mixture. Fat should contain 5–10% linoleic acid and 0.6–1.2% α-linolenic acid.
Vitamins		
Vitamin A	300–900 μg RAE[1]	Could be added as preformed vitamin A or provitamin A carotenoids.
Vitamin C	180–400 mg	Highly labile in processed food. If added to foods, encapsulation should be considered to prevent degradation through interaction with pro-oxidants.
Vitamin D	12.5–15 μg	Estimates of dietary intake are not available. Range based on ensuring serum levels of 25-hydroxy-vitamin D.
Vitamin E (α-tocopherol)	15–20 mg	Should be added to foods since natural foods are mainly sources of γ- rather than α-tocopherol.
Vitamin K	No recommended level	Amount in foods would be adequate provided ration is at least 50% whole foods.[2]

TABLE 3-1 Continued

Nutrient or Energy Intake	Recommended Amount	Comments
Thiamin	1.6–3.4 mg	Dependent on energy use and intake. Amount in foods would be adequate provided ration is at least 50% whole foods.
Riboflavin	2.8–6.5 mg	Dependent on energy use.
Niacin	28–35 mg	Dependent on energy use. The amount added to the ration should not be over 35 mg.
Vitamin B_6	2.7–3.9 mg	Dependent on negative energy balance and loss of lean tissue. If a higher protein level is provided, the amount of vitamin B_6 should be increased proportionally.
Folate	400–560 µg	Fortification may be needed.
Vitamin B_{12}	No recommended level	Amount in foods would be adequate provided ration is at least 50 % whole foods.
Biotin	No recommended level	Amount in foods would be adequate provided ration is at least 50% whole foods.
Pantothenic Acid	No recommended level	Amount in foods would be adequate provided ration is at least 50% whole foods.
Choline	No recommended level	Amount in foods would be adequate provided ration is at least 50% whole foods.
Minerals		
Calcium	750–850 mg	Major concern for higher levels is the potential formation of kidney stones.
Chromium	No recommended level	Amount in foods would be adequate provided ration is at least 50% whole foods.
Copper	900–1,600 µg	If added to foods, encapsulation should be considered due to its pro-oxidant activity.
Iodine	150–770 µg	Could be added as iodized salt.
Iron	8–18 mg	If added to foods, encapsulation should be considered due to its pro-oxidant activity. Palatability should determine the amount in ration foods.

continued

TABLE 3-1 Continued

Nutrient or Energy Intake	Recommended Amount	Comments
Magnesium	400–550 mg	No more than 350 mg of magnesium salts should be present to meet the minimum daily amount of magnesium recommended. The rest should come from food sources. Also, if salt needs to be added and taste becomes objectionable, encapsulation should be considered.
Manganese	No recommended level	Amount in foods would be adequate provided ration is at least 50% whole foods.
Molybdenum	No recommended level	Amount in foods would be adequate provided ration is at least 50% whole foods.
Phosphorus	700–2,500 mg	Because inorganic phosphates may cause diarrhea, it is recommended that they are added only up to 700 mg. Intakes above this amount should come from food sources only.
Potassium	Aim to 3.3–4.7 g	Foods naturally high in potassium should be included in ration; if added to foods to achieve recommended levels, taste problems might be encountered.
Selenium	55–230 μg	No clear evidence of effects as an enhancer of immune function or performance.
Sodium	≥3 g up to 12 g as supplement	For individuals who lose salt in excess or when in extremely hot or strenuous situations, sodium could be supplemented up to 12 g total. Part of this amount should be included in the form of candy, gels, or powder to add to fluids. Palatability will limit addition of sodium to these products; therefore, salt tablets should also be provided under medical guidance.
Zinc	11–25 mg	If it needs to be added and taste becomes objectionable, encapsulation should be considered.
Ergogenics Caffeine	100–600 mg	Not more than 600 mg in a single dose. There is no evidence of dehydration at this level.

[1] RAE = retinol activity equivalents.

[2] Whole foods = food items prepared to preserve natural nutritive value.

that last for a maximum total period of one month and that include recovery periods between missions of about 24–72 hours.

Energy and Macronutrients

To develop the recommendation on the total caloric intake of the ration, the committee integrated information from several sources. First, the committee considered health risks and benefits of a high, medium, and low energy intake diet. Second, information provided to the committee regarding the eating behavior in the field was reviewed. The data included food preferences, degree of satisfaction, and actual consumption of the current rations. Finally, past studies demonstrating that soldiers do not eat enough when exposed to the high-stress situations in the field (IOM, 1995) were considered. This undereating is attributed to an array of psychological factors that are difficult to control. In fact, data collected during training exercises of various military groups (e.g., special operation forces, marines) indicate that under stressful field conditions soldiers consume an average energy intake of 2,400 kcal (see Montain, 2004 in Appendix B). This level of intake is not enough to maintain body weight; however, the weight loss is moderate if the period of low energy intake is not sustained. Taking this information into account, the committee concluded that a ration with a caloric content of 2,400 kcal—if designed with adequate macronutrients and micronutrients, and eaten entirely and for short periods of time such as three to seven days up to a month—would not pose any health risks. With the expected energy expenditures of 4,500 kcal/day during the missions, it is possible that some soldiers might lose as much as 10 percent body weight before the end of the month, even with refeeding between missions; this degree of weight loss could result in adverse but mild performance defects. Therefore, it is recommended that weight loss be measured after one month of use; if weight loss is higher than 10 percent for a soldier, he should not be sent on assault missions until weight is regained to within 5 percent of initial weight.

The committee emphasizes that the ration nutrient contents recommended here are meant to be consumed for the short-term missions assumed in this report (three- to seven-day missions that last for a maximum total period of one month), not to substitute for longer periods in which Meals, Ready-to-Eat (MREs) or menus from food services constitute a more appropriate diet.

The distribution, level, and type of macronutrients for the ration (see Box 3-1) were established by considering the major health risks that might be posed by eating a hypocaloric diet in a combat situation. One major health risk that needs remediation is the excessive weight loss that occurs when the energy intake is below the energy output. The typical energy deficit of 50 percent seen in combat operations leads to a negative nitrogen balance that can result in muscle loss, fatigue, and loss of performance. To minimize these potential consequences, the committee recommends a protein level of 1.2–1.5 g/kg of body weight per day,

BOX 3-1
General Design of the Recommended Assault Ration

Basic Ration:

Protein	100–120 g (400–480 kcal; 17–20% kcal)
Carbohydrate	350 g (1,400 kcal; 58 % kcal)
Fat	58–67 g (520–600 kcal; 22–25% kcal)
Water	105 g (assuming an average of 17% moisture)
Total weight (kcal)	613–642 g (2,400 kcal)

Carbohydrate (and Electrolyte) Supplement:

Carbohydrate	100 g (400 kcal)
Water	17 g (assuming an average of 17% moisture)
Sodium	up to 12 g (based on palatability)
Potassium	up to 3.3–4.7 g (based on palatability)
Total Weight (kcal)	117 g (400 kcal)

Salt Tablets (Available Through Medical Personnel):

Sodium	up to 12 g
Potassium	up to 4.7 g
Total Weight	16.7 g

Packaging: 181 g

Total Weight   **0.95 kg**
Total Energy Content **2,800 kcal**

NOTE: This ration is intended for use over three- to seven-day missions for up to a month. Prolonged and continuous use of these rations as a sole source of sustenance may lead to substantial weight loss. Constraints: weight of 3 lbs (1.36 kg) and volume of 0.12 cubic feet.

or 100–120 g of total protein per day. This level of protein would spare muscle protein and decrease net nitrogen loss; in addition, it would maintain an adequate level of serum proteins needed as, for example, antioxidant enzymes as well as potentially maintain immune and cognitive functions.

The carbohydrate content of the ration is an important energy source and also plays a role in maintaining gastrointestinal health. Strong evidence that carbohydrate enhances cognitive function is still lacking; therefore optimizing physical performance was the rationale for the 350 g of carbohydrate recommended for the basic ration. Numerous data, however, suggest that supplementing the diet with carbohydrate throughout periods of continuous physical exercise and stress not only increases energy intake but also helps maintain and optimize physical performance. The supplementation of the basic ration with additional carbohydrate (up to 100 g or 400 kcal) is therefore deemed critical to optimizing performance; therefore, the committee recommends such carbohydrate supplementation in the form of gels, candy, or dry powder (to add to water) be available during combat missions. To maintain gastrointestinal health, a range of 15–17 g of a mix of both viscous, nonfermentable and nonviscous, fermentable fiber is recommended.

The primary reason to add fat to the ration is to provide a readily digestible food source of high energy density. Fat is also critical for the palatability of the ration and to permit absorption of fat-soluble vitamins. Because this ration is meant to be completely consumed, it is important that the acceptability of the ration be optimized; therefore, a minimum amount of fat is required in the ration to provide palatability. In general, surveys show that high-fat foods are not preferred by soldiers in the field (personal communication, A. Young, USARIEM, August 9, 2004). The committee concluded that, among the macronutrients, adequate levels of protein and carbohydrate were a priority and that the remainder of the macronutrients (up to the energy level of 2,400 kcal) should be provided as fat. Considering published data on preferences of athletes and the energy constraints of the ration, the committee recommends providing between 58 and 67 g of fat and distributing it across a variety of foods.

Micronutrients

In making its recommendations for levels of micronutrients in the ration, the committee followed a general approach, which is described here. The levels recommended here are primarily based on Recommended Dietary Allowance (RDA) or Adequate Intake (AI) for 19- to 30-year-old males from DRI reports (IOM, 2004) and then modified by the committee after considering data in the literature about sweat losses and utilization under high energy expenditure and stress. Food developers designing these rations might encounter difficulties in adhering to a single level of a nutrient due to organoleptic issues, food technology issues, or the presence of certain micronutrients in foods in limited amounts. Therefore, to provide food developers flexibility, a range is recommended for most micronutrients. For most cases, the ranges are based on the RDA or AI and the 95th percentile of intake of the US population as reported in the National Health and Nutrition Examination Survey (NHANES) III, a recent population-based survey, or other surveys if NHANES III data were unavailable. To avoid adverse effects when the 95th percentile dietary intake is higher than the Tolerable Upper Intake Level (UL), then the UL is included as the upper limit of the recommended range.

Unless deemed necessary to maintain health or improve performance and to avoid the addition of supplements to the extent possible, the committee recommends micronutrient levels that could be naturally occurring in foods feasible for this ration; fortification of foods may result in adverse sensory effects, promote interactions with other nutrients, and, in addition, is costly. In cases such as potassium, however, it was recognized that food alone would not provide enough of a particular nutrient and that some form of supplementation might be needed. In other cases, such as for the trace elements molybdenum, manganese, and chromium, no recommendation is made because those minerals are widely distributed in foods and a deficiency is not anticipated during the short period of intake of these rations.

Exceptions to this general approach are described for each particular micronutrient in Chapter 2 and include the following: (1) for the B vitamins, the committee considered the importance of energy expenditure when setting the recommendations, while for vitamin B_6, negative energy balance and loss of protein were considered; (2) for vitamin C, the committee added 25 mg to account for the needs of smokers; and (3) for vitamin A, the committee recommends a minimum of 300 μg RAE (retinol activity equivalents) to minimize the risk of night blindness.

In making recommendations for micronutrient requirements for soldiers during high-intensity physical activity, one factor that needs to be accounted for is micronutrient loss in the sweat or urine or both. Among factors causing increased sweat volume are exercise intensity and environmental temperature, both of which are relevant for this report. As noted in Chapter 2, data on micronutrient losses are lacking in most cases and research is needed. Although data are limited, these factors cannot be ignored when making recommendations. When specific data for additional micronutrient losses in sweat or urine during intense exercise in the heat (e.g., zinc and copper) was available, then the amount was added to the upper end level of the range recommended. In other cases, such as for sodium, an estimation of the maximum losses for intense exercise under hot climates and for salt losers was calculated from the data available on sweat sodium concentrations for different ambient conditions and activities and estimated total sweat volume.

Where necessary, the committee cautions about the potential for nutrient oxidation, or interactions with other nutrients in the ration. Therefore, it advises that chemical analysis be performed on the final ration following appropriate shelf-life studies. The importance of nutrient stability and interactions is further discussed later in this chapter under the section entitled Food Matrix Considerations.

In summary, in recommending levels of micronutrients, the committee considered DRIs, dietary intakes for the US population, health concerns specific to the circumstances (see below), cognitive and physical performance, heat stress, and sweat and other losses. For a summary of the recommendations for micronutrients, see Table 3-1.

Other Bioactives

The committee reviewed (see Chapter 2) the effects of several bioactive substances due to their potential benefits in physical or cognitive performance. The reader is also referred to Costello (Costello and Chrousos, 2004 in Appendix B). Other bioactives is a broad category of components that are not considered essential nutrients but that have been suggested to function in particular cells or as performance enhancers. Caffeine is the only component for which there is compelling data showing effectiveness for combat soldiers and therefore only caffeine received the endorsement of the committee. Caffeine is often consumed in the field and its use for physical and cognitive performance was recommended in a recent Committee on Military Nutrition Research report (IOM, 2001).

Some other bioactives are already consumed at liberty in either the sports community (e.g., L-carnitine, creatine, neurotransmitter precursors) or the general population (e.g., *Ginkgo biloba* and Ginseng extracts). Soldiers also consume these types of bioactives with the goal of increasing physical endurance. For the most part, neither the evidence for improving physical performance nor the potential adverse effects of their use or interactions with other nutrients is clear. One reason for these inconclusive results might be that the studies have not been conducted in a randomized and blinded manner. For example, it is uncertain whether creatine actually builds muscle tissue or simply increases muscle bulk due to water accumulation (Tarnopolsky et al., 2004). However, the literature is fairly compelling regarding the benefit of creatine supplementation in the enhancement of muscle strength during resistance training as well as improvement of repetitive bouts of high-intensity activity (Terjung et al., 2000). Due to its usage, the committee suggests pursuing randomized, blinded trials to elucidate the risks, including withdrawal effects, and potential benefits of taking creatine; ideally, these trials should be conducted under conditions that mimic combat situations.

Flavonoids are a subclass of polyphenols that might provide some benefit as antioxidants against the oxidative stress occurring during intense exercise and mental activities. It is believed that the antioxidant properties of these compounds might act in a synergistic manner with other dietary antioxidants (e.g., vitamin C, vitamin E) or antioxidant enzyme system (Liu, 2004) but most of the research has been done in vitro. More in vivo studies are needed to explore this possibility. In the meantime, and consistent with previous statements in this report, the committee recommends including foods such as fruits, vegetables, tea, and chocolate that contain significant amounts of flavonoids.

Supplementary Carbohydrate and Electrolytes

As mentioned above, the supplementation of the basic ration with additional carbohydrate is critical to optimizing performance. Therefore, the committee recommends that such supplementation in the form of gels, dry powder to add to water, or candy be available during combat missions. In this way, small amounts of carbohydrate will be supplied as an extra source of energy.

Similarly, small amounts of extra sodium can be added in the form of powders to add to fluids or in candy or gels. Additional sodium can be made available in salt tablets under medical guidance. The extra sodium will ensure that, in cases of excessive salt loss such as under conditions of hot climate or for excessive salt losers, sodium balance is not compromised.

HEALTH CONCERNS

General Gastrointestinal Tract Considerations

Among the possible effects on gut function by specific ration nutrients, the following were considered:

Potential Effects on Diarrhea

Literature reports indicate that diets very high in fructose may cause gastrointestinal distress and osmotic diarrhea. It is important to limit the use of fructose as a monosaccharide to less than 25 g (see Chapter 2) and measure its level in the final product, since there is some indication of high levels of fructose in the ration beverages.

Potential Effects on Nausea

There have been some reports on nausea caused by high amounts of dietary zinc; however, the levels recommended in the assault ration are unlikely to be high enough to cause nausea. Also, high amounts of potassium, particularly in the form of potassium chloride, are linked to unpleasant taste, nausea, gastrointestinal inflammation, and gut distress. Potassium is less likely to cause such effects in a food matrix. Although further research needs to be done on these points, the committee concludes that the levels of these nutrients in the assault ration are not excessive.

Addition of Prebiotics or Probiotics

Various probiotics were also considered for possible inclusion in the ration. The extremely long shelf-life required by the ration specifications precludes the use of any probiotic, since their stability to fulfill elements of long shelf-life is insufficient at this time.

General Immune Considerations

Certain essential nutrients (vitamins A, C, B_6, B_{12}, E, pantothenic acid, folate, and minerals such as selenium, zinc, copper, iron, and phosphorus) are known to cause immunodeficiency when provided for prolonged periods (e.g., weeks or months) in less than required amounts. The proposed assault ration is designed to contain adequate amounts of each of these nutrients. Other nutrients (e.g., arginine, glutamine, vitamin C and E in large amounts, ω-3 fatty acids and β-glucan) and other bioactives (e.g., Echinacea extracts) have been proposed to enhance immune function. As described in this report, the current evidence does not support a recommendation to include them in the assault ration.

General Dehydration Considerations

Although the committee was not asked to consider water requirements in its recommendations for the proposed assault ration, certain hydration issues were considered important to the optimal composition of the ration. For example, since the sodium content would be closely linked to water needs, the committee recommends a dietary sodium content that would accommodate moderate sweat losses of 6.5–10.5 L/day. For those that lose salt in excess, supplemental salt would be required. Furthermore, the committee supports continued use of the camel-back to provide water and also recommends that a mechanism be developed to provide the option of flavoring the water so as to encourage fluid intake.

Another important facet of diet design related to hydration is the potential for renal stone formation. Although the most important variable to reduce the risk of renal stone formation is water intake sufficient to meet sweat losses, sodium, calcium, and oxalate content of the proposed assault ration were also considered to minimize this complication. The effect of specific macronutrient levels, namely carbohydrate and protein, on water needs was also discussed. The importance of providing enough water during these missions so that water needs due to sweat losses and the nature of the ration are met, cannot be overemphasized.

Finally, gastrointestinal fluid and electrolyte losses due to diarrhea illness can also severely stress water balance. Providing a palatable assault ration that will likely meet anticipated levels of energy intake under these short-term combat conditions should limit the use of local foods which might increase the risk of diarrheal disease. In addition, the recommendation of using fiber, both viscous and nonviscous, should support better gastrointestinal function.

FOOD MATRIX CONSIDERATIONS

Food rations meant for short-term, high-intensity operations use present a unique challenge to the product developer and nutritionist. With careful planning, it should be possible to provide complete nutritional needs in a restricted volume and weight (0.12 cubic feet; 1.36 kg) with long shelf-life (two to three years) and nutrient stability. From a practical standpoint, military studies show that troops entering combat will selectively choose food from existing rations, such as MREs, in quantities sufficient to achieve low-level energy intakes (approximately 2,400 kcal). First Strike Rations (FSRs), rations in their testing phase, were strategically designed at the Natick Soldier Center to be consumed in the initial stages of combat. In contrast to the MREs, which can provide about 3,600 kcal/day, current FSRs provide approximately 2,400–2,800 kcal if all components are eaten. Tests conducted during training indicate that selective eating is less likely to occur with an FSR that contained about 2,400 kcal.

Therefore, the committee makes these assumptions:

- Providing a ration with a minimal energy content of 2,400 kcal would be appropriate for the short term (repeated periods of three to seven days up to a month);
- Equally distributing macronutrients and micronutrients among all food items of the ration would minimize nutrient deficiencies in the event soldiers discard selective ration items and would also provide a steady nutrient intake;
- Including the recommended amounts of micronutrients for a daily diet of approximately 4,500 kcal would be necessary for metabolic efficiency;
- Adding calories in the form of beverage powder supplements, carbohydrate-rich gels, or fruit-flavored candies would be beneficial;
- Providing a mechanism to make flavored or sweetened water or both would be likely to increase fluid intake, when fluid intake is desirable.

Ration Components

Foods that are included in a ration should have variety in flavors, colors, and textures and should be both sweet and savory. Current FSRs and MREs already have such variety. The restricted volume and weight of the proposed ration must be coupled with packaging needs for stability and protection. Individual portions that can be easily distributed in backpacks and uniform pockets are needed. It is unlikely that troops will consume all items at a single sitting; thus, each portion should aim to provide a designated percentage of calories and other nutrients.

Consumption studies done by the military over many years suggest that a ration composed solely of candy, high-energy, or high-protein bars is unlikely to be satisfying after a few days. Results from the survey of troops in Afghanistan (personal communication, C. Koenig, USARIEM, November 19, 2004) indicated that some items currently in the FSR were consumed less; namely, tuna, wheat snack bread, and energy-rich, glucose-optimized drink were the least popular. Ease of consumption, as well as taste, were most important to the soldiers.

The savory items, such as sandwiches, wraps, cheese spreads, and jerked meats, fulfill the desire for an "entrée." Addition of more fruit-based products, such as fruit rolls or bars, could enhance the micronutrient intakes as well as provide fiber. Flavor variety is also needed. Familiar flavors and products based on popular fast food items, such as pizza-based products, would be appropriate.

Ration development should capitalize on existing technologies for food processing whenever possible. Familiar products or facsimiles thereof with enhanced nutrient content can be used. For example, power bar products already come in a variety of forms, from high-energy to high-protein bars to bite-size pieces and gels. Repackaging of commercial products to fit military needs is also sometimes feasible. Dried fruits, including raisins, figs, apricots, cranberries, cherries, and banana chips, can be included for variety, as well as for potassium, fiber, micronutrient, and flavonoid supplementation. The existing HOOAH!® bar might be fortified with more protein and other nutrients.

Savory entrées, sandwiches, or wraps present the largest challenges to the product developers. FSRs already include shelf-stable pocket sandwiches with savory fillings (e.g., barbecue, chicken, Italian beef), as well as cheese spread, jerky, and dairy bar, all of which provide protein. Potato crisps, sturdy crackers (e.g., Wheat Thins® and rye crisp), and dense breads can be considered as possible additions, although the latter may not meet soldiers' expectations for bread.

Foods packaged in tubes are common in Europe, but not widely seen in the United States. This form of packaging can be used for peanut butter, cheese and other spreads, and presents a vehicle for introducing micronutrients.

Gels that provide carbohydrate and electrolytes are used by highly trained athletes, such as bicyclists and marathon runners. In a small package, they can deliver energy boosts as well as electrolytes. Powdered drink mixes with similar carbohydrate and electrolytes can be used to flavor water and increase fluid intake. Commercially available gels and powders have minimal amounts of electrolytes but could be fortified.

Constraints on Ration Components

The proposed nutrient composition of the ration (see Table 3-1) places some constraints on the food forms and matrixes used. The recommendations suggest the use of whole foods as much as possible, as opposed to fortification of foods or use supplements or tablets. This would influence nutrient content and contribute to variability in the products. The recommended levels of some nutrients may also dictate the use of fortification with labile vitamins such as vitamin C as well as with other nutrients such as folate that are likely to be low in the ration due to the types of foods included. Food developers need to carefully consider the shelf-life of the ration to ensure that levels of labile micronutrients are neither above (if storage period is shorter than anticipated) nor below (due to interactions with other components) the range of recommended levels. To minimize the potential decreased bioavailability due to interactions, the use of encapsulated forms for some nutrients may be necessary. Electrolytes (sodium and potassium) and other minerals (zinc and magnesium) are known to have objectionable tastes to some, possibly at the levels recommended.

Palatability of the ration components is a primary concern. The ration is intended for short-term consumption, that is, during repetitive missions that last for three to seven days, possibly over a relatively short period of time, such as a month. Safe use of the ration is an important consideration. Although the rations could provide sufficient nutritional value for longer term if more than one ration is eaten, the committee does not recommend consuming two or more rations per day. Because the foods that will be included are highly processed, they may not provide as complete an array of food components as a regular diet. Also, the distribution of the energy-providing nutrients is atypical for US diets. Therefore, the committee's recommendations assume a short-term consumption regimen. Monotony, induced by limited food choice, is known to reduce the amount of food consumed, as well as lower acceptability of the items (Kramer et al., 2001). Thus, providing a variety of acceptable products for the short term is necessary.

Taste

An important consideration under the high-intensity physical activity of combat situations is that rehydration must occur with replenishment of electrolytes. The high levels of electrolytes sodium and potassium recommended by the committee will affect the taste and flavor of the ration components. Most of the published work on taste quality and preference of electrolytes has been done on sodium. Very high or very low levels of salt in foods are generally liked less, but there is a strong dependence on the food matrix (Beauchamp et al., 1983; Drewnowski et al., 1996). The preferred level of salt in soups is about 200 mmol/L (approximately 500 mg sodium/100 mL). Processed foods, such as canned soups, can contain as much as 1,000 mg sodium per serving (240 mL).

Addition of sodium and potassium salts via sports drinks or gels provides less than 50–100 mg per serving. The recommended level of sodium in a rehydration beverage is at least 50 mmol/L (Maughan and Shirreffs, 1997; Maughan et al., 1997). Palatability does not appear to be a problem with concentrations from 40–60 mmol/L (Passe, 2001; Shirreffs et al., 1996).

Little research has been done on the taste sensations elicited by potassium, magnesium, or zinc in foods. Potassium chloride (KCl) is the most common form of potassium used in foods, primarily as a salt substitute. This compound has a bitter, soapy taste at high concentrations. Bertino et al. (1986) reported that palatability decreased for KCl in soup and crackers at 0.13 mol/L and 1.8 percent, respectively. Fortification with potassium salts is possible in baked products and liquid solutions, if the concentration is kept under 400 mg potassium/100 g and salts other than KCl (e.g., potassium bicarbonate and various potassium phosphates) are used (Mentavlos, 2002). Magnesium also has a bitter taste that seems to be detectable at similar concentrations (0.3 mol/L; Delwiche et al., 2001). Zinc salts that are often included in nutritional supplements and mouth care products are known to produce astringent sensations, but not strong sour, bitter, sweet, or salty tastes (Keast, 2003). Calcium salts generally do not have objectionable tastes and may minimize other mineral taste sensations (Lawless et al., 2003).

Nutrient Density and Satiety

Much of the research on the impact of nutrient density on food intake is related to its potential link to obesity. The consumption of high-energy-density, high-fat foods is associated with increased total intake of calories (de Castro, 2004). How nutrient density affects the satiety value of various foods or food components is an important concept in formulating military rations. Factors affecting eating behaviors that lead to food underconsumption, an ongoing problem for troops in combat situations, were described in *Not Eating Enough* (IOM, 1995). The effects of food composition and nutrient density and their impact on satiety are recognized and detailed in that publication.

From a biological standpoint, food consumption is driven by a feeling of hunger, which stimulates eating. Satiation occurs when the feeling of hunger dissipates, usually due to a feeling of fullness (Blundell et al., 1996). Satiety occurs after food is eaten, and this tends to delay the next eating bout. Merrill et al. (2004) considered satiety to be the result of both biological and psychological effects resulting from food consumption. Gerstein et al. (2004) point out that studies of macronutrient effects on satiety suggest that, when in isolation, protein is the most satiating macronutrient, followed by carbohydrates and fat. A number of recent studies, however, indicated that greater satiety results from consumption of foods higher in protein and carbohydrate than fat (see, for example, Blundell and MacDiarmid, 1997; Holt et al., 1999; Marmonier et al., 2000). Anderson and Moore (2004) reviewed studies of protein effects on food intake regulation in humans, and although they came to the same conclusion, these authors pointed out that further research is needed. Many of the observations of macronutrient impact on satiety were made with pure sources of the energy-providing nutrients, and not foods, which are mixtures of several of these and other nutrients (Bell et al., 1998; Rolls, 1995; Rolls and Shide, 1992).

Some research shows that energy-dense foods that are rich in fat tend to have lower ability to lead to satiety (Holt et al., 1995). On the other hand, high-fat foods tend to be well liked, and because they are less likely to contribute to a feeling of fullness or satiation, they will be overconsumed (Blundell et al., 1996; Nasser et al., 2001). Foods high in sucrose have high satiety value (Holt et al., 1995), which suggests that a mix of carbohydrate-rich and fat-rich foods is needed to provide a balance in the assault ration. The satiety value of a variety of

Army rations was assessed by Merrill and coworkers (2002, 2004). Their research focus has been on "the perceptual consequences of eating" in an attempt to measure and predict the perceived satiety of meal ration components, including some from the FSR and MREs. These provide a preliminary database that could assist in further development of foods that will stimulate consumption of more calories and counter the underconsumption and weight loss observed under combat operations.

Nutrient Stability and Possible Nutrient Interactions

Vitamin stability and degradation in processed food and has been reviewed extensively (Gregory and Kirk, 1981; Karmas and Harris, 1988; Labuza and Riboh, 1982; Villota and Hawkes, 1992). Heat, light, ultraviolet and gamma radiation, oxidation, water content, and activity all influence the rate of loss (Gregory, 1996; Labuza, 1980; Nelson and Labuza, 1994). In addition, specific vitamins exhibit different rates of destruction. Water-soluble vitamins, such as ascorbic acid and folate, are subject to degradation in higher water content and water activity foods (Gregory, 1996; IOM, 2002). Fat-soluble vitamins, such as vitamins A, D, E, and K, are subject to oxidation, which is often accelerated by light and heat (Ottaway, 1993).

When vitamins are added as fortificants, they are often encapsulated or coated. This technology provides a physical barrier, primarily to prevent nutrients from oxidation, catalytic reactions, and degradation and to prevent changes in flavor, color, or texture that might be affected by oxidation products. Numerous patented processes for doing this have been developed in recent years (Brazel, 1999; Risch and Reineccius, 1995). The actual procedure used for vitamin coating or encapsulation will depend on the vitamin's properties, as well as the presence of pro-oxidants. Fat-soluble vitamins may be stabilized by antioxidants, including dl-α-tocopherol or butylated hydroxyanisole or butylated hydroxytoluene. Vitamin C can be coated with various substances, such as ethyl cellulose, cyclodextrins, or lipids, to prevent contact with iron, copper, or nickel. Encapsulation of vitamin C slows its degradation under high heat and moisture conditions (Uddin et al., 2001). It should also protect it from oxidation by metals, such as iron. Because vitamin C can enhance nonheme iron absorption from foods and improve absorption of nonchelated iron used for fortification, the interactions between these two nutrients has been considered in fortification programs (Hurrell, 2002b; IOM, 2000).

The questions of iron absorption and iron bioavailability from iron fortificants has been addressed extensively in the context of alleviating global iron deficiency anemia (Foege, 2002; Hurrell, 2002a). Embedded in these discussions are references to the undesirable changes in color, flavor, and texture, as well as shelf-life stability due to lipid oxidation, caused by various iron fortificants. Sensory changes due to the various classes of iron compounds, however, are not well documented, as reviewed by Bovell-Benjamin and Guinard (2003). Hurrell (2002b) pointed out that "the most soluble and absorbable iron compounds often cause unacceptable color and flavor changes when added to foods."

In a review of iron fortification, Hurrell et al. (2002) noted that iron is the most difficult mineral to add to food. Ferrous sulfate is the most common water-soluble form of iron used in infant formulas, bread, and pasta; however, fat oxidation catalyzed by this compound can cause loss of shelf-life due to flavor and color changes. Other less soluble forms such as ferrous fumarate and ferric saccharate can be used and they cause slightly less change in flavor, but have lower bioavailability. Elemental iron powder, specifically electrolytic iron powder, is often used for infant cereal fortification, but it, too, can cause color changes visible to the mother, but accepted by infants (Bovell-Benjamin and Guinard, 2003; Hurrell et al., 2002). Sodium iron ethylenediaminetetraacetic acid (Hurrell, 1997) and ferrous bisglycinate (Bovell-Benjamin et al., 2000) are among newer, more expensive forms of iron fortification that are being studied, and even they cause color changes. Encapsulated ferrous salts are available (Zlotkin et al., 2001) but not widely used due to the heat instability of some coatings and lack of information about bioavailability. In formulating the FSRs, encapsulation of vitamin C and use of various soluble forms of iron should be considered.

Compared with vitamins, minerals are much more stable, even under extreme conditions of heat and humidity. Although some minerals are water-soluble, the likely food products will be relatively low in water content and water activity. When iron is added for fortification, care must be taken to protect vitamins A and C and thiamin, due to the possibility of accelerated degradation. Iron also catalyzes oxidative rancidity of polyunsaturated oils and fats, which can produce undesirable changes in color and flavor. Fortification of food with copper could accelerate vitamin C degradation and interfere with bioavailability of other minerals, such as zinc; however, copper is naturally present in food and would probably not be added. Zinc-copper interactions are not envisioned to present a concern at the levels recommended here.

Iodine is stable in foods, and can be added to the ration in the form of iodized salt. Although some food manufacturers have had concerns about the use of iodized salt in processing due to possible effects on flavor and color, there is little evidence to support this concern (West et al., 1995).

Shelf-Life Stability

Standard procedures for shelf-life testing should be employed during the development and testing of the ration components. As noted in an earlier IOM report on an emergency relief food product (IOM, 2002), shelf-life testing is an integral part of the development process. Most commercial products do not have the extended storage life expected of either military or emergency foods. Accelerated shelf-life testing is often used to predict stability over long time periods under extreme conditions (Labuza and Schmidl, 1985, 1988). Other prediction models have also been proposed (Cardelli and Labuza, 2001; Gacula and Singh, 1984; Nelson and Labuza, 1994).

Decisions about shelf-life and length of storage are made based on changes in at least one characteristic of the food, such as sensory quality, vitamin content, or lipid oxidation. Changes due to aging include texture deterioration, browning due to Maillard Browning or oxidation, staling, and off-flavor development (Lawless and Heymann, 1999). Carefully planned shelf-life studies can lead to prediction models for storage stability (Labuza and Schmidl, 1988).

Acceptable analytical techniques are critical to the success of conducting shelf-life studies and to guaranteeing specific levels of nutrients in the ration at the end of the projected storage period. The analysis of each ration component for vitamin and mineral content should be part of the routine quality control program. Sensory testing should also be integral to quality assurance.

General Concerns and Recommendations

- An assault ration must provide a concentrated source of designated nutrients in foods that are highly acceptable to trained soldiers in physically and psychologically stressful situations.
- The military should continue to evaluate food preferences of soldiers when they are under stress and in strenuous circumstances and to reformulate or replace products accordingly.
- Existing food products already in the marketplace should be considered for inclusion when they meet nutritional and sensory needs and stability requirements.
- Specific foods that are high in needed nutrients, such as potassium in fruits, can be included to formulate rations, in lieu of relying upon vitamin or mineral fortification.
- The ration is expected to be stable for long periods of time (up to three years) and to retain its sensory quality and nutritional value; the stability of the ration must be monitored carefully by planned analytical testing.
- Product developers should capitalize on existing and innovative processing technologies for future products and for fortification.

MONITORING RATION PERFORMANCE AND USE

The ration recommended here was designed with the best available data. Some of the data, however, derive from studies in which the environment or the subjects were substantially different from the ones for which this ration is to be utilized. For example, much of the data on optimizing physical performance come from studies performed with athletes; to extrapolate the conclusions regarding athletes to highly trained soldiers deployed in short combat missions is generally not ideal. The committee believes that further work needs to be conducted to confirm that the current ration provides optimal performance and maintains health or to have the opportunity of improving the ration by making necessary adjustments. Additionally, little is known about food preferences of subjects under such stress. The military should consider conducting studies to test the performance and acceptability of the ration under the real circumstances of combat and under different environments (e.g., cold versus hot versus high altitude) with attention to actual duration of use of such rations.

The military should closely monitor the actual use of the ration. This ration was designed for the rigorous operational conditions assumed, specifically, short-term missions to which highly trained male soldiers are deployed. For health reasons, it should not be used as a substitute for other rations when military personnel are in garrison or in other types of extended missions.

The committee's recommendations on adding carbohydrate and salt supplements are critical to maintaining the health and performance of soldiers. They are particularly important for individuals who lose salt in excess, for missions in hot climates, or during strenuous exercise. Due to the stressful circumstances or other factors, some soldiers may not be always aware or knowledgeable of their health status or nutrient requirements. Soldiers required instructions on the use of these carbohydrate and salt supplements and should be reminded of their use at appropriate times.

The military should be attentive to the quality of the ration from both a microbiological and a chemical composition standpoint. For some of the nutrients, such as fructose, a change in the recipe (i.e., a substantial increase in fructose) may have adverse gastrointestinal tract effects on a number of individuals. It is critical not only to advise the food manufacturer to carefully follow the formulation of a food as prescribed but also to perform in-house nutrient analysis of the products. Tests to determine the microbiological stability of the products for safety and quality reasons are also indispensable in all food quality control operations.

FUTURE NEEDS

The committee finds that gaps in knowledge exist and that additional data in the following general areas of investigation should prove particularly beneficial to future development and refinement of an optimal ration for the military operations envisioned: (1) additional knowledge regarding nutrient requirements and food technology issues; (2) deeper understanding of food preferences under high-stress situations; (3) more information on conditions under which the ration is actually used; and (4) development of methods to identify individuals at risk of losing excess electrolytes or developing kidney stones. Specific suggestions for future research needs can be found for each individual nutrient in Chapter 2. The following are specific areas of research that the committee considers of priority to continue the efforts in developing rations to enhance physical and cognitive performance during high-stress, short-term situations.

The committee emphasizes the importance of conducting studies under conditions that approximate the combat situations for which the ration is required; in addition, the physical and cognitive performance outcome measurements should be relevant and appropriate for those conditions (e.g., shot pattern tightness, complex reaction time, vigilance rather than objective or self-reported measurements of mood states).

Research on Nutrient Requirements

- Conduct research to determine whether the hypocaloric status of soldiers reported in combat has an effect on physical and cognitive performance measures that are relevant in combat situations.
- Confirm the effects of high-carbohydrate and high-protein diets on performance under hypocaloric conditions and stress on physical and cognitive performance; the effects of a high-protein diet on muscle loss and immune function should be specifically tested under those scenarios and under various climates (e.g., hot and cold temperatures).
- Study the potential benefits of carbohydrate supplementation for soldiers under hypocaloric conditions and stress on cognitive and physical performance; to minimize the confounding effects of energy intake, these studies should be conducted at the same energy intake level for all subjects.
- Conduct further research on the potential benefits of adding specific amino acids in addition to protein when subjects are consuming a hypocaloric diet under the environmental conditions and high-stress situations of combat missions. There is suggestive evidence obtained under significantly different conditions that warrants continuing research, specifically with arginine for immune enhancement and wound healing, and glutamine for intestinal function and immune function.
- Investigate the potential synergistic effects of a mixture of antioxidants (e.g., vitamin C, vitamin E, and flavonoids) from antioxidant-rich foods and fortified foods on physical performance and immune function in a randomized trial. Before such studies are conducted, valid markers of antioxidant activity that will permit comparison of studies across laboratories are needed.
- Determine the requirements of certain micronutrients (e.g., vitamins C and E, B vitamins, zinc, selenium, iron, copper) when individuals are consuming a hypocaloric diet under the environmental conditions and high-stress situations of combat missions (e.g., intense physical activity, high energy expenditure and reduced caloric intake, and hot and humid conditions). This would include evaluating the losses of minerals through sweat, urine and feces, as appropriate. This would also include assessing

the potential benefits of supplementing some nutrients in maintaining or improving health and performance.

- Pursue randomized, well-controlled trials to elucidate the risks (e.g., withdrawal effects) and potential benefits (e.g., cognitive performance) of taking selected bioactives that are often consumed in the field, such as creatine; these trials should be conducted under conditions that mimic combat situations.
- Investigate and document the feasibility of using such rations in emergency disaster, high-stress situations when adequate rations to sustain energy balance may be impossible to provide.

Research on Food and Ration Development and Field Use

The committee concludes that the US Army Research Institute of Environmental Medicine and the Natick Soldier Center should continue the existing systematic approach to ration development for combat missions. As currently practiced, in addition to the required nutrients, such an approach should incorporate early in the design process issues of palatability and food preferences of end-users. Other critical factors to consider are the required long shelf-life of the rations, nutrient interactions, and packaging considerations.

- Study the combined effects of intense physical activity, acute stress, and energy deficit on hunger and appetite.
- Evaluate the acceptability of the assault ration under field conditions to determine percentage eaten and food preferences. The extent of selectively trading and discarding ration items under combat conditions needs to be evaluated by surveys.
- Monitor the actual use of rations with respect to duration and frequency of use under actual field conditions.
- Create innovative ways of adding certain nutrients to foods without compromising palatability; specifically, pursue research to improve palatability characteristics of foods with the high concentrations of sodium and potassium recommended. In addition, develop ingredients to hide bitterness qualities of metals and other nutrients.
- Test the safety and quality of products in the ration throughout their shelf-life. This should include chemical analysis of the recommended nutrients.

REFERENCES

Anderson GH, Moore SE. 2004. Dietary proteins in the regulation of food intake and body weight in humans. *J Nutr* 134(4):974S–979S.

Beauchamp GK, Bertino M, Engelman K. 1983. Modification of salt taste. *Ann Intern Med* 98(5 Pt 2):763–769.

Bell EA, Castellanos VH, Pelkman CL, Thorwart ML, Rolls BJ. 1998. Energy density of foods affects energy intake in normal-weight women. *Am J Clin Nutr* 67(3):412–420.

Bertino M, Beauchamp GK, Engelman K. 1986. Increasing dietary salt alters salt taste preference. *Physiol Behav* 38(2):203–213.

Blundell JE, MacDiarmid JI. 1997. Fat as a risk factor for overconsumption: Satiation, satiety, and patterns of eating. *J Am Diet Assoc* 97(7 Suppl):S63–S69.

Blundell JE, Lawton CL, Cotton JR, Macdiarmid JI. 1996. Control of human appetite: Implications for the intake of dietary fat. *Ann Rev Nutr* 16:285–319.

Bovell-Benjamin AC, Guinard JX. 2003. Novel approaches and application of contemporary sensory evaluation practices in iron fortification programs. *Crit Rev Food Sci Nutr* 43(4):379–400.

Bovell-Benjamin AC, Viteri FE, Allen LH. 2000. Iron absorption from ferrous bisglycinate and ferric triglycinate in whole maize is regulated by iron status. *Am J Clin Nutr* 71(6):1563–1569.

Brazel CS. 1999. Microencapsulation: Offering solutions for the food industry. *Cereal Foods World* 44(6):388–393.

Cardelli C, Labuza TP. 2001. Application of Weibull hazard analysis to the determination of the shelf-life of roasted and grounded coffee. *Lebbensmitten Wiss u Tech* 34(5):273–278.

Costello RB, Chrousos GP. 2004 (August 9). *Other Bioactive Food Components and Dietary Supplements.* Paper presented at the Institute of Medicine Workshop on Optimization of Nutrient Composition of Military Rations for Short-Term, High-Stress Situations, Natick, MA. Institute of Medicine Committee on Optimization of Nutrient Composition of Military Rations for Short-Term, High-Stress Situations.

de Castro JM. 2004. Dietary energy density is associated with increased intake in free-living humans. *J Nutr* 134(2):335–341.

Delwiche JF, Buletic Z, Breslin PA. 2001. Covariation in individuals' sensitivities to bitter compounds: Evidence supporting multiple receptor/transduction mechanisms. *Percept Psychophys* 63(5):761–776.

Drewnowski A, Henderson SA, Driscoll A, Rolls BJ. 1996. Salt taste perceptions and preferences are unrelated to sodium consumption in healthy older adults. *J Am Diet Assoc* 96(5):471–474.

Foege W. 2002. Keynote address: Issues in overcoming iron deficiency. *J Nutr* 132(4 Suppl):790S–793S.

Gacula MC Jr, Singh J. 1984. *Statistical Methods in Food and Consumer Research.* Orlando, FL: Academic Press.

Gerstein DE, Woodward-Lopez G, Evans AE, Kelsey K, Drewnowski A. 2004. Clarifying concepts about macronutrients' effects on satiation and satiety. *J Am Diet Assoc* 104(7):1151–1153.

Gregory JF III. 1996. Vitamins. In: Fennema OR, ed. *Food Chemistry.* 3rd ed. New York: Marcel Dekker. Pp. 531–616.

Gregory JF III, Kirk JR. 1981. The bioavailability of vitamin B_6 in foods. *Nutr Rev* 39(1):1–8.

Holt SH, Delargy HJ, Lawton CL, Blundell JE. 1999. The effects of high-carbohydrate vs high-fat breakfasts on feelings of fullness and alertness, and subsequent food intake. *Int J Food Sci Nutr* 50(1):13–28.

Holt SH, Miller JC, Petocz P, Farmakalidis E. 1995. A satiety index of common foods. *Eur J Clin Nutr* 49(9):675–690.

Hurrell RF. 1997. Preventing iron deficiency through food fortification. *Nutr Rev* 55(6):210–222.

Hurrell RF. 2002a. Fortification: Overcoming technical and practical barriers. *J Nutr* 132(4 Suppl):806S–812S.

Hurrell R. 2002b. How to ensure adequate iron absorption from iron-fortified food. *Nutr Rev* 60(7 Pt 2):S7–S15.

Hurrell R, Bothwell T, Cook JD, Dary O, Davidsson L, Fairweather-Tait S, Hallberg L, Lynch S, Rosado J, Walter T, Whittaker P. 2002. The usefulness of elemental iron for cereal flour fortification: A SUSTAIN Task Force report. Sharing United States technology to aid in the improvement of nutrition. *Nutr Rev* 60(12):391–406.

IOM (Institute of Medicine). 1995. *Not Eating Enough*. Washington, DC: National Academy Press.

IOM. 2000. *Dietary Reference Intakes for Vitamin C, Vitamin E, Selenium, and Carotenoids*. Washington, DC: National Academy Press.

IOM. 2001. *Caffeine for the Sustainment of Mental Task Performance. Formulations for Military Operations*. Washington, DC: National Academy Press.

IOM. 2002. *High-Energy, Nutrient-Dense Emergency Relief Food Product*. Washington, DC: National Academy Press.

IOM. 2004. *Dietary Reference Intakes Tables—The Complete Set*. [Online]. Available: http://www.iom.edu/Object.File/Master/21/372/0.pdf [accessed February 24, 2005].

Karmas E, Harris RS, eds. 1988. *Nutritional Evaluation of Food Processing*. 3rd ed. New York: Van Nostrand Reinhold.

Keast RSJ. 2003. The effect of zinc on human taste perception. *J Food Sci* 68(5):1871–1877.

Kramer FM, Lesher LL, Meiselman HL. 2001. Monotony and choice: Repeated serving of the same item to soldiers under field conditions. *Appetite* 36(3):239–240.

Labuza TP. 1980. The effect of water activity on reaction kinetics of food deterioration. *Food Tech* 34(4):36–41, 59.

Labuza TP, Riboh D. 1982. Theory and application of arrhenius kinetics to the prediction of nutrient losses in foods. *Food Tech* 36(10):66–74.

Labuza TP, Schmidl MK. 1985. Accelerated shelf-life testing of foods. *Food Tech* 39(9):57–64.

Labuza TP, Schmidl MK. 1988. Use of sensory data in the shelf-life testing of foods: Principles and graphical methods for evaluation. *Cereal Foods World* 33(2):193–206.

Lawless HT, Heymann H. 1999. *Sensory Evaluation of Food. Principles and Practices*. Gaithersburg, MD: Aspen Publishers.

Lawless HT, Rapacki F, Horne J, Hayes A. 2003. The taste of calcium and magnesium salts and anionic modifications. *Food Qual Pref* 14(4):319–325.

Liu RH. 2004. Potential synergy of phytochemicals in cancer prevention: Mechanism of action. *J Nutr* 134(12 Suppl):3479S–3485S.

Marmonier C, Chapelot D, Louis-Sylvestre J. 2000. Effects of macronutrient content and energy density of snacks consumed in a satiety state on the onset of the next meal. *Appetite* 34(2):161–168.

Maughan RJ, Shirreffs SM. 1997. Recovery from prolonged exercise: Restoration of water and electrolyte balance. *J Sports Sci* 15(3):297–303.

Maughan RJ, Leiper JB, Shirreffs SM. 1997. Factors influencing the restoration of fluid and electrolyte balance after exercise in the heat. *Br J Sports Med* 31(3):175–182.

Mentavlos AA. 2002. *Sensory Perceptions of Potassium Salts in Liquid and Solid Model Systems*. Ph.D. dissertation. University of Illinois at Urbana-Champaign.

Merrill EP, Cardello AV, Kramer FM, Lesher LL, Schutz HG. 2004. The development of a perceived satiety index for military rations. *Food Quality Preference* 15(7–8):859–870.

Merrill EP, Kramer FM, Cardello A, Schutz H. 2002. A comparison of satiety measures. *Appetite* 39(2):181–183.

Montain SJ. 2004 (August 9). *Physiological Demands of Combat Operations*. Paper presented at the Institute of Medicine Workshop on the Optimization of Nutrient Composition of Military Rations for Short-Term, High-Stress Situations, Natick, MA. Institute of Medicine Committee on Optimization of Nutrient Composition of Military Rations for Short-Term, High-Stress Situations.

Nasser JA, Kissileff HR, Boozer CN, Chou CJ, Pi-Sunyer FX. 2001. PROP taster status and oral fatty acid perception. *Eat Behav* 2(3):237–245.

Nelson KA, Labuza TP. 1994. Water activity and food polymer science: Implications of state on arrhenius and WLF models in predicting shelf-life. *J Food Eng* 22:271–289.

Ottaway PB. 1993. Stability of vitamins in food. In: Ottaway PB, ed. *The Technology of Vitamins in Food*. New York: Chapman and Hall. Pp. 90–113.

Passe DH. 2001. Physiological and psychological determinants of fluid intake. In: Maughan RJ, Murray R, eds. *Sports Drinks. Basic Science and Practical Aspects*. Boca Raton, FL: CRC Press. Pp. 45–87.

Risch SJ, Reineccius GA, eds. 1995. *Encapsulation and Controlled Release of Food Ingredients*. ACS Symposium Series 590. Washington, DC: American Chemical Society.

Rolls BJ. 1995. Carbohydrates, fats, and satiety. *Am J Clin Nutr* 61(4 Suppl):960S–967S.

Rolls BJ, Shide DJ. 1992. The influence of dietary fat on food intake and body weight. *Nutr Rev* 50(10):283–290.

Shirreffs SM, Taylor AJ, Leiper JB, Maughan RJ. 1996. Post-exercise rehydration in man: Effects of volume consumed and drink sodium content. *Med Sci Sports Exerc* 28(10):1260–1271.

Tarnopolsky M, Mahoney D, Thompson T, Naylor H, Doherty TJ. 2004. Creatine monohydrate supplementation does not increase muscle strength, lean body mass, or muscle phosphocreatine in patients with myotonic dystrophy type 1. *Muscle Nerve* 29(1):51–58.

Terjung RL, Clarkson P, Eichner ER, Greenhaff PL, Hespel PJ, Israel RG, Kraemer WJ, Meyer RA, Spriet LL, Tarnopolsky MA, Wagenmakers AJ, Williams MH. 2000. American College of Sports Medicine roundtable. The physiological and health effects of oral creatine supplementation. *Med Sci Sports Exerc* 32(3):706–771.

Uddin MS, Hawlader MN, Zhu HJ. 2001. Microencapsulation of ascorbic acid: Effect of process variables on product characteristics. *J Microencapsul* 18(2):199–209.

US Departments of Army, Navy, and Air Force. 2001. *Nutrition Standards and Education*. AR 40-25/BUMEDINST 10110.6/AFI 44-141. Washington, DC: US Department of Defense Headquarters.

Villota R, Hawkes JG. 1992. Reaction kinetics in food systems. In: Heldman DR, Lund DB, eds. *Handbook of Food Engineering*. New York: Marcel Dekker. Pp. 39–144.

West CE, de Koning FLHA, Merx RJHM. 1995. *Effect of Iodized Salt on the Colour and Taste of Food*. New York: UNICEF.

Zlotkin S, Arthur P, Antwi KY, Yeung G. 2001. Treatment of anemia with microencapsulated ferrous fumarate plus ascorbic acid supplied as sprinkles to complementary (weaning) foods. *Am J Clin Nutr* 74(6):791–795.

A

Workshop Agenda

Nutrient Composition of Military Rations for Short-Term, High-Stress Combat Operations

Committee on Military Nutrition Research

Food and Nutrition Board

Institute of Medicine

The National Academies

US Army Research Institute of Environmental Medicine, Natick, MA
August 9-11, 2004

August 9, 2004

1:00 pm   **WELCOME AND INTRODUCTORY REMARKS**
John Erdman, Chair, Committee on Military Nutrition Research (CMNR)

1:10 pm   **INTRODUCTION TO COMBAT RATIONS**
(Moderator: Wayne Askew, CMNR)

1:15   Specifying Optimal Nutrient Composition for Military Assault
              Rations
              Andrew Young, US Army Research Institute of Environmental
              Medicine(USARIEM)

1:35   Physiological Demands of Combat Operations
              Scott Montain, USARIEM

1:55   Medical Consequences of Combat Operations
              MAJ Sangeeta Kaushik, USARIEM

2:15   Discussion on Rations

2:45 pm   **OPTIMIZATION OF MACRONUTRIENT COMPOSITION**
              (Moderator: Robin Kanarek, Tufts University)

2:50   Carbohydrate and Fat Intake: What is the Optimal Balance?
              Jorn Helge, Copenhagen Muscle Research Center

3:10   Carbohydrate-Protein Balance for Muscle Performance
              Kevin Tipton, University of Birmingham, UK

3:30   Carbohydrate Ingestion During Intense Activity
              Edward Coyle, University of Texas at Austin

3:50   BREAK

4:05   Macronutrient Composition of Military Rations for Cognitive
              Performance in Short-Term, High-Stress Situations
              Randall Kaplan, Canadian Sugar Institute

4:25   Do Structured Lipids Offer Advantages for Negative Energy
              Balance Stress Conditions?
              Ronald Jandacek, University of Cincinnati

4:45   Optimum Protein Intake in Hypocaloric States
              L. John Hoffer, Jewish General Hospital

5:05   Discussion on Optimization of Macronutrient Composition

6:00   End of Day

August 10, 2004

8:00 am   Breakfast

**8:30 am   OPTIMIZATION OF MICRONUTRIENT COMPOSITION
            AND ADDITION OF OTHER BIOACTIVE COMPOUNDS**
            *(Moderator: Rob Russell, Committee on Nutrient Composition of
            Rations)*

8:35   Vitamins C and E in the Prevention of Oxidative Stress,
            Inflammation and Fatigue from Exhaustive Exercise
            Maret Traber, Oregon State University

8:55   Zinc, Magnesium, Copper, Iron, Selenium, and Calcium in Assault
            Rations: Roles in Promotion of Physical and Mental Performances
            *Henry Lukaski, USDA-ARS Grand Forks Human Nutrition
            Research Center*

9:15   Effect of Inadequate B Vitamin Intake and Extreme Physical Stress
            Lynn Bailey, University of Florida

9:35   Optimization of the Nutrient Composition in Military Rations for
            Short-Term, High-Intensity Situations: Sodium, Potassium, and
            Other Electrolytes
            Susan Shirreffs, Loughborough University, UK

9:55   Other Bioactive Food Components and Dietary Supplements
            Becky Costello, National Institutes of Health

10:15   BREAK

10:30   Discussion of Micronutrient Composition and Addition of
            Bioactive Compounds

12:00 pm   LUNCH

1:00 pm   OPTIMIZATION OF THE IMMUNE SYSTEM
            (Moderator: Esther Sternberg, CMNR)

1:05   Effect of Physical Activity and Other Stressors on Appetite:
            Overcoming Underconsumption of Military Operational Rations
            James Stubbs, Rowett Research Institute

1:30   Optimization of Immune Function in Military Personnel
            *Simin Meydani, Jean Mayer USDA Human Nutrition Research
            Center on Aging at Tufts University*

1:50   Optimization of Nutrient Composition for Assault Rations:
            Interaction of Stress with Immune Function
            Ronenn Roubenoff, Tufts University

2:10   BREAK

2:25   Discussion of Immune/Stress

3:15 pm   NUTRITIONAL PREVENTIVE MEDICINE
            (Moderator: Bruce Bistrian, CMNR)

3:20   The Potential Impact of Prebiotics and Probiotics on
            Gastrointestinal and Immune Health of Combat Soldiers
            Mary Ellen Sanders, Food Culture Technologies

3:40   Development of a Low Residue Diet
            Joanne Slavin, University of Minnesota

4:00   Diet and Kidney Stones: Optimizing Military Field Rations
            Linda Massey, Washington State University

4:20   Discussion of Immune/Stress and Gastrointestinal Gut Barrier

5:30   End of Day

August 11, 2004

8:00 am   Breakfast

8:30 am   FOOD PRODUCT DEVELOPMENT
            *(Moderator: Brian Wansink, University of Illinois at Urbana-
            Champaign)*

8:35   Assault Rations: Organoleptic, Satiability, and Engineering
            Challenges
            Dennis Passe, Scout Consulting, LLC

8:55	Foods for People under Stress: Special Considerations *Steven Wood, Abbott Laboratories*
9:15	Food Intake Regulation: Diurnal and Dietary Composition Components *Rick Mattes, Purdue University*
9:35	A General Model of Intake Regulation: Diurnal and Dietary Composition Components *John de Castro, University of Texas at El Paso*
9:55	Discussion of Food Product Development
11:30	Adjourn

B

Workshop Papers

Specifying Optimal Nutrient Composition for Military Assault Rations

Andrew J. Young, US Army Research Institute of Environmental Medicine
Gerald A. Darsch, US Army Soldier Systems Center

INTRODUCTION

This report summarizes expert panel deliberations during a workshop organized by the Committee on Military Nutrition Research (CMNR) of the Food and Nutrition Board of the Institute of Medicine (IOM). The CMNR organized the workshop to address questions raised by the US Army Research Institute of Environmental Medicine (USARIEM) regarding optimal nutritional content for a new individual combat ration, First Strike Ration (FSR), being developed by Department of Defense (DoD) Combat Feeding Directorate at the US Army Natick Soldier Center. This new restricted ration was developed for highly mobile soldiers in high-intensity conflict by providing foods that can be eaten "on the move." As a result, the FSR is smaller and lighter than the main individual operational ration, the Meal, Ready-to-Eat (MRE). In addition to their practicality, the FSR received high customer acceptance during recent deployments (Operation Enduring Freedom, Operation Iraqi Freedom). However, constraints imposed by ration design factors on the range of food components suitable for inclusion in an FSR might limit intake of certain nutrients needed to maintain soldier performance during sustained combat operations. The IOM ad hoc committee, charged with evaluating those concerns and recommending optimal nutrient content for future versions of the ration, convened a workshop to gather information regarding the nutritional needs of individuals doing high-intensity activities for a short term while under stress.

OPERATIONAL RATIONS AND MILITARY OPERATIONS

US Army Field Feeding Doctrine (i.e., fundamental principles by which the military forces guide their actions) calls for supporting soldiers by providing them with "the right meal at the right place at the right time" (US Department of the Army, 1996). To accomplish this, Natick Soldier Center's DoD Combat Feeding Directorate conducts research, development, testing, evaluation and engineering support for combat rations, field food service equipment and total combat feeding systems for the military services and the Defense Logistics Agency. To that end, the Combat Feeding Directorate has developed an appropriate range of combat rations that are available for requisition through the military supply system. Each of these rations is designed to meet the Military Reference Dietary Intakes (MDRIs) as established in AR 40-25 (US Departments of the Army, Navy, and Air Force, 2001). Detailed descriptions, including menus, nutrient content, and packaging information for the entire spectrum of these operational rations, are documented elsewhere (US Department of Defense, 2004). Table B-1 briefly summarizes key features for several of the most widely used rations.

In those instances when operational conditions preclude serving hot, cafeteria-style rations, military personnel are provided individual operational rations, of which the MRE is the flagship ration. The nutrient requirements of most deployed soldiers can be satisfied when they are provided MREs or other appropriate rations listed in Table B-1. However, due to several factors explained below, the current rations may not completely satisfy nutritional requirements of soldiers in some situations (i.e., during the assault phase of combat operations, certain Special Operations Forces missions, and missions anticipated to be conducted by Future Force Soldiers).

First, daily energy expenditures of personnel engaged in these types of military missions are so high (Tharion et al., 2005) that these soldiers will not maintain an energy balance even when they consume three complete MREs per day, which could lead to adverse physiological effects and detriments in health and performance (see also next section on "Physiological Demands of Combat Operations"). Moreover, in some cases during combat operations, soldiers receive only two MREs, which further exacerbates the situation.

Second, soldiers who must carry heavy loads or engage in strenuous military duties (e.g., light infantry, US Marine Corps, and Special Operation Forces) compound their energy balance problem by "field-stripping" the MREs. To lighten their heavy loads, soldiers often open the individual meal packages, select certain components based on individual preference, and discard the remainder.

TABLE B-1 Principle Types of Operational Rations Fielded by the US Department of Defense

Ration	Purpose	Nutrition (Average Meal)	Key Characteristics
Unit Group Ration/Heat & Serve	Group Feeding (50 meal/module)	1,450 kcal 14% protein 32% fat 54% carbohydrate	21 menus (14 lunch/dinner, 7 breakfast) Includes semi perishables 18 month shelf-life 113 lb, 5 ft^3/module Organized food service required
Unitized Group Ration, A	Group Feeding (50 meal/module)	1,450 kcal 14% protein 32% fat 54% carbohydrate	21 menus (same as above) Includes perishables 3 month shelf life (made-to-order) 113 lb, 5 ft^3/module Organized food service required
Meal, Ready-to-Eat (MRE)	Individual Feeding (3 MREs/day)	1,300 kcal 13% protein 34% fat 53% carbohydrate	24 menus Heat processed foods in flexible retort pouches 36 month shelf-life 1.5 lb, 0.052 ft^3/meal Ready-to-Eat
Meal, Cold-Weather/ Food Packet, Long Range Patrol (MCW/LRP)	Individual Feeding (1 to 3 MCW/LRP per day) during cold-weather or special operation forces and marine corps	1,540 kcal 15% protein 35% fat 50% carbohydrate	12 menus Dehydrated and dried food components, 28–40 oz water needed to fully rehydrate 36 month shelf life 1 lb/meal, 0.04 ft^3/meal Individually prepared

SOURCE: US Department of Defense (2004).

Because MREs and other rations were designed to meet the nutritional needs of deployed soldiers who consume the entire daily ration (in which the nutrients are not evenly distributed), such selective consumption will further decrease total intake of energy and/or will compromise adequate intake of specific nutrients. Although field-stripping does, in fact, lighten a soldier's load, the cost of the discarded components can approach $34 over a three-day period. More importantly, studies at USARIEM and elsewhere have documented a variety of adverse biomedical and performance consequences (Lieberman, 2003; Montain and Young,

2003) when such semistarvation is coupled with other physiological stressors encountered during sustained combat operations (e.g., sleep deprivation, anxiety, dehydration).

The need for a specialized ration for high-tempo, assault-type missions has been recognized since the end of World War II (Samuels et al., 1947) when military planners recommended development of an "Assault Candy Ration." To better meet the individual's nutritional needs during these high-intensity operations, Natick Soldier Center's Combat Feeding Directorate have developed a new smaller, lighter, individual operational ration comprised of eat-on-the-move food components, the FSR. The FSR is intended for use during specific missions such as those described above when soldiers must operate for periods of three days, or possibly longer, with minimal resupply. This ration will serve to "bridge the gap" until operational tempo abates and more nutritionally complete rations can provided. Because of the relevance of the operations for which FSRs are envisioned, their full implementation in the field may occur in an accelerated fashion; in fact, it is estimated that the FSR, pending the military services' approval, will enter the procurement system in the first part of 2007. Through the use of spiral development generated under an Army Technology Objective (ATO) entitled "Nutritionally Optimized FSR" (IV.MD.2005.02), jointly sponsored by USARIEM and the Natick Soldier Center Combat Feeding Program, science and technology innovations are planned for insertion as part of a preplanned product improvement program. The objective of this ATO is to develop and utilize novel nutrient delivery systems, food formulations, and field feeding strategies to provide on-demand access to specific nutrients to best sustain performance. The specific strategies, when identified, will improve overall energy and nutrient intake by 20 percent and enhance cognitive and physical performance by 20 percent. The DOD asked the IOM committee to provide recommendations that will guide the design of the ration for sustained combat operations and will identify nutritional research to accomplish this objective.

WORKSHOP TASKING: RECOMMENDATIONS FOR NUTRITIONAL OPTIMIZATION OF THE FIRST-STRIKE RATION

Overall Approach

The Committee on Optimization of Nutrient Composition of Military Rations for Short-Term, High-Stress Situations asked the workshop participants to consider the specific requirements for the FSR (size, volume, weight) that constrain the ration's design such that the ration is unlikely to provide enough energy to match the daily energy expenditures of the soldiers. Table B-2 lists important design features and performance objectives for the FSR development effort. The workshop's primary objective was to gather information and provide recommendations regarding nutritional strategies suitable for implementation to

TABLE B-2 Field Feeding Approaches During Assault Phase Operations

	Current			Future
Existing/ Desired Characteristic	3 MREs/day	3 MRE's, Field- Stripped	FSR (prototype)	FSR Goals
Size	0.25 ft^3	0.16 ft^3	0.13 ft^3	TBD
Weight	4.75 lb	3.2 lb	2.51 lb	TBD
Nutritional Content	3,900 kcal	Unknown	2,855 kcal	TBD kcal
	489 g carbohydrate		370 g carbohydrate	TBD g carbohydrate
	132 g protein		101 g protein	TBD g protein
	12 mg zinc		? zinc	TBD g zinc
Nutrient Delivery (% consumed)	60	Unknown	90	95
Performance		Unknown		
Cognitive/Vigilance	Sustained		Sustained	Enhanced
Physical	Sustained		Sustained	Enhanced

NOTE: FSR = First Strike Ration; MRE = Meal, Ready-to-Eat; TBD = to be determined.

make an FSR that would best sustain health and performance despite semi-starvation arising from high daily energy expenditure and constrained energy intake. Box B-1 details several specific questions that the workshop was directed to address. The overall question was the following: Given the fact that weight and size limitations preclude the FSR from completely preventing negative energy balance in soldiers subsisting on the ration, would health and performance best be preserved by a nutrient composition that *maximizes energy density* (i.e., minimize energy deficit) or, alternatively, *by a micro- and macronutrient composition that specifically optimizes health status and performance*, potentially at the expense of a less than maximum energy density?

Besides addressing nutrient content, the speakers at the workshop were also asked to consider ration design approaches to enhance overall consumption of the ration. The problem of ration underconsumption during field training and operational deployments is well documented and was the focus of an earlier report (IOM, 1995). The CMNR previously concluded that five broad categories of factors contributed to ration under consumption.

The first four categories of factors related to the environment and to behavior that potentially impairs appetite and/or limits food consumption were identified as the following: exposure to harsh climate and danger (environment); social interactions during meals; appropriateness of the meal to time of day (eating situation); and the attitudes toward field-feeding systems held by soldiers and

---

BOX B-1
Questions to Be Addressed by CMNR Workshop on Optimization of Nutrient Composition of Military Rations for Short-Term, High-Stress Situations

1. Should energy content (energy density) of the First Strike Ration (FSR) be maximized so as to minimize the energy debt, or is there a more optimal "mix" of macronutrients and micronutrients, not necessarily producing maximal energy density?
2. What is the optimal macronutrient distribution (protein, fat, and carbohydrate) for the FSR to best sustain and/or enhance performance during combat missions?
3. What are the specific types and amounts of macronutrients (e.g., complex verses simple carbohydrates, proteins with specific amino acid profiles, type of fat, etc) to optimize such FSR to enhance performance during combat missions?
4. What are the specific types and levels of micronutrients (antioxidants, cofactors, vitamins, minerals, pre- and probiotics or other bioactives that could/should be added to the FSR to enhance performance during combat missions?
5. What strategies (passive or active) could increase FSR consumption and enhance nutritional status of soldiers conducting combat operations? Consideration should include but not be restricted to:
   i. Component packaging, types, sizing, flavors
   ii. Bioavailability factors
6. Recommendations must be feasible, practical, and physiologically meaningful.

---

their leaders (individual). Based on the CMNR recommendations, technical reports and commanders' guides have been prepared and distributed providing guidance to minimize the effect of those negative factors; however, from a practical standpoint, commanders conducting combat operations are permitted little flexibility to mitigate those kinds of stressors. The fifth category is underconsumption factors, related to a ration's characteristics that influence customer acceptability and for which the committee offered more practical recommendations to improve consumption. These recommendations included the following: to enhance menu variety; to improve food sensory features, packaging, and ease of use for the rations and components; and to provide smaller snacking or "nibbling" food items as well as energy- and nutrient-rich beverages that could be carried in pockets and consumed quickly while on the move.

Clearly, those recommendations should be the driving focus behind the FSR. All of those approaches have already been incorporated into the newest versions of the MRE and other operational rations during the continuous product improvement programs that Combat Feeding Directorate conducts and they have been recognized by troops who consume combat rations. For this workshop, the panel of experts was asked to consider how similar, practical approaches could be used to further enhance consumption of the FSR, thereby better satisfying the nutritional needs of soldiers during assault type operations.

Workshop Overview

Under the auspices of the CMNR, the Committee on Optimization of Nutrient Composition of Military Rations for Short-Term, High-Stress Situations and the IOM organized a workshop to address the questions posed by USARIEM. The workshop was hosted by USARIEM and the Natick Soldier Center in Natick, MA, in August 2004. USARIEM scientists provided the workshop participants with their tasks, overviews of military ration systems, and background briefings on the physiological and medical consequences of combat operations on military personnel. For the remainder of the workshop, invited scientific experts presented information on topics organized into five major categories: optimization of macronutrient composition; optimization of micronutrients and other bioactive compounds; nutritional optimization of the immune system; nutritional preventive medicine; and food product development. Those presentations are the basis for the remainder of this report.

REFERENCES

IOM (Institute of Medicine). 1995. *Not Eating Enough*. Washington, DC: National Academy Press.
Lieberman HR. 2003. Nutrition, brain function and cognitive performance. *Appetite* 40(3):245–254.
Montain SJ, Young AJ. 2003. Diet and physical performance. *Appetite* 40(3):255–267.
Samuels JP, McDevitt RP, Bollman MC, Maclinn W, Richardson LM, Voss LG. Conway HA. 1947. In: Meyer AI, eds. *Ration Development*. Operational Studies 1(12). Fort Lee, VA: Office of the Quartermaster General.
Tharion WJ, Lieberman HR, Montain SJ, Young AJ, Baker-Fulco CJ, Delany JP, Hoyt RW. 2005. Energy requirements of military personnel. *Appetite* 44(1):47–65.
US Department of the Army. 1996. *Basic Doctrine for Army Field Feeding and Class 1 Operations Management*. FM 10-23. Washington, DC: Department of the Army.
US Department of Defense. 2004. *Operational Rations of the Department of Defense*. Natick PAM 30-25. Natick, MA: US Army Natick Soldier Center.
US Departments of Army, Navy, and Air Force. 2001. *Nutrition Standards and Education*. AR 40-25/BUMEDINST 10110.6/AFI 44-141. Washington, DC: US Department of Defense Headquarters.

Physiological Demands of Combat Operations

Scott J. Montain, US Army Research Institute of Environmental Medicine

INTRODUCTION

The combat foot soldiers within the light infantry and special operations units are the military populations targeted for use of next-generation assault rations. These soldiers are required to carry or transport all of the supplies, sometimes exceeding 50 kg, they will need for the operation. Missions often are of the continuous type termed "sustained operations" (SUSOPS) lasting from two to seven days or longer that consist of near-continuous physical work, restricted sleep, and limited breaks for meals. While the energy cost of any single task is not necessarily high, total daily energy expenditures can reach extremely high levels because of long hours of wakefulness. Thus, these soldiers are faced with sustained environmental exposure, exertional fatigue, sleep deprivation, and energy deficits.

The lightweight and small assault ration being developed specifically for these soldiers must be capable of sustaining their performance while in repeated SUSOPS missions lasting for three days when energy expenditures exceed 18 MJ (4,300 kcal)/day, and up to seven days during which daily energy expenditures are expected to be less. This chapter describes the physiological challenges facing combat foot soldiers to facilitate defining their nutritional requirements. This topic has been discussed in greater depth in other publications (Friedl, 2003; Tharion et al., 2005), and the reader is referred to these papers for additional information.

ENERGY COST OF SOLDIER ACTIVITIES

The total daily energy expenditures of combat units during training exercises has ranged from 15.5 to 29.8 MJ (3,700 to 7,120 kcal)/day (Figure B-1); with the highest values occurring during cold-weather operations. The tasks performed typically have included long, sustained periods of low to moderate intensity work (expected metabolic rates of 250 to 450 Watts), with short periods of relatively high-intensity work (expected metabolic rates in excess of 600 Watts). Factors contributing to these high daily energy expenditures have been the relatively long periods of work (> 15 h/day), traversing rough terrain or soft surfaces (e.g., snow, mud, or sand), and carrying heavy loads.

Much of what we know regarding the energy cost of soldier activities comes from investigations of soldiers performing simulated combat missions as part of training courses. In these scenarios, total daily energy expenditures (TDEE) are often quite high. For example, airmen participating in the US Air Force Combat Survival Course averaged 19.7 MJ (4,700 kcal)/day of TDEE (Jones et al., 1992),

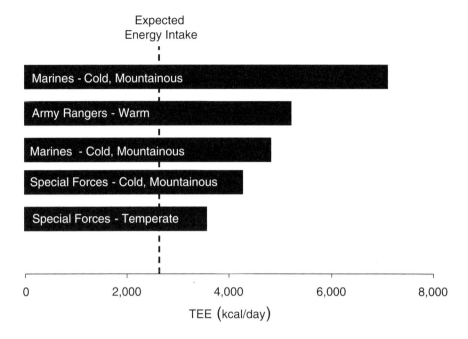

FIGURE B-1 Measured troop energy expenditures during military field operations.
NOTE: TEE = total energy expenditure.
SOURCE: Tharion et al. (2005).

soldiers attending the US Army Special Forces Assessment School averaged 21.7 MJ (5,180 kcal)/day (Fairbrother et al., 1995), and marines at the US Marine Corps Infantry Officer Course averaged 22.5 MJ (4,700 kcal)/day of TDEE during cold-weather operations (Hoyt et al., 2001) and 16 to17 MJ (3,820 to 4,060 kcal)/day during hot weather (author's unpublished results; personal communication, R. Hoyt, US Army Research Institute of Environmental Medicine, 1999). The US Air Force Combat Survival Course is a 5-day course that trains aircrew members in parachuting and survival, evasion, resistance, and escape procedures, as well as simulated prisoner of war interrogations. The US Army Special Forces Assessment School conducts 20-day training and includes activities such as physical fitness tests, battle marches, and long-range movements carrying backpacks, weapons, and other field equipment. In the Marine Corps Infantry Officer Course, marines perform a series of simulated combat operations using dismounted infantry, mounted infantry, and amphibious tactics. In each of these courses, night operations are included, leading to near-continuous physical work, with marines active 16 to 22 h/day.

Students enrolled in the US Army Ranger training course perform a series of physically demanding field exercises intermittently over a 60-day period. While total energy expenditures averaged over the 60-day course are lower than those for many of the shorter, more intense military training courses, they are still quite high, averaging 16.8 MJ (4,010 kcal)/day (Moore et al., 1992) and 17.1 MJ (4,090 kal)/day (Shippee et al., 1994) for more than two months. Combat fundamentals taught during the course include patrolling; squad reconnaissance and ambush; mountaineering; small boat operations; and attack, ambush, and raid drills. The unique aspect of this course is repeated, periodic food restriction and sleep deprivation as one of the intentional stressors—making it a model for studying the physiological strain likely to be imposed on soldiers performing repeated SUSOPS missions during combat, which is the subject of interest in this workshop.

As noted in the introduction, combat foot soldiers carry their own supplies at high energy expenditure costs. The loads they carry can be very heavy depending on what phase of a mission they are performing. A recent study (Dean and Dupont, 2003) in which soldier loads were measured during actual operations in Afghanistan revealed that soldiers in the traveling phase of a mission carried an average of 59.3 kg (131 lb). Their approach load averaged 45.7 kg (101 lb), and their fighting load averaged 28.5 kg (63 lb). When normalized to body weight, these loads were equivalent to carrying 77 percent, 57 percent, and 35 percent of body mass, respectively. Current soldier development efforts are exploring methods to dramatically lower the soldier load, but soldier load remains a major physical stressor during combat execution.

PHYSIOLOGICAL CONSEQUENCES OF COMBAT OPERATIONS

The massive load each soldier carries limits the amount of space and weight that soldiers are willing to reserve for food. The nature of SUSOPS missions also means that food is consumed on the go. These two factors lead to soldiers stripping their personal rations of items that they don't like or will be unlikely to eat. When voluntary intake has been measured, it typically averages between 10 and 12 MJ (2,390 to 2,870 kcal) (Baker-Fulco, 1995). Since energy expenditure is often much higher than intake, there is demand placed on endogenous energy stores to meet energy demands of the mission.

Metabolic Status and Body Composition Changes

Blood glucose levels typically decrease over SUSOPS missions, but the average values generally only fall 10 mg/dL (0.5 to 0.6 mM) from baseline values. There are soldiers, however, who demonstrate much higher reductions. In a recent investigation (author's unpublished results), during which marines consumed 1,600 kcal/day and 210 g of carbohydrate/day while expending

3,850 kcal/day, it was observed that 12 to 23 percent of volunteers had blood glucose values below 76 mg/dL (< 4.2 mM) after four to eight days of SUSOPS. Concomitant with these metabolic changes were substantial increases in blood ketone and free fatty acid concentrations.

The underfeeding accompanying SUSOPS is accompanied by reductions of both fat and lean body mass. For example, Nindl and colleagues (2002) reported fat and lean tissues losses of 1.2 and 1.5 kg, respectively, over a 72 h SUSOPS. Similarly, Moore and colleagues (1992) reported that 38 percent of the 12 kg body mass loss that occurred during Ranger training (when severely underfed) was attributable to nonfat tissue loss.

Cognitive Performance

Opstad and colleagues (1978) found that visual vigilance decreased 4 to 28 percent after three to four days of sustained operations activity. Reaction time and coding declined 12 to 30 percent over the same time period, while prone marksmanship declined 10 percent. Inclusion of three to six hours of continuous sleep once during the five-day operation partially or fully reversed these declines. There was large interindividual variability, but general deterioration occurred due to omissions, not mistakes. Similar results have been reported by others, as Bugge and colleagues (1979) observed, decreased logical reasoning (46 percent), letter cancellation attempts (40 percent), and code test scores (45 percent) after four days of sustained operations. More recently, Tharion and colleagues (1997) reported a reduction in visual vigilance (44 percent), slower processing (21 percent), and fewer correct responses (17 percent) on a four-choice reaction test, and compromised performance on a match to sample task after 73 to 74 h of sleep deprivation and operational stress. Associated with the impaired cognitive performance were increased levels of fatigue, confusion, tension, and depression. Shippee and colleagues (1994) evaluated decoding, memory, reasoning, and pattern recognition during the eight-week US Army Ranger Course. Soldiers maintained near perfect accuracy at decoding and reasoning at the expense of speed (7 to 10 percent fewer attempts). Memory accuracy declined over time. Both speed and accuracy were impaired on the pattern recognition task—particularly during the desert and jungle phases.

Physical Performance

Prolonged operations lasting several weeks' duration and associated with substantial losses of lean body mass (Moore et al., 1992; Shippee et al., 1994) have resulted in reductions (20 percent) in maximal lifting capacity and vertical jump height (15 to 16 percent). Shorter duration studies with minimal lean body mass loss generally showed little or no decrement in muscle strength, power, or fatigability (Bulbulian et al., 1996; Guezennec et al., 1994; Vanhelder and

Radomski, 1989); however, this is not universal (Legg and Patton, 1987). Sustained operations scenarios lasting less than one week have resulted in reduced maximal aerobic power and endurance (Guezennec et al., 1994) as have sleep-deprivation studies (Vanhelder and Radomski, 1989).

Performance of simple and well-learned motor tasks (e.g., weapon handling) do not appear to be compromised by sustained operational stress (Haslam, 1984). However, endurance time is frequently impaired during aerobic exercise tasks (Vanhelder and Radomski, 1989), and there is an increased perception of effort to perform the same task. Nindl and colleagues (2002) recently reported 25 percent lower work productivity on a physical persistence task; in agreement with the hypothesis that SUSOPS compromises prolonged and monotonous tasks (Figure B-2). Independent of energy intake (Rognum et al., 1986), operational effectiveness is also affected if sleep is inadequate.

Marksmanship can be compromised by sustained operation activities particularly when very little restorative sleep is obtained. Tharion and colleagues

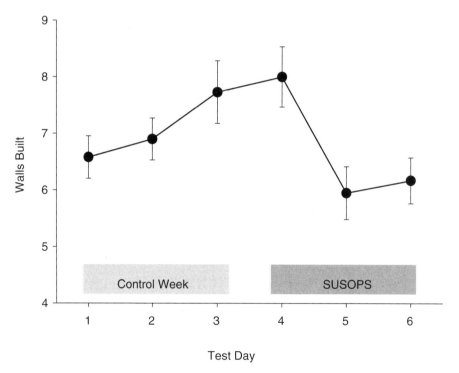

FIGURE B-2 Work productivity on a physical persistence task over 72 h of simulated military sustained operations (SUSOPS) training as well as a control week without near-continuous work and underfeeding.
SOURCE: Nindl et al. (2002).

(2003) reported significantly impaired marksmanship after 73 to 74 hours of total sleep deprivation during Navy Seal training. Specifically, they observed greater distance from center of mass (38 percent) increased dispersion of shot groups (235 percent), as well more missed targets (37 percent), all indicative of reduced marksmanship. These adverse findings occurred despite a 53 percent slowei sighting time. In contrast, Johnson and colleagues (2001) reported that despite soldiers rating the marksmanship task as more difficult to perform after 48 and 72 h of SUSOPS (2 h of sleep per night), there was no reduction in the number of randomly appearing targets hit during the test. Haslam (1984) reported no negative results during nine days of sustained operations and sleeping either 1.5 or 3 h daily on shot group clustering when troops fired in the prone supported position. However, their ability to acquire and accurately hit a randomly appearing target declined during the course. The group receiving only 1.5 h of daily sleep performed 50 percent below baseline from days 5–9 of the field exercise, whereas the group receiving 3 h of daily sleep had a more modest reduction (the number of hits fell from 6–7 to 4–5).

Similarly, the caloric deficit associated with sustained operations scenarios appears to have inconsistent effects on soldier performance (Montain and Young, 2003). Rognum and colleagues (1986) reported no difference either in time to complete an assault course or in prone marksmanship performance when students were provided 1,500 or 8,000 kcal/day during a five-day scenario. However, Guezennec and colleagues (1994) observed 8 percent reductions in maximal aerobic power when soldiers were restricted to 1,800 kcal/day but no reduction in maximal aerobic power when soldiers were fed 3,200 or 4,200 kcal/day. Similarly, Tharion and Moore (1993) reported reductions in shot group tightness on a marksmanship task after sustained road marching soldiers were fed 250 g of carbohydrate per day, but no change when soldiers consumed a diet with 400 or 550 g of carbohydrate.

Time and content of the previous meal may be an explanation for the divergent results. Montain and colleagues (1997) reported a relationship in that an increase in energy (or carbohydrate) intake sustains uphill run time over three days of physically demanding field training. Moreover, 11 of 13 soldiers who best sustained uphill-run performance had eaten 70 to 378 g of carbohydrate during the four h preceding the uphill run, while 10 of the 13 soldiers with the greatest decrement had eaten none of their rations since the previous night's meal. All participants in this study were provided with two Meals, Ready-to-Eat each day or approximately 2,600 kcal and 300 g of carbohydrate per day. These data suggest that soldiers subsisting on diets with these energy and carbohydrate levels during high-tempo operations are receiving near the minimum energy necessary to sustain performance, necessitating good food discipline (i.e., eating the food provided), and good food choices (i.e., eat the carbohydrate-containing foods) to preserve physical performance.

Endocrine Changes

Dramatic changes in the blood hormonal milieu arise during sustained operations protocols and persist during both rest and exercise. In the five day Norwegian Ranger Course, in which food and sleep are kept to a minimum, there was a progressive increase in catecholamine concentration (Rognum et al., 1981) as well as cortisol, growth hormone, and aldosterone levels (Opstad, 1992; Opstad and Aakvaag, 1981) and a reciprocal fall in testosterone and prolactin (Opstad and Aakvaag, 1982) as well as other adrenal and testicular androgens (Opstad, 1992). The increase in catecholamine concentration is associated with a downregulation of adrenergic receptors on white blood cells (Opstad et al., 1994). Similar observations have been reported for soldiers participating in the US Army Ranger Selection Course (Moore et al., 1992; Shippee et al., 1994).

The decline in testosterone (up to 70 percent from baseline) and other anabolic hormones may be due in part to the caloric and/or protein restriction imposed during the courses. Short periods of refeeding quickly reverse declines in insulin-like growth factor-1 (IGF-1) (Friedl et al., 2000) (Figure B-3). When additional energy of a mixed diet of protein, fat, and carbohydrate have been provided (400 and 1,400 kcal), reductions in IGF-1 and testosterone were attenuated (Friedl et al., 2000; Guezennec et al., 1994). However, when additional calories (4,900 kcal) have been provided predominately by carbohydrate alone, testosterone reductions were only modestly lowered (Opstad and Aakvaag, 1982), suggesting that the testosterone and IGF-1 changes may have been consequent to energy deficit and possibly insufficient amino acid intake (Sanchez-Gomez et al., 1999).

Immune Function

The effects of sustained operations on immune function remain poorly understood. The outbreak of infectious disease among soldiers participating in US Army Ranger and Special Forces Assessment Schools suggests that multistress environments can compromise immune defense mechanisms (Moore et al., 1992). Changes in immune cell parameters and in vitro responses to stress have varied from study to study, but they appear related to the duration and severity of the sustained operations stress.

The five day Norwegian Ranger Course produced a general leukocytosis, predominantly due to two- to threefold increase in neutrophils and monocytes (Boyum et al., 1996). Lymphocyte numbers decreased as did CD4 T cells, CD8 T cells, CD16 natural killer cells, and CD19 B cells. Neutrophil chemotaxis and oxidative burst capacity increased during the course before returning to baseline levels (or below) after five days of training (Wiik et al., 1996). These changes have been attributed to sleep deprivation and appear relatively insensitive to changes in caloric (carbohydrate) intake (Wiik et al., 1996). Immunoglobulin M

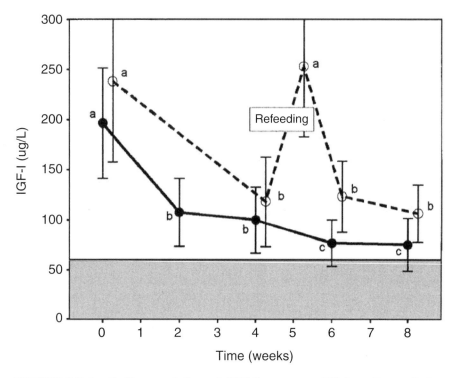

FIGURE B-3 Insulin-like growth factor-1 (IGF-1) response to US Army Ranger Training under two levels of underfeeding and response to several days of refeeding during the course. Letters indicate means that are not significantly different (Scheffe's test).
NOTE: Different letters indicate a significant difference in IGF-1 response (e.g., a versus b).
SOURCE: Friedl et al. (2000).

and immunoglobulin A decrease 20 to 30 percent during the course, while mitogenic responses to antigen exposure have not been consistent from course to course (Boyum et al., 1996).

The activities of the eight week US Army Ranger School appear to modify immune function, although the magnitude varies among the type of response. For example, Moore and colleagues (1992) found a similar percentage of positive delayed hypersensitivity responses to streptococcus and tetanus over the course despite relatively severe sleep deprivation and a 16 percent drop in body mass. There was no change in immunoglobulin concentrations during the course. However, as lymphocyte proliferation to mitogen stimulation declined during the course, an increasing number of students became pneumonia carriers, and 25 percent of the students sought medical attention for infections during the final portion of the course (swamp and desert phases).

Additional ranger studies (Bernton et al., 1995) revealed reductions in cell mediated immunity responses among the trainees. Shippee and colleagues (1994) examined immunological responses after students were provided additional calories during the course. Only 2 to 8 percent of the students required medical attention during the mountain and swamp phases. Immunoglobulin levels did not change, and neutrophil oxidative burst capability increased during the course. There was a general leukocytosis, due primarily to increased granulocytes, but lymphocyte concentrations fell. The ability of leukocytes to proliferate in response to mitogen stimulation was suppressed but was less than reported in previous courses when underfeeding was more severe (Moore et al., 1992). These latter responses suggest a possible shift in proportion of lymphocytes of the T-helper type 1 (T_{H1}) phenotype (cell-mediated) to the T-helper type 2 (T_{H2}) phenotype (antibody-mediated). This immune system adaptation occurs after trauma (Decker et al., 1996; Mack et al., 1997; O'Sullivan et al., 1995) and with disease (Raziuddin et al., 1998) and can immunocompromise the host to certain types of infectious agents (Mack et al., 1997; O'Sullivan et al., 1995).

SUMMARY

The goal of the US military developmental assault ration, currently called the First Strike Ration, is to sustain troop health and performance for at least 96 h of unsupported military operations. To accomplish this objective, the nutritional components must sustain a soldier commonly expending in excess of 18 MJ (4,300 kcal) of energy per day and carrying loads in excess of 45 to 50 kg during while exposed to environmental extremes. It is well documented that the mission stress can challenge immune and neuroendocrine homeostasis and if sutained too long or repeated too frequently, that troop health and performance can be compromised. Likewise, there is evidence that nutritional support can reduce the physiological strain. The challenge is in defining the proper mix of macro- and micro-nutrients to sustain the soldier within a ration system the soldiers will choose to carry and consume during mission execution.

ACKNOWLEDGMENTS

The views, opinions and/or findings in this report are those of the authors, and should not be construed as an official Department of the Army position, policy, or decision, unless so designated by other official documentation.

REFERENCES

Baker-Fulco CJ. 1995. Overview of dietary intakes during military exercises. In: Marriott BM, ed. *Not Eating Enough*. Washington, DC: National Academy Press. Pp. 121–149.

Bernton E, Hoover D, Galloway R, Popp K. 1995. Adaptation to chronic stress in military trainees. Adrenal androgens, testosterone, glucocorticoids, IGF-1, and immune function. *Ann N Y Acad Sci* 774:217–231.

Boyum A, Wiik P, Gustavsson E, Veiby OP, Reseland J, Haugen AH, Opstad PK. 1996. The effect of strenuous exercise, calorie deficiency and sleep deprivation on white blood cells, plasma immunoglobulins and cytokines. *Scand J Immunol* 43(2):228–235.

Buggc JF, Opstad PK, Magnus PM. 1979. Changes in the circadian rhythm of performance and mood in healthy young men exposed to prolonged, heavy physical work, sleep deprivation, and caloric deficit. *Aviat Space Environ Med* 50(7):663–668.

Bulbulian R, Heaney JH, Leake CN, Sucec AA, Sjoholm NT. 1996. The effect of sleep deprivation and exercise load on isokinetic leg strength and endurance. *Eur J Appl Physiol Occup Physiol* 73(3–4):273–277.

Dean CE, Dupont F. 2003. *Modern Warrior's Combat Load. Dismounted Operations in Afghanistan. April–May 2003.* Letter Report. Ft. Leavenworth, KS: US Army Center for Army Lessons Learned.

Decker D, Schondorf M, Bidlingmaier F, Hirner A, von Ruecker AA. 1996. Surgical stress induces a shift in the type-1/type-2 T-helper cell balance, suggesting down-regulation of cell-mediated and up-regulation of antibody-mediated immunity commensurate to the trauma. *Surgery* 119(3):316–325.

Fairbrother B, Kramer T, Mays M, Kramer M, Tulley R, Delany J, Marchitelli L, Tessicini M, Shippee RL, Askew S, Popp K, Hoyt R, Rood J, Frykman P, Arsenault J, Jezior D. 1995. *Nutritional and Immunological Assessment of Soldiers During the Special Forces Assessment and Selection Course.* Technical Report No. T95-22. Natick, MA: US Army.

Friedl KE. 2003. Military studies and nutritional immunology: Undernutrition and susceptibility to illness. In: Hughes DA, Darlington LG, Bendich A, eds. *Diet and Human Immune Function.* Towtown, NJ: Humana Press, Inc. Pp. 381–396.

Friedl KE, Moore RJ, Hoyt RW, Marchitelli LJ, Martinez-Lopez LE, Askew EW. 2000. Endocrine markers of semistarvation in healthy lean men in a multistressor environment. *J Appl Physiol* 88(5):1820–1830.

Guezennec CY, Satabin P, Legrand H, Bigard AX. 1994. Physical performance and metabolic changes induced by combined prolonged exercise and different energy intakes in humans. *Eur J Appl Physiol Occup Physiol* 68(6):525–530.

Haslam DR. 1984. The military performance of soldiers in sustained operations. *Aviat Space Environ Med* 55(3): 216-221.

Hoyt RW, Buller MJ, DeLany JP, Stultz D, Warren K, Hamlet MP, Shantz D, Matthew WT, Tharion WJ, Smith P, Smith B. 2001. *Warfighter Physiological Status Monitoring (WPSM): Energy Balance and Thermal Status during a 10-day Cold Weather US Marine Corps Infantry Officer Course Field Exercise.* Technical Report No. T02-02. Natick, MA: US Army Research Institute of Environmental Medicine.

Johnson RF, Merullo DJ, Montain SJ, Castellani JW. 2001. Marksmanship during simulated sustained operations. *Proceedings of the Human Factors and Ergonomics Society. 45th Annual Meeting.* 45:1382–1385.

Jones TE, Mutter SH, Aylward JM, DeLany JP, Stephens RL, Caretti DM, Jezior DA, Cheema B, Lester LS, Askew EW. 1992. *Nutrition and Hydration Status of Aircrew Members Consuming the Food Packet, Survival, General Purpose, Improved During a Simulated Survival Scenario.* Technical Report No. T1-93. Natick, MA: US Army Research Institute of Environmental Medicine.

Legg SJ, Patton JF. 1987. Effects of sustained manual work and partial sleep deprivation on muscular strength and endurance. *Eur J Appl Physiol Occup Physiol* 56(1):64–68.

Mack VE, McCarter MD, Naama HA, Calvano SE, Daly JM. 1997. Candida infection following severe trauma exacerbates Th2 cytokines and increases mortality. *J Surg Res* 69(2):399–407.

Montain SJ, Young AJ. 2003. Diet and physical performance. *Appetite* 40(3):255–267.

Montain SJ, Shippee RL, Tharion WJ. 1997. Carbohydrate-electrolyte solution effects on physical performance of military tasks. *Aviat Space Environ Med* 68(5):384–391.

Moore RJ, Friedl KE, Kramer TR, Martinez-Lopez LE, Hoyt RW, Tulley RE, DeLany JP, Askew EW, Vogel JA. 1992. *Changes in Soldier Nutritional Status & Immune Function During the Ranger Training Course.* Technical Report No. T13-92. Natick, MA: US Army Medical Research & Development Command.

Nindl BC, Leone CD, Tharion WJ, Johnson RF, Castellani JW, Patton JF, Montain SJ. 2002. Physical performance responses during 72 h of military operational stress. *Med Sci Sports Exerc* 34(11):1814–1822.

O'Sullivan ST, Lederer JA, Horgan AF, Chin DH, Mannick JA, Rodrick ML. 1995. Major injury leads to predominance of the T helper-2 lymphocyte phenotype and diminished interleukin-12 production associated with decreased resistance to infection. *Ann Surg* 222(4):482–490.

Opstad PK. 1992. Androgenic hormones during prolonged physical stress, sleep, and energy deficiency. *J Clin Endocrinol Metab* 74(5):1176–1183.

Opstad PK, Aakvaag A. 1981. The effect of a high calory diet on hormonal changes in young men during prolonged physical strain and sleep deprivation. *Eur J Appl Physiol Occup Physiol* 46(1):31–39.

Opstad PK, Aakvaag A. 1982. Decreased serum levels of oestradiol, testosterone and prolactin during prolonged physical strain and sleep deprivation, and the influence of a high calorie diet. *Eur J Appl Physiol Occup Physiol* 49(3):343–348.

Opstad PK, Ekanger R, Nummestad M, Raabe N. 1978. Performance, mood, and clinical symptoms in men exposed to prolonged, severe physical work and sleep deprivation. *Aviat Space Environ Med* 49(9):1065–1073.

Opstad PK, Haugen AH, Sejersted OM, Bahr R, Skrede KK. 1994. Atrial natriuretic peptide in plasma after prolonged physical strain, energy deficiency and sleep deprivation. *Eur J Appl Physiol Occup Physiol* 68(2):122–126.

Raziuddin S, al-Dalaan A, Bahabri S, Siraj AK, al-Sedairy S. 1998. Divergent cytokine production profile in Behcet's disease. Altered Th1/Th2 cell cytokine pattern. *J Rheumatol* 25(2):329–333.

Rognum TO, Vaage O, Hostmark A, Opstad PK. 1981. Metabolic responses to bicycle exercise after several days of physical work and energy deficiency. *Scand J Clin Lab Invest* 41(6):565–571.

Rognum TO, Vartdal F, Rodahl K, Opstad PK, Knudsen-Baas O, Kindt E, Withey WR. 1986. Physical and mental performance of soldiers on high- and low-energy diets during prolonged heavy exercise combined with sleep deprivation. *Ergonomics* 29(7):859–867.

Sanchez-Gomez M, Malmlof K, Mejia W, Bermudez A, Ochoa MT, Carrasco-Rodriguez S, Skottner A. 1999. Insulin-like growth factor-I, but not growth hormone, is dependent on a high protein intake to increase nitrogen balance in the rat. *Br J Nutr* 81(2):145–152.

Shippee R, Friedl K, Kramer T, Mays M, Popp K, Askew E, Fairbrother B, Hoyt R, Vogel J, Marchitelli L, Frykman P, Martinez-Lopez L, Bernton E, Kramer M, Tulley R, Rood J, Delany J, Jezior D, Arsenault J. 1994. *Nutritional and Immunological Assessment of Ranger Students with Increased Caloric Intake.* Technical Report No. T95-5. Fort Detrick, MD: US Army Medical Research and Materiel Command.

Tharion WJ, Moore RJ. 1993. *Effects of Carbohydrate Intake and Load Bearing Exercise on Rifle Marksmanship Performance.* Technical Report No. T5-93. Natick, MA: US Army Medical Research and Development Command.

Tharion WJ, Lieberman HR, Montain SJ, Young AJ, Baker-Fulco CJ, Delany JP, Hoyt RW. 2005. Energy requirements of military personnel. *Appetite* 44(1):47–65.

Tharion WJ, Shukitt-Hale B, Coffey B, Desai M, Strowman SR, Tulley R, Lieberman HR. 1997. *The Use of Caffeine to Enhance Cognitive Performance, Reaction Time, Vigilance, Rifle Marksmanship, and Mood States in Sleep-Deprived Navy SEAL (BUD/S) Trainees.* T98-4. Natick, MA: US Army Research Institute of Environmental Medicine.

Tharion WJ, Shukitt-Hale B, Lieberman HR. 2003. Caffeine effects on marksmanship during high-stress military training with 72 hour sleep deprivation. *Aviat Space Environ Med* 74(4):309–314.

VanHelder T, Radomski MW. 1989. Sleep deprivation and the effect on exercise performance. *Sports Med* 7(4):235–247.

Wiik P, Opstad PK, Boyum A. 1996. Granulocyte chemiluminescence response to serum opsonized zymosan particles ex vivo during long-term strenuous exercise, energy and sleep deprivation in humans. *Eur J Appl Physiol Occup Physiol* 73(3–4):251–258.

Carbohydrate and Fat Intake: What is the Optimal Balance?

Jørn Wulff Helge, Copenhagen Muscle Research Center

INTRODUCTION

This paper addresses the optimal distribution of fat and carbohydrate to be included in the macronutrient composition of military assault rations as well as the specific types of fat to be used in these rations, and describes possible related performance and health issues. The purpose of this paper is to provide guidance regarding questions that may be used to make recommendations for an optimal ration composition, the task of the Committee on Optimization of Nutrient Composition of Military Rations for Short-Term, High-Stress Situations. To provide practical guidance for the complex and broad issues when improving fat and carbohydrate composition of assault rations, this paper focuses on these specific questions:

What is the optimal fat–carbohydrate balance in the ration?

- Is it possible to perform strenuous physical tasks/training on a high-fat diet?
- Is there a performance enhancement under short-term exposure to a fat-rich diet?
- What do we know about the effects of energy deficit and heavy physical demand on the carbohydrate/fat balance–substrate stores?

Are there specific types of fat that are optimal for the ration?

- Do specific fatty acids affect performance?
- Do specific fatty acids affect health issues?

These questions are addressed using the assumptions specified for the military assault situation: The ration is targeted for well-trained male soldiers, with an average weight of 80 kg, undergoing average daily energy expenditures of

4,000 to 4,500 kcal, and deployed to repeatable three- to seven-day missions with recovery periods of one to three days. During these missions, they are carrying a heavy load while engaged in prolonged, low- to moderate-intensity activity (up to 20 h/day) interspersed with brief, high-intensity activity.

OPTIMAL FAT–CARBOHYDRATE BALANCE IN THE RATION

Strenuous Physical Tasks and Training on a High-Fat Diet

It is well known that work performed at higher exercise intensities requires a large contribution of carbohydrates (Brooks and Mercier, 1994). Furthermore, there is evidence that short-term, high-fat diet adaptation can be used to spare muscle glycogen and decrease carbohydrate oxidation during exercise and, hypothetically, increase high-intensity exercise capacity (Burke and Hawley, 2002; Helge, 2000). Unfortunately, such carbohydrate sparing after short-term, high-fat diet adaptation is often accompanied by a reduced muscle (Phinney et al., 1983) and liver (Hultman and Nilsson, 1971) glycogen storage in comparison with the results from consumption of a short-term, high-carbohydrate diet. It is, therefore, pertinent to know whether high-intensity exercise capacity can be upheld when dietary fat contribution is high.

Stepto and colleagues (2002) studied seven elite trained endurance athletes who underwent two four-day dietary periods consuming either a high-carbohydrate diet (70 to 75 percent carbohydrate) or a high-fat diet (> 65 percent fat) in a crossover design with an 18-day washout period in between. During the dietary adaptation period, subjects performed two controlled exercise sessions on days one and four, during which they exercised for 20 minutes at 65 percent of VO_2max and subsequently performed eight 5-minute exercise bouts at 86 percent of VO_2max interspersed with 60-second breaks. In addition to the training performed in the laboratory, the subjects also undertook training outside, but no difference in duration of training was apparent between dietary adaptation periods. The subjects were capable of performing the training, except during one high-intensity exercise bout, while consuming the fat-rich diet. Despite these results, the subjective rating of perceived exertion was higher on day four in the last few bouts after a fat-rich diet when compared with the results of a carbohydrate-rich diet (Table B-3). These results indicate that, for at least four days, elite athletes are capable of performing training at a reasonably high intensity while consuming a fat-rich diet but with a higher subjective rate of perceived exertion.

Consistent with these data, we noted that in our studies involving moderately untrained male subjects during long-term training and high-fat diet adaptation, the subjects on a high-fat diet were able to train and exercise at moderate and high intensities but perceived increased mental effort as compared with subjects on a high-carbohydrate diet (Helge, 2002). There is currently no explanation for this higher mental effort, but previous studies of subjects on a short-

TABLE B-3 Comparing the Effects of a High-Carbohydrate Diet versus a High-Fat Diet on Elite Trained Athletes

Day 4	High-Carbohydrate Diet	High-Fat Diet
VO_2 (L/minute)		
Bout 1	4.3 ± 0.4	4.3 ± 0.4
Bout 4	4.3 ± 0.4	4.4 ± 0.3
Bout 8	4.3 ± 0.3	4.5 ± 0.2
RER		
Bout 1	0.94 ± 0.03	0.86 ± 0.03
Bout 4	0.91 ± 0.03[a]	0.85 ± 0.03
Bout 8	0.90 ± 0.04[a]	0.85 ± 0.02
RPE	13.8 ± 1.8	16.00 ± 1.3[a]

NOTE: Values are mean ± standard error of the means. RER = respiratory exchange ratio; RPE = rate of perceived exertion; VO_2 = oxygen uptake during exercise at 80 percent of peak power output (86 percent VO_2max).
[a]($p < 0.05$) high carbohydrate versus high fat.
SOURCE: Stepto et al. (2002).

term adaptation to a fat-rich diet (Galbo et al., 1979; Jansson et al., 1982) found a higher catecholamine response and heart rate during submaximal exercise as compared with subjects on a carbohydrate-rich diet. The possible influence of a high-fat diet adaptation on the sympathetic nervous system response during exercise might cause mental strain; however, the mechanistic coupling between the increase in sympathetic response induced by a high-fat diet and the increased perception of exertion during submaximal exercise remains to be explained.

Effects of Short-Term Consumption of a Fat-Rich Diet on Performance

The coupling between muscle glycogen storage and endurance exercise capacity, which was demonstrated by Bergstrom and colleagues (1967), spurred researchers to investigate means to manipulate glycogen storage and use or both. One approach was a fat-rich diet adaptation, which induces markedly higher fat oxidation during exercise and reduced carbohydrate use (Christensen and Hansen, 1939; Phinney et al., 1983). This higher fat oxidation, however, occurs at the expense of a muscle glycogen concentration that is, at best, maintained and, in many cases, lower than that in those consuming a carbohydrate-rich diet (Helge et al., 1998b; Phinney et al., 1983). Despite these conflicting adaptations, a number of studies have manipulated the dietary fat content to achieve an improved performance capacity. In this context, short-term exposure to fat-rich diets is defined as adaptation periods lasting less than eight days and having a fat content contributing more than 40 percent of total energy in the diet. The studies are listed in Table B-4, and overall, only one study shows an increased capacity to perform exercise after short exposure to a fat-rich diet. This study, by Muoio and colleagues (1994), has been extensively criticized in the literature due to a nonrandomized use of diet adaptation. The remaining ten studies found either an unchanged (three studies) or decreased (seven studies) exercise capacity after a short-term, fat-rich diet, indicating a lack of performance enhancement after such consumption and, in the worst case, a decreased performance. However, because of the number of variables influencing these findings (such as the content of fat:carbohydrate in the diet, the subjects' training background, the exercise intensity, and the type of exercise test applied to test performance enhancement [Helge et al., 1998b]), caution should be used when drawing final conclusions. A more detailed discussion on the effects of short-term, high-fat adaptation can be found elsewhere (Burke and Hawley, 2002; Helge, 2000).

Effects of Energy Deficit and Intense Physical Activity on the Carbohydrate–Fat Balance and Substrate Stores

An essential goal for the assault ration is to enable soldiers to perform prolonged, low-intensity activity interspersed with high-intensity activity, with a daily energy deficit estimated to be approximately 2,000 kcal.

Only few studies are available in which the conditions mimicked those experienced by the soldiers. At the Copenhagen Muscle Research Centre, we have studied two groups of moderately to well-trained men who, fully self-supported and on cross-country skis pulling heavy sledges, traversed the Greenland ice cap (Helge et al., 2003; unpublished results). The dietary macronutrient compositions and basic subject characteristics are given in Table B-5. The two groups crossed the ice cap in 42 and 32 days and experienced a weight loss of approximately 6 and 7 kg, respectively, of which the majority was fat and the remainder, lean body mass (Figure B-4). Based on standard calculations, these losses are equivalent to a daily energy deficit of approximately 1,000 to 1,500 kcal. Albeit the differences in study design (e.g., the two interventions are for longer terms than those for the assault rations), the results may provide useful information for developing assault rations. The skiers' maximal oxygen uptake remained unchanged in upper-body exercise (arm cranking), but it decreased in lower-body exercise (normal bicycle) (Helge et al., 2003; unpublished results). Accordingly, the muscle biopsy data, enzyme activities, and capillarization data indicated that the arm muscle response tended to be positive, whereas the leg muscle response was neutral or negative. Overall, this would suggest that despite the energy deficit and the type and large amount of physical work, the macronutrient compositions did provide sufficient substrate to almost fully fuel and retain the capacity for physical activity. Based on the available evidence, the fat content could probably be increased up to 50 percent without causing adverse effects. Unfortunately, due to the study design and the timing of muscle biopsies,

TABLE B-4 Short-Term Adaptation for High-Fat Diets and High-Carbohydrate Diets in Humans: Effects on Endurance Performance

		Dietary Content		Exercise Intensity	
	Duration (days)	Fat (% of energy)	Carbohydrate (% of energy)	% of VO$_2$max	Performance Reference measure† (min)
Christensen and	3	94	4	176 Watt^a	88 ± 4
Hansen, 1939	3	3	83	176 Watt	240 (n = 2)
Bergstrom et al.,	3	46	5	75	57 ± 2*
1967	3	0	82	75	167 ± 18*
Martin et al., 1978	3	—	< 10	72	33 ± 3
	3	—	> 75	72	78 ± 5*
Galbo et al., 1979	4	76	10, 5	70	64 ± 6
	4	76	10, 5	70	59 ± 6
	4	9, 5	77	68	106 ± 5*
O'Keeffee et al.,	7	59	13	80	60 ± 5
1989	7	—	72	80	113 ± 12*
Williams et al., 1992	7	48	37	71	135 ± 5‡
	7	35	56	71	127 ± 5‡
Muoio et al., 1994	7	38	50	75–80	91 ± 10*
	7	24	61	75–80	69 ± 7
	7	15	73	75–80	76 ± 8
Starling et al., 1997	1	68	16	75^b	139 ± 7‡
	1	5	83	75	117 ± 3*‡
Pitsiladis and	3	65	9	70 (10°C)^c	89.2 [78–130]^d
Maughan, 1999	3	9	82	70 (10°C)	158 [117–166]*
	3	65	9	70 (10°C)	44 [32–51]
	3	6	82	70 (10°C)	53 [50–82] *
Burke et al., 2000	5 + 1^e	68	19	TT^f	31 ± 1‡
	5 + 1	13	74	TT	34 ± 3‡
Carey et al., 2001	6 + 1^e	69	16	TT^g	44 ± 1 km
	6 + 1	15	70	TT	42 ± 1 km

NOTE: Data are mean values; however, for exercise performance mean ± standard error of the means; n = number in sample.

*p < 0.05 different from other diets (same exercise intensity).

†Performance measure is time (min) to exhaustion unless otherwise noted.

‡Performance mesure is time (min) to complete task.

^{a}Exercise performance at 1,080 kJ (VO$_2$ during exercise was 2.6 L).

^{b}Performance was measured as a 1,600 kJ, self-paced cycling bout.

^{c}Room temperature.

^{d}Mean and range.

^{e}High-fat diet followed by one day of high-carbohydrate diet.

^{f}Time trial (TT) (7 kJ/kg body mass).

^{g}Time trial (TT) (60 min).

TABLE B-5 Subject Characteristics and Dietary Composition

Study	Study 1	Study 2
Subject Number	4	7
BMI	26 ± 0.6	26 ± 0.7
Crossing time (days)	42	32
Exercise per day (hours)	5–6	5.5
Energy intake (kcal)	4,500 ± 300	4,300 ± 200
Fat (% of energy)	31 ± 1	39 ± 1
Protein (% of energy)	9 ± 1	11 ± 1
Carbohydrate (% of energy)	60 ± 1	50 ± 1

NOTE: Values are mean ± standard error of the means; BMI = body mass index.
SOURCE: Author's unpublished results.

muscle substrates during the traverse are unavailable. Of particular interest in this context, however, is whether the muscle triacylglycerol stores, a main substrate source during prolonged, low- to moderate-intensity exercise in well-trained soldiers, are replenished by the ration. Several research groups recently have suggested that repletion of muscle triacylglycerol stores after physical activity could be important to optimize muscle recovery and exercise capacity (Berggren et al., 2004; Johnson et al., 2004; Spriet and Gibala, 2004). Decombaz and colleagues (2001) suggested that daily consumption of fat at a level of 2 g/kg of body mass would be sufficient to fully restore muscle triacylglycerol levels. This would imply that an average soldier at 80 kg would need to consume fat at a level of 160 g/day, which is achieved if the ration contains approximately 55 percent of total energy as fat. The macronutrient composition in the ration must be optimized such that the replenishment of both muscle glycogen and triacylglycerol is sufficiently increased within the given energy limitation of the ration.

SPECIFIC FATS FOR THE ASSAULT RATION

Fatty Acids and Optimal Performance

In the literature, animal studies have demonstrated preferential mobilization (Raclot and Groscolas, 1993) and oxidation (Jones et al., 1992; Leyton et al., 1987; Shimomura et al., 1990) of unsaturated versus saturated fatty acids. As mentioned, interventions that spare carbohydrate use may benefit performance capacity. The available evidence showing that a difference in dietary fatty acid composition will affect endurance is, however, sparse. In rats, endurance performance, measured in vitro in rat extensor digitorum longus muscle after intermit-

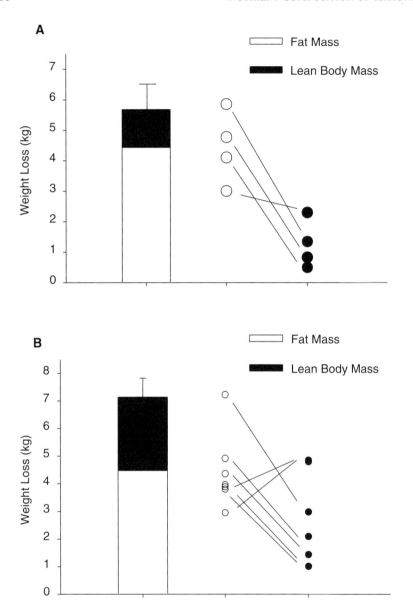

FIGURE B-4 Mean and individual changes in body composition in (A) four male subjects (data from Helge et al., 2003) and (B) seven male subjects (authors unpublished results) after crossing the Greenland ice cap on cross-country skis in 42 (A) and 32 (B) days.

tent, low-frequency stimulation, was lower after nine weeks' adaptation to a diet rich in *n*-6 fatty acids as compared with adaption to a diet rich in *n*-3 fatty acids; both diets contained 10 percent fat (w/w) (Ayre and Hulbert, 1996). Another study in rats found no effect of dietary fatty acid composition on endurance performance in trained or sedentary animals after high-fat diet adaptation, but substrate oxidation was affected (higher oxidation) by the dietary fatty acid composition (Helge et al., 1998a, see Figure B-5). Studies in salmon (McKenzie et al., 1998; Wagner et al., 2004) have also addressed the effects of dietary fatty acid composition on performance capacity, but the data show no consistent trends. In humans, the evidence is limited: A study (*n* = 3) found that endurance performance measured at 70 to 75 percent VO_2max decreased after consumption

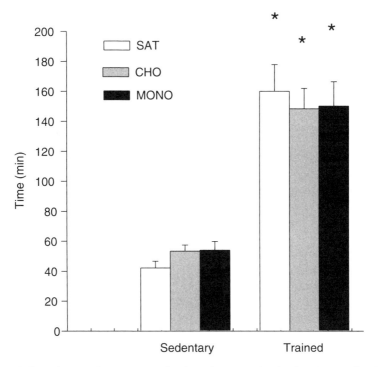

FIGURE B-5 Endurance time to exhaustion in sedentary and trained male rats after four weeks' adaptation to one of two fat-rich diets containing either unsaturated or saturated fatty acids or to a carbohydrate-rich diet.

NOTE: Values are means ± standard error (n = 7–11). CHO = carbohydrate; MONO = monounsaturated fat; n = number in sample; SAT = saturated fat.

* = significantly different from the sedentary groups (p < 0.05).

SOURCE: Helge et al. (1998a).

of a polyunsaturated fat-rich diet as compared with a saturated-fat diet (Lukaski et al., 2001). The author's unpublished observations found that the consumption of a saturated-fat diet, versus a polyunsaturated-fat diet, had no effect on endurance performance. Thus, insufficient data are available to support a role for dietary fatty acid composition on exercise performance.

Fatty Acids and Health Considerations

Are there adverse or positive effects of including different fatty acids in the ration? This question includes a number of complex issues that are incompletely resolved; space limitations prevent their being addressed here, but the following list of potential roles for dietary fatty acids should be considerd for further research:

- The influence of dietary fatty acid composition on membrane function (Pan et al., 1994).
- The influence of dietary fatty acid composition (particularly the content of n-3 and n-6 fatty acids) on immune function (Venkatraman et al., 2000).
- The potential hypolipedemic effects of n-3 fatty acids (Harris, 1997).
- The effects of saturated fatty acids on decreasing insulin sensitivity (Pan et al., 1994).
- The interactions with and effects of specific fatty acids on gene expression in muscle (Spriet and Gibala, 2004; Venkatraman et al., 2000).

The amount of physical activity performed by these soldiers as well as their good training status suggests that shorter term modifications of dietary fatty acid composition and dietary fat content would have insignificant effects on their general health and function.

SUMMARY

The following arguments confer positive and negative aspects of adding increased amounts of fat to the ration. The positive effects of adding more fat include an increased energy content of the ration and a faster repletion of muscle triacylglycerol stores. The negative effects of adding more fat include increased rates of perceived exertion and mental strain during physical activity and a potential lowering of muscle glycogen stores (possibly liver glycogen). There may be an additional increased risk of inducing higher ketone levels but, in my opinion, such a risk does not pose a problem in this situation.

Insufficient evidence exists to verify the effects of specific dietary fatty acids on performance capacity. Some data suggest health and metabolic benefits from the consumption of specific fatty acids. However, in fit and healthy younger men exposed to intense physical activity, these effects, if indeed present, would have more influence on long-term health status rather than on short-term exercise capacity and health. Therefore, the fatty acid composition in the ration should adhere to the requirements established by the Institute of Medicine (IOM, 2002).

Based on the issues addressed above the recommendations for the ration are the following:

- The fat content in the ration can be between 30 to 50 percent (of total energy) without reducing physical capacity; however, increasing the fat content may lead to slightly higher mental strain.
- When protein requirements are met and sufficient carbohydrate for high-intensity tasks is given, fat can be used to increase the energy content of the ration.
- While no specific fatty acid types improve performance, adequate essential fatty acids must be included in the ration at the current recommended levels (IOM, 2002).

ACKNOWLEDGMENTS

The author is affiliated with the Copenhagen Muscle Research Centre, which is supported by grants from the University of Copenhagen, from the faculties of science and of health sciences at this university, and from the Copenhagen Hospital Corporation.

REFERENCES

Ayre KJ, Hulbert AJ. 1996. Effects of changes in dietary fatty acids on isolated skeletal muscle functions in rats. *J Appl Physiol* 80(2):464–471.

Berggren JR, Hulver MW, Dohm GL, Houmard JA. 2004. Weight loss and exercise: Implications for muscle lipid metabolism and insulin action. *Med Sci Sports Exerc* 36(7):1191–1195.

Bergstrom J, Hermansen L, Hultman E, Saltin B. 1967. Diet, muscle glycogen and physical performance. *Acta Physiol Scand* 71(2):140–150.

Brooks GA, Mercier J. 1994. Balance of carbohydrate and lipid utilization during exercise: The "crossover" concept. *J Appl Physiol* 76(6):2253–2261.

Burke LM, Hawley JA. 2002. Effects of short-term fat adaptation on metabolism and performance of prolonged exercise. *Med Sci Sports Exerc* 34(9):1492–1498.

Burke LM, Angus DJ, Cox GR, Cummings NK, Febbraio MA, Gawthorn K, Hawley JA, Minehan M, Martin DT, Hargreaves M. 2000. Effect of fat adaptation and carbohydrate restoration on metabolism and performance during prolonged cycling. *J Appl Physiol* 89(6):2413–2421.

Carey AL, Staudacher HM, Cummings NK, Stepto NK, Nikolopoulos V, Burke LM, Hawley JA. 2001. Effects of fat adaptation and carbohydrate restoration on prolonged endurance exercise. *J Appl Physiol* 91(1):115–122.

Christensen EH, Hansen O. 1939. Arbeitsfähigkeit und ernärung. *Skand Archiv Physiol* 81:160–171.

Decombaz J, Schmitt B, Ith M, Decarli B, Diem P, Kreis R, Hoppeler H, Boesch C. 2001. Postexercise fat intake repletes intramyocellular lipids but no faster in trained than in sedentary subjects. *Am J Physiol Regul Integr Comp Physiol* 281(3):R760–R769.

Galbo H, Holst JJ, Christensen NJ. 1979. The effect of different diets and of insulin on the hormonal response to prolonged exercise. *Acta Physiol Scand* 107(1):19–32.

Harris WS. 1997. n-3 Fatty acids and serum lipoproteins: Human studies. *Am J Clin Nutr* 65(5 Suppl):1645S–1654S.

Helge JW. 2000. Adaptation to a fat-rich diet. Effects on endurance performance in humans. *Sports Med* 30(5):347–357.

Helge JW. 2002. Long-term fat diet adaptation effects on performance, training capacity, and fat utilization. *Med Sci Sports Exerc* 34(9):1499–1504.

Helge JW, Ayre K, Chaunchaiyakul S, Hulbert AJ, Kiens B, Storlien LH. 1998a. Endurance in high-fat-fed rats: Effects of carbohydrate content and fatty acid profile. *J Appl Physiol* 85(4):1342–1348.

Helge JW, Lundby C, Christensen DL, Langfort J, Messonnier L, Zacho M, Andersen JL, Saltin B. 2003. Skiing across Greenland icecap: Divergent effects on limb muscle adaptations and substrate oxidation. *J Exp Biol* 206(Pt 6):1075–1083.

Helge JW, Wulff B, Kiens B. 1998b. Impact of a fat-rich diet on endurance in man: Role of the dietary period. *Med Sci Sports Exerc* 30(3):456–461.

Hultman E, Nilsson L. 1971. Liver glycogen in man. Effect of different diets and muscular exercise. In: Pernow B, Saltin B, eds. *Muscle Metabolism During Exercise. Proceedings of a Karolinska Institutet Symposium held in Stockholm, Sweden, September 6–9, 1970.* New York: Plenum. Pp. 143–151.

IOM (Institute of Medicine). 2002. *Dietary Reference Intakes. Energy, Carbohydrates, Fiber, Fat, Fatty Acids, Cholesterol, Protein, and Amino Acids.* Washington, DC: The National Academies Press.

Jansson E, Hjemdahl P, Kaijser L. 1982. Diet induced changes in sympatho-adrenal activity during submaximal exercise in relation to substrate utilization in man. *Acta Physiol Scand* 114(2):171–178.

Johnson NA, Stannard SR, Thompson MW. 2004. Muscle triglyceride and glycogen in endurance exercise: Implications for performance. *Sports Med* 34(3):151–164.

Jones PJ, Ridgen JE, Phang PT, Birmingham CL. 1992. Influence of dietary fat polyunsaturated to saturated ratio on energy substrate utilization in obesity. *Metabolism* 41(4):396–401.

Leyton J, Drury PJ, Crawford MA. 1987. Differential oxidation of saturated and unsaturated fatty acids in vivo in the rat. *Br J Nutr* 57(3):383–393.

Lukaski HC, Bolonchuk WW, Klevay LM, Milne DB, Sandstead HH. 2001. Interactions among dietary fat, mineral status, and performance of endurance athletes: A case study. *Int J Sport Nutr Exerc Metab* 11(2):186–198.

Martin B, Robinson S, Robertshaw D. 1978. Influence of diet on leg uptake of glucose during heavy exercise. *Am J Clin Nutr* 31(1):62–67.

McKenzie DJ, Higgs DA, Dosanjh BS, Deacon G, Randall DJ. 1998. Dietary fatty acid composition influences swimming performance in Atlantic salmon (*Salmo salar*) in seawater. *Fish Physiol Biochem* 19(2):111–122.

Muoio DM, Leddy JJ, Horvath PJ, Awad AB, Pendergast DR. 1994. Effect of dietary fat on metabolic adjustments to maximal VO_2 and endurance in runners. *Med Sci Sports Exerc* 26(1):81–88.

O'Keeffe KA, Keith RE, Wilson GD, Blessing DL. 1989. Dietary carbohydrate intake and endurance exercise performance of trained female cyclists. *Nutr Res* 9:819–830.

Pan DA, Hulbert AJ, Storlien LH. 1994. Dietary fats, membrane phospholipids and obesity. *J Nutr* 124(9):1555–1565.

Phinney SD, Bistrian BR, Evans WJ, Gervino E, Blackburn GL. 1983. The human metabolic response to chronic ketosis without caloric restriction: Preservation of submaximal exercise capability with reduced carbohydrate oxidation. *Metabolism* 32(8):769–776.

Pitsiladis YP, Maughan RJ. 1999. The effects of exercise and diet manipulation on the capacity to perform prolonged exercise in the heat and in the cold in trained humans. *J Physiol* 517(Pt 3):919–930.

Raclot T, Groscolas R. 1993. Differential mobilization of white adipose tissue fatty acids according to chain length, unsaturation, and positional isomerism. *J Lipid Res* 34(9):1515–1526.

Shimomura Y, Tamura T, Suzuki M. 1990. Less body fat accumulation in rats fed a safflower oil diet than in rats fed a beef tallow diet. *J Nutr* 120(11):1291–1296.

Spriet LL, Gibala MJ. 2004. Nutritional strategies to influence adaptations to training. *J Sports Sci* 22(1):127–141.

Starling RD, Trappe TA, Parcell AC, Kerr CG, Fink WJ, Costill DL. 1997. Effects of diet on muscle triglyceride and endurance performance. *J Appl Physiol* 82(4):1185–1189.

Stepto NK, Carey AL, Staudacher HM, Cummings NK, Burke LM, Hawley JA. 2002. Effect of short-term fat adaptation on high-intensity training. *Med Sci Sports Exerc* 34(3):449–455.

Venkatraman JT, Leddy J, Pendergast D. 2000. Dietary fats and immune status in athletes: Clinical implications. *Med Sci Sports Exerc* 32(7 Suppl):S389–S395.

Wagner GN, Balfry SK, Higgs DA, Lall SP, Farrell AP. 2004. Dietary fatty acid composition affects the repeat swimming performance of Atlantic salmon in seawater. *Comp Biochem Physiol A Mol Integr Physiol* 137(3):567–576.

Williams C, Brewer J, Walker M. 1992. The effect of a high carbohydrate diet on running performance during a 30-km treadmill time trial. *Eur J Appl Physiol Occup Physiol* 65(1):18–24.

Carbohydrate–Protein Balance for Physical Performance

Kevin D. Tipton, University of Birmingham, UK

INTRODUCTION

Proper nutrition for military personnel has long been an important consideration for military planners. Nutrition may be especially important for military combat personnel performing duties that entail short-term, strenuous physical tasks in high-stress situations. Stress during military operations results from a combination of increased energy expenditure, decreased energy intake, and a lack of sleep for extended periods. These multiple stressors on mental and physical capabilities may decrease muscle performance enough to compromise both lives and military success. Sufficiently effective nutrients in combat rations would enhance the soldiers'capabilities and reduce both the loss of combat effectiveness and the number of casualties. Protein and carbohydrate consumption may contribute to optimal muscle performance during these situations.

The unique circumstances in the field make it difficult for soldiers to consume sufficient protein and carbohydrate as well as overall energy during their missions. For example, weight and size that soldiers can carry is limited and evidence shows that high-stress combat can suppress appetite (Popper et al., 1989). These factors lead to large energy deficits and macronutrient deficiencies for the three- to seven-day periods of these operations. These energy and macronutrient deficits could lead to metabolic disturbances that impair muscular performance during demanding and intense military operations.

The combination of stressors—decreased energy and protein intake, sleep deprivation, extreme physical activity, and high stress levels—that soldiers face during these missions represents a complex and unique situation. Unfortunately, little, if any, direct information is available about muscular metabolic response to these stressors and about the appropriate nutrient intake that would be optimal for these capabilities.

This review uses data collected during periods of physiological stress to develop strategies to enhance protein and carbohydrate intake during sustained military operations. Because of a paucity of such data, however, this review provides a speculative guideline for recommendations. The following are specific questions that this review addresses:

- What would be the optimal macronutrient balance between protein and carbohydrate for an assault ration to enhance muscle performance during combat missions? Does the intensity of activity (i.e., high-tempo, stressful, repetitive combat missions) alter the optimal balance?
- What protein intake is recommended to best sustain homeostasis while people are eating reduced calories and exercising?
- What are the types and levels of macronutrients (e.g., complex versus simple carbohydrates, proteins with specific amino acid profiles, other sources of nitrogen, etc.) that would optimize such an assault ration to enhance muscle performance during combat missions?

ENERGY INTAKE AND PHYSICAL ACTIVITY

Energy intake plays a major role in body protein metabolism. Operational requirements, as noted above, limit the intake of available energy in rations during short-term, high-stress missions. Such limitations in energy intake, combined with high levels of physical activity, ensure that participants are in an energy deficit for the three- to seven-day duration of a mission. Measurements made during simulated sustained operations do not clearly demonstrate muscle loss (Montain and Young, 2003; Nindl et al., 2002); however, body composition measures may not have the sensitivity to detect small changes over a short time. Nevertheless, the evidence provided below suggests that energy deficits that occur during these missions will lead to muscle loss.

Many classic studies from the laboratory of Calloway and Butterfield have demonstrated the importance of energy balance to maintain body nitrogen balance. Todd and colleagues (1984) clearly demonstrated that nitrogen balance is better maintained when energy balance is positive or, at least, zero (Figure B-6). Nitrogen balance could not be maintained when energy intake was 15 percent less than energy output. Presumably, the body's predominant and accessible source, muscle protein, would also be the major site of this nitrogen loss. Energy restriction over longer periods (e.g., 10 weeks) results in the loss of lean mass during very low calorie dieting (Layman et al., 2003); however, the metabolic mechanisms for this loss remain unexplained.

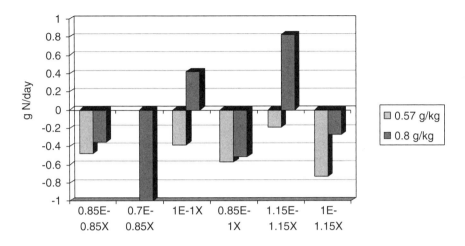

FIGURE B-6 Nitrogen (N) balance during differing levels of energy intake (E) and physical activity (X) at two different levels of protein intake. Each bar is at either energy balance or 15 percent deficit due to increased exercise. These data illustrate that nitrogen balance is negative during energy deficits and improved by low-intensity exercise. Nitrogen balance is not positive in any combination of energy intake and exercise on the lowest $(0.57 \text{ g·kg}^{-1}\text{·d}^{-1})$ level.
SOURCE: Adapted from Todd et al. (1984).

Muscle protein synthesis is reduced by 65 percent in food-deprived rats (Anthony et al., 2000), and perturbations in muscle metabolism from energy deficits could occur very rapidly. Recently, Tipton et al. (2003) demonstrated that the release of amino acids from leg muscle in healthy volunteers occurred in the first 24 h of energy restriction (80 percent of their weight maintenance levels). In that study, the volunteers were resting and consumed their habitual level of dietary protein. It seems that reducing energy intake by only 20 percent immediately stimulates a catabolic situation in muscle, suggesting that soldiers participating in missions where their energy intake is half of their energy output would be losing nitrogen, most likely from muscle. Unfortunately, it is not clear how the energy restriction and negative energy balance inherent for these sustained operations reduces muscle performance (Friedl, 1995).

A portion of the uncertainty about the effects of energy balance on muscle performance in short-term military missions with concomitant stressors, such as high-physical activity, sleep loss, and dietary restrictions, can be attributed to the complexity of the situation and the lack of information from studies. Protein use can be improved by physical activity (Butterfield and Calloway, 1984; Todd et al., 1984) (Figure B-6). Increased energy intake to support increased physical activity improves the nitrogen balance, and the physical activity improves nitro-gen retention (Butterfield and Calloway, 1984; Todd et al., 1984). Following an acute bout of resistance exercise, muscle protein synthesis and net muscle pro-tein balance are increased, even in trained individuals (Biolo et al., 1995; Phillips et al., 1997, 1999). Muscle protein synthesis was increased following four hours of walking (Carraro et al., 1990), but no balance data are available for that type of activity.

Whereas these data could be interpreted to suggest that the physical activity common during military maneuvers may improve protein balance and have a good effect on muscle protein, there are reasons to believe otherwise. There is typically a period of adaptation to physical activity in which nitrogen balance is diminished (Butterfield, 1987; Butterfield and Calloway, 1984; Gontzea et al., 1975). This transient increase in protein loss peaks at four to ten days following initiation of the exercise program; easily encompassing the time typically used for these missions. However, these data are from untrained individuals initiating physical activity, so the applicability of these data to the situations being dis-cussed for soldiers is unclear. It is easy to accept that the habitual level of training before participating in difficult missions could be protective, but there are no data to support this contention. Furthermore, the data supporting a benefit to nitrogen balance from activity were obtained during an energy balance (Todd et al., 1984). Positive nitrogen balance could not be maintained when energy balance was negative, despite increased physical activity (Figure B-6). Thus, it seems that the conditions intrinsic to the sustained operations missions will result in negative nitrogen balance and loss of muscle protein.

The intensity of the activity necessary for successful completion of the mis-sions may increase the loss of muscle protein and, thus, exacerbate the effects of the negative energy balance. Given that the logistical limitations to the rations for these missions preclude carrying additional rations to accommodate the increased activity, any increase in activity will result in increased energy deficits. Furthermore, there is evidence that high-intensity exercise is debilitating for muscle protein metabolism. Whereas muscle protein synthesis has been demon-strated to increase following both resistance (Biolo et al., 1995; Phillips et al., 1997, 1999) and endurance (Carraro et al., 1990) exercise in humans, it is depressed following prolonged, high-intensity exercise in rats (Anthony et al., 1999; Gautsch et al., 1998). It is possible that species-specific differences in the response of muscle to exercise may explain the differential. On the other hand, the response of muscle protein synthesis to resistance exercise in rats (Farrell et al., 1999; Hernandez et al., 2000) is similar to that for humans (Biolo et al., 1995; Phillips et al., 1997, 1999). It is more likely that the intensity of the exercise during the treadmill running was severe and resulted in decreased muscle protein synthesis. The rats ran at approximately 80 percent of VO_2max for approximately two hours, roughly equivalent to the effort that only an elite runner could maintain for a marathon. Furthermore, if relative life span is taken into account, two hours on a treadmill for a rat could be considered equivalent to the effort of several days for humans. Thus, it is conceivable that this intense physical exercise would also result in reduced muscle protein synthesis in humans. The evidence presented suggests that, rather than increasing protein use, the physical activity involved in prolonged military missions may be detrimental to muscle protein metabolism. The energy deficit, combined with high-tempo, stressful physical activity, suggests that muscle protein metabolism will be altered during missions of this type.

Protein Intake

As with energy intake, protein intake during these missions can be limited by operational factors. There is a great deal of controversy in the sports science community about the protein requirements for athletes and active individuals; however, little question remains that increased protein intake would be advantageous in an energy deficit made worse by high levels of physical activity. Todd and colleagues (1984) demonstrated that, at low levels of protein intake (0.57 g/kg per day), nitrogen balance was negative during both energy balance and energy deficit. Increasing protein intake from 0.57 to 0.85 g/kg per day improved nitrogen balance when energy intake was 15 percent less than energy output (Figure B-6). Either way, nitrogen balance was negative during both intakes. At this time, there is way to determine if the loss of body protein could be ameliorated by higher protein intakes and, if so, what would constitute the optimal level of protein intake. A question also remains of a ceiling effect whereby no further improvement is possible with increased protein intake. Unknown as well is whether positive balance is feasible during the conditions inherent to military operations. In addition, it is impossible to determine whether eliminating negative nitrogen balance is necessary to improve the performance and health of the military. A recent study demonstrated that a greater proportion of weight lost during energy restriction comes from fat, rather than lean, mass when protein intake is increased (Layman et al., 2003). Data from this study suggest that increasing protein intake spares body protein during periods of negative energy balance. However, the applicability to soldiers during sustained operations is limited because this study was conducted on obese female subjects in weight-loss situations and did not involve exercise.

Loss of nitrogen likely is exacerbated by the combination of higher protein intakes before missions and lower protein intake during missions. Millward and colleagues demonstrated that body protein is lost when dietary protein intake is decreased (Pacy et al., 1994; Price et al., 1994; Quevedo et al., 1994). Data from these studies suggest an adaptation period that takes several days (often the time expected for most of these missions) (Figure B-7). These data also suggest that the sudden decline in protein intake expected when soldiers undertake these missions would contribute to a loss of body proteins, most likely from muscle.

However, in these studies, the subjects were in energy balance and did not exercise, so it is unclear how applicable these data are to sustained operations.

The available information suggests that decreasing protein intake during these missions will be detrimental to muscle protein metabolism. The recommendation to maximize protein intake during the missions seems prudent; however, there are sufficient questions to prevent a specific recommendation from being made with any confidence.

Carbohydrate and Lipid Intake

There is no question that carbohydrate intake is critical for optimal muscle performance during strenuous activity. Maintenance of blood glucose and glycogen for muscle fuel are important for muscular performance (Burke et al., 2004; Coyle, 2004; Hargreaves et al., 2004). Several studies have demonstrated that increased carbohydrate intake improved performance in military tasks (Montain and Young, 2003; Montain et al., 1997). Severe muscle glycogen depletion has been shown during four- to five-day field operations (Jacobs et al., 1983). Although provision of extra carbohydrates did not increase the glycogen levels in these soldiers (Jacobs et al., 1983) sufficient carbohydrate intake seems important for performance maintenance during sustained military operations (Montain and Young, 2003).

Carbohydrate intake may also enhance muscle protein metabolism. Acute provision of carbohydrates increases net muscle protein balance following exercise,

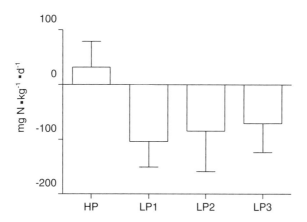

FIGURE B-7 Change in nitrogen (N) balance due to change from the first three days of high-protein (HP) to low-protein (LP) intake.
SOURCE: Quevedo et al. (1994).

presumably through the action of insulin (Borsheim et al., 2004b). Nevertheless, any increase in net muscle protein balance from ingestion of carbohydrate is much less than that from ingestion of an amino acid source (Borsheim et al., 2004a; Miller et al., 2003). On a whole body level, Gaudichon and colleagues (1999) demonstrated that carbohydrate ingestion increased postprandial use of dietary protein to a greater extent than did lipids. It is likely that increased use of available nutrients by the body is especially important in situations of limited nutrient availability. Replacing carbohydrate with fat has been demonstrated to increase nitrogen balance during hypocaloric situations (Richardson et al., 1979). On the other hand, Boirie and colleagues have presented a series of studies (Boirie et al., 1997; Dangin et al., 2003) suggesting that, after protein ingestion, amino acids released slowly into the blood provide a superior anabolic response. Given that lipids do slow the digestion of nutrients, it could be argued that lipids may improve the anabolic response in the muscle. We recently tested this notion in our laboratory, and despite equivalent protein ingestion during two small, separate meals, net muscle protein balance was greater from proteins when fat was included in the meal (Elliot et al., unpublished data). Thus, including both carbohydrates and lipids in the ration should maximize the accretion of ingested protein into muscle when nutrients are limited. The exact composition of such nutrients remains unknown.

Intake of Amino Acids

Amino acids provided by protein ingestion stimulate the accretion of muscle protein. Evidence from acute metabolic studies suggests that increased muscle protein synthesis and net muscle protein synthesis result only from the provision of essential amino acids; that is, nonessential amino acids are unnecessary to stimulate muscle protein accretion (Borsheim et al., 2002; Tipton and Wolfe, 2001; Tipton et al., 1999, 2003). Furthermore, the response of muscle protein balance to essential amino acids seems dose dependent (Borsheim et al., 2002). Aside from increasing amino acid availability for protein synthesis, essential amino acids may act as signals for stimulating protein synthesis. Essential amino acids, particularly leucine, activate translational signaling (Anthony et al., 2000; Kimball and Jefferson, 2001; Kimball et al., 2002). In rats, leucine stimulates muscle protein synthesis that was diminished by severe exercise (Anthony et al., 1999), but feeding carbohydrates only did not (Gautsch et al., 1998). Essential amino acids may be particularly effective during sustained operations when physical activity is extreme.

More evidence for the potential efficacy of essential amino acids during sustained military operations comes from acute metabolic studies performed in our laboratory. Following resistance exercise, ingesting 12 g of essential amino acids resulted in an amino acid uptake that was more than double that from ingesting 20 g of whole proteins (Borsheim et al., 2002; Tipton et al., 2004)

(Figure B-8). Consuming only 60 percent of the volume more than doubled the anabolic response, which means a superior response was obtained for less mass/volume. Furthermore, essential amino acids, combined with exercise, ameliorated the amino acid release from muscle in response to a 20 percent energy deficit (Tipton et al., 2003). These factors suggest that essential amino acids could be important for ration design.

SUMMARY

The metabolic demands endured by soldiers on sustained military operations are severe and unique. Very little research exists that specifically examines the results from missions that involve underfeeding and high-activity levels as well as high stress on muscle metabolism and performance. The indirectly available information suggests that optimal ration development should include maximizing the energy and protein content within the operational limits. Carbohydrate and fat are clearly important, but it is unclear what quantity each should represent in the overall composition. Recent evidence from acute metabolic studies suggests that essential amino acids may be an important component of a ration for sustained missions. The anabolic response to essential amino acids seems to be superior to a larger amount of intact protein, thus offering higher efficiency. Further research is necessary to determine the effects of these various nutrients on muscle metabolism and performance in specific situations experienced during sustained military operations.

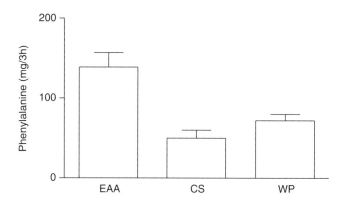

FIGURE B-8 Phenylalanine uptake during three hours (h) following ingestion of 12 g of free essential amino acids (EAA), 20 g of casein (CS), or 20 g of whey proteins (WP). SOURCE: Borsheim et al. (2002); Tipton et al. (2004).

REFERENCES

Anthony JC, Anthony TG, Kimball SR, Vary TC, Jefferson LS. 2000. Orally administered leucine stimulates protein synthesis in skeletal muscle of postabsorptive rats in association with increased eIF4F formation. *J Nutr* 130(2):139–145.

Anthony JC, Anthony TG, Layman DK. 1999. Leucine supplementation enhances skeletal muscle recovery in rats following exercise. *J Nutr* 129(6):1102–1106.

Biolo G, Maggi SP, Williams BD, Tipton KD, Wolfe RR. 1995. Increased rates of muscle protein turnover and amino acid transport after resistance exercise in humans. *Am J Physiol* 268(3 Pt 1):E514–E520.

Boirie Y, Danglin M, Gachon P, Vasson M, Maubois JL, Beaufrere B. 1997. Slow and fast dietary proteins differently modulate postprandial protein accretion. *Proc Natl Acad Sci USA* 94(26):14930–14935.

Borsheim E, Tipton KD, Wolf SE, Wolfe RR. 2002. Essential amino acids and muscle protein recovery from resistance exercise. *Am J Physiol Endocrinol Metabol* 283(4):E648–E657.

Borsheim E, Aarsland A, Wolfe RR. 2004a. Effect of an amino acid, protein, and carbohydrate mixture on net muscle protein balance after resistance exercise. *Int J Sport Nutr Exerc Metab* 14(3):255–271.

Borsheim E, Cree MG, Tipton KD, Elliott TA, Aarsland A, Wolfe RR. 2004b. Effect of carbohydrate intake on net muscle protein synthesis during recovery from resistance exercise. *J Appl Physiol* 96(2):674–678.

Burke LM, Kiens B, Ivy JL. 2004. Carbohydrates and fat for training and recovery. *J Sports Sci* 22(1):15–30.

Butterfield GE. 1987. Whole-body protein utilization in humans. *Med Sci Sports Exerc* 19(5 Suppl):S157–S165.

Butterfield GE, Calloway DH. 1984. Physical activity improves protein utilization in young men. *Br J Nutr* 51(2):171–184.

Carraro F, Stuart CA, Hartl WH, Rosenblatt J, Wolfe RR. 1990. Effect of exercise and recovery on muscle protein synthesis in human subjects. *Am J Physiol* 259(4 Pt 1):E470–E476.

Coyle EF. 2004. Fluid and fuel intake during exercise. *J Sports Sci* 22(1):39–55.

Dangin M, Guillet C, Garcia-Rodenas C, Gachon P, Bouteloup-Demangc C, Reiffers-Magnani K, Fauquant J, Ballevre O, Beaufrere B. 2003. The rate of protein digestion affects protein gain differently during aging in humans. *J Physiol* 549(Pt 2):635–644.

Farrell PA, Fedele MJ, Vary TC, Kimball SR, Lang CH, Jefferson LS. 1999. Regulation of protein synthesis after acute resistance exercise in diabetic rats. *Am J Physiol* 276(4 Pt 1):E721–E727.

Friedl KE. 1995. When does energy deficit affect soldier physical performance? In: Marriott BM, ed. *Not Eating Enough*. Washington, DC: National Academy Press. Pp. 253–283.

Gaudichon C, Mahe S, Benamouzig R, Luengo C, Fouillet H, Sare S, van Oycke M, Ferriere F, Rautureau J, Tome D. 1999. Net postprandial utilization of [^{15}N]-labeled mild protein nitrogen is influenced by diet composition in humans. *J Nutr* 129(4):890–895.

Gautsch TA, Anthony JC, Kimball SR, Paul GL, Layman DK, Jefferson LS. 1998. Availability of eIF4E regulates skeletal muscle protein synthesis during recovery from exercise. *Am J Physiol* 274(2 Pt 1):C406–C414.

Gontzea I, Sutzescu P, Dumitrache S. 1975. The influence of adaptation to physical effort on nitrogen balance in man. *Nutr Rept Intern* 11:231–236.

Hargreaves M, Hawley JA, Jeukendrup A. 2004. Pre-exercise carbohydrate and fat ingestion: Effects on metabolism and performance. *J Sports Sci* 22(1):31–38.

Hernandez JM, Fedele MJ, Farrell PA. 2000. Time course evaluation of protein synthesis and glucose uptake after acute resistance exercise in rats. *J Appl Physiol* 88(3):1142–1149.

Jacobs I, Anderberg A, Schele R, Lithell H. 1983. Muscle glycogen in soldiers on different diets during military field manoeuvres. *Aviat Space Environ Med* 54(10):898–900.

Kimball SR, Jefferson LS. 2001. Regulation of protein synthesis by branched-chain amino acids. *Curr Opin Clin Nutr Metab Care* 4(1):39–43.

Kimball SR, Farrell PA, Jefferson LS. 2002. Invited review: Role of insulin in translational control of protein synthesis in skeletal muscle by amino acids or exercise. *J Appl Physiol* 93(3):1168–1180.

Layman DK, Boileau RA, Erickson DJ, Painter JE, Shiue H, Sather C, Christou DD. 2003. A reduced ratio of dietary carbohydrate to protein improves body composition and blood lipid profiles during weight loss in adult women. *J Nutr* 133(2):411–417.

Miller SL, Tipton KD, Chinkes DL, Wolf SE, Wolfe RR. 2003. Independent and combined effects of amino acids and glucose after resistance exercise. *Med Sci Sports Exerc* 35(3):449–455.

Montain SJ, Young AJ. 2003. Diet and physical performance. *Appetite* 40(3):255–267.

Montain SJ, Shippee RL, Tharion WJ. 1997. Carbohydrate-electrolyte solution effects on physical performance of military tasks. *Aviat Space Environ Med* 68(5):384–391.

Nindl BC, Leone CD, Tharion WJ, Johnson RF, Castellani JW, Patton JF, Montain SJ. 2002. Physical performance responses during 72 h of military operational stress. *Med Sci Sports Exerc* 34(11):1814–1822.

Pacy PJ, Price GM, Halliday D, Quevedo MR, Millward DJ. 1994. Nitrogen homeostasis in man: The diurnal responses of protein synthesis and degradation and amino acid oxidation to diets with increasing protein intakes. *Clin Sci* 86(1):103–118.

Phillips SM, Tipton KD, Aarsland A, Wolf SE, Wolfe RR. 1997. Mixed muscle protein synthesis and breakdown after resistance exercise in humans. *Am J Physiol* 273(1 Pt 1):E99–E107.

Phillips SM, Tipton KD, Ferrando AA, Wolfe RR. 1999. Resistance training reduces the acute exercise-induced increase in muscle protein turnover. *Am J Physiol* 276(1 Pt 1):E118–E124.

Popper R, Smits G, Meiselman HL, Hirsch E. 1989. Eating in combat: A survey of US Marines. *Mil Med* 154(12):619–623.

Price GM, Halliday D, Pacy PJ, Quevedo MR, Millward DJ. 1994. Nitrogen homeostasis in man: Influence of protein intake on the amplitude of diurnal cycling of body nitrogen. *Clin Sci* 86(1):91–102.

Quevedo MR, Price GM, Halliday D, Pacy PJ, Millward DJ. 1994. Nitrogen homoeostasis in man: Diurnal changes in nitrogen excretion, leucine oxidation and whole body leucine kinetics during a reduction from a high to a moderate protein intake. *Clin Sci* 86(2):185–193.

Richardson DP, Wayler AH, Scrimshaw NS, Young VR. 1979. Quantitative effect of an isoenergetic exchange of fat for carbohydrate on dietary protein utilization in healthy young men. *Am J Clin Nutr* 32(11):2217–2226.

Tipton KD, Wolfe RR. 2001. Exercise, protein metabolism, and muscle growth. *Int J Sport Nutr Exerc Metab* 11(1):109–132.

Tipton KD, Borsheim E, Wolf SE, Sanford AP, Wolfe RR. 2003. Acute response of net muscle protein balance reflects 24-h balance after exercise and amino acid ingestion. *Am J Physiol Endocrinol Metab* 284(1):E76–E89.

Tipton KD, Elliott TA, Cree MG, Wolf SE, Sanford AP, Wolfe RR. 2004. Ingestion of casein and whey proteins result in muscle anabolism after resistance exercise. *Med Sci Sports Exerc* 36(12):2073–2081.

Tipton KD, Ferrando AA, Phillips SM, Doyle D Jr, Wolfe RR. 1999. Postexercise net protein synthesis in human muscle from orally administered amino acids. *Am J Physiol* 276(4 Pt 1):E628–E634.

Todd KS, Butterfield GE, Calloway DH. 1984. Nitrogen balance in men with adequate and deficient energy intake at three levels of work. *J Nutr* 114(11):2107–2118.

Carbohydrate Ingestion During Intense Activity

Edward F. Coyle, University of Texas at Austin

INTRODUCTION

The Committee on Optimization of Nutrient Composition of Military Rations for Short-Term, High-Stress Situations was charged with making recommendations on the composition of a food ration (assault ration) that will best sustain physical and cognitive performance for short-term use by highly-trained soldiers during high-tempo, stressful, repetitive combat missions; in addition, the food ration will also prevent possible adverse health consequences under the conditions of a hypocaloric diet. Stress may be due to high physical and cognitive workloads such as exercise, extreme environmental temperature, dehydration, heat exhaustion, threat to personal safety, sleep deprivation, and other operational demands. Important health concerns for soldiers during combat missions are the optimization of gastrointestinal processes and prevention of diarrhea, dehydration, hyperthermia, kidney stones; optimization of the function of immune system; and prevention of infections. The expected daily expenditure of these soldiers is approximately 4,000 to 4,500 kcal/day. The assault ration will provide approximately 2,400 kcal/day for three to seven days with one to three days of recovery.

This paper focuses on several aspects of the design of such a ration. Although a lot of the literature presented is from the sports and exercise community, their conclusions can be used to support recommendations for the assault ration described above. This paper attempts to answer the following questions:

- What would be the optimal amount of carbohydrates for an assault ration to enhance performance during combat missions?
- What are the types and levels of macronutrients (e.g., complex verses simple carbohydrates) that would optimize an assault ration to enhance performance during combat missions?
- How much is performance going to decline when there is a reduction in both carbohydrates and calories?

CARBOHYDRATE INTAKE DURING EXERCISE

Despite long-ago evidence that carbohydrate ingestion during exercise improved athletic performance, the discovery in the 1960s and 1970s of muscle glycogen's importance as a source of carbohydrate energy for athletes (Bergstrom et al., 1967) seemed to have overshadowed, until the mid-1980s, the potential energy contribution from carbohydrate ingested during the period of exercise (Coggan and Coyle, 1991; Coyle et al., 1986; Hargreaves, 1996). Costill and

Miller (1980) emphasized the need for fluid intake during exercise but recommend against ingesting very much carbohydrate. This recommendation is understandable for that period of time, given that the physiological benefits of fluid replacement were beginning to be established, as reflected in the 1975 American College of Sports Medicine (ACSM) position-statement, whereas the physiological benefits of carbohydrate ingestion for blood glucose supplementation as well as the physiological mechanisms explaining this benefit were not yet established (Hargreaves, 1996). In the 1980s, the observation that adding carbohydrate to water temporarily slowed the gastric emptying rate was interpreted to suggest that fluid replacement solutions should not contain much carbohydrate (Coyle et al., 1978). It was also thought, albeit mistakenly, that "ingested glucose contributes very little to the total energy utilized during exercise" (Costill and Miller, 1980). Therefore, the prevailing recommendation in 1980 was that "under conditions that threaten the endurance athlete with dehydration and hyperthermia, fluid replacement solutions should contain little sugar (> 25 g/L or > 2.5 percent) and electrolytes" (Costill and Miller, 1980).

Later in the 1980s, it was established that ingested carbohydrate and blood glucose can indeed be oxidized at rates of approximately 1 g/minute and that this exogenous carbohydrate becomes the predominant source of energy late in a bout of prolonged, continuous exercise (Convertino et al., 1996). Carbohydrate ingestion can delay muscle fatigue during prolonged cycling and running, and it also improves the power output that can be maintained (Hargreaves, 1996; Millard-Stafford, 1992; Millard-Stafford et al., 1997). It is now understood that the slight slowing of gastric emptying caused by solutions containing up to 8 percent of carbohydrate is a relatively minor factor in fluid replacement rate compared with the large influence of increased fluid volume for increasing gastric emptying and fluid replacement rate (Coyle and Montain, 1992a, b; Maughan, 1991; Maughan and Noakes, 1991; Maughan et al., 1993). Therefore, it is generally recommended that endurance athletes ingest carbohydrate at a rate of 30 to 60 g/h (Casa et al., 2000; Convertino et al., 1996). The type of carbohydrate can be glucose, sucrose, maltodextrins, or some high-glycemic starches. Fructose intake should be limited to amounts that do not cause gastrointestinal discomfort (Casa et al., 2000; Convertino et al., 1996). This rate of carbohydrate ingestion can be met by drinking solutions containing 4 to 8 percent of carbohydrates (4 to 8 g/100 mL) (Casa et al., 2000; Convertino et al., 1996; Rehrer, 1994; Rehrer et al., 1993).

Performance During Short-Term, Intermittent High-Intensity Exercise

Benefits of carbohydrate ingestion during performance of high-intensity, intermittent exercise attempted after at least 60 minutes of continuous moderate-intensity exercise (i.e., 65 to 80 percent VO_2max) was the focus of study beginning in the late 1980s. Power output measured over 5 to 15 minutes of high-intensity and predominantly aerobic exercise has been generally observed to increase by ingesting carbohydrate (Coggan and Coyle, 1988; Mitchell et al., 1989; Murray et al., 1987; Sugiura and Kobayashi, 1998) In the 1996 ACSM position statement on *Exercise and Fluid Replacement*, it was concluded that "During intense exercise lasting longer than 1 h, it is recommended that carbohydrates be ingested at a rate of 30–60 g/h to maintain oxidation of carbohydrates and delay fatigue" (Convertino et al., 1996).

During the past decade, attention has focused on determining if carbohydrate intake during sporting events such as soccer and tennis improves various indices of performance. As discussed below, carbohydrate ingestion appears to frequently benefit performance as demonstrated in tests of "shuttle-running" ability, which simulates the stop-and-start nature of many sports requiring bursts of speed and some fatigue resistance (Nicholas et al., 1995). Physiological mechanisms for this ergogenic effect of carbohydrate ingestion are not clear and have been theorized to involve more than simply skeletal muscle metabolism, implying a neuromuscular component. The challenges now are identifying the types of physical activity and sporting situations during which carbohydrate ingestion is advisable and those during which such a recommendation is not effective or even counterproductive.

Conditions During Which Carbohydrate Ingestion During Exercise Does Not Appear to Improve Performance

Performance or fatigue resistance can be governed by numerous physiological factors involving, primarily, the skeletal muscle, the cardiovascular system, and the nervous system. Some primary causes of fatigue are not influenced by carbohydrate ingestion during exercise; for example, the negative effects of hyperthermia on performing prolonged exercise in a hot environment [e.g., 33°C to 35°C (91.4°F to 96°F)] do not appear to be lessened by carbohydrate ingestion (Febbraio et al., 1996; Fritzsche et al., 2000). However, during exercise in a cool environment [i.e., 5°C (41°F)] (Febbraio et al., 1996) that is not limited by hyperthermia, or when subjects drink fluids during exercise in a hot environment and also do not become hyperthermic (Fritzsche et al., 2000), carbohydrate ingestion improves performance. Under conditions not eliciting hyperthermia, the most important factor for performing prolonged, intense exercise appears to be maintaining carbohydrate availability and thus carbohydrate oxidation, especially from blood glucose oxidation as muscle glycogen concentration declines. This goal was better achieved by ingesting 7 percent carbohydrate solutions as compared with a 14 percent solution (Febbraio et al., 1996).

Another example of a condition when carbohydrate ingestion during exercise would not be expected to improve performance is when the cause of fatigue is the accumulation of hydrogen ion in skeletal muscle (e.g., low muscle pH), as occurs during a single bout of intense exercise performed continuously for 2 to

30 minutes. Performing exercise that is not sufficiently stressful to cause fatigue, as evidenced by reduced power production, or that does not require high levels of effort to maintain power, as reflected, for example, by high levels of various stress hormones, would not benefit from carbohydrate ingestion. Furthermore, carbohydrate intake is not generally recommended during events, performed either continuously or intermittently, that are completed in 30 to 45 minutes or less. Although this last concept has not been extensively studied to date, it is a valid assumption based on the practices of athletes competing in events lasting only 30 to 45 minutes. As discussed, carbohydrate ingestion does not appear to lessen fatigue from hyperthermia or dehydration-induced hyperthermia, even when the durations of exercise are prolonged (e.g., one to three hours) (Febbraio et al., 1996; Fritzsche et al., 2000). Thus, there does not appear to be any benefit of adding carbohydrate to fluid replacement solution under these conditions. Accordingly, people who exercise at moderate intensity for less than one hour and do not experience fatigue do not appear to benefit from carbohydrate ingestion during exercise. Yet ingesting carbohydrate at a rate of 30 to 60 g/h does not appear to present a general physiological risk to people who do not experience gastrointestinal discomfort.

Conditions During Which Carbohydrate Ingestion Improves Performance through Unexplained Physiological Mechanisms

Carbohydrate ingestion during prolonged exercise can benefit performance if inadequate carbohydrate energy from blood glucose is the cause of fatigue (Coggan and Coyle, 1991; Febbraio et al., 1996). This effect on performance is a well-documented physiological mechanism by which the ergogenic benefit of carbohydrate ingestion during exercise can be explained. However, carbohydrate ingestion has been observed to improve performance under conditions in which fatigue is not clearly caused by a lack of aerobic or anaerobic carbohydrate energy. For example, when the duration of continuous exercise is extended to approximately 60 minutes and thus the intensity is 80 to 90 percent VO_2max, carbohydrate ingestion during exercise has been shown to improve power output by 6 percent during the 50- to 60-minute period (Below et al., 1995).

Other recent studies have also reported a performance benefit of carbohydrate feeding when the total duration of the performance bout is approximately 60 minutes or more by breaking the time into shorter exercise durations, thereby simulating the demands of many sports (basketball, soccer, hockey) in which high-intensity exercise is interspersed with periods of recovery (Mitchell et al., 1989; Murray et al., 1987). Carbohydrate ingestion is ergogenic during 15-minute bouts of intermittent "shuttle running," performed numerous times (e.g., five times) as well as during repeated high-intensity intervals of one minute's duration and a three-minute recovery (Davis et al., 1997, 1999, 2000; Nicholas et al., 1995; Welsh et al., 2002). The total duration of these work–rest bouts was more than 60 minutes. The physiological mechanisms responsible for these performance benefits from carbohydrate ingestion are not clear and have been theorized to involve the central nervous system, skeletal muscle, and the cardiovascular system. It is likely that carbohydrate feeding influences the interactions of all three systems, possibly through the actions of neurotransmitters, hormones, and peptides that are already known (e.g., insulin, catecholamines, and serotonin), that are newly recognized (e.g., interluken-6), or that have yet to be discovered. Regardless, sufficient evidence is accumulating to recommend carbohydrate ingestion during exercise bouts of continuous or intermittent exercise that lasts for 60 minutes or longer and cause fatigue from factors other than hyperthermia.

Can Carbohydrate Ingestion During Exercise Be Counterproductive?

It is recommended that carbohydrate be ingested at a rate of 30 to 60 g/h during exercise (Convertino et al., 1996), recognizing that ingesting more does not increase oxidation rate but can produce gastrointestinal discomfort in many people (Rehrer et al., 1992; Wagenmakers et al., 1993). In the latter case, carbohydrate feeding can be counterproductive when ingested in amounts (> 60 to 90 g/h) or concentrations (> 7 to 8 percent) that are too large (Febbraio et al., 1996; Galloway and Maughan, 2000).

If it produced gastrointestinal discomfort, carbohydrate ingestion at 30 to 60 g/h during exercise can impair performance as compared with no carbohydrate ingestion, a factor that is likely to vary from sport to sport and athlete to athlete. Carbohydrate ingestion should be used with caution during events lasting approximately 15 to 45 minutes and requiring repeated bouts of intense exercise lasting several minutes followed by several minutes of rest because these events may cause large swings in blood glucose and insulin concentration. Feeding plans must be specific to the varied intensity and time demands of the event. Those feeding schedules might be more than those described below, yet without data or experience to make more specific recommendations; all that can be done at present, besides recognizing these limitations, is to encourage systematic trial and error.

From a practical perspective, the recommendation of ingesting 30 to 60 g/h of carbohydrate during exercise should emphasize that this be accomplished by taking feedings every 10 to 30 minutes, as allowed by the event. The goal of the feeding schedule should be to create a steady flow of carbohydrate into the blood stream, which will then provide a steady flow of exogenous glucose into the blood. In other words, if carbohydrate feeding is begun during an event, it should be continued throughout the event in a manner that allows for a steady flow of exogenous glucose into the blood with minimal gastrointestinal discomfort. Avoid giving a large bolus of carbohydrate (i.e., more than 30 to 60 g) early in an event and then discontinuing carbohydrate feeding. This practice will prime the body for glucose metabolism, reduce fat oxidation, and then deprive the body of the fuel it has been primed to metabolize.

Summary and Recommendations for
Carbohydrate Intake During Exercise

During exercise that lasts longer than one hour and that causes fatigue, physically active people are advised to ingest 30 to 60 g/h of carbohydrate that can be rapidly converted to blood glucose because doing so generally improves performance. There is not a clear physiological need to consume any fluid or fuel when beginning exercise while reasonably hydrated and proceeding to exercise at low or moderate intensity for less than one hour without experiencing undo fatigue. However, there is no apparent reason for people to avoid fluid or carbohydrate intake if this is their preference and is well tolerated.

ACKNOWLEDGMENTS

The author is a member of the Sports Medicine Review Board of the Gatorade Sports Science Institute. Portions of this manuscript are similar to a recent review by the author published in 2004. Coyle EF. 2004. Fluid and fuel intake during exercise. *Journal of Sports Sciences* 22:39–55.

REFERENCES

Below PR, Mora-Rodriguez R, Gonzalez-Alonso J, Coyle EF. 1995. Fluid and carbohydrate ingestion independently improve performance during 1 h of intense exercise. *Med Sci Sports Exerc* 27(2):200–210.

Bergstrom J, Hermansen L, Hultman E, Saltin B. 1967. Diet, muscle glycogen and physical performance. *Acta Physiol Scand* 71(2):140–150.

Casa DJ, Armstrong LE, Hillman SK, Montain SJ, Reiff RV, Rich BSE, Roberts WO, Stone JA. 2000. National Athletic Trainers' Association Position Statement: Fluid replacement for athletes. *J Athlet Train* 35(2):212–224.

Coggan AR, Coyle EF. 1988. Effect of carbohydrate feedings during high-intensity exercise. *J Appl Physiol* 65(4):1703–1709.

Coggan AR, Coyle EF. 1991. Carbohydrate ingestion during prolonged exercise: Effects on metabolism and performance. *Exerc Sport Sci Rev* 19:1–40.

Convertino VA, Armstrong LE, Coyle EF, Mack GW, Sawka MN, Senay LC, Sherman WM. 1996. American College of Sports Medicine Position Stand on exercise and fluid replacement. *Med Sci Sports Exerc* 28(1):i–vii.

Costill D, Miller J. 1980. Nutrition for edurance sports. Carbohydrate and fluid balance. *Int J Sports Med* 1:2–14.

Coyle EF, Montain SJ. 1992a. Benefits of fluid replacement with carbohydrate during exercise. *Med Sci Sports Exerc* 24(9 Suppl):S324–S330.

Coyle EF, Montain SJ. 1992b. Carbohydrate and fluid ingestion during exercise: Are there trade-offs? *Med Sci Sports Exerc* 24(6):671–678.

Coyle EF, Coggan AR, Hemmert MK, Ivy JL. 1986. Muscle glycogen utilization during prolonged strenuous exercise when fed carbohydrate. *J Appl Physiol* 61(1):165–172.

Coyle EF, Costill DL, Fink WJ, Hoopes DG. 1978. Gastric emptying rates for selected athletic drinks. *Res Q* 49(2):119–124.

Davis JM, Jackson DA, Broadwell MS, Queary JL, Lambert CL. 1997. Carbohydrate drinks delay fatigue during intermittent, high-intensity cycling in active men and women. *Int J Sport Nutr* 7(4):261–273.

Davis JM, Welsh RS, Alerson NA. 2000. Effects of carbohydrate and chromium ingestion during intermittent high-intensity exercise to fatigue. *Int J Sport Nutr Exerc Metab* 10(4):476–485.

Davis JM, Welsh RS, De Volve KL, Alderson NA. 1999. Effects of branched-chain amino acids and carbohydrate on fatigue during intermittent, high-intensity running. *Int J Sports Med* 20(5):309–314.

Febbraio MA, Murton P, Selig SE, Clark SA, Lambert DL, Angus DJ, Carey MF. 1996. Effect of CHO ingestion on exercise metabolism and performance in different ambient temperatures. *Med Sci Sports Exerc* 28(11):1380–1387.

Fritzsche RG, Switzer TW, Hodgkinson BJ, Lee SH, Martin JC, Coyle EF. 2000. Water and carbohydrate ingestion during prolonged exercise increase maximal neuromuscular power. *J Appl Physiol* 88(2):730–737.

Galloway SD, Maughan RJ. 2000. The effects of substrate and fluid provision on thermoregulatory and metabolic responses to prolonged exercise in a hot environment. *J Sports Sci* 18(5):339–351.

Hargreaves M. 1996. Carbohydrates and exercise performance. *Nutr Rev* 54(4 Pt 2):S136–S139.

Maughan RJ. 1991. Fluid and electrolyte loss and replacement in exercise. *J Sports Sci* 9 (Spec No):117–142.

Maughan RJ, Noakes TD. 1991. Fluid replacement and exercise stress. A brief review of studies on fluid replacement and some guidelines for the athlete. *Sports Med* 12(1):16–31.

Maughan RJ, Goodburn R, Griffin J, Irani M, Kirwan JP, Leiper JB, MacLaren DP, McLatchie G, Tsintsas K, Williams C, Wellington P, Wilson WM, Wootton S. 1993. Fluid replacement in sport and exercise—A consensus statement. *Br J Sport Med* 27(1):34.

Millard-Stafford M. 1992. Fluid replacement during exercise in the heat. Review and recommendations. *Sports Med* 13(4):223–233.

Millard-Stafford M, Rosskopf LB, Snow TK, Hinson BT. 1997. Water versus carbohydrate-electrolyte ingestion before and during a 15-km run in the heat. *Int J Sport Nutr* 7(1):26–38.

Mitchell JB, Costill DL, Houmard JA, Fink WJ, Pascoe DD, Pearson DR. 1989. Influence of carbohydrate dosage on exercise performance and glycogen metabolism. *J Appl Physiol* 67(5):1843–1849.

Murray R, Eddy DE, Murray TW, Seifert JG, Paul GL, Halaby GA. 1987. The effect of fluid and carbohydrate feedings during intermittent cycling exercise. *Med Sci Sports Exerc* 19(6):597–604.

Nicholas CW, Williams C, Lakomy HK, Phillips G, Nowitz A. 1995. Influence of ingesting a carbohydrate-electrolyte solution on endurance capacity during intermittent, high-intensity shuttle running. *J Sports Sci* 13(4):283–290.

Rehrer NJ. 1994. The maintenance of fluid balance during exercise. *Int J Sports Med* 15(3):122–125.

Rehrer NJ, Beckers EJ, Brouns F, Saris WH, Ten Hoor F. 1993. Effects of electrolytes in carbohydrate beverages on gastric emptying and secretion. *Med Sci Sports Exerc* 25(1):42–51.

Rehrer NJ, Wagenmakers AJ, Beckers EJ, Halliday D, Leiper JB, Brouns F, Maughan RJ, Westerterp K, Saris WH. 1992. Gastric emptying, absorption, and carbohydrate oxidation during prolonged exercise. *J Appl Physiol* 72(2):468–475.

Sugiura K, Kobayashi K. 1998. Effect of carbohydrate ingestion on sprint performance following continuous and intermittent exercise. *Med Sci Sports Exerc* 30(11):1624–1630.

Wagenmakers AJ, Brouns F, Saris WH, Halliday D. 1993. Oxidation rates of orally ingested carbohydrates during prolonged exercise in men. *J Appl Physiol* 75(6):2774–2280.

Welsh RS, Davis JM, Burke JR, Williams HG. 2002. Carbohydrates and physical/mental performance during intermittent exercise to fatigue. *Med Sci Sports Exerc* 34(4):723–731.

Macronutrient Composition of Military Rations for Cognitive Performance in Short-Term, High-Stress Situations

Randall J. Kaplan, Canadian Sugar Institute

INTRODUCTION

The importance of nutrition for cognitive performance in military settings has long been recognized. The Committee on Military Nutrition Research (CMNR) of the Food and Nutrition Board, Institute of Medicine (IOM) of the National Academies has published several volumes on this topic, including reports on the cognitive effects of performance-enhancing food components (IOM, 1994); inadequate energy intakes (IOM, 1995); protein and amino acids (IOM, 1999); and caffeine (IOM, 2001).

Cognitive performance refers to intellectual behaviors such as memory, reasoning, attention, vigilance, and choice reaction time. Mood (e.g., happy, sad, calm, tense) and psychomotor performance (e.g., sensation, perception, agility) are distinct from cognitive performance, but they can have a considerable influence on it (Mays, 1995; Spring et al., 1994) and are therefore relevant to this discussion. The aspects of cognition that are important in combat settings include the ability to perceive, attend to, and respond appropriately to cues; make prompt decisions; and sustain vigilance (IOM, 1994; Mays, 1995).

The Committee on Optimization of Nutrient Composition of Military Rations for Short-Term, High-Stress Situations, an ad hoc committee of the CMNR, has been given the task of recommending the nutrient composition of a ration for combat missions to optimize physical and cognitive performance and to prevent adverse health consequences.

This daily ration is intended for repeated short-term use (three to seven days followed by one to three days of ad libitum recovery) by fit male soldiers during high-tempo, stressful combat missions. Stress may be caused by physical and cognitive workloads, extreme temperature, threats to safety, and sleep deprivation, all of which can interfere with cognitive performance (Lieberman et al., 2002b; Owen et al., 2004).

The purpose of this report is to briefly review relevant evidence on the effects of energy and macronutrients (i.e., carbohydrate, protein, and fat) on cognitive performance and mood, and to provide recommendations for the macronutrient composition of the assault ration, including types of each macronutrient, to enhance cognitive performance. Because factors associated with combat operations are likely to lead to cognitive deficits relative to normal functioning, the realistic goal in optimizing the nutrient composition of the ration should be to decrease these deficits, rather than to enhance performance beyond normal bounds.

To address this task this paper discusses the following specific questions:

- Should the energy content of the ration (energy density) be maximized so as to minimize the energy debt, or is there a more optimal "mix" of macronutrients and micronutrients, not necessarily producing maximal energy density?
- What would be the optimal macronutrient balance between carbohydrate, protein, and fat for such an assault ration to enhance cognitive performance during combat missions?
- What are the types and levels of macronutrients (e.g., complex verses simple carbohydrates, proteins with specific amino acid profiles, type of fat, etc.) that would optimize such an assault ration to enhance cognitive performance during combat missions?

For the purpose of this paper, it has been assumed that other nutrional requirements of the soldiers (e.g., water, micronutrients) will be met. If these other requirements are not met, the results could override the importance of macronutrient requirements. For instance, it is well established that hypohydration (Wilson and Morley, 2003) and iron deficiency (Sandstead, 2000) present significant detriments to cognitive performance. In the combat situation, particularly during extreme temperatures, the highest priority for reducing cognitive impairment is adequate hydration (IOM, 1995).

The maximum weight of the macronutrient component of a 1,360 gram-ration is approximately 500 g [calculated from a standard, approximately 2,400-kcal ration, comprising 50 percent of energy as carbohydrate (300 g), 30 percent as fat (80 g), and 20 percent as protein (120 g)], with the remaining 860 g comprised of noncaloric components, including moisture, fiber, and micronutrients. Theoretically, 500 g could provide between 2,000 kcal (i.e., entirely protein and carbohydrate) and 4,500 kcal (i.e., entirely fat), in which case the energy needs of the soldiers (4,000 to 4,500 kcal/day) could be met within the weight limitation of the ration if energy density were increased as much as possible. The question is: Should the energy content of the ration be maximized, or is there a more optimal ratio of macronutrients for cognitive performance?

ENERGY INGESTION AND COGNITIVE PERFORMANCE

Acute Effects

The acute effects (hours) of energy ingestion on cognitive performance have been examined in a number of studies in healthy, nonstressed subjects. Several reviews of the literature have concluded that the provision of energy in the morning (breakfast) generally improves cognitive performance over the next 30 minutes to 2 h, compared with no energy provision, with more robust effects on tests of memory and less consistent effects on tests of attention or vigilance (Bellisle et al., 1998; Dye and Blundell, 2002; Kanarek, 1997; Leigh Gibson and

Green, 2002; Pollitt and Matthews, 1998). The mechanism for these results has not been elucidated, but likely both gut-mediated and centrally acting post-absorptive signals are involved (Kaplan et al., 2001).

By contrast to the breakfast studies, large meals provided at mid-day (lunch) consistently impair cognitive performance (e.g., memory, vigilance, and reaction time) and mood (e.g., alertness and fatigue) over the next one to two hours, compared with the effects of those consuming no lunch or a light lunch. This phenomenon is known as the "post-lunch dip" and is likely related to normal changes in daily circadian rhythm as well as changes to habitual intake patterns (Bellisle et al., 1998; Dye et al., 2000; Kanarek, 1997; Leigh Gibson and Green, 2002).

A few studies have examined the short-term effects of energy intake on cognitive performance and mood under stressful conditions, showing the benefits of increased energy intake. One study found no changes in mood after low-energy intake during breakfast and lunch (264 kcal) as compared with a higher energy intake (1,723 kcal; consistent with energy needs of the subjects) during a nonstressful condition (Macht, 1996). However, when participants were subjected to emotionally stressful white noise, those with a low-energy intake experienced a degradation in mood (i.e., more irritability and less relaxation), whereas those with a higher energy intake did not.

Another study strongly supports a beneficial effect of increased energy ingestion on cognitive performance and mood under stressful conditions (Lieberman et al., 2002a). In this study, 143 male subjects from an elite combat unit were tested during periods of intense physical activity over 10 h, during which energy needs were not met with regular meals (approximately 765 kcal) (Lieberman et al., 2002a). Energy supplementation (carbohydrate-containing drink) throughout the day improved vigilance and mood (i.e., increased vigor, decreased confusion) in a dose-dependent manner compared with the effects of a noncaloric placebo drink. The strongest effects on performance resulted from the highest energy drink (approximately 1,309 kcal), followed by the medium-energy drink (approximately 654 kcal), and the placebo (0 kcal) (Figure B-9). It is impossible to determine from this study whether the beneficial effects were caused by an increase in energy ingestion or an increase in carbohydrate ingestion.

Medium-Term Effects

The medium-term effects (days) of dieting to lose weight consistently impair cognitive performance and mood (Leigh Gibson and Green, 2002). The effects are attributed to the act of dieting, rather than to inherent differences between dieters and nondieters because the impedence on performance is not observed when the same individuals are not dieting (Green and Rogers, 1995). It has been suggested that this impairment is caused more by a psychological pre-occupation with food and feelings of hunger than by a physiologic effect of low

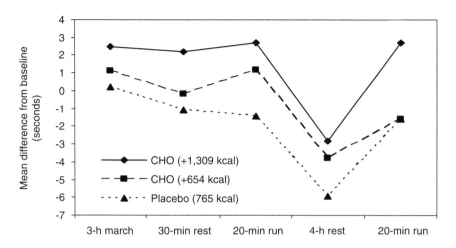

FIGURE B-9 Vigilance performance of soldiers who received carbohydrate (CHO) beverages or placebo in addition to regular meals (providing approximately 765 kcal) while engaging in various activities over 10 h.
NOTE: A higher number on the y-axis represents improved performance.
SOURCE: Adapted from Lieberman et al. (2002a) with permission by the *American Journal of Clinical Nutrition © Am J Clin Nutr.* American Society for Clinical Nutrition.

energy intake (Leigh Gibson and Green, 2002). This conclusion is based on evidence that (1) individuals perform worse on cognitive tests when they are dieting, even when no actual weight is lost; (2) the magnitude and structure of the deficits is comparable to those caused by anxiety and depression; and (3) performance is not clearly affected by weight loss in the absence of other stress. It has been hypothesized that task-irrelevant feelings of hunger and thoughts of food may impair performance by interfering with normal working memory function. Working memory can be conceptualized as "the fundamental cognitive processing system, in that it serves to allocate limited cognitive processing capacity to other ongoing cognitive operations in order of their relevance or importance to an individual" (Leigh Gibson and Green, 2002).

A study using a similar eating pattern as would be consumed by combat soldiers (several days of hypocaloric intake followed by ad libitum intake) supports the hypothesis that energy restriction impedes performance in the absence of significant weight loss (Laessle et al., 1996). In this study, healthy female subjects consumed a low-calorie diet (approximately 651 kcal/day) for four days, followed by ad libitum intake (approximately 2,876 kcal/day) for three days each week for four weeks. During the low-calorie periods, subjects reported stronger feelings of hunger and thoughts about food as well as demonstrating worse moods, more irritability, difficulties concentrating, and greater fatigue than during the ad libitum periods even though weight loss was minimal. Repeated episodes of low energy intakes over the 4 weeks did not reduce feelings of hunger. The implication of this study is that the negative effects of hunger are unlikely to be reduced during periods of low energy intake when soldiers repeatedly eat hypocaloric diets followed by ad libitum recovery periods. In other words, it may be very difficult to train soldiers to ignore their hunger feelings. It should be noted, however, that this study was performed with women and not under the unique added stressors of combat missions.

The hypothesis presented suggests that psychological feelings of hunger contribute to cognitive deficits during periods of low energy intake; however, the physiologic consequences of low energy intake and negative energy balance cannot be ruled out as contributing factors because other acute evidence (presented earlier) and longer term evidence under the stressful conditions presented below do not clearly indicate the mechanism involved. Most likely, both psychological and physiological factors associated with low energy intake, particularly under stressful conditions, contribute to the performance deficit.

The evidence that increased appetite interferes with the ability to perform optimally suggests that reducing hunger may be beneficial for mood and cognitive performance. Indeed, declining hunger sensations have been associated with being more energetic, lively, calm, and relaxed (Fischer et al., 2004). The macronutrient composition of foods can play an important role in minimizing hunger. Protein consistently and robustly induces greater satiety than carbohydrate or fat on a per calorie basis (Westerterp-Plantenga, 2003) and has a greater effect on satiety than do substantially higher energy intakes from the other macronutrients (Stubbs and Whybrow, 2004; Stubbs et al., 2000) (Figure B-10). Carbohydrate appears to induce greater satiety than fat does on a per calorie basis (Stubbs et al., 2000), but the differences are minimal when palatability and energy density of foods are matched (Rolls and Bell, 1999). Thus, to reduce the negative effects of hunger on cognitive performance and mood, it may be beneficial to increase the protein content of hypocaloric military rations and to reduce the fat content.

Various types of each macronutrient also have different effects on satiety (Stubbs et al., 2000). A review concluded that high glycemic index carbohydrates (i.e., rapidly raise blood glucose concentration) have a greater effect on satiety than low glycemic index carbohydrates over the short term (up to one hour after carbohydrate ingestion), whereas lower glycemic index carbohydrates have a stronger effect on satiety over the longer term (i.e., up to 6 h after carbohydrate ingestion) (Anderson and Woodend, 2003). However, these effects are not likely caused entirely by changes in blood glucose (Kaplan and Greenwood, 2002). The data implicating different effects of fat type on satiety are mixed, with some suggesting that polyunsaturated fatty acids have a stronger effect on increasing satiety than monounsaturated or saturated fatty acids do (French and Robinson, 2003; Lawton et al., 2000), whereas others have found no differences between

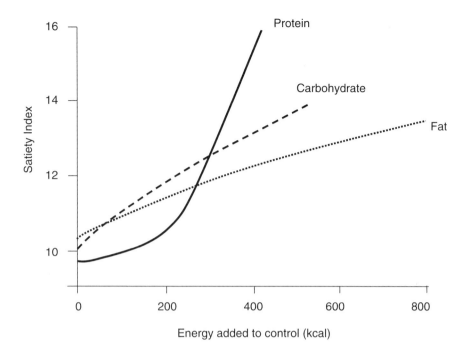

FIGURE B-10 Effect of increasing energy content of macronutrient loads on satiety over 3.25 h.
NOTE: Data were collated from a number of studies.
SOURCE: Adapted from Stubbs and Whybrow (2004).

the two (Alfenas and Mattes, 2003; Flint et al., 2003). Medium-chain triglycerides, which are rapidly metabolized, have been shown to exert a stronger effect on satiety than long-chain triglycerides do; however, only a few human studies are available and the results are inconclusive (French and Robinson, 2003; St-Onge and Jones, 2002). Research on the effects of protein type on satiety is also limited because evidence in human studies suggesting that some proteins might suppress appetite more than others is inconsistent (Anderson and Moore, 2004; Westerterp-Plantenga, 2003).

It is important to note that, although it is argued here that reducing hunger in soldiers consuming hypocaloric rations may be beneficial for cognitive performance, this may not be relevant if appetite is suppressed by hypohydration, physical activity, or stress to the extent that feelings of hunger and thoughts of food are eliminated. It is well documented that soldiers tend to underconsume foods, and this may be partially due to a suppression of appetite (IOM, 1995). Thus, it is important to determine whether the expected increase in appetite associated with the hypocaloric intake of combat soldiers is stronger or weaker than the suppression of appetite that will be caused by other factors. There is evidence, however, that when military rations provide only 60 percent of energy needs (i.e., energy intake and energy expenditure was 1,946 kcal and 3,200–3,300 kcal, respectively), the entire rations are consumed (Shukitt-Hale et al., 1997), suggesting that soldiers' appetites are strong under these circumstances. These data would support the argument that strong feelings of hunger will be present in combat soldiers consuming assault rations containing approximately 2,400 kcal/day when their needs are > 4,000 kcal/day.

Long-Term Effects

The long-term effects (weeks or months) of energy intake on cognitive performance are not relevant if soldiers are able to consume enough excess energy during the one- to- three-day ad libitum recovery period to make up for the negative energy balance during the three to seven days, such that they do not lose weight. By contrast, if soldiers are in a state of negative energy balance over weeks and months because of repeated consumption of hypocaloric diets and inadequate recovery periods, then the long-term effects of low energy intake are relevant.

Evidence on the long-term effects of low energy intake on cognitive performance shows that those effects are minimal in the absence of significant stress but are significant if stress is present. In a review of the effects of underconsumption of military rations on cognitive performance, Mays (1995) concluded that underconsumption leading to weight loss up to 6 percent over 10 to 45 days does not affect performance in the absence of significant stress. A more recent study over a 30-day trial supports this conclusion (Shukitt-Hale et al., 1997). However, consistent with the long-term dieting data (e.g., Kretsch et al., 1997), underconsumption combined with stress during military operations (e.g., exercise, sleep deprivation, and danger) significantly degrades performance within a few days (Mays, 1995). Based on the available data, Mays proposed a relationship between long-term negative energy balance and cognitive performance (Figure B-11). These data suggest that consumption levels of 75 to 90 percent of requirements may actually enhance performance in the first 3 to 15 days, whereas consumption of 50 percent or less of requirements degrades performance, particularly under stressful conditions. Over the longer term, performance continues to degrade along with negative energy balance. Thus, if repeated short-term periods of low energy intake during combat operations lead to long-term negative energy balance, deficits in cognitive performance can be expected.

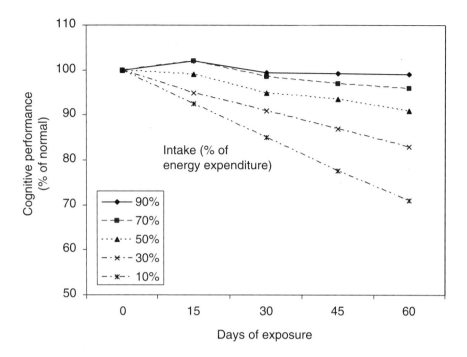

FIGURE B-11 Proposed relationship between energy intake as a percentage of energy expenditure and cognitive performance over two months, based on the results of several studies.
SOURCE: Adapted from Mays (1995).

CARBOHYDRATE INGESTION AND COGNITIVE PERFORMANCE

Glucose Compared with a Noncaloric Placebo

For the purposes of this paper, "carbohydrate" refers to digestible or glycemic carbohydrates that provide energy (primarily sugars and starches). It does not include dietary fiber, resistant starch, or other nondigestible carbohydrates that do not provide energy as a carbohydrate.

A large number of studies conducted over the past 20 years have shown beneficial effects of glucose ingestion on cognitive performance as compared with noncaloric sweetened placebos (e.g., aspartame, saccharin) in animals and humans over the short term—from 15 minutes to 3 h after ingestion (Greenwood, 2003; Korol, 2002; Korol and Gold, 1998; Messier, 2004). Cognitive impairments associated with hypoglycemic episodes have also been a consistent finding

(McCall, 1992). Early studies suggested that the cognitive-enhancing effects of glucose were only evident when an existing deficit was present, such as in elderly subjects and in patients with Alzheimer's disease, schizophrenia, and Down syndrome, but not in healthy young adults (Korol and Gold, 1998). Since that time, others have shown that consuming glucose can improve performance in young adults if cognitive tasks are sufficiently demanding (Benton, 2001); however, the magnitude of the effects depends on glucose regulation and baseline cognitive abilities (Awad et al., 2002; Greenwood, 2003; Kaplan et al., 2000; Messier, 2004).

The beneficial effects of consuming glucose are dependent on the type of cognitive test, task difficulty, and glucose dose (Greenwood, 2003; Messier, 2004). In contrast with the data showing the benefits of eating breakfast and the detriments of eating lunch, the effects of consuming glucose appear to be positive in both the morning and the afternoon (Sunram-Lea et al., 2001). The effects of glucose are strongest on functions mediated by the medial temporal lobe and surrounding areas, including long-term verbal memory, and less robust for other tasks, including short-term memory, attention, and reaction time. Glucose consumption can, however, improve performance on a wide range of tasks as long as the tasks are of sufficient difficulty. For instance, Kennedy and Scholey (2000) found glucose ingestion improved performance in young adults on a difficult test (serial sevens, which requires subjects to count backwards by sevens), but not on two easier tests (Figure B-12). These findings suggest that an increased brain requirement for glucose is needed before benefits of glucose ingestion can be observed. Conditions for which glucose could reverse deficits in performance caused by increased brain requirements for glucose include those of aging (McNay and Gold, 2001), increased cognitive demand (Fairclough and Houston, 2004), and physical activity (Brun et al., 2001; Grego et al., 2004; Nybo and Secher, 2004). Thus, carbohydrate ingestion is likely to benefit cognitive performance during combat operations for which brain glucose requirements would likely be increased because of the demanding nature of the tasks and high levels of physical activity.

The dose of glucose that enhances cognitive performance follows an inverted U-shaped response in humans and animals. Consistently, low doses have no effect on performance, intermediate doses (25 to 75 g) improve performance, and high doses have no effect or impair performance (Greenwood, 2003; Greenwood et al., 2003; Messier, 2004; Parsons and Gold, 1992) (Figure B-13). Taken together, these findings suggest that a moderate amount of glucose improves performance on a range of demanding cognitive tests in young adults, or on tasks in demanding situations (e.g., stress, physical activity), but glucose is unlikely to improve performance on simpler tasks under nonstressful conditions.

There is no consensus on the mechanism that explains the effects of glucose on cognitive performance, but several hypotheses have been proposed. The following effects of glucose ingestion have been most commonly suggested as

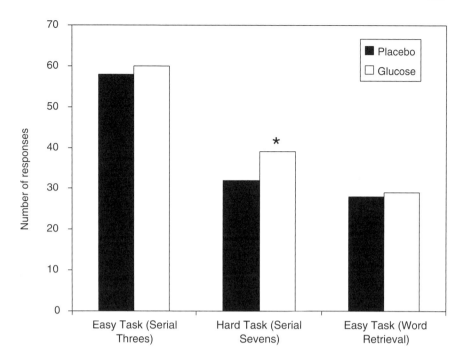

FIGURE B-12 Mean number of responses (subtractions or words produced) made on each of three tasks after ingestion of noncaloric saccharin-sweetened placebo or of 25 g glucose drinks.
*p < 0.01 compared with corresponding placebo group.
SOURCE: Adapted from Kennedy and Scholey (2000).

possible mechanisms: replenishes brain extracellular glucose that declines during difficult tasks; increases synthesis of the brain neurotransmitter acetylcholine; increases central insulin; or influences peripheral signals that are relayed to the brain via the vagus nerve (Greenwood, 2003; Messier, 2004; Park, 2001).

Carbohydrate Foods

As noted earlier, one study found that a carbohydrate-containing beverage provided in addition to regular hypocaloric meals benefited vigilance and mood during combat training (Figure B-9), but it is impossible to determine whether the benefits were due to increased energy intake or to carbohydrate intake (Lieberman et al., 2002a). The authors suggested that the benefits could have been due to an increased supply of glucose to the brain, which could have helped

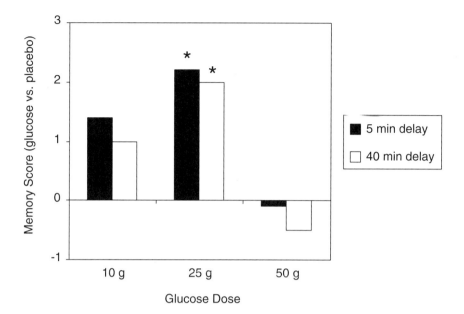

FIGURE B-13 Logical memory scores in elderly subjects 5 and 40 minutes after glucose ingestion, presented as differences from placebo (saccharin). Significant memory enhancement was observed after 25 g glucose, but not at the higher or lower doses.
* $p < 0.05$ versus placebo.
SOURCE: Adapted from Parsons and Gold (1992), used with permission from Elsevier.

prevent a reduction in the synthesis of neurotransmitters protecting the brain from the consequences of an energy deficit.

Other studies suggest that carbohydrate, independent of energy intake, benefits performance under hypocaloric (Wing et al., 1995) and physically demanding (Achten et al., 2004) circumstances that are relevant for combat operations. Wing and colleagues (1995) found that a low-energy (549 kcal/day), low-carbohydrate–high-fat diet was associated with impaired performance on a test of general brain function after one week as compared with the results of an equal-energy, high-carbohydrate–low-fat diet. In addition, during 11 days of intense running training, Achten and colleagues (2004) found that higher carbohydrate–lower fat diets improved overall mood and reduced fatigue as compared with the results of equal-energy (approximately 3,900 kcal/day), low-carbohydrate–high-fat diets.

Under nonexercise, adequate energy situations, carbohydrate ingestion has been associated with both better and worse moods (Benton, 2002; Leigh Gibson and Green, 2002), which may be dependent on the testing time after ingestion. Carbohydrate may improve mood up to 30 minutes after ingestion, but it is associated with a sedative effect after about 2 h (Benton, 2002). The sedating effect may be caused by a carbohydrate-induced increased tryptophan/large neutral amino acid ratio, which increases both the brain tryptophan levels and the synthesis of the neurotransmitter serotonin (Spring et al., 1994). However, the effect of carbohydrate on serotonin is abolished with the ingestion of as little as 4-percent protein (Benton, 2002; Benton and Donohoe, 1999; Benton and Nabb, 2003; Spring et al., 1994), so these findings are likely not relevant for military rations with mixed macronutrient composition. Another hypothesis suggests that beneficial effects of carbohydrate on mood are related to an increased release of endorphins relevant to the ingestion of any palatable food, rather than to carbohydrate per se (Benton, 2002).

Carbohydrate Type

The type of carbohydrate may be important for cognitive performance although research in this area is limited to two studies. In one study in healthy elderly subjects, 50 g of carbohydrate from glucose, potato (high glycemic index), or barley (low glycemic index) all improved performance on memory and a test of general brain function up to one hour after ingestion, particularly in subjects with poorer baseline memory and glucose regulation (Kaplan et al., 2000). The cognitive-enhancing effects of barley, which raised blood glucose to 6 mmol/L, were novel because it had previously been believed that blood glucose must be at a concentration of 8 to 10 mmol/L for a benefit to be observed. These findings were supported by a recent study that found that a high-carbohydrate meal with a lower glycemic index improved memory in young adults up to 3 h after ingestion, but a higher glycemic index meal did not (Benton et al., 2003). The findings could not be related to blood glucose levels, but these data, along with the evidence showing an inverted U-shaped dose response for glucose, suggest that a prolonged increase in blood glucose and insulin levels, rather than rapid fluctuations, may be beneficial.

It is noteworthy that virtually all studies examining the effects of carbohydrate on cognitive performance or mood have used glucose or glucose polymers (e.g., starches). A few studies have examined the effects of fructose which is metabolized differently from glucose, in rats, but the evidence is mixed (Messier, 2004). Until evidence to the contrary is available in humans, it should be assumed that the beneficial effects of carbohydrate are limited to sources of glucose or glucose polymers.

PROTEIN, FAT, MACRONUTRIENT BALANCE, AND COGNITIVE PERFORMANCE

Protein has the potential to influence cognitive performance because several amino acids, including tryptophan, tyrosine, phenylalanine, arginine, histadine, and threonine, are precursors of neurotransmitters or neuromodulators and can influence their synthesis (Lieberman, 2003). Indeed, individual amino acids have been shown to influence cognitive performance; however, these effects are likely not relevant when examining the effects of protein consumed as part of a food ration (Greenwood, 1994). In particular, tyrosine benefits cognitive performance in sleep deprived, stressed subjects, likely by its role as a precursor for the neurotransmitters norepinephrine and dopamine (Lieberman, 2003). Tryptophan may be beneficial as a sleep aid, by way of its effects on increasing synthesis of serotonin, and it improves vigilance by way of increasing the release of melatonin (Lieberman, 2003). However, any potential benefits of these amino acids would likely be as between-meal supplements, rather than as part of normal meals (Greenwood, 1994).

As noted in the carbohydrate section above, several reports have concluded that high-carbohydrate–low-protein meals are sedating because they cause an increase in serotonin synthesis, whereas protein-rich meals are arousing and can improve reaction time and vigilance (Dye and Blundell, 2002; IOM, 1994; Leigh Gibson and Green, 2002). However, as noted, these findings are likely not relevant for mixed macronutrient military rations because as little as 4 percent protein prevents the effect on serotonin. Moreover, other data do not support a negative influence on mood by consumption of a high-carbohydrate–low-protein diet. A review by Benton and Donohoe (1999) concluded that diets higher in carbohydrate and lower in protein are associated with less depression, anger, and tension and with being more energetic.

Although the fat content of diets can have an effect on cognitive performance over the long term (i.e., months or years) (Greenwood and Young, 2001; Kaplan and Greenwood, 1998), fat likely only has limited effects over the short term (i.e., hours or days), possibly related to the fact that rates of fat and carbohydrate oxidation are not influenced by the fat content of a meal (Flatt et al., 1985). Nevertheless, some studies have found acute effects of fat on performance and mood, but the data are inconsistent. Recent reviews concluded that in general, high-fat–low-carbohydrate meals can lead to declines in alertness and reaction time, particularly when they differ from habitual fat intake (Dye and Blundell, 2002; Leigh Gibson and Green, 2002).

Few direct comparisons between pure macronutrients have been made. Kaplan and colleagues (2001) found that in healthy elderly persons, pure protein, carbohydrate, and fat could all improve memory performance 15 minutes after ingestion compared with a noncaloric placebo, suggesting a general benefit of energy ingestion, likely mediated by a peripheral mechanism, which could include gut peptides or signals to the brain by way of the vagus nerve. However, it was also found that each macronutrient had unique effects on performance. For instance, as shown in Figure B-14, only glucose tended to improve memory 60 minutes after ingestion, and performance on a visual-motor task; and protein was the only macronutrient to slow the rate of forgetting. Various peripheral and

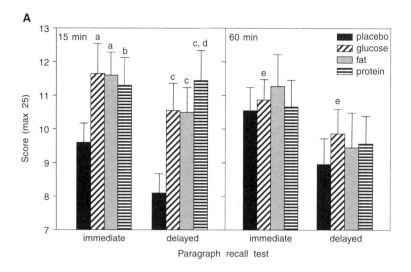

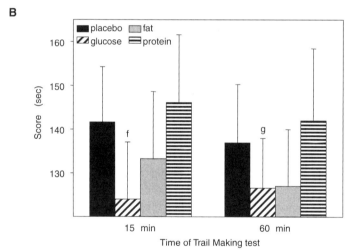

FIGURE B-14 (A) Mean (± standard error of means) scores on immediate and delayed paragraph recall 15 and 60 minutes after consumption of placebo, glucose, fat, and protein test drinks. (B) Mean (± standard error of means) scores on Trail Making Test (parts A + B) in men (n = 10) at 15 and 60 minutes after ingestion of placebo, glucose, fat, and protein test drinks.

NOTE: Lower scores represent better performance. (A) a, b, c, d, e = significantly different from placebo: a = p ≤ 0.02; b = p for trend = 0.04; c = p ≤ 0.001; d = p = 0.002 (rate of forgetting, immediate + delayed); e = p for trend = 0.09 (for composite score, immediate + delayed). (B) f, g = significantly different from placebo; f = p for trend = 0.04; g = p = 0.02.
SOURCE: Adapted from Kaplan et al. (2001) with permission by the *American Journal of Clinical Nutrition* © *Am J Clin Nutr.* American Society for Clinical Nutrition.

central mechanisms could account for these specific effects. Another study also found unique effects of each macronutrient in healthy young adults (Fischer et al., 2001). Carbohydrate improved choice reaction and short-term memory time after one hour; protein improved choice reaction time after two hours; fat improved performance on short-term memory and attention.

Taken together, several reviews have concluded that, although macronutrients have been shown to have different effects on cognitive performance, the effects have been inconsistent, and few overall conclusions can be made at this time about an optimal ratio of macronutrients for cognitive performance (Bellisle et al., 1998; Dye and Blundell, 2002; Dye et al., 2000; Kanarek, 1997; Lieberman, 2003).

CONCLUSIONS

Despite discrepancies in the literature, some conclusions can be made about the effects of energy ingestion on cognitive performance. (1) Energy ingestion approaching the level of energy needs generally improves cognitive performance and mood over the short term (several hours) compared with no energy or very low energy ingestion; the fact that benefits seem to be independent of weight loss suggest that feelings of hunger and thoughts of food contribute to the cognitive and mood deficits. Thus, minimizing hunger may minimize the negative effects on performance. Hunger can be minimized with higher protein and lower fat ingestion. (3) Over longer periods (weeks or months), there is a gradual impairment in cognitive performance associated with negative energy balance and weight loss, with greater and more rapid deficits associated with very low energy intakes (< 50 percent of energy requirements), particularly under stressful conditions.

The review of the research presented in this paper shows that the scientific literature in this area is inconsistent and contradictory; therefore, it is difficult to make definitive recommendations regarding the questions posed in the introduction. The research, although not conclusive, supports the following conclusions described below.

The following are desired characteristics of an assault ration designed for cognitive performance:

- Adequate and sustained glucose supply to the brain. The provision of glucose or carbohydrate to the brain improves mood and performance when brain glucose requirements increase, which appears to occur during cognitively demanding tasks, particularly under hypocaloric, stressful, or physically demanding conditions.
- Moderate fluctuations in blood glucose. Consistent evidence shows that both hypoglycemia and hyperglycemia impair cognitive performance; that intermediate, but not high or low, doses of glucose improve performance;

and that limited evidence shows that low glycemic index carbohydrates improve performance over a longer period than do higher glycemic index carbohydrates. Thus moderate, rather than extreme, fluctuations in blood glucose are desirable.

- Minimize feelings of hunger. Hypocaloric intakes are associated with deficits in cognitive performance and mood, and this is caused, in part, by feelings of hunger and thoughts of food interfering with normal cognitive processes. Reducing feelings of hunger is desirable.
- Minimize long-term negative energy balance. Sufficient data indicate that long-term energy deficits resulting in negative energy balance and weight loss are associated with deficits in cognitive performance and mood under stressful situations. Long-term negative energy balance should be minimized.

The optimal composition of the assault ration for cognitive performance would be characterized by the following:

- A maximized carbohydrate content of the ration to provide an adequate and sustained supply of glucose to the brain, because of their hypocaloric nature and the fact that substantial carbohydrate will be required to sustain physical activity. The carbohydrate source should ideally provide glucose (e.g., glucose, sucrose, starch) rather than other monosaccharides (e.g., fructose) as the beneficial effects of carbohydrate have only been shown with glucose. The effect of the ration on blood glucose should be moderate for optimal and sustained cognitive performance and should also reduce feelings of hunger. Importantly, the carbohydrate source may have a high or low glycemic index to give the overall ration a moderate effect on blood glucose, because the other components of the ration could affect blood glucose. For instance, both protein (increases insulin release) and fiber can lower blood glucose. Higher protein and fiber content rations may necessitate higher glycemic index carbohydrates to obtain a ration with a moderate effect on blood glucose.
- If feelings of hunger are strong and long-term energy balance is not a major problem (i.e., energy balance can be maintained by high energy intakes during the recovery periods between combat operations), then protein content of the ration should be increased and fat content should be decreased to increase satiety and reduce feelings of hunger. In this case, the energy density of the ration will not be maximized. Not enough evidence exists to recommend a specific amino acid or fatty acid profile that will optimize cognitive performance compared with any other profile. It seems prudent to supply minimum amino acid requirements.
- If feelings of hunger are weak because of stress or hypohydration outweighing the effects on appetite of the low calorie diet, and long-term

negative energy balance and weight loss are expected, then minimum protein requirements should be met for nitrogen balance, and fat content should be increased to maximize energy intake over the long term. In this case, additional protein to reduce hunger would be less important than increasing long-term energy intake by maximizing fat content and energy density of the ration.

- To reduce long-term negative energy balance, high-energy intake should be encouraged during the recovery periods. Thus, intake during recovery should consist of energy-dense foods with minimal effects on satiety (i.e., high-fat, low-protein foods).

REFERENCES

Achten J, Halson SL, Moseley L, Rayson MP, Casey A, Jeukendrup AE. 2004. Higher dietary carbohydrate content during intensified running training results in better maintenance of performance and mood state. *J Appl Physiol* 96(4):1331–1340.

Alfenas RC, Mattes RD. 2003. Effect of fat sources on satiety. *Obes Res* 11(2):183–187.

Anderson GH, Moore SE. 2004. Dietary proteins in the regulation of food intake and body weight in humans. *J Nutr* 134(4):974S–979S.

Anderson GH, Woodend D. 2003. Effect of glycemic carbohydrates on short-term satiety and food intake. *Nutr Rev* 61(5):S17–S26.

Awad N, Gagnon M, Desrochers A, Tsiakas M, Messier C. 2002. Impact of peripheral glucoregulation on memory. *Behav Neurosci* 116(4):691–702.

Bellisle F, Blundell JE, Dye L, Fantino M, Fern E, Fletcher RJ, Lambert J, Roberfroid M, Specter S, Westenhofer J, Westerterp-Plantenga MS. 1998. Functional food science and behaviour and psychological functions. *Br J Nutr* 80(Suppl 1):S173–S193.

Benton D. 2001. The impact of the supply of glucose to the brain on mood and memory. *Nutr Rev* 59(1 Pt 2):S20–S21.

Benton D. 2002. Carbohydrate ingestion, blood glucose and mood. *Neurosci Biobehav Rev* 26(3):293–308.

Benton D, Donohoe RT. 1999. The effects of nutrients on mood. *Public Health Nutr* 2(3A):403–409.

Benton D, Nabb S. 2003. Carbohydrate, memory, and mood. *Nutr Rev* 61(5):S61–S67.

Benton D, Ruffin MP, Lassel T, Nabb S, Messaoudi M, Vinoy S, Desor D, Lang V. 2003. The delivery rate of dietary carbohydrates affects cognitive performance in both rats and humans. *Psychopharmacology (Berl)* 166(1):86–90.

Brun JF, Dumortier M, Fedou C, Mercier J. 2001. Exercise hypoglycemia in nondiabetic subjects. *Diabetes Metab* 27(2 Pt 1):92–106.

Dye L, Blundell J. 2002. Functional foods: Psychological and behavioural functions. *Br J Nutr* 88(Suppl 2):S187–S211.

Dye L, Lluch A, Blundell JE. 2000. Macronutrients and mental performance. *Nutrition* 16(10):1021–1034.

Fairclough SH, Houston K. 2004. A metabolic measure of mental effort. *Biol Psychol* 66(2):177–190.

Fischer K, Colombani PC, Langhans W, Wenk C. 2001. Cognitive performance and its relationship with postprandial metabolic changes after ingestion of different macronutrients in the morning. *Br J Nutr* 85(3):393–405.

Fischer K, Colombani PC, Wenk C. 2004. Metabolic and cognitive coefficients in the development of hunger sensations after pure macronutrient ingestion in the morning. *Appetite* 42(1):49–61.

Flatt JP, Ravussin E, Acheson KJ, Jequier E. 1985. Effects of dietary fat on postprandial substrate oxidation and on carbohydrate and fat balances. *J Clin Invest* 76(3):1019–1024.

Flint A, Helt B, Raben A, Toubro S, Astrup A. 2003. Effects of different dietary fat types on postprandial appetite and energy expenditure. *Obes Res* 11(12):1449–1455.

French S, Robinson T. 2003. Fats and food intake. *Curr Opin Clin Nutr Metab Care* 6(6):629–634.

Green MW, Rogers PJ. 1995. Impaired cognitive functioning during spontaneous dieting. *Psychol Med* 25(5):1003–1010.

Greenwood CE. 1994. Performance-enhancing effects of protein and amino acids. In: Marriott BM, ed. *Food Components to Enhance Performance*. Washington, DC: National Academy Press. Pp. 263–275.

Greenwood CE. 2003. Dietary carbohydrate, glucose regulation, and cognitive performance in elderly persons. *Nutr Rev* 61(5):S68–S74.

Greenwood CE, Young SN. 2001. Dietary fat intake and the brain: A developing frontier in biological psychiatry. *J Psychiatry Neurosci* 26(3):182–184.

Greenwood CE, Kaplan RJ, Hebblethwaite S, Jenkins DJ. 2003. Carbohydrate-induced memory impairment in adults with type 2 diabetes. *Diabetes Care* 26(7):1961–1966.

Grego F, Vallier JM, Collardeau M, Bermon S, Ferrari P, Candito M, Bayer P, Magnie MN, Brisswalter J. 2004. Effects of long duration exercise on cognitive function, blood glucose, and counterregulatory hormones in male cyclists. *Neurosci Lett* 364(2):76–80.

IOM (Institute of Medicine) 1994. *Food Components to Enhance Performance*. Washington, DC: National Academy Press.

IOM. 1995. *Not Eating Enough*. Washington, DC: National Academy Press.

IOM. 1999. *The Role of Protein and Amino Acids in Sustaining and Enhancing Performance*. Washington, DC: National Academy Press.

IOM. 2001. *Caffeine for the Sustainment of Mental Task Performance: Formulations for Military Operations*. Washington, DC: National Academy Press.

Kanarek R. 1997. Psychological effects of snacks and altered meal frequency. *Br J Nutr* 77(Suppl 1):S105–S118.

Kaplan RJ, Greenwood CE. 1998. Dietary saturated fatty acids and brain function. *Neurochem Res* 23(5):615–626.

Kaplan RJ, Greenwood CE. 2002. Influence of dietary carbohydrates and glycaemic response on subjective appetite and food intake in healthy elderly persons. *Int J Food Sci Nutr* 53(4):305–316.

Kaplan RJ, Greenwood CE, Winocur G, Wolever TM. 2000. Cognitive performance is associated with glucose regulation in healthy elderly persons and can be enhanced with glucose and dietary carbohydrates. *Am J Clin Nutr* 72(3):825–836.

Kaplan RJ, Greenwood CE, Winocur G, Wolever TM. 2001. Dietary protein, carbohydrate, and fat enhance memory performance in the healthy elderly. *Am J Clin Nutr* 74:687–693.

Kennedy DO, Scholey AB. 2000. Glucose administration, heart rate and cognitive performance: Effects of increasing mental effort. *Psychopharmacology (Berl)* 149(1):63–71.

Korol DL. 2002. Enhancing cognitive function across the life span. *Ann N Y Acad Sci* 959:167–179.

Korol DL, Gold PE. 1998. Glucose, memory, and aging. *Am J Clin Nutr* 67(Suppl):764S–771S.

Kretsch MJ, Green MW, Fong AK, Elliman NA, Johnson HL. 1997. Cognitive effects of a long-term weight reducing diet. *Int J Obes Relat Metab Disord* 21(1):14–21.

Laessle RG, Platte P, Schweiger U, Pirke KM. 1996. Biological and psychological correlates of intermittent dieting behavior in young women. A model for bulimia nervosa. *Physiol Behav* 60(1):1–5.

Lawton CL, Delargy HJ, Brockman J, Smith FC, Blundell JE. 2000. The degree of saturation of fatty acids influences post-ingestive satiety. *Br J Nutr* 83(5):473–482.

Leigh Gibson E, Green MW. 2002. Nutritional influences on cognitive function: Mechanisms of susceptibility. *Nutr Res Rev* 15(1):169–206.

Lieberman HR. 2003. Nutrition, brain function and cognitive performance. *Appetite* 40(3):245–254.

Lieberman HR, Falco CM, Slade SS. 2002a. Carbohydrate administration during a day of sustained aerobic activity improves vigilance, as assessed by a novel ambulatory monitoring device, and mood. *Am J Clin Nutr* 76(1):120–127.

Lieberman HR, Tharion WJ, Shukitt-Hale B, Speckman KL, Tulley R. 2002b. Effects of caffeine, sleep loss, and stress on cognitive performance and mood during US Navy SEAL training. *Psychopharmacology (Berl)* 164:250–261.

Macht M. 1996. Effects of high- and low-energy meals on hunger, physiological processes and reactions to emotional stress. *Appetite* 26(1):71–88.

Mays MZ. 1995. Impact of underconsumption on cognitive performance. In: Marriott BM, ed. *Not Eating Enough*. Washington, DC: National Academy Press. Pp. 285–302.

McCall AL. 1992. The impact of diabetes on the CNS. *Diabetes* 41(5):557–570.

McNay EC, Gold PE. 2001. Age-related differences in hippocampal extracellular fluid glucose concentration during behavioral testing and following systemic glucose administration. *J Gerontol A Biol Sci Med Sci* 56(2):B66–B71.

Messier C. 2004. Glucose improvement of memory: A review. *Eur J Pharmacol* 490(1–3):33–57.

Nybo L, Secher NH. 2004. Cerebral perturbations provoked by prolonged exercise. *Prog Neurobiol* 72(4):223–261.

Owen G, Turley H, Casey A. 2004. The role of blood glucose availability and fatigue in the development of cognitive impairment during combat training. *Aviat Space Environ Med* 75(3): 240–246.

Park CR. 2001. Cognitive effects of insulin in the central nervous system. *Neurosci Biobehav Rev* 25(4):311–323.

Parsons MW, Gold PE. 1992. Glucose enhancement of memory in elderly humans: An inverted-U dose-response curve. *Neurobiol Aging* 13(3):401–404.

Pollitt E, Mathews R. 1998. Breakfast and cognition: An integrative summary. *Am J Clin Nutr* 67(Suppl):804S–813S.

Rolls BJ, Bell EA. 1999. Intake of fat and carbohydrate: Role of energy density. *Eur J Clin Nutr* 53(Suppl 1):S166–S173.

Sandstead HH. 2000. Causes of iron and zinc deficiencies and their effects on brain. *J Nutr* 130(2 Suppl):347S–349S.

Shukitt-Hale B, Askew EW, Lieberman HR. 1997. Effects of 30 days of undernutrition on reaction time, moods, and symptoms. *Physiol Behav* 62(4):783–789.

Spring BJ, Pingitore R, Schoenfeld J. 1994. Carbohydrates, protein and performance. In: Marriott BM, ed. *Food Components to Enhance Performance*. Washington, DC: National Academy Press. Pp. 321–350.

St-Onge MP, Jones PJ. 2002. Physiological effects of medium-chain triglycerides: Potential agents in the prevention of obesity. *J Nutr* 132(3):329–332.

Stubbs RJ, Whybrow S. 2004. Energy density, diet composition and palatability: Influences on overall food energy intake in humans. *Physiol Behav* 81(5):755–764.

Stubbs J, Ferres S, Horgan G. 2000. Energy density of foods: Effects on energy intake. *Crit Rev Food Sci Nutr* 40(6):481–515.

Sunram-Lea SI, Foster JK, Durlach P, Perez C. 2001. Glucose facilitation of cognitive performance in healthy young adults: Examination of the influence of fast-duration, time of day and pre-consumption plasma glucose levels. *Psychopharmacology (Berl)* 157(1):46–54.

Westerterp-Plantenga MS. 2003. The significance of protein in food intake and body weight regulation. *Curr Opin Clin Nutr Metab Care* 6(6):635–638.

Wilson MM, Morley JE. 2003. Impaired cognitive function and mental performance in mild dehydration. *Eur J Clin Nutr* 57(Suppl 2):S24–S29.

Wing RR, Vazquez JA, Ryan CM. 1995. Cognitive effects of ketogenic weight-reducing diets. *Int J Obes Relat Metab Disord* 19(11):811–816.

Do Structured Lipids Offer Advantages for Negative Energy Balance Stress Conditions?

R. J. Jandacek, University of Cincinnati

INTRODUCTION AND REVIEW

The objective of this paper is to address the question of whether structured lipids offer advantages as a source of energy for hypocaloric, high-energy expenditure stress conditions of short-term combat operations (repetitive three- to seven-day missions with recovery periods of one to three days). A review of structured lipids and their metabolism is followed by a discussion of the question provided and the recommendation.

Ingested Energy Sources

Virtually all of the fat that we consume is in the form of triacylglcyerols, three long-chain fatty acids bonded to glycerol. The chain length of most dietary fatty acids is 16 and 18 carbon atoms.

It was found by Rubner (1885) and Atwater and Bryant (1900) that the energy in food that is available to support metabolic and other activity is equivalent to that produced by oxidation of the carbon and hydrogen atoms of the compounds in food macronutrients. In a bomb calorimeter, the oxidation of carbohydrates generates 4 kcal/g (16.7 kJ/g). The oxidation of fatty acids with 18-carbon chains yields 9.5 kcal/g (39.7 kJ/g). Fatty acids of shorter chain length contain a higher fraction of carbon atoms bonded to oxygen and therefore give off less energy when oxidized. Heat produced by the oxidation of octanoic acid is 8 kcal/g (33.4 kJ/g).

Although we have understood this concept for a century, the equivalence of the bomb calorimeter and the human body is a remarkable discovery. The β-oxidation of palmitic acid that produces acetyl CoA and carbon dioxide (CO_2) via the TCA (tricarboxylic acid) cycle provides the same amount of heat and work as the bomb calorimeter. The sum of the reactions in the body is the same as that in the bomb calorimeter: fat plus oxygen produces heat, CO_2, and water.

The chemical energy contained in the C-C and C-H bonds of fatty acids is the densest source of energy available in foods, where C is carbon and H is hydrogen. The energy of ingested fat is stored if total caloric intake exceeds energy expenditure, or it is used to meet energy needs. The sections that follow briefly review the types of dietary fat and the unique properties of fats made with medium-chain fatty acids.

Types of Dietary Fat

Dietary fat comprises triacylglycerols, phospholipids, and sterols. Phospholipids and sterols are important in health, but triacylglycerols provide essentially all of the energy in dietary lipids.

A triacylglycerol molecule contains an asymmetric carbon atom (carbon 2 of the glycerol) if the fatty acids in the 1 and 3 positions are different. Fatty acid positions in the 1 and 3 positions are hydrolyzed by pancreatic lipase. The chemical structure of a triacylglycerol molecule (trilaurin) is shown in Figure B-15.

Figure B-16 shows dietary fatty acids in animal and vegetable triacylglycerols. The long-chain fatty acids account for a majority of the fat consumed by people. Docosahexaenoic acid is found in fatty fish such as salmon and tuna.

Medium-Chain Fatty Acids and Structured Lipids

In addition to these long-chain fatty acids in common foods, small quantities of shorter fatty acids are part of the triacylglycerols of butterfat. These fatty acids include butyric, hexanoic (caproic), octanoic (caprylic), decanoic (capric), and dodecanoic (lauric) acids. Octanoic and decanoic acids make up approximately 4 percent of butterfat fatty acids.

Octanoic and decanoic acids account for approximately 13 percent of the fatty acids in coconut oil. They became commercially available as byproducts of coconut oil fractionation to obtain lauric acid, an ingredient for detergent products. These byproducts made it possible to synthesize medium-chain fatty acid triacylglycerols (MCT, MCT oil).

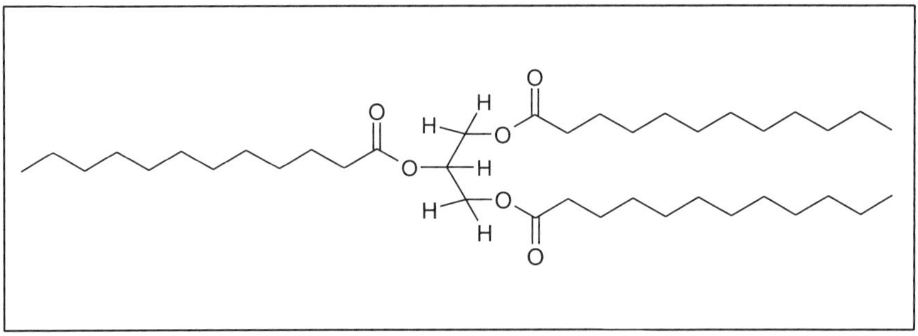

FIGURE B-15   A triacylglycerol, trilaurin ($C_{39}H_{74}O_6$).

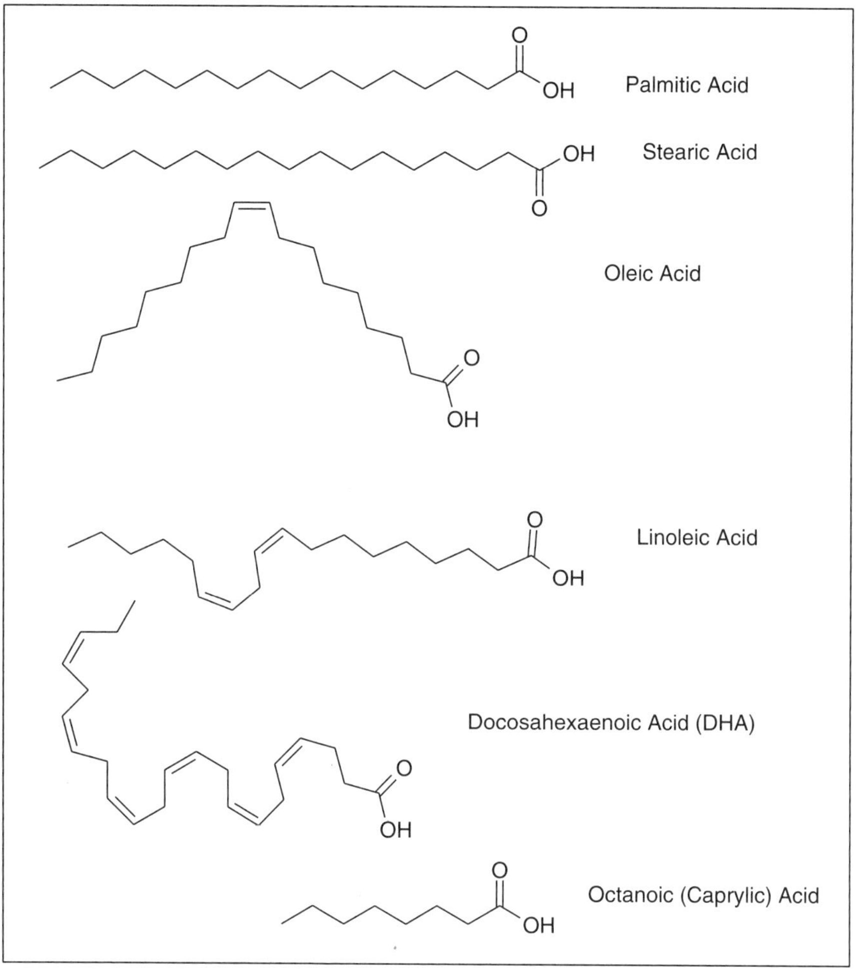

FIGURE B-16 Principal long-chain fatty acids found in dietary fat. Octanoic acid is a medium-chain fatty acid that is a principal component of structured lipids.

Structure

Synthetic triacylglycerols were also made from mixtures of long-chain and medium-chain fatty acids; these esters were termed "structured lipids," even though the fatty acid distribution in the three positions of the glycerol was completely random and unstructured. More recently, enzymatic techniques have made it possible to synthesize triacylglycerols with medium-chain fatty acids in the 1 and 3 positions, and long-chain fatty acids in the 2 position.

Absorption

MCT oil was found to have therapeutic advantages in cases of pancreatic insufficiency because its intestinal hydrolysis is more rapid than that of long-chain fats. MCT oil is absorbed from the intestine in subjects with subnormal pancreatic lipase, such as patients with cystic fibrosis. The hydrolysis products are transported via the portal vein rather than via the lymphatic route. MCT does not provide the essential fatty acids linoleic and α-linolenic acids.

Utilization

Structured lipids were proposed to have benefits in providing energy to patients who were not able to consume food through the gastrointestinal tract and therefore required intravenous nutritional support (i.e., total parenteral nutrition, TPN). The provision of intravenous energy has successfully used emulsions of fat in small particles. It was found that these particles in blood circulation acquire surface lipoproteins (e.g., apolipoprotein C-II, C-III, E) from high-density lipoproteins. The lipid is hydrolyzed by endothelial lipoprotein lipase and the lipolytic products are used by peripheral tissues.

Medium-chain fatty acids are rapidly hydrolyzed from triacylglycerol and do not require carnitine for tissue uptake; however, acidosis can result from this high rate of hydrolysis. For this reason, physical mixtures of MCTs or structured lipids with medium-chain fatty acids and long-chain fatty acids (including essential fatty acids) bonded to the same glycerol molecule may have advantages for TPN compared with long-chain triacylglycerols (Bellantone et al., 1999; Rubin et al., 2000). Some reported advantages of structured lipids in TPN were summarized previously (Jandacek, 1994).

In addition to use in TPN, another hypothetical nutritional advantage for medium-chain fatty acids (and therefore for structured lipids) was explored. This hypothesis suggests that the rapid absorption of medium-chain fatty acids via the portal vein to the liver results in rapid mitochondrial oxidation of these acids that can then reduce the body's use of glycogen as a fuel. It was also suggested that the use of MCTs in place of carbohydrate would reduce insulin elevation and hypoglycemia. As reviewed previously (Jandacek, 1994), studies did not support these hypotheses in human exercise trials, and a more recent trial also found no performance improvement with a specific structured lipid (Vistisen et al., 2003).

A further refinement to structured lipids was the synthesis of "truly structured" lipids, in which the positions of the medium- and long-chain fatty acids were specific rather than random. The advantage of this kind of structure is that the placement of the medium-chain fatty acids in the exterior 1 and 3 positions would result in their rapid lipase-catalyzed hydrolysis (Jandacek et al., 1987). Specific position structured lipids would be capable of providing essential fatty acids (in the 2 position) with rapidly hydrolyzed octanoic or decanoic acid in the

1 and 3 positions. This kind of molecule could therefore be advantageous in providing fat in patients with pancreatic insufficiency.

The isomerization of monoacylglycerols may affect the metabolism of structured lipids. The preferred (low energy) form of monoacylglycerols is the 1(3)-monoacylglycerol. Isomerization of the 2-monoacylglycerol to the 1(3) isomer is accelerated by heat is rapid for short- and medium-chain fatty acids and for long-chain polyunsaturated fatty acids. It is likely that a significant fraction of 2-monoacylglycerols of medium-chain fatty acids formed in the intestine is isomerized (and then hydrolyzed) within the time frame of intestinal transit. A comparison of the absorption of long-chain fatty acid triacylglycerols, MCTs, and structured lipids is shown in Figure B-17. The structured lipid is shown as a "specific" triacylglycerol.

DISCUSSION OF QUESTIONS

Based on the physical properties and metabolism of structured fatty acids, three areas of discussion address the question of whether or not structured lipids have any of the following advantages in energy deficit status during high stress circumstances: (1) intestinal absorption, (2) energy content, (3) energy utilization, and (4) appetite.

Is There an Advantage in Intestinal Absorption?

Current data indicate that there is no advantage in the absorption of medium-chain fatty acids in structured lipids, as long as the subjects have normal levels of pancreatic lipase. There is no need to optimize the hydrolysis rate in the small intestine of normal healthy individuals. There is a 20-fold excess capacity for the absorption of fat, suggesting that there are more than adequate levels of lipase, bile salts, enterocyte capacity, and chylomicron formation. Evidence for this is supported by the work of Kinsell and colleagues (1953). They fed vegetable oil as the entire diet to subjects for a week and observed not only that there were no ill effects, but also that there were reductions in serum cholesterol. Work by Kasper (1970) found that when dietary fat was raised to three times the normal consumption at a level of 300 g/day, the body was able to compensate, and this level of fat was well absorbed. He then pushed the system further with a diet of 639 g fat/day. This amount also was well tolerated by a subject during a 20-day trial, further confirming that normal humans have an excess capacity for the absorption of fat. These results negate the need to optimize the hydrolysis rate in the small intestine of healthy individuals. Furthermore, there is no evidence that subjects stressed by several days of caloric deficit will absorb less than normal levels of dietary fat. The use of a fat that is hydrolyzed rapidly will therefore not enhance caloric use relative to normal, well-absorbed, long-chain fats in people with normal pancreatic lipase levels.

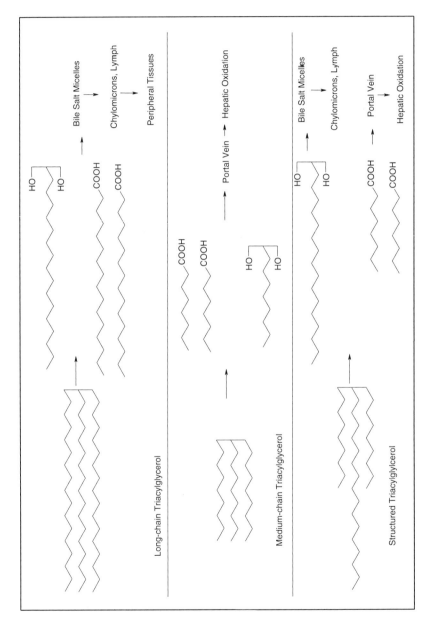

FIGURE B-17 Intestinal absorption of triacylglcyerols of long- and medium-chain fatty acids.

Is There an Advantage in Energy Content?

As discussed above, the maximum energy content of macronutrients available to a person is the heat of combustion. For long-chain fats this value is 9.5 kcal (39.7 kJ)/g. The caloric energy of the fatty acids is dependent on chain length, and the energy that can be used from octanoic acid is 8 kcal (33.5 kJ)/g. Although the difference in caloric density of long-chain and medium-chain fatty acids is small, it seems prudent to maximize the energy provided per unit weight of the food provided in anticipated caloric deprivation.

Is There an Advantage in Energy Utilization?

The energy provided by macronutrient metabolism results in storage, work, or heat. In the case of excessive caloric intake, a portion of the energy is directed toward storage, principally in the form of triacylglycerol fatty acids in adipose tissue. In negative caloric balance, ingested energy is converted to heat and work. In a situation of energy stress in a high-temperature environment, it would be desirable to maximize ingested energy as work (ATP production).

A study of high relevance to this topic was reported by Bendixen and co-workers (2002). They compared four types of triacylglycerol fats in 11 normal, healthy men ranging in age from 22 to 28 years. The fats included a conventional long-chain triacylglcyerol; a positionally specific structured fat (octanoic acid in the 1(3) position); a randomly structured lipid; and a mixture of MCT with long-chain triacylglycerols. All three fats that included medium-chain fatty acids resulted in higher postprandial energy expenditure than did the long-chain dietary fat. This result is consistent with rapid absorption of medium-chain fatty acids via the portal vein and, because elongation is not favored, they are directed toward mitochondrial oxidation. If this oxidation is not entirely coupled to the production of ATP (e.g., peroxisomal oxidation) then the result would be a negative energy balance. In this study there was no difference among fats in subjective appetite measures or ad libitum energy consumption. Total energy expenditure was smaller after the conventional fat meal, relative to the other fats. Diet-induced thermogenesis was lower after the conventional fat than after the random structured lipid. In the 5-hour postprandial period there was a (non-significant) trend toward lower oxidation of fat from the long-chain fat (1.65 g/5 h versus 3.1–3.5 g/5 h), and a trend toward higher carbohydrate oxidation in this group (13.9 versus 11.1–13.1 g/5 h). The authors concluded that "structured fats do not change short-term postprandial appetite sensations or ad libitum energy intakes, but do result in higher postprandial energy expenditure than do conventional fats and hence promote negative energy and fat balance" (Bendixen et al., 2002).

Is There an Advantage in Appetite?

During hypocaloric stress it is possible that a nutrient that provides satiety would be advantageous. There was no difference in the satiating effect of the different fats in the Bendixen study in terms of subjective tests and in terms of ad libitum caloric intake (Bendixen et al., 2002). However, in some reports long-chain fatty acids have been reported to be more satiating than medium-chain fatty acids (Cox et al., 2004; Feltrin et al., 2004).

CONCLUSION

There is no reason to substitute structured lipids for long-chain fatty acid triacylglycerols to meet the needs of stress resulting from high energy expenditure and low energy intake. Maximizing caloric density is the optimal approach. During a relatively short duration of five to ten days, essential fatty acids are not limiting factors. In terms of the fat composition, triacylglycerols that are oxidatively stable, high in energy density, and readily digested are recommended. Oils high in oleic acid and low in polyunsaturated acids (e.g., high oleic oils from cultivars of sunflower and safflower oils) meet these criteria.

REFERENCES

Atwater WO, Bryant AP. 1900. The availability and fuel value of food materials. *Connecticut Storrs Agricultural Extension Station Annual Report, 1899.* Pp. 73–110.

Bellantone R, Bossola M, Carriero C, Malerba M, Nucera P, Ratto C, Crucitti P, Pacelli F, Doglietto GB, Crucitti F. 1999. Structured versus long-chain triglycerides: A safety, tolerance, and efficacy randomized study in colorectal surgical patients. *J Parenter Enteral Nutr* 23(3):123–127.

Bendixen H, Flint A, Raben A, Hoy CE, Mu H, Xu X, Bartels EM, Astrup A. 2002. Effect of 3 modified fats and a convential fat on appetite, energy intake, energy expenditure, and substrate oxidation in healthy men. *Am J Clin Nutr* 75(1):47–56.

Cox JE, Kelm GR, Meller ST, Randich A. 2004. Suppression of food intake by GI fatty acid infusions: Roles of celiac vagal afferents and cholecystokinin. *Physiol Behav* 82(1):27–33.

Feltrin KL, Little TJ, Meyer JH, Horowitz M, Smout AJ, Wishart J, Pilichiewicz AN, Rades T, Chapman IM, Feinle-Bisset C. 2004. Effects of intraduodenal fatty acids on appetite, antropyloroduodenal motility, and plasma CCK and GLP-1 in humans vary with their chain length. *Am J Physiol Regul Integr Comp Physiol* 287(3):R524–R533.

Jandacek RJ. 1994. Structured lipids: An overview and comments on performance enhancement potential. In: Marriott BM, ed. *Food Components to Enhance Performance.* Washington, DC: National Academy Press. Pp. 351–379.

Jandacek RJ, Whiteside JA, Holcombe BN, Volpenhein RA, Taulbee JD. 1987. The rapid hydrolysis and efficient absorption of triglycerides with octanoic acid in the 1 and 3 positions and long-chain fatty acid in the 2 position. *Am J Clin Nutr* 45(5):940–945.

Kasper H. 1970. Faecal fat excretion, diarrhea, and subjective complaints with highly dosed oral fat intake. *Digestion* 3(6):321–330.

Kinsell LW, Michaels GD, Partridge FW, Boling LA, Balch HE, Cochrane GC. 1953. Effect upon serum cholesterol and phospholipids of diets containing large amounts of vegetable fat. *Am J Clin Nutr* 1(3):224–231.

Rubin M, Moser A, Vaserberg N, Greig F, Levy Y, Spivak H, Ziv Y, Lelcuk S. 2000. Structured triacylglycerol emulsion, containing both medium- and long-chain fatty acids, in long-term home parenteral nutrition: A double-blind randomized cross-over study. *Nutrition* 16(2):95–100.

Rubner M. 1885. Calorimetrische Untersuchungen. *Zeitsch Biol* 21:377.

Vistisen B, Nybo L, Xu X, Hoy CE, Kiens B. 2003. Minor amounts of plasma medium-chain fatty acids and no improved time trial performance after consuming lipids. *J Appl Physiol* 95(6):2434–2443.

Optimum Protein Intake in Hypocaloric States

L. John Hoffer, Jewish General Hospital

INTRODUCTION

The goal of this workshop is to advise the military in developing a hypocaloric ration that maximizes physical and mental performance. As currently envisioned, rations of 2,400 kcal per day will be consumed by soldiers expending approximately 4,000 to 4,500 kcal per day for three to seven days followed by one to three days of recovery. What is the optimum protein content of such a ration? Should the energy deficit be minimized, or are other aspects of the ration more important?

The main concerns when a person's energy expenditure consistently exceeds intake—that is, when he or she is starving—are depletion of the fat store and loss of muscle mass and function. The 32 young men who participated in the famous Minnesota human starvation experiment (Keys et al., 1950) consumed approximately 1,500 kcal per day and, during the subsequent 26 weeks, they lost approximately 25 percent of their lean tissue mass. This occurred despite their consumption of 50 g of protein per day, an amount that exceeded the average protein requirement of 0.6 g/kg of body weight and was close to the current Recommended Dietary Allowance (RDA) of 0.8 g/kg (IOM, 2002). By the 24th week of the study, physiologic adaptation had restored energy and nitrogen equilibrium despite continuing starvation. This adaptation is crucial for survival during starvation (Hoffer, 1999a, b).

The Minnesota experiment illustrates what has long been known (Elwyn et al., 1979; Munro, 1964; Pellett and Young, 1992) and recently reemphasized (IOM, 2002; Millward, 2004; Tipton and Wolfe, 2004): starvation induces body protein loss. For a variety of reasons analyzed earlier by the Committee on Military Nutrition Research (CMNR) (IOM, 1995), soldiers in a stressful, high-energy-expenditure environment typically fail to increase their energy intake enough to match their energy expenditure. This situation fits the definition of starvation, and in keeping with its cardinal features, these soldiers lose fat and lean tissue mass. Their physiologic state appears to be the same as that of starvation that is induced simply by low food consumption. Thus, despite ample carbohydrate intake, circulating concentrations of insulin-like growth factor-1 and 3,5,3'-triiodothyronine are decreased as occurs in conventional starvation, and they increase when the energy gap is narrowed, even if there is no other change in the stressful environment (Friedl et al., 2000).

Carbon oxidation always equals energy expenditure, and when energy expenditure exceeds food energy consumption, the body draws on endogenous fat, its chief energy store. Fat loss is therefore an essential feature of starvation. But the situation with regard to protein loss is unclear. Why does it occur? How avoidable is it? Factors that affect its magnitude are enumerated below.

Micronutrient Status

Mineral deficiencies, particularly those of potassium (Rudman et al., 1975), phosphorus (Rudman et al., 1975), zinc (Khanum et al., 1988; Wolman et al., 1979), and, presumably, magnesium, impair the normal protein-sparing adaptation to starvation.

Absence of a Catabolic State

Tissue injury, inflammation, and systemic infection reverse the physiologic adaptation to starvation and increase body nitrogen loss (Hoffer, 1999b).

Magnitude of the Energy Deficit

This phenomenon is illustrated by a study in which male volunteers with a body mass index (BMI) of 24.5 kg/m^2 participated in an 8-week US Army Ranger course (Friedl, 1997; Friedl et al., 2000). The program consisted of four periods of an initial several days of ad libitum feeding followed by seven to ten days of food restriction in a setting of daily energy expenditures of 4,000 to 4,500 kcal, thermal stress, and sleep deprivation. In the first of two studies, food intake was restricted to 1,400 kcal, with 52 g of protein per day (similar to the Minnesota study). In the second study, supplemental food provided an additional 400 kcal and 15 g of protein. In both experiences food intake during the brief recovery periods did not fully compensate for the deficits incurred during the restriction periods. The greater intake of energy (but also of protein; see below) by the second group produced marked benefits. In particular, the better-fed group experienced less weight loss and their percentage of fat-free mass (FFM) was significantly greater at the end of the study (Friedl et al., 2000).

Fat Store

Some experts claim that very obese, starving people lose body nitrogen more slowly (and have a slower rate of nitroten loss as a fraction of total weight loss) than starving people of normal weight (Elia et al., 1999; Van Itallie and Yang, 1977). Since severely obese people invariably lose FFM during therapeutic starvation, it would seem that starving, nonobese soldiers must inevitably experience FFM loss. It should be borne in mind, however, that severe obesity increases the lean tissue compartment (Drenick, 1975; Henry et al., 1986), and at least some of the lean tissue loss during therapeutic starvation occurs simply because a smaller body requires less muscle to be lifted and moved. From this perspective, normal-weight or only mildly obese people may actually conserve body protein more effectively than severely obese ones during starvation.

It is certainly true that very obese people tolerate starvation with a greater sense of well-being and survive it for longer time. Adults of normal weight die after fasting for approximately 2 months, whereas severely obese people have survived fasts lasting many months (Barnard et al., 1969; Thomson et al., 1966). The longest monitored fast on record was by a 27-year-old man who initially weighed 207 kg and survived 382 days of uninterrupted fasting (Stewart and Fleming, 1973). Friedl and colleages (1994) cite a description of the starvation that occurred among the British forces during the Turkish siege of Kut from December 1915 to April 1916. Soldiers who began with superabundant fat stores survived, whereas those who began with a smaller fat reserve soon died in the cold winter climate (Hehir, 1922).

A study by Friedl and colleagues (1994) provides important insight into this phenomenon. The body composition of 55 men was determined before and after their successful completion of an 8-week US Army Ranger course in which energy intake was unusually low (1,300 kcal per day during the restriction periods). Body fat was an average of 14.3 percent at the start and decreased to an average of 5.8 percent at the end of the course. The remarkable finding was that, during progressive starvation, body fat stabilized at a minimum of 5 percent. The men who reached this limit continued to lose weight, but the source of the weight loss was now FFM. This observation suggests that 5 percent body fat represents a biological limit that is essential for successful adaptation to starvation. US Army data reviewed by Friedl (1995) suggest the contribution of lean tissue loss to total weight loss increases gradually as body fat falls below 10 percent. Nevertheless, the 5 percent limit appears to represent a "metabolic floor" that also approximately coincides with the psychological limit of voluntary participation (Friedl, 1995). As long as body fat remains above this critical level, a high-protein intake can spare body protein, but once it falls below it, protein-sparing is no longer possible. Obese people therefore survive prolonged starvation longer than lean ones because it takes longer to deplete their fat store to the critical level below which protein catabolism accelerates and disability becomes marked.

Comparison has been made between the Minnesota study and modern calorie-restriction studies like the Biosphere 2 study which involved normal-weight individuals (Heilbronn and Ravussin, 2003). This comparison is complicated by the fact that the average BMI of the Minnesota volunteers was only 21.4 when they embarked on their starvation regimen. Thus, even before they began to starve, the Minnesota volunteers had BMIs comparable to modern adults who would be considered calorie restricted. The BMIs of most fit young men of the 21st century typically range from 23 to 25. The crucial determinant of well-being and physical function is more likely to be the absolute lean tissue mass that exists for a given body structure than a percentage reduction. At the end of the starvation phase of the Minnesota study, the average BMI had fallen to 16.3; this was associated with a severity of fat and lean tissue depletion that was incompatible with normal physiologic function. Had the baseline BMI of the Minnesota volunteers been greater, their final BMI would presumably have been closer to the range reported in modern calorie-restriction experiences. Taken together, these considerations suggest that elite soldiers being considered for extended hypocaloric field maneuvers should have normal fat and muscle stores as indicated by a normal physical examination, a BMI not less than approximately 23, and body fat not less than an appropriate minimum, such as 15 percent.

Protein Intake

While it is true that energy deficiency worsens nitrogen balance, it is also true that an increase in protein intake improves nitrogen balance over a wide range of energy intakes from deficient to maintenance (Munro, 1964; Shaw et al., 1983). It was not at first appreciated that a high protein intake protects the lean tissue store during starvation because the early studies were of short duration. Short-duration studies are confounded by a transient loss of body nitrogen, called "labile protein," that occurs immediately after energy (or protein) intake is reduced, and by the failure to allow sufficient time for physiologic adaptation to the new diet. When nitrogen balance studies are carried out long enough for the transient effect of labile protein loss to end and metabolic adaptation to take effect—a process that requires several days (Hoffer, 1999a, b)—high protein intakes are protein sparing in many energy-deficient states (Hoffer, 2003).

The protein-sparing effect of increased dietary protein is not necessarily limited to obese persons. In one study, nonobese men were calorie restricted for 10 weeks while consuming 93 g of protein per day. The men lost 7.4 kg (BMI fell from 24.9 to 22.6), 83 percent of which was fat (Velthuis-te Wierik et al., 1995). This is the composition of adipose tissue, which is approximately 85 percent fat and 15 percent FFM (Garrow, 1982; Grande and Keys 1980; Waki et al., 1991). In the Biosphere 2 experiment, eight normal men and women starved for 6 months, then remained in energy equilibrium for 18 months during which they consumed 2,200 kcal per day including 82 g of protein (Walford et al., 2002; Weyer et al., 2000). The men's BMI decreased from 23.7 to 19.3 and the women's from 21.2 to 18.5 (Walford et al., 2002). In the five persons in whom it was measured, body fat fell to 10 percent (significantly less than the 20 percent body fat in a matched normal comparison group), but their FFM was normal

(Weyer et al., 2000). Several studies in the obesity field have demonstrated zero nitrogen balance in normally active, moderately obese people adhering to very low energy diets supplying 1.5 g of protein per kg of ideal body weight per day (Gelfand and Hendler, 1989; Piatti et al., 1994). The proposition that lean tissues need not be lost during starvation is further supported by data from military trainees who lost body fat (i.e., starved) during basic training without food restriction. In one study, moderately obese female army trainees lost 2.2 kg of fat but simultaneously gained 1.7 kg of FFM (Friedl, 1995). In a study of obese male army recruits, basic training was associated with an average of loss of 12.5 kg within the first 3 months, virtually all of it as fat (Lee et al., 1994). Protein intakes in all these studies were substantially greater than in the Minnesota study and in published US Army Ranger field studies. One may conclude that important protein sparing may well be achievable in starving, normal-weight soldiers by increasing the protein content of their rations.

Another issue to be considered is whether the high level of physical activity required during maneuvers increases the protein requirement. Sports experts advise athletes to consume approximately 1.5 g of protein per kg of body weight every day. This is nearly twice the RDA (IOM, 2002) and nearly three times the average minimum requirement (Fielding and Parkington, 2002; Tipton and Wolfe, 2004). Could the increased protein requirement incurred by exercise add to the high-protein requirement induced by starvation? This issue was addressed by the CMNR (IOM, 1999), who found there was insufficient evidence to conclude that high-level physical activity increases the normal protein requirement. More recent reviews have come to the same conclusion (Fielding and Parkington, 2002; Tipton and Wolfe, 2004). Since the increased food intake necessary to meet a high-energy requirement automatically increases protein intake, the most cogent reason for advising athletes to consume a lot of protein is that this is what they naturally do.

In summary, lean tissues can be conserved during starvation by four mechanisms: (1) the only modest adipose tissue unloading—and hence less absolute weight loss and less disuse muscle atrophy—that occurs when baseline fat stores are normal or only moderately increased; (2) a high, or at least maintained, level of physical activity (Ballor and Poehlman 1994; Prentice et al., 1991); (3) the prevention of a severe depletion of the fat reserve; and (4) substantially greater protein intake than in the Minnesota experiment. Despite the common assumption that protein wasting is unavoidable in the presence of energy deficiency (IOM, 1995), there are good reasons to predict that the lean tissue stores of soldiers in the field can in fact be largely, if not completely, protected by increasing their protein intake. The daily ration currently under consideration provides 2,400 kcal. If, like other US Army rations (Cline and Warber, 1999), 15 percent of the energy is from protein, this ration will provide 90 g of protein per day, or 1.15 g of protein per kilogram of body weight for the average 78 kg US male soldier (IOM, 1999). This may be sufficient to prevent starvation-induced lean tissue loss. Indeed, US Army Ranger course participants who consumed considerably less than 90 g/day suffered only modest losses of FFM and their physical performance appeared to be maintained (Friedl, 1995, 1997). In the Ranger study described earlier, in which daily energy and protein intakes during restriction periods were 1,800 kcal and 67 g of protein, respectively, FFM decreased by 6 percent or 4 kg (Friedl et al., 2000). Upper arm muscle cross-sectional area decreased from 68 to 60 cm^2, but 60 cm^2 remains at the upper 85th percentile for normal age-matched men. Will 90 g of protein per day prevent even these losses? Would 120 g of protein per day (1.5 g of protein per kg) be even more effective? This larger amount of protein would be provided by a 2,400 kcal ration with 20 percent of energy from protein and would conform to the current expert recommendation of 1.5 g/kg for athletes (Fielding and Parkington, 2002; Tipton and Wolfe, 2004). Although 120 g of protein per day seems to exceed the military protein RDA (MRDA) of 100 g per day, first established in 1947, it actually does not. In 1947 the average male soldier weighed only 68 kg (IOM, 1999); the original MRDA was therefore equivalent to a protein intake of 1.5 g/kg of body weight.

Potential drawbacks to a high-protein diet include unpalatability, early satiety, and increased obligatory urine volume to eliminate the additional urea osmoles (Friedl, 1999). However, an increase of protein intake from 90 to 120 g per day would not increase obligatory urine volume because urea is an "ineffective osmole" (Kamel et al., 2004). With regard to satiety and palatability, it is worth recalling that protein comprised 30 to 35 percent of the daily energy intake of paleolithic humans. This is equivalent to 2.5 to 3.5 g/kg (Eaton and Cordain, 1997; Eaton et al., 1996). It seems very likely that a palatable diet providing a "mere" 1.5 g/kg of protein could be devised.

CONCLUSIONS

If soldiers are required to starve for only three to seven days before refeeding, it does not matter how much protein they consume, and the design of the ration should focus on features such as palatability. Field studies do show, however, that ad libitum feeding over the few days following seven to ten days of food restriction is insufficient to make up the energy deficit incurred, so soldiers returning too quickly to the field will experience progressive starvation (Friedl et al., 1994). It is also possible that a highly successful ration could be put to use for longer periods than initially planned for. The following conclusions and suggestions are offered with these possibilities in mind.

Contrary to what is commonly assumed, it is very likely that the lean tissue store of normal-weight persons can be largely conserved during starvation through a combination of a high-protein intake, physical activity, and avoidance of severe body fat loss. This hypothesis has not been tested in a field situation. The prediction is that a hypocaloric ration providing 2,400 kcal and 90 g of protein per day will spare the lean tissue store of soldiers on extended stressful maneuvers. It would be interesting and useful to determine whether a ration providing 2,400 kcal and 120 g of protein is even more effective, as well as practical and palatable. The protein-sparing effect of high-protein intakes will not be demonstrable unless balance studies are long enough to allow for metabolic adaptation.

The energy deficit should be minimized. Protein sparing is only possible when body fat is above a minimum of approximately 5 percent of body weight. Energy-deficient states are psychologically very unpleasant and appear to be increasingly so as the lower fat limit is approached (Friedl, 1997). The psychological unpleasantness of hypocaloric rations may well be their most debilitating short-term feature (Keys et al., 1950). As has already been pointed out (Friedl, 1995; Friedl et al., 1994), it is important, when selecting elite soldiers for stressful missions, to consider their starting body composition. Under starvation conditions, very lean and muscular does not translate into better.

REFERENCES

Ballor DL, Poehlman ET. 1994. Exercise-training enhances fat-free mass preservation during diet-induced weight loss: A meta-analytical finding. *Int J Obes Relat Metab Disord* 18(1):35–40.

Barnard DL, Ford J, Garnett ES, Mardell RJ, Whyman AE. 1969. Changes in body composition produced by prolonged total starvation and refeeding. *Metabolism* 18(7):564–569.

Cline AD, Warber JP. 1999. Overview of garrison, field, and supplemental protein intake by US military personnel. In: *The Role of Protein and Amino Acids in Sustaining and Enhancing Performance.* Washington, DC: National Academy Press. Pp. 93–108.

Drenick EJ. 1975. Weight reduction by prolonged fasting. In: Bray GA, ed. *Obesity in Perspective: A Conference.* John E. Fogarty International Center for Advanced Study in the Health Sciences, October 1–3, 1973. DHEW Publication No. NIH 75-708. Washington, DC: US Government Printing Office. Pp. 341–360.

Eaton SB, Cordain L. 1997. Evolutionary aspects of diet: Old genes, new fuels. Nutritional changes since agriculture. *World Rev Nutr Diet* 81:26–37.

Eaton SB, Eaton SB 3rd, Konner MJ, Shostak M. 1996. An evolutionary perspective enhances understanding of human nutritional requirements. *J Nutr* 126(6):1732–1740.

Elia M, Stubbs RJ, Henry CJ. 1999. Differences in fat, carbohydrate, and protein metabolism between lean and obese subjects undergoing total starvation. *Obes Res* 7(6):597–604.

Elwyn DH, Gump FE, Munro HN, Iles M, Kinney JM. 1979. Changes in nitrogen balance of depleted patients with increasing infusions of glucose. *Am J Clin Nutr* 32(8):1597–1611.

Fielding RA, Parkington J. 2002. What are the dietary protein requirements of physically active individuals? New evidence on the effects of exercise on protein utilization during post-exercise recovery. *Nutr Clin Care* 5(4):191–196.

Friedl KE. 1995. When does energy deficit affect soldier physical performance? In: Marriott BM, ed. *Not Eating Enough.* Washington, DC: National Academy Press. Pp. 253–283.

Friedl KE. 1997. Variability of fat and lean tissue loss during physical exertion with energy deficit. In: Kinney JM, Tucker HN, eds. *Physiology, Stress, and Malnutrition: Functional Correlates, Nutritional Intervention.* Philadelphia: Lippincott-Raven. Pp. 431–450.

Friedl KE. 1999. Protein and amino acids: Physiological optimization for current and future military operational scenarios. In: *The Role of Protein and Amino Acids in Sustaining and Enhancing Performance.* Washington, DC: National Academy Press. Pp. 85–91.

Friedl KE, Moore RJ, Hoyt RW, Marchitelli LJ, Martinez-Lopez LE, Askew EW. 2000. Endocrine markers of semistarvation in healthy lean men in a multistressor environment. *J Appl Physiol* 88(5):1820–1830.

Friedl KE, Moore RJ, Martinez-Lopez LE, Vogel JA, Askew EW, Marchitelli LJ, Hoyt RW, Gordon CC. 1994. Lower limit of body fat in healthy active men. *J Appl Physiol* 77(2):933–940.

Garrow JS. 1982. New approaches to body composition. *Am J Clin Nutr* (5):1152–1158.

Gelfand RA, Hendler R. 1989. Effect of nutrient composition on the metabolic response to very low calorie diets: Learning more and more about less and less. *Diabetes Metab Rev* 5(1):17–30.

Grande F, Keys A. 1980. Body weight, body composition and calorie status. In: Goodhart RS, Shils ME, eds. *Modern Nutrition in Health and Disease*. 6th ed. Philadelphia: Lea & Febiger. Pp. 3–34.

Hehir P. 1922. Effects of chronic starvation during the siege of Kut. *Br Med J* 1:865–869.

Heilbronn LK, Ravussin E. 2003. Calorie restriction and aging: Review of the literature and implications for studies in humans. *Am J Clin Nutr* 78(3):361–369.

Henry RR, Wiest-Kent TA, Scheaffer L, Kolterman OG, Olefsky JM. 1986. Metabolic consequences of very-low-calorie diet therapy in obese non-insulin-dependent diabetic and nondiabetic subjects. *Diabetes* 35(2):155–164.

Hoffer LJ. 1999a. Evaluation of the adaptation to protein restriction in humans. In: El-Khoury AE, ed. *Methods for the Investigation of Amino Acid and Protein Metabolism*. Boca Raton, FL: CRC Press. Pp. 83–102.

Hoffer LJ. 1999b. Metabolic consequences of starvation. In: Shils ME, Olson JA, Shike M, Ross AC, eds. *Modern Nutrition in Health and Disease*. Baltimore, MD: Williams & Wilkins. Pp. 645–665.

Hoffer LJ. 2003. Protein and energy provision in critical illness. *Am J Clin Nutr* 78(5):906–911.

IOM (Institute of Medicine). 1995. In: Marriott BM, ed. *Not Eating Enough*. Washington, DC: National Academy Press. Pp. 41–54.

IOM. 1999. *The Role of Protein and Amino Acids in Sustaining and Enhancing Performance*. Washington, DC: National Academy Press.

IOM. 2002. *Dietary Reference Intakes for Energy, Carbohydrate, Fiber, Fat, Fatty Acids, Cholesterol, Protein, and Amino Acids*. Washington, DC: The National Academies Press.

Kamel KS, Cheema-Dhadli S, Shafiee MA, Halperin ML. 2004. Dogmas and controversies in the handling of nitrogenous wastes: Excretion of nitrogenous wastes in human subjects. *J Exp Biol* 207(Pt 12):1985–1991.

Keys A, Brozek J, Henschel A, Mickelsen O, Taylor HL. 1950. *The Biology of Human Starvation*. Minneapolis, MN: The University of Minnesota Press.

Khanum S, Alam AN, Anwar I, Akbar Ali M, Mujibur Rahaman M. 1988. Effect of zinc supplementation on the dietary intake and weight gain of Bangladeshi children recovering from protein-energy malnutrition. *Eur J Clin Nutr* 42(8):709–714.

Lee L, Kumar S, Leong LC. 1994. The impact of five-month basic military training on the body weight and body fat of 197 moderately to severely obese Singaporean males aged 17 to 19 years. *Int J Obes Relat Metab Disord* 18(2):105–109.

Millward DJ. 2004. Macronutrient intakes as determinants of dietary protein and amino acid adequacy. *J Nutr* 134(6 Suppl):1588S–1596S.

Munro HN. 1964. General aspects of the regulation of protein metabolism by diet and hormones. In: Munro HN, Allison JB, eds. *Mammalian Protein Metabolism*. Vol. 1. New York: Academic Press. Pp. 381–481.

Pellett PL, Young VR. 1992. The effects of different levels of energy intake on protein metabolism and of different levels of protein intake on energy metabolism: A statistical evaluation from the published literature. In: Scrimshaw NS, Schurch B, eds. *Protein-Energy Interactions. Proceedings of an I/D/E/C/G Workshop, Held in Waterville Valley, NH, USA, October 21 to 25, 1991*. Lausanne, Switzerland: Nestlé Foundation. Pp. 81–121.

Piatti PM, Monti F, Fermo I, Baruffaldi L, Nasser R, Santambrogio G, Librenti MC, Galli-Kienle M, Pontiroli AE, Pozza G. 1994. Hypocaloric high-protein diet improves glucose oxidation and spares lean body mass: Comparison to hypocaloric high-carbohydrate diet. *Metabolism* 43(12):1481–1487.

Prentice AM, Goldberg GR, Jebb SA, Black AE, Murgatroyd PR, Diaz EO. 1991. Physiological responses to slimming. *Proc Nutr Soc* 50(2):441–458.

Rudman D, Millikan WJ, Richardson TJ, Bixler TJ 2nd, Stackhouse J, McGarrity WC. 1975. Elemental balances during intravenous hyperalimentation of underweight adult subjects. *J Clin Invest* 55(1):94–104.

Shaw SN, Elwyn DH, Askanazi J, Iles M, Schwarz Y, Kinney JM. 1983. Effects of increasing nitrogen intake on nitrogen balance and energy expenditure in nutritionally depleted adult patients receiving parenteral nutrition. *Am J Clin Nutr* 37(6):930–940.

Stewart WK, Fleming LW. 1973. Features of a successful therapeutic fast of 382 days' duration. *Postgrad Med J* 49(569):203–209.

Thomson TJ, Glasg MB, Runcie J, Miller V. 1966. Treatment of obesity by total fasting for up to 249 days. *Lancet* 2(7471):992–996.

Tipton KD, Wolfe RR. 2004. Protein and amino acids for athletes. *J Sports Sci* 22(1):65–79.

Van Itallie TB, Yang MU. 1977. Diet and weight loss. *N Engl J Med* 297(21):1158–1161.

Velthuis-te Wierik EJ, Westerterp KR, van den Berg H. 1995. Impact of a moderately energy-restricted diet on energy metabolism and body composition in non-obese men. *Int J Obes Relat Metab Disord* 19(5):318–324.

Waki M, Kral JG, Mazariegos M, Wang J, Pierson RN Jr, Heymsfield SB. 1991. Relative expansion of extracellular fluid in obese vs. nonobese women. *Am J Physiol* 261(2 Pt 1):E199–E203.

Walford RL, Mock D, Verdery R, MacCallum T. 2002. Calorie restriction in biosphere 2: Alterations in physiologic, hematologic, hormonal, and biochemical parameters in humans restricted for a 2-year period. *J Gerontol* 57A(6):B211–B224.

Weyer C, Walford RL, Harper IT, Milner M, MacCallum T, Tataranni PA, Ravussin E. 2000. Energy metabolism after 2 y of energy restriction: The biosphere 2 experiment. *Am J Clin Nutr* 72(4):946–953.

Wolman SL, Anderson GH, Marliss EB, Jeejeebhoy KN. 1979. Zinc in total parenteral nutrition: Requirements and metabolic effects. *Gastroenterology* 76(3):458–467.

Vitamins C and E in the Prevention of Oxidative Stress, Inflammation, and Fatigue from Exhaustive Exercise

Maret G. Traber, Oregon State University
Angela Mastaloudis, Pharmanex

INTRODUCTION

This paper attempts to address the effects of exercise on oxidative stress and immune function and whether increasing the intake of antioxidants would reduce this stress, first in energy balance conditions and then in energy deficit conditions. Findings from our studies in ultramarathon runners may help answer this and the specific following questions:

1. What are the types and levels of direct antioxidants (e.g., vitamins C and E, carotenoids) that could be added to rations for short-term use by soldiers during high-tempo, stressful, repetitive combat missions to enhance performance and/or improve recovery during combat missions?
2. Would certain nonvitamin antioxidants help performance?
3. What is the impact of exercise on oxidative stress and immune function? Will increasing the intake of antioxidants reduce this stress in energy balance conditions and then in energy deficit conditions?
4. Is there any concern with megadoses of antioxidants—should soldiers be already taking supplements? For example, could megadoses of antioxidants negatively affect performance or adaptation?

OXIDATIVE STRESS GENERATED DURING EXERCISE

The human body continuously produces reactive oxygen species (ROS) as a result of normal metabolism in the mitochondria (Halliwell and Gutteridge, 1999). ROS are an unavoidable but necessary byproduct of cellular respiration. ROS also have a beneficial role in that leukocytes use radicals to help kill bacteria. This action produces a large increase in oxygen use, called a "respiratory burst," to catalyze hydrogen peroxide with chloride ions to create a strongly antiseptic hypochlorite ion. Unfortunately, hypochlorite is also a strong oxidizing agent and can produce free radicals.

In response to endurance exercise, the body's oxygen consumption can increase 10 to 20 times (Åstrand and Rodahl, 1986), while skeletal muscle oxygen consumption can increase 100 to 200 times (Halliwell and Gutteridge, 1999). This increased oxygen consumption may produce ROS in amounts that exceed the body's antioxidant supplies. Clearly, exercise can cause oxidative stress resulting in lipid peroxidation (Alessio, 2000; Child et al., 1998; Duthie et al., 1990; Hessel et al., 2000; Marzatico et al., 1997; Mastaloudis et al., 2001; Rokitzki et al., 1994), DNA damage (Hartmann and Niess, 2000), and, possibly, protein oxidation (Alessio, 2000; Tirosh and Reznick, 2000).

Electrons "leaking" from the mitochondria during exercise are considered a main source of oxidative stress (Halliwell and Gutteridge, 1999). Other potential sources of ROS during exercise include enhanced purine oxidation, damage to iron-containing proteins, disruption of Ca^{2+} homeostasis (Jackson, 2000), and NADPH oxidase (Hessel et al., 2000). These exercise-induced ROS are also thought to modulate acute phase inflammatory responses (Cannon and Blumberg, 2000).

We found that during an ultramarathon race (32-mile forest trail through hilly terrain), as compared with a sedentary trial, deuterium-labeled vitamin E disappeared from the plasma faster (disappearance rates of 2.8×10^{-4} versus 2.3×10^{-4}, p < 0.03) and lipid peroxidation increased (75 ± 7 pg/ml at prerace to 131 ± 17 at postrace (p < 0.02) (Mastaloudis et al., 2001). Lipid peroxidation was assessed by measuring plasma F_2-isoprostanes (F_2-IsoPs), prostaglandin-like compounds produced by free-radical catalyzed lipid peroxidation of arachidonic acid (20:4 *n*-6, a long-chain polyunsaturated fatty acid) (Morrow et al., 1990). F_2-IsoPs are widely accepted as sensitive and reliable measures of in vivo lipid peroxidation (Roberts, 1997). Importantly, F_2-IsoPs have proatherogenic biological activity, including vasoconstriction and activation of platelet aggregation (Nieman et al., 2002; Roberts and Morrow, 2000). Moreover, they have been shown to recruit proatherogenic monocytes and induce monocyte adhesion (Leitinger et al., 2001). Thus, endurance exercise not only increases oxidative stress, but also increases a proatherogenic response.

MODULATION OF OXIDATIVE STRESS DURING AN ULTRAMARATHON BY VITAMINS C AND E

Based on our findings that an ultramarathon race increases oxidative stress (Mastaloudis et al., 2001), we hypothesized that prior supplementation with anti-oxidants (vitamins C and E) would decrease oxidative stress during distance running (Mastaloudis, 2004; Mastaloudis et al., 2004a, b). If the antioxidant supplements decreased oxidative stress, they should decrease lipid peroxidation and inflammation, slow α-tocopherol use, decrease DNA damage, decrease muscle damage, and improve recovery. To test these hypotheses, we carried out a randomized, double-blind study in ultramarathon runners (n = 11 women, 11 men) who consumed either (1) antioxidants (AO) [1,000 mg vitamin C (500 mg twice daily) and 300 mg vitamin E (400 IU *RRR*-α-tocopheryl acetate)] or (2) matching placebos (PL) for seven weeks (six weeks before through one week after the race). The race was a 50 km (32 mile) ultramarathon that took place in the hills of Corvallis, Oregon. The study design is shown in Figure B-18.

Subject Characteristics and Plasma Antioxidant Concentrations

Subjects were approximately 40 years of age and were recreationally trained endurance runners. Complete descriptions of the subjects have been published (Mastaloudis, 2004; Mastaloudis et al., 2004b). Plasma α-tocopherol and ascorbic acid concentrations were similar in the two groups before supplementation (Mastaloudis, 2004). Following six weeks of supplementation, the PL-group plasma concentrations were unchanged. In contrast, the AO-group α-tocopherol plasma concentrations increased from 28 ± 2 to 45 ± 3 μM (p < 0.0001) and were higher than in the PL group (p < 0.0007). Similarly, the AO group had a higher ascorbic acid plasma concentration, 121 ± 9 μM, than did the PL group, 78 ± 9 μM (p < 0.0007) following supplementation. Note that in both the PL and AO groups the ascorbic acid concentrations are well into the range for repleted subjects (Levine et al., 1996, 2001).

All subjects completed the race. Run times and intensity were similar among

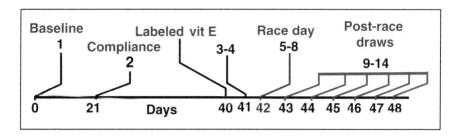

FIGURE B-18 Study Design. Subjects (n = 22) were randomly assigned in a double-blind fashion to one of two groups: (1) PL [(1,000 mg of citric acid (500 mg twice daily) and 300 mg of soybean oil] or (2) AO [1,000 mg ascorbic acid (500 mg twice daily) and 300 mg *RRR*-α-tocopheryl acetate]. Blood samples were obtained before supplementation (baseline); after three weeks of supplementation (compliance); 24, 12, and 1 hours before the race. Samples were also taken at mid-race at kilometer 27 (~ 5 h), immediately postrace, 2 h postrace (approximately 10 h), and daily for six days postrace (1–6 days, 24–144 h). All samples were fasting morning blood draws except 12 h, mid-, post-, and two h post-race.
NOTE: AO = antioxidant; PL = placebo.
SOURCE: Summarized from Mastaloudis (2004); Mastaloudis et al. (2004a), used with permission from Elsevier.

treatment groups and genders: 7.1 ± 0.2 h at a pace of 13.7 ± 0.4 minutes per mile and a heart rate of 146 ± 2 beats per minute. Energy expenditure was calculated based on the average heart rate during the run and the corresponding oxygen consumption (VO_2), multiplied by the time it took each subject to finish the race (Mastaloudis et al., 2004b). Energy expenditure was approximately 7,000 kcal for men and 5,000 kcal for women; both consumed about 2,000 kcal on race day and were in caloric deficit (Table B-6).

TABLE B-6 Race Results

	Women		Men	
	AO (n = 6)	PL (n = 5)	AO (n = 6)	PL (n = 5)
Run Time (hr)	7.1 ± 0.4	7.3 ± 0.6	6.8 ± 0.4	6.8 ± 0.2
Energy Expenditure (kcal)	4,997 ± 207	4,958 ± 187	6,928 ± 558	7,006 ± 297
Energy Intake[a] (kcal)	1,844 ± 137	2,040 ± 221	2,530 ± 325	2,468 ± 279
Vitamin E Intake (mg)	3 ± 1	2 ± 1	3 ± 1	4 ± 1
Vitamin C Intake (mg)	39 ± 14	32 ± 9	28 ± 5	17 ± 5

NOTE: AO = antioxidant ; PL = placebo.
[a]Women versus men p < 0.05.
SOURCE: Mastaloudis et al. (2004b), used with permission from Elsevier.

Vitamins C and E intakes from foods consumed during race day were compiled. During the run vitamin C intake was < 50 mg for most subjects, and vitamin E intake was < 5 mg.

Vitamin C, Vitamin E, and Lipid Peroxidation

Plasma F_2-isoprostanes (F_2-IsoP) concentrations increased in the PL group in response to the race, but prior supplementation with vitamins C and E completely suppressed the increase in the AO group (Figure B-19) (Mastaloudis et al., 2004a). At postrace, when oxidative stress was maximal, F_2-IsoP concentrations were inversely correlated with both the ratio for α-tocopherol:lipids ($R = -0.61$, $p < 0.003$) and with ascorbic acid ($R = -0.41$, $p = 0.05$) (Mastaloudis et al., 2004a), providing further documentation that antioxidants were responsible for preventing lipid peroxidation.

Both men and women in the PL group responded to the run with similar F_2-IsoP concentration increases (Mastaloudis et al., 2004a). However, men's and

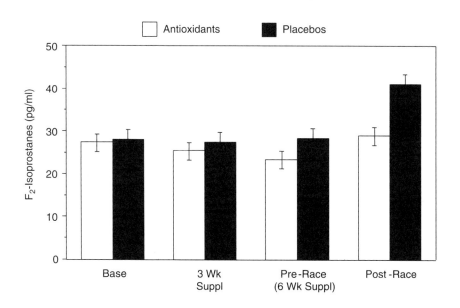

FIGURE B-19 Antioxidant supplementation prevents the increase in lipid peroxidation as observed in ultramarathon runners. Plasma F_2-isoprostanes concentrations increased from pre- to postrace only in the placebo (PL) group (28 ± 2 to 41 ± 3 pg/ml; $p < 0.01$). Additionally, postrace F_2-isoprostanes concentrations were significantly higher in the PL group than in the antioxidant group ($p < 0.001$).
SOURCE: Mastaloudis et al. (2004a), used with permission from Elsevier.

women's responses were markedly different during recovery. In PL women, F_2-IsoP concentrations returned to baseline within two hours postrace, while in PL men, higher F_2-IsoP concentrations persisted for the duration of the study (six days) (Mastaloudis et al., 2004a). This difference in oxidative stress in men and women has been observed previously. Healthy young men compared with age-matched women had greater concentrations of markers of oxidative stress (plasma TBARS [thiobarbituric acid reactive substances] and urinary 8-Iso-PGF_2). Following antioxidant supplementation (600 mg vitamin C and 300 mg vitamin E daily for 4 weeks), levels of lipid peroxidation markers were normalized to concentrations similar to those observed in the women (Ide et al., 2002). Thus, men in comparison with women are subjected to continued higher oxidative stress in the absence of antioxidant supplementation.

Cytokine Levels after the Race

Very few studies have examined the effects of antioxidants on both exercise-induced oxidative stress and inflammation (Childs et al., 2001; Nieman et al., 2002). We found that AO supplementation had no effect on exercise-induced increases in tumor necrosis factor (TNF)-a, interleukin (IL)-6, C-reactive protein (CRP), or IL-1, despite the finding that increases in lipid peroxidation were prevented (Mastaloudis et al., 2004a). Similarly, ascorbic acid (1,500 mg/day) consumption for one week before an ultramarathon did not prevent exercise-induced increases in plasma F_2-IsoPs, lipid hydroperoxides, or IL-6 (pro-inflammatory cytokine) (Nieman et al., 2002). Postexercise supplementation with vitamin C (approximately 1,000 mg/day) and n-acetyl-cysteine for one week also had no effect on exercise-induced IL-6 increases (Childs et al., 2001). Army recruits that participated in an intensive 48-hour final military endurance exercise were also shown to have increased CRP, but the effect of antioxidants were not tested (Brull et al., 2004). In general, antioxidants do not modulate increases in cytokine concentrations in response to exercise.

Assessing DNA Damage

The ultramarathon was a sufficiently strenuous exercise that, by mid-race, the runners exhibited DNA damage as assessed with the comet assay (a whole-cell electrophoresis assay that estimates DNA damage) (Mastaloudis et al., 2004b). However, the proportion of cells with DNA damage returned to baseline by the end of the race, declined below baseline values two days after the race, and remained low for six days after the race (Mastaloudis et al., 2004b). Both men and women within each treatment group had similar circulating AO levels, but the women had a higher proportion of DNA damage after the race. In addition, the women in the AO group were more protected, showing a decrease in the proportion of DNA damage on the day following the ultramarathon race, while men experienced little benefit.

Overall, this exercise appeared to induce a temporary increase in DNA damage. This increase, however, has no apparent adverse effects and may be beneficial because it appears to induce the replacement of damaged cells.

Muscle Damage Following Running

Runners experienced muscle damage after the ultramarathon: deficits in maximal force production by the knee extensors and flexors were documented (Mastaloudis et al., in press). Prior supplementation with vitamins C and E did not prevent muscle damage or fatigue or improve recovery. The ultramarathon run may have been so damaging that it overwhelmed the protective effects of the antioxidants. For example, vitamin C was found to be protective in a more moderate exercise protocol (60 minutes of box-stepping exercise), in which supplementation enhanced the rate of recovery from maximal force deficit (Jakeman and Maxwell, 1993).

Plasma markers of muscle damage were increased by the endurance exercise in our study (Mastaloudis et al., in press) and were unaffected by AO supplementation. Both lactate dehydrogenase (LDH) and creatine kinase (CK) increased in response to the race; LDH peaked at postrace and CK reached maximal values 2 h and 1 day postrace; neither was affected by AO treatment. These observations are in agreement with others. There was no influence on increased CK concentrations in response to a 90 minute treadmill run by two weeks prior supplementation with 500 mg vitamin C and 400 mg vitamin E (Petersen et al., 2001). Our findings are in contrast, however, with other studies (Rokitzki et al., 1994) that reported prior supplementation with 200 mg vitamin C and 400 IU vitamin E for 4.5 weeks diminished increases in CK following a 90 km ultramarathon.

Our study also showed that vitamins C and E did not prevent LDH increases after distance running. However, daily supplementation with 1,200 IU α-tocopherol for four weeks prior to running diminished LDH increases following six successive days of running (Itoh et al., 2000), suggesting that a larger dose of vitamin E is required to reduce muscle damage resulting from endurance exercise. The results seem influenced not only by the level of exercise but also by the amount, duration, and type of supplemental AO.

Endogenous Mechanisms to Increase Antioxidant Defenses

Plasma ascorbic acid concentrations increased in both the AO and PL groups during the 50 km ultramarathon run, with significant increases at mid-race, and at postrace compared with levels measured prerace; levels returned to prerace values two hours after the race (Mastaloudis et al., 2004a, b). Increases in plasma ascorbic acid in response to vigorous exercise have been reported in some (Duthie et al., 1990; Kaikkonen et al., 1998; Mastaloudis et al., 2001; Petersen et al., 2001; Rokitzki et al., 1994; Viguie et al., 1993), but not all (Meydani et al., 1993; Peters et al., 2001a, b) studies. Exercise-related increases in circulating cortisol has been suggested to promote efflux of ascorbic acid from the adrenal gland and the mobilization of ascorbic acid from other tissue sites such as leukocytes or erythrocytes (Gleeson et al., 1987). Similarly, some (Nieman et al., 2000; Peters et al., 2001a, b), but not all (Nieman et al., 2002), studies demonstrated that exercise-related increases in circulating cortisol diminish with vitamin C supplementation. Taken together, these findings suggest that oxidative stress may regulate cortisol secretion.

Plasma uric acid concentrations also increased in response to the run, consistent with the findings of others (Hellsten et al., 1997; Liu et al., 1999; Rokitzki et al., 1994), and the increase may be explained by enhanced purine oxidation resulting from exercise (Hellsten et al., 1997; Liu et al., 1999; Rokitzki et al., 1994).

Concurrent increases in plasma ascorbic and uric acids may reflect the body's response to extreme exercise by enhancing AO defenses, including increased AO enzymes (Marzatico et al., 1997) and AO nutrients (Child et al., 1998; Rokitzki et al., 1994; Viguie et al., 1993).

Some studies investigating the effects of vitamin E supplementation on endurance runners have reported increases in plasma α-tocopherol concentrations in both the AO and the PL groups following exercise (Buchman et al., 1999; Rokitzki et al., 1994; Vasankari et al., 1997). We (Mastaloudis et al., 2004a) observed increased plasma α-tocopherol concentrations during exercise in the AO group only. Plasma tocopherols are transported entirely within lipoproteins and fluctuate with lipoprotein concentrations (Traber and Jialal, 2000) and after correcting α-tocopherol for lipids, no significant changes in α-tocopherol/lipid concentrations were observed in either group (Mastaloudis et al., 2004a). In the only other study to report both α-tocopherol and α-tocopherol/lipid concentrations (Buchman et al., 1999), fluctuations in lipoproteins explained the differential responses in the AO and PL groups. Thus, the increase in plasma α-tocopherol concentrations during the exercise may be a result of fluctuations in lipoprotein concentrations rather than an actual increase due to exercise.

Increases and Depletions of Plasma Lipids

Plasma lipids (total cholesterol plus triglycerides) increased during the race, but decreased to below prerace levels two hours after the race and remained low for three days (Figure B-20). These data suggest that extreme endurance exercise depletes lipid stores that subsequently remain depleted for several days. Rations should provide adequate fat content and total kcals to ensure that tissue stores of lipids are maintained for endurance and multi-day physical work in the field.

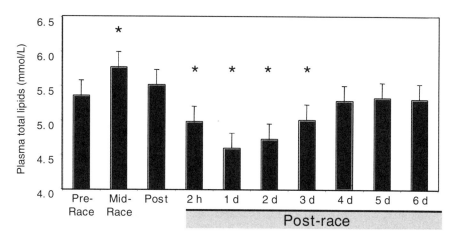

FIGURE B-20 Plasma lipids increase during the race but are depleted for three days postrace. No differences in plasma total lipids (total cholesterol plus triglycerides) were observed between genders or among treatment groups within each gender.

NOTE: *Compared with prerace levels, plasma total lipids were higher at mid-race ($p < 0.004$), but were lower two hours ($p < 0.01$), one day ($p < 0.0001$), two days ($p < 0.0001$), and three days ($p < 0.01$) postrace.

SOURCE: Adapted from Mastaloudis (2004), used with permission.

Conclusions

ROS generated in response to exercise cause oxidative damage (Mastaloudis et al., 2001, 2004a), stimulate an inflammatory response (Vassilakopoulos et al., 2003), and damage skeletal muscle (Cannon and Blumberg, 2000; Sjodin et al., 1990). Hypothetically, AO supplementation could prevent exercise-induced oxidative damage, inflammation, and muscle damage. We found, however, that while supplementation with vitamins C and E prevented increases in lipid peroxidation in response to endurance exercise (Mastaloudis et al., 2004a), they had no apparent effect on DNA damage (Mastaloudis et al., 2004b), inflammation (Mastaloudis et al., 2004a), or muscle damage (Mastaloudis et al., in press). These results suggest that the mechanism of oxidative damage is operating independently of the inflammatory and muscle damage responses (Nieman et al., 2002).

Preventing production and enhancing clearance of F_2-IsoPs may be more beneficial than preventing inflammation. F_2-IsoPs have demonstrated pro-atherogenic biological activity, including vasoconstriction and activation of platelet aggregation (Nieman et al., 2002; Roberts and Morrow, 2000). In addition, they are known to recruit proatherogenic monocytes and induce monocyte adhesion (Leitinger et al., 2001). In contrast, the muscle damage-induced inflammatory response stimulates recovery from exercise by inducing regeneration of damaged tissue and recruitment of satellite cell proliferation (Malm, 2001). In our studies, AO supplementation proved to prevent the damaging increase in lipid peroxidation without influencing inflammation. This is especially important because preventing exercise-induced inflammation could inhibit muscular adaptation to physical activity, the so-called "training effect" of exercise.

Supplementation of both vitamins C and E appears beneficial in exercise. Certainly, the ultramarathon runners were adequately nourished with respect to vitamin C, but studies in cigarette smokers suggest that vitamin C is necessary to maintain vitamin E concentrations (Bruno et al., 2005). Prior supplementation with vitamin E alone may be possible, but the assault ration should contain vitamin C not only for its own benefits but also for maintaining vitamin E concentrations.

In healthy adults, there are no obvious adverse effects of either vitamin C or E supplements alone or in combination (Hathcock et al., 2005), and the Tolerable Upper Intake Levels are 2,000 and 1,000 mg, respectively (IOM, 2000). A recent meta-analysis assessed the combined results of 19 clinical trials of vitamin E supplementation for various diseases reported that patients who took supplements of 400 IU/day or more were 6 percent more likely to die from any cause than those who did not take vitamin E supplements (Miller et al., 2005). However, three other meta-analyses that combined the results of randomized controlled trials designed to evaluate the efficacy of vitamin E supplementation in cardiovascular disease found no evidence that vitamin E supplementation up to 800 IU/day significantly increased or decreased cardiovascular disease mortality or all-cause mortality (Eidelman et al., 2004; Shekelle et al., 2004; Vivekananthan et al., 2003). At present, there is no convincing evidence that vitamin E itself increases the risk of death from cardiovascular disease or other causes. Therefore, AO vitamin supplements could be added to assault rations to prevent the adverse increase in lipid peroxidation as described in the ultramarathon runners in our study (Mastaloudis et al., 2004a).

ACKNOWLEDGMENTS

We thank the runners and the support from National Institute of Environmental Health Sciences Grant ES11536 and National Institutes of Health Grant DK59576. The following individuals provided supplements and ergogenic aids: Jim Clark, Cognis Health and Nutrition; Klaus Krämer, BASF; Tim Corliss, Clif Bar; Jeff Zachwieja, Gatorade.

The following individuals played key roles in our study: Dawn W. Hopkins, The Department of Exercise and Sport Science, Linus Pauling Institute, Oregon State University, Corvallis; Scott Leonard, Linus Pauling Institute, Oregon State University, Corvallis; David Yu, Linus Pauling Institute, Oregon State University, Corvallis; Robert P. O'Donnell, Statistics, Oregon State University, Corvallis; Roderick H. Dashwood, Linus Pauling Institute, Oregon State University, Corvallis; Balz Frei, Linus Pauling Institute, Oregon State University, Corvallis; Jason D. Morrow, Departments of Medicine and Pharmacology, Vanderbilt University School of Medicine, Nashville, Tennessee; and Sridevi Devaraj, Department of Pathology, the University of California Medical Center, Sacramento; Jeffrey J. Widrick, The Department of Exercise and Sport Science, Oregon State University, Corvallis.

REFERENCES

Alessio HM. 2000. Lipid peroxidation in healthy and diseased models: Influence of different types of exercise. In: Sen CK, Packer L, Hanninen, O, eds. 1st ed. *Handbook of Oxidants and Antioxidants in Exercise*. New York: Elsevier. Pp. 115–128.

Åstrand P-O, Rodahl K. 1986. *Textbook of Work Physiology: Physiological Basis of Exercise*. 3rd ed. New York: McGraw Hill.

Brull DJ, Serrano N, Zito F, Jones L, Montgomery HE, Rumley A, Sharma P, Lowe GDO, World MJ, Humphries SE, Hingorani AD. 2004. Human CRP gene polymorphism influences CRP levels: Implications for the prediction and pathogenesis of coronary heart disease. *Arterioscler Thromb Vasc Biol* 23(11):2063–2069.

Bruno RS, Ramakrishnan R, Montine TJ, Bray TM, Traber MG. 2005. α-Tocopherol disappearance is faster in cigarette smokers and is inversely related to their ascorbic acid status. *Am J Clin Nutr* 81(1):95–103.

Buchman AL, Killip D, Ou C, Rognerud CL, Pownall H, Dennis K, Dunn JK. 1999. Short-term vitamin E supplementation before marathon running: A placebo-controlled trial. *Nutr* 15(4):278–283.

Cannon JG, Blumberg JB. 2000. Acute phase immune responses in exercise. In: Sen CK, Packer L, Hanninen O, eds. *Handbook of Oxidants and Antioxidants in Exercise*. 1st ed. New York: Elsevier. Pp. 177–194.

Child RB, Wilkinson DM, Fallowfield JL, Donnelly AE. 1998. Elevated serum antioxidant capacity and plasma malondialdehyde concentration in response to a simulated half-marathon run. *Med Sci Sports Exerc* 30(11):1603–1607.

Childs A, Jacobs C, Kaminski T, Halliwell B, Leeuwenburgh C. 2001. Supplementation with vitamin C and N-acetyl-cysteine increases oxidative stress in humans after an acute muscle injury induced by eccentric exercise. *Free Radic Biol Med* 31(6):745–753.

Duthie GG, Robertson JD, Maughan RJ, Morrice PC. 1990. Blood antioxidant status and erythrocyte lipid peroxidation following distance running. *Arch Biochem Biophys* 282(1):78–83.

Eidelman RS, Hollar D, Herbert PR, Lamas GA, Hennekens CH. 2004. Randomized trials of vitamin E in the treatment and prevention of cardiovascular disease. *Arch Intern Med* 164(14):1552–1556.

Gleeson M, Robertson JD, Maughan RJ. 1987. Influence of exercise on ascorbic acid status in man. *Clin Sci* 73(5):501–505.

Halliwell B, Gutteridge JMC. 1999. *Free Radicals in Biology and Medicine*. 3rd ed. New York: Oxford University Press Inc.

Hartmann A, Niess AM. 2000. Oxidative DNA damage in exercise. In: Sen CK, Packer L, Hanninen O, eds. *Handbook of Oxidants and Antioxidants in Exercise*. 1st ed. New York: Elsevier. Pp. 195–217.

Hathcock JN, Azzi A, Blumberg J, Bray T, Dickinson A, Frei B, Jialal I, Johnston CS, Kelly FJ, Krämer K, Packer L, Parthasarathy S, Sies H, Traber MG. 2005. Vitamins E and C are safe across a broad range of intakes. *Am J Clin Nutr* 81(4):736–745.

Hellsten Y, Tullson PC, Richter EA, Bangsbo J. 1997. Oxidation of urate in human skeletal muscle during exercise. *Free Radic Biol Med* 22(1/2):169–174.

Hessel E, Haberland A, Muller M, Lerche D, Schimke I. 2000. Oxygen radical generation of neutrophils: A reason for oxidative stress during marathon running? *Clin Chim Acta* 298(1-2): 145–156.

Ide T, Tsutsui H, Ohashi N, Hayashidani S, Suimatsu N, Tsuchihashi M, Tamai II, Takeshita A. 2002. Greater oxidative stress in healthy young men compared with premenopausal women. *Arterioscler Thromb Vasc Biol* 22(3):438–442.

IOM (Institute of Medicine). 2000. *Dietary Reference Intakes for Vitamin C, Vitamin E, Selenium and Carotenoids*. Washington, DC: National Academy Press.

Itoh H, Ohkuwa T, Yamazaki Y, Shimoda T, Wakayama A, Tamura S, Yamamoto T, Sato Y, Miyamura M. 2000. Vitamin E supplementation attenuates leakage of enzymes following 6 successive days of running training. *Int J Sports Med* 21(5):369–374.

Jackson M. 2000. Exercise and oxygen radical production by muscle. In: Sen C, Packer L, Hanninen O, eds. 1st ed. *Handbook of Oxidants and Antioxidants in Exercise*. 1st ed. New York: Elsevier. Pp. 57–68.

Jakeman P, Maxwell S. 1993. Effect of antioxidant vitamin supplementation on muscle function after eccentric exercise. *Eur J Appl Physiol Occup Physiol* 67(5):426–430.

Kaikkonen J, Kosonen L, Nyyssonen K, Porkkala-Sarataho E, Salonen R, Dorpela H, Salonen JT. 1998. Effect of combined coenzyme Q10 and d-a-tocopheryl acetate supplementation on exercise-induced lipid peroxidation and muscular damage: A placebo-controlled double-blind study in marathon runners. *Free Radic Res* 29(1):85–92.

Leitinger N, Huber J, Rizza C, Mechtcheriakova D, Bochkov V, Koshelnick Y, Berliner JA, Binder BR. 2001. The isoprostane 8-iso-PGF(2α) stimulates endothelial cells to bind monocytes: Difference to thromboxane-mediated endothelial activation. *FASEB J* 15(7):1254–1256.

Levine M, Conry-Cantilena C, Wang Y, Welch RW, Washko PW, Dhariwal KR, Park JB, Lazarev A, Graumlich JF, King J, Cantilena LR. 1996. Vitamin C pharmacokinetics in healthy volunteers: Evidence for a recommended dietary allowance. *Proc Natl Acad Sci USA* 93(8):3704–3709.

Levine M, Wang Y, Padayatty SJ, Morrow J. 2001. A new recommended dietary allowance of vitamin C for healthy young women. *Proc Natl Acad Sci USA* 98(17):9842–9846.

Liu ML, Bergholm R, Makimattila S, Lahdenpera S, Valkonen M, Hilden H, Yki-Jarvinen H, Taskinen MR. 1999. A marathon run increases the susceptibility of LDL to oxidation in vitro and modifies plasma antioxidants. *Am J Physiol* 276(6 Pt 1):E1083–E1091.

Malm C. 2001. Exercise-induced muscle damage and inflammation: Fact or fiction? *Acta Physiol Scand* 171(3):233–239.

Marzatico F, Pansarasa O, Bertorelli L, Somenzini L, Della Valle G. 1997. Blood free radical antioxidant enzymes and lipid peroxides following long-distance and lactacidemic performances in highly trained aerobic and sprint trained athletes. *J Sports Med Phys Fitness* 37(4):235–239.

Mastaloudis A. 2004. *Inhibition of Exercise-Induced Oxidative Stress, Inflammation and Muscle Damage by Prior Supplementation with the Antioxidant Vitamins E and C*. Ph.D. dissertation. Oregon State University, Corvallis.

Mastaloudis A, Leonard SW, Traber MG. 2001. Oxidative stress in athletes during extreme endurance exercise. *Free Radic Biol Med* 31(7):911–922.

Mastaloudis A, Morrow JD, Hopkins DW, Deveraj S, Traber MG. 2004a. Antioxidant supplementation prevents exercise-induced lipid peroxidation, but not inflammation, in ultramarathon runners. *Free Radic Biol Med* 36(10):1329–1341.

Mastaloudis A, Traber MG, Carstensen K, Widrick J. In press. Antioxidants do not prevent muscle damage in response to an ultramarathon run. *Med Sci Sports Exerc* Jan. 2006.

Mastaloudis A, Yu TW, Frei B, Dashwood RH, Traber MG. 2004b. Endurance exercise results in DNA damage as detected by the comet assay. *Free Radic Biol Med* 36(8):966–975.

Meydani M, Evans WJ, Handelman G, Biddle L, Fielding RA, Meydani SN, Burrill J, Fiatarone MA, Blumberg JB, Cannon JG. 1993. Protective effect of vitamin E on exercise-induced oxidative damage in young and older adults. *Am J Physiol* 33(5 Pt 2):R992–R998.

Miller ER 3rd, Paston-Barriuso R, Dalal D, Riemersma RA, Appel LJ, Guallar E. 2005. Meta-analysis: High-dosage vitamin E supplementation may increase all-cause mortality. *Ann Intern Med* 142(1):37–46.

Morrow J, Hill K, Burk R, Nammour T, Badr K, Roberts J. 1990. A series of prostaglandin F_2-like compounds are produced in vivo in humans by a non-cyclooxygenase, free radical catalyzed mechanism. *Proc Natl Acad Sci USA* 87(23):9383–9387.

Nieman DC, Henson DA, McAnulty SR, McAnulty L, Swick NS, Utter AC, Vinci DM, Opiela SJ, Morrow JD. 2002. Influence of vitamin C supplementation on oxidative and immune changes after an ultramarathon. *J Appl Physiol* 92(5):1970–1977.

Nieman DC, Peters EM, Henson DA, Nevines EI, Thompson MM. 2000. Influence of vitamin C supplementation on cytokine changes following an ultramarathon. *J Interferon Cytokine Res* 20(11):1029–1030.

Peters EM, Anderson R, Nieman DC, Fickl H, Iogessa V. 2001a. Vitamin C supplementation attenuates the increases in circulating cortisol, adrenaline, and anti-inflammatory polypeptides following ultramarathon running. *Int J Sports Med* 22(7):537–543.

Peters EM, Anderson R, Theron AJ. 2001b. Attenuation of increase in circulating cortisol and enhancement of the acute phase protein response in vitamin C-supplemented ultramarathoners. *Int J Sports Med* 22(2):120–126.

Petersen EW, Ostrowski K, Ibfelt T, Richelle M, Offord E, Halkjaer-Kristensen J, Pedersen BK. 2001. Effect of vitamin supplementation on cytokine response and on muscle damage after strenuous exercise. *Am J Physiol* 280(6):C1570–C1575.

Roberts J. 1997. The generation and actions of isoprostanes. *Biochim Biophys Acta* 1345(2):121–135.

Roberts JL II., Morrow JD. 2000. Measurement of F_2-isoprostanes as an index of oxidative stress in vivo. *Free Radic Biol Med* 28(4):505–513.

Rokitzki L, Logemann E, Sagredos AN, Murphy M, Wetzel-Roth W, Keul J. 1994. Lipid peroxidation and antioxidative vitamins under extreme endurance stress. *Acta Physiol Scand* 151(2):149–158.

Shekelle PG, Morton SC, Jungvig LK, Udani J, Spar M, Tu W, M JS, Coulter I, Newberry SJ, Hardy M. 2004. Effect of supplemental vitamin E for the prevention and treatment of cardiovascular disease. *J Gen Intern Med* 19(4):380–389.

Sjodin B, Hellsten Westing Y, Apple F. 1990. Biochemical mechanisms for oxygen free radical formation during exercise. *Sports Med* 10(4):236–254.

Tirosh O, Reznick O. 2000. Chemical bases and biological relevance of protein oxidation. In: Sen CK, Packer L, Hanninen O, eds. *Handbook of Oxidants and Antioxidants in Exercise*. 1st ed. New York: Elsevier. Pp. 89–114.

Traber M, Jialal I. 2000. Measurement of lipid-soluble vitamins-further adjustment needed? *Lancet* 355(9220):2013–2014.

Vasankari TJ, Kujala UM, Vasankari TM, Vuorimaa T, Ahotupa M. 1997. Increased serum and low-density-lipoprotein antioxidant potential after antioxidant supplementation in endurance athletes. *Am J Clin Nutr* 65(4):1052–1056.

Vassilakopoulos T, Karatza MH, Katsaounou P, Kollintza A, Zakynthinos S, Roussos C. 2003. Antioxidants attenuate the plasma cytokine response to exercise in humans. *J Appl Physiol* 94(3):1025–1032.

Viguie C, Frei B, Shigenaga M, Ames B, Packer L, Brooks G. 1993. Antioxidant status and indexes
    of oxidative stress during consecutive days of exercise. *J Appl Physiol* 75(2):566–572.
Vivekananthan DP, Penn MS, Sapp SK, Hsu A, Topol EJ. 2003. Use of antioxidant vitamins
    for the prevention of cardiovascular disease: Meta-analysis of randomised trials. *Lancet*
    361(9374):2017–2023.

Zinc, Magnesium, Copper, Iron, Selenium, and Calcium in Assault Rations: Roles in Promotion of Physical and Mental Performance

Henry C. Lukaski and James G. Penland,
USDA-ARS Grand Forks Human Nutrition Research Center

INTRODUCTION

Military personnel are exposed to environmental, physical, and mental stressors during combat and require adequate dietary intakes of energy, water, and micronutrients for optimal performance. During deployment, soldiers decrease food consumption up to 50 percent, resulting in a suboptimal intake of energy and micronutrients (Baker-Fulco, 1995). Thus, reduced food intake and increased losses of minerals during assault operations suggest the need to evaluate mineral nutrition of military personnel (Shippee, 1993).

Only male soldiers participate in first-strike assault operations. These missions occur for repetitive brief periods (three to seven days), followed by short recovery periods (one to three days) that can last for months. Under these circumstances, it is unlikely that such brief durations of reduced micronutrient intake will elicit severe mineral deficiencies. However, repeated bouts of first-strike assaults without adequate replenishment of minerals may predispose soldiers to a reduced mineral nutritional status and result in impaired physiological and psychological function and performance.

This review addresses the mineral needs of male soldiers. It does so by comparing the prevalence of inadequate mineral intakes of civilian and military men and summarizing the effects of restricted and supplemental mineral intakes on their performance. Additionally, it provides a strategy for increasing food and nutrient intake to promote optimal performance of the male combat soldier. Findings from studies of women with documented mineral depletion are described to highlight impairments in performance that would be applicable to men with similarly reduced mineral nutritional status.

The following are specific questions that this review attempts to answer:

- Which of the minerals might reach deficit levels, given the high-stress, high-intensity scenario? Given existing information that suggests that soldiers probably consume insufficient amounts of zinc during military operations, and that they could become zinc deficient, are there potential effects on health or performance?

- What are the types and levels of cofactors in antioxidant and other biochemical reactions with high metabolic flux (e.g., zinc, manganese, copper, selenium, or others) that could be added to assault rations to enhance performance during combat missions? Does the presence of preexisting malnutrition make a difference?
- Is there any concern with taking megadoses of minerals; should soldiers be already taking supplements?

LIMITING MINERALS IN THE DIET

Estimating a group's adequate intake of a nutrient is achieved through comparison with the Estimated Average Requirement (EAR). If an EAR is not available, then the Adequate Intake (AI) is used. The Recommended Dietary Allowance (RDA) is not used to assess the adequacy of nutrient intakes by groups (IOM, 2000a).

Inadequate Dietary Mineral Intakes in Adults

Epidemiological surveys using dietary recall reveal (NHANES III, Continuing Survey of Food Intake of Individuals, and US Food and Drug Administration Total Diet Study) that intakes of some minerals by the US population do not meet the Dietary Recommended Intake (DRI) recommendations. Among men ages 19 to 50 years, 50 percent did not meet the AI for calcium or the EAR for magnesium (Table B-7). Inadequate zinc intakes were found among 10 percent of men, but iron intakes generally met the EAR (6 mg) (IOM, 1997, 2000b, 2001).

Nutritional surveys reveal wide-ranging estimates of possible copper deficiency in the US population (IOM, 2001). Although findings of the NHANES III and Continuing Survey of Food Intake of Individuals showed no men with copper intakes less than the EAR, the US Food and Drug Administration Total Diet Study revealed that 25 percent of men consume less than the EAR for copper. Analyses of diets from ten multinational studies indicated that copper intakes were less than the EAR in 11 percent of the population (Klevay et al., 1993). Another study analyzed duplicate diets of randomly selected adults in Baltimore, Maryland, and found that 36 percent of the adults had dietary copper intakes less than the EAR (Pang et al., 2001).

Inadequate Dietary Mineral Intakes in Military Personnel

Based on observation of the foods soldiers consume (Rose et al., 1987), soldiers frequently have inadequate intakes of certain minerals. Zinc and magne-

TABLE B-7 Dietary Reference Intakes of Minerals in Diets of American Men Ages 19–50 Years and Actual Intakes

Mineral	Dietary Reference Intake		Not Attaining (%)	
	RDA	EAR or AI	RDA	EAR or AI
Calcium		1,000 mg[a]		50[a]
Copper	900 mg	700 mg	5	0
Iron	8 mg	6 mg	10	0
Magnesium	400–420 mg	350 mg	50	50
Selenium	55 mg	45 mg	0	0
Zinc	11 mg	9.4 mg	20	10

NOTE: The percentage of men not attaining the RDA/EAR/AI has been assessed using the US national survey intake data found in the appendices of the source below. An RDA is set from an EAR; calcium does not have an EAR therefore also no RDA. AI = Adequate Intake; EAR = Estimated Average Requirement; RDA = Recommended Dietary Allowance.
[a]Indicates the value is an AI rather than an EAR.
SOURCE: IOM (1997, 2000b, 2001).

sium intakes of male marine engineers fed standard rations were less than the recommended amounts (Tharion et al., 2000). The addition of hot meals to standard rations, compared with provision of only standard rations, promoted adequate mineral intakes for the soldiers (Thomas et al., 1995). However, feeding a customized, high-carbohydrate diet, compared with standard rations, during training in a hot, humid environment decreased the proportion of elite male soldiers with inadequate intakes of calcium (50 versus 95 percent) but not magnesium (75 versus 75 percent) or zinc (20 versus 25 percent) (personal communication, S. Montain, USARIEM, August 9, 2004; Savannah Ranger Study, 1996). Male hospital personnel were studied during operational training to compare the effects of meal-based versus standard rations on the resulting adequacy of mineral intakes (Baker-Fulco et al., 2002). Compared with the standard ration, the high-carbohydrate, meal-based ration was associated with more soldiers consuming adequate calcium, similar percentages consuming adequate magnesium, but fewer consuming adequate zinc (Table B-8). Thus, magnesium, zinc, and calcium intake levels are limited in civilian and military men, and data on copper and selenium in soldiers are lacking.

FUNCTIONAL RESPONSES TO DIFFERENCES IN MINERAL INTAKES

Mineral intakes affect human biological functions. Controlled studies of restriction and supplementation of mineral intakes reveal deficits and enhance-

TABLE B-8 Male Hospital Workers During Training Consumption[a] of Limiting Minerals

Mineral	Dietary Plan	
	Concept	MRE XVII
Calcium	31	44
Iron	0	2
Magnesium	38	43
Zinc	100	21

NOTE: MRE = Meal, Ready-to-Eat.
[a]Percentage of soldiers consuming less than 70 percent of the military standards for adequacy of nutrient intake.
SOURCE: Baker-Fulco et al. (2002).

ments, respectively, in measures of physiological and psychological function and performance.

Zinc

Zinc is required for the structure and activity of more than 300 enzymes (Vallee and Falchuk, 1993). Because zinc functions in all physiological systems, adequate zinc status is needed for optimal physiological and psychological performance.

Low zinc status impairs muscle and cardiorespiratory functions (Table B-9). Adolescent gymnasts with decreased serum zinc concentrations, compared with age-matched, nonathletic controls, experienced reduced muscle strength (Brun et al., 1995). Male athletes with low, in contrast with normal, serum zinc concentrations had decreased power output (physical work capacity, watts) and increased blood lactate concentrations during peak exercise tests (Khaled et al., 1997).

Controlled feeding studies with low zinc intakes show adverse physiological function. Men fed severely zinc deficient diet (< 1 versus 12 mg/day of zinc) had decreased muscle strength and work capacity (Van Loan et al., 1999). Physically active men fed a moderately low zinc diet (5 versus 18 mg/day) had impaired cardiorespiratory function during peak and prolonged submaximal exercise (Lukaski, 2005).

Low zinc intakes and status have been related to deficits in memory, perception, attention, and motor skills, while zinc supplementation has improved memory (Table B-10). Low serum zinc in otherwise well-nourished men fed 5, compared with 15, milligrams per day of zinc was associated with faster, but less accurate, performance on memory for digits and several perceptual tasks (Tucker and Sandstead, 1984). Contrasted to a control period when men were fed adequate zinc (10 mg/day), low zinc intakes (1, 2, 3, or 4 mg/day) resulted in

TABLE B-9 Effects of Selected Minerals on Measures of Physical Function and Performance

Mineral	Subjects	Study Design	Outcome	Reference
Zinc	Adolescents	Observation	↓Strength	Brun et al., 1995
	Men	Observation	↓Power	Khaled et al., 1997
	Men	5 vs. 18 mg/day	[a]↓Aerobic capacity, ↑Ventilation, ↑HR	Lukaski, 2005
	Men	<1 vs. 12 mg/day as zinc sulfate	[a]↓Strength	Van Loan et al., 1999
Magnesium	Men	+250 mg/day as magnesium oxide	[b]↑Endurance, ↓Oxygen use	Brilla and Gunther, 1995
	Men	+250 mg/day as magnesium oxide	[b]↑Strength	Brilla and Haley, 1992
	Men	+370 mg/day as magnesium pidolinate	[b]↓Oxygen use, ↓Lactate	Golf et al., 1994
Copper	Men	0.9 vs. 2 mg/day as copper amino acid chelate	[b]↑Oxygen use, ↑HR, ↑Lactate, ↓Muscle cytochrome c oxidase activity	Lukaski and Johnson, 2005
Iron	Women	+100 mg/day as ferrous sulfate	↑Training	Brownlie et al., 2002
	Women	+100 mg/day as ferrous sulfate	↑Strength	Brutsaert et al., 2003
	Women	+100 mg/day as ferrous sulfate	↓Time trial	Hinton et al., 2000

NOTE: See text for details.
[a]Effect of lower, compared with higher, intake.
[b]Effect of supplement.

decreased performance on psychomotor (tracking and connect-the-dots), attention (orienting and misdirection), memory (letter, shape, and cube recognition), perceptual (search-count), and spatial (maze) tasks. However, there was no evidence of a "dose–response" effect of dietary zinc on cognitive performance (Penland, 1991). Reaction times during word recall were significantly slower when men were fed low amounts of zinc (5 versus 14 mg/day) (Kretsch et al., 2000).

Magnesium

Magnesium, a cofactor in more than 300 enzyme reactions in which food is metabolized and new products are formed, regulates many biological functions (Shils, 1997). Thus, it is a potentially limiting nutrient for human performance.

TABLE B-10 Effects of Selected Minerals on Measures of Psychological Function and Performance

Mineral	Subjects	Study Design	Outcome	Reference
Zinc	Men	5 vs. 15 mg/day	[a]↓Memory, ↓Perception	Tucker and Sandstead, 1984
	Men	5 vs. 14 mg/day	↓Memory	Kretsch et al., 2000
	Men	1, 2, 3, 4 vs. 10 mg/day[a]	[a]↓Psychomotor, ↓Attention, ↓Perception, ↓Memory	Penland, 1991
Magnesium	Men	Observation	↓EEG alpha activity	Delorme et al., 1992
Copper	Women	1 vs. 3 mg/day	[a]↑Sleep time, ↑Confusion, ↑Latency to sleep, ↑Depression, ↓Feeling rested	Penland, 1988
	Women	1 vs. 3 mg/day	[a]↓Short-term memory, ↑Distraction	Penland et al., 2000
Iron	Women	+90 mg/day of ferrous fumarate	[b]↑Attention, ↑Memory	Groner et al., 1986
	Women	Not reported	↑Learning, ↑Memory	Murray-Kolb et al., 2004
	Women	5 vs. 15 mg	[a]↑Sleep duration, ↑Awakenings	Penland, 1988
	Men	Not reported	↓Alertness, ↓Visual detection	Tucker et al., 1981, 1982, 1984
Selenium	Women	+100 mg/day	[b]↓Anxiety, ↓Depression	Benton and Cook, 1991
	Men	30 vs. 230 μg/day	[b]↓Confusion, ↓Depression	Penland and Finley, 1995
			↑Positive mood	Finley and Penland, 1998

NOTE: See text for details.
[a]Effect of lower, compared with higher, intake.
[b]Effect of supplement.

The dietary restriction of magnesium reduced the magnesium status and impaired physiological function and performance in untrained adults. As shown in Table B-9, physically active men supplemented with magnesium (250 mg/day for four weeks) experienced increased endurance and decreased oxygen use during submaximal exercise (Brilla and Gunter, 1995).

Supplementation with magnesium salts improved cellular function. Men receiving 370 mg of magnesium daily for four weeks had reduced serum lactate concentration and oxygen uptake during a progressive rowing test (Golf et al., 1994). Magnesium supplementation (250 mg/day for seven weeks) increased muscle strength and power in men participating in a strength training regimen (Brilla and Haley, 1992). Although modest strength gains occurred with magnesium intakes of 540 mg/day (290 mg from diet and 250 mg from supplements), increases were achieved at intakes greater than the RDA of 420 mg/day (IOM, 1997).

Whereas severe magnesium deficiency has been associated with numerous neurological and psychological disturbances (Dubray and Rayssiguier, 1997), few reports have described neuropsychological effects from marginal magnesium restriction (Delorme et al., 1992; Table B-10). Male athletes with low, compared with normal, erythrocyte magnesium had significantly less alpha activity in the right occipital region as recorded by an electroencephalogram (EEG) (Delorme et al., 1992), which suggests that magnesium is involved in regulating cortical activity related to motor function.

Copper

Copper is a cofactor of many metalloenzymes and, thus, copper status may affect diverse biological functions. It regulates iron absorption, neurotransmitter metabolism, antioxidant defense, and oxygen use. Longitudinal studies of diet and physical training showed an adaptation in antioxidant protection (Table B-9). Collegiate swimmers training for competition increased dietary copper from 1 to 1.4 mg/day, resulting in an increased erythrocyte superoxide dismutase activity and no change in plasma copper, whereas nontraining control subjects did not change enzyme activity at the same intakes of copper (Lukaski et al., 1989, 1990). Adequate copper intake is needed for adaptation in antioxidant protection during physical training.

Marginal copper intake reduces energy metabolism. Men fed less (0.9 versus 1.6 mg/day) dietary copper showed increased oxygen use, heart rate, and post-exercise lactate concentrations during submaximal exercise (Lukaski and Johnson, 2005). Muscle cyctochrome c oxidase activity decreased with the marginal dietary copper (Table B-9). Thus, restricted copper intake appears to increase energy use during low-level work.

Many of the studies to measure cognition and behavioral effects of copper deficiencies have been conducted with women. Restricted dietary copper has been associated with impaired verbal memory, and disrupted sleep and mood states in women (Table B-10). Increased sleep times, longer latency to sleep, and feeling less rested upon awakening as well as increased confusion, depression, and total mood disturbances were reported when dietary copper was low (0.8 versus 2 mg/day) (Penland, 1988). Short-term memory and immediate recall of verbally presented words (list recall) worsened with low dietary copper (1 versus

3 mg) (Penland et al., 2000). Low copper intakes were also associated with increased difficulty in discriminating between relevant and irrelevant responses. Sufficient plasma copper and ceruloplasmin are associated with improved verbal and long-term memory, increased clustering of verbal material (strategy), and fewer distractions (Penland et al., 2000).

Iron

Iron is needed to deliver oxygen to tissues and to use oxygen at the cellular level. It serves as a functional component of iron-containing proteins needed for efficient energy use as well as for catecholamine metabolism.

Whereas the adverse effects of iron deficiency anemia on work capacity and endurance are well established (Tobin and Beard, 1997), there is growing interest in the functional effects of tissue iron depletion without anemia. Iron deficiency anemia in men is rare, except with excessive blood loss. Estimates of tissue iron depletion in men range from 5 to 15 percent despite only a 5 percent prevalence of low iron intake (IOM, 2001). Accumulating evidence shows that a low-iron status without anemia (e.g., low serum ferritin or transferrin saturation) elicits impaired physical performance, including time used to complete standard running distance (Hinton et al., 2000), endurance training adaptation (Brownlie et al., 2002), and muscle function (Brutsaert et al., 2003) that are all ameliorated with increased iron intake.

Male soldiers participating in Ranger training maintained normal hematology with increased ferritin and decreased serum iron (Shippee, 1993). Various measures of muscle strength and endurance decreased with the training. Because food intake as well as body and fat-free mass concomitantly decreased, one may conclude that reduced iron status contributed to the impaired physical performance.

Iron status has been related to attention, memory, and learning. Iron supplementation in young women (180 mg/day for 30 days) improved attention and short-term memory (Groner et al., 1986), while verbal learning and memory improved significantly in nonanemic, iron-deficient women supplemented similarly with iron (Bruner et al., 1996). Accuracy and reaction times on tasks measuring attention, memory, and learning were improved in women with the highest, compared with the lowest, ferritin and transferrin saturation in the absence of anemia (Murray-Kolb et al., 2004).

Sleep and mood disturbances have been related to dietary iron restriction. Nonanemic women and menstruating women fed low dietary iron (5 versus 15 mg/day) reported more frequent night-time awakenings and more total sleep duration (Penland, 1988). This low iron intake also increased reports of depression, fatigue, and total mood disturbances (Penland, 1989).

Select patterns of cortical activity (measured by EEG) have been predicted by iron status in nonanemic men. Consistent with depressed alertness, lower serum iron and ferritin were associated with more low-frequency EEG activity and lower amplitude-evoked potentials in response to visual stimuli (Tucker and Sandstead, 1981; Tucker et al., 1982, 1984).

Selenium

Selenium acts through its association with proteins as an antioxidant and a regulator of thyroid hormone metabolism. The independent role of selenium in exercise performance and metabolism is not well understood because of its inter-dependence with vitamin E and other nutrients in antioxidant defense.

Endurance-trained men supplemented with selenium (180 µg/day as selenomethionine versus a placebo) significantly increased plasma selenium and glutathione peroxidase activity with no effect on performance (Tessier et al., 1995b). Improvements in peak oxygen uptake were significantly correlated with glutathione peroxidase activity only in the men supplemented with selenium. Young men supplemented with 240 µg/day of selenium (selenomethionine) and trained for endurance had no performance benefit but a significant increase in muscle glutathione peroxidase activity (Tessier et al., 1995a). Thus, supplemental selenium upregulates biochemical markers of selenium status without enhancing performance.

Several studies have shown an effect of selenium intakes and status on mood states in both men and women (Table B-10). Women and men supple-mented with selenium (100 µg/day) reported less anxiety and depression and more energy (Benton and Cook, 1991). Men fed supplemental selenium (230 versus 30 µg/day) reported less confusion and depression (Penland and Finley, 1995). Activity of glutathione peroxidase, a selenium enzyme, in platelets was positively correlated with all mood states (Finley and Penland, 1998).

Calcium

Although its role in bone metabolism is emphasized, calcium acts in mediating vascular, muscular, and nerve functions. Adverse effects of inadequate calcium intake on physical performance are not well studied. However, calcium is required to regulate glycolysis and glycogenolysis and to control protein break-down. Studies of the effects of calcium restriction or supplementation on human metabolism are lacking despite evidence that calcium intake for 50 percent of adult men is less than the AI (IOM, 1997).

DIETARY INTAKE, NUTRITIONAL STATUS, AND PERFORMANCE IN FIELD STUDIES

Military personnel participating in training and operational exercises consis-tently decrease food intake, thus consuming inadequate amounts of minerals. Blood biochemical markers of nutritional status, however, do not reveal overt mineral deficiencies although assessments of hormonal and immune functions show decreases (Booth et al., 2003; Shippee, 1993). Failure to detect nutritional deficiencies is explained by a lack of sensitive biochemical markers of mineral status, brief durations of restricted intakes, and mineral mobilization from stores into the blood with increased metabolic demands and loss of body weight.

Measurable impairments in aerobic capacity or muscle power occur when body weight decreases about 10 percent with a 5 percent loss in muscle mass (Friedl, 1995). Cognitive function declines when significant weight loss (> 6 percent) occurs (Mays, 1995). When energy restriction (50 percent decrease) occurs with strenuous activity, sleep deprivation and mental stress, cognitive performance may fall by more than 33 percent within a few days (Mays, 1993). Decreased food intake plus physical and mental stressors for 12 days increase reports of fatigue and sleep impairment, even at modest levels of weight loss (3 percent) (Booth et al., 2003). Thus, brief and prolonged periods of exposure to nutritional, environmental, physical, and mental stressors impair cognitive performance, including attention, perception, memory, and reasoning (Mays, 1993).

Some reports describe decreased nutritional status during military operations. Shippee (1993) found decreased iron and altered copper and zinc status in Ranger II. Also, Booth and colleagues (2003) reported a decline in iron status in both 12- and 23-day training activities. It is unclear if these findings reflect a response to stress and inflammation or to inadequate intakes of these minerals.

Repeated assault operations may result in mineral depletion because of inadequate intake, and increased turnover and losses of minerals may promote marginal deficiencies under stressful conditions. Also, entry into operations with marginal mineral status may predispose individuals to deficiency status and functional deficits, particularly with repetitive assaults without replenishment of depleted mineral reserves.

FOOD QUALITY AND NUTRIENT DENSITY

Replacing standard combat rations with fresh food and hot meals may alleviate the adverse effects on body weight, physical performance, and cognitive function (Booth et al., 2003; Tharion et al., 2004). This approach, however, is not feasible for soldiers in assault operations. Therefore, new strategies are needed to provide soldiers with proper nutrition.

One approach is to increase the nutrient density of assault rations. Mineral nutrient densities should meet the military standards for reduced-energy rations for men (Baker-Fulco et al., 2001; US Departments of the Army, Navy, and Air Force, 2001). Thus, with reduced energy intake, soldiers would still have adequate mineral intakes.

Steps to improve food intake should be further explored (Hirsch and Kramer, 1993). These include adding new, fortified foods and using stages of change models to foster healthful nutrition habits (Veverka et al., 2003). Increasing emphasis on maintaining adequate hydration and sleep, particularly during recovery periods, will support these efforts.

Active efforts to prevent marginal mineral depletion should be employed. Some suggestions include:

- Develop and support an active nutrition education program.
- Provide palatable, mineral-rich food items in the rations, including on-the-go foods.
- Increase the availability of mineral-rich foods during recovery periods.
- Encourage unit leaders and peers to be models of healthful eating behaviors.

SUMMARY AND CONCLUSIONS

Evidence shows that military personnel fail to consume adequate amounts of magnesium, zinc, and calcium. These minerals, as well as copper, selenium, and iron, play key roles in promoting optimal physiological and psychological function and performance. Limited data on mineral intakes and the resulting status of soldiers in various types of training do not provide evidence of overt nutritional deficiencies. A lack of sensitive biochemical markers of nutritional status hinders interpretation of available data. It is difficult to discriminate the independent effect of severely restricted energy intake on potential micronutrient impairments. Nevertheless, physiological and psychological impairments found in civilians with marginal mineral deficits are consistent with perturbations reported in soldiers during operations and suggest similarities, particularly when the low mineral intakes have been noted in the soldiers.

Based on limited evidence of inadequate intakes of zinc and magnesium, and the presumption of increased zinc losses associated with increased physical activity and elevated rates of sweat, zinc and magnesium status may be compromised. With repeated bouts of these conditions and inadequate replenishment of zinc and magnesium stores, soldiers may manifest marginal zinc and magnesium depletion and experience limitations in work capacity, recovery after deployment, perception, and attention. Furthermore, zinc depletion may attenuate immune function and increase the potential for acute bouts of gastrointestinal distress. Evidence of reduced antioxidant defense is generally lacking in military personnel during short-term assault missions. However, recurrent intermittent periods of inadequate intakes of copper, selenium, zinc, and manganese without adequate intakes during recovery may lead to decreased activity of protective antioxidant enzymes.

Generalized use of multiple vitamin and mineral supplements at intakes not exceeding recommended levels should not be hazardous to soldiers participating in assault missions. The use of single nutrient supplements in amounts exceeding the recommended intake should be avoided to eliminate potential adverse interactions with other nutrients, particularly mineral elements.

Initiating a proactive approach to decrease the potential of adverse effects of limited mineral intakes is recommended. Increasing the mineral densities of assault rations should be advantageous. Adopting an active nutrition education program with palatable, mineral-rich foods and encouraging leaders to model healthy eating behaviors also should be useful to reverse the high rates of low-mineral intakes of soldiers.

RESEARCH NEEDS

There is a need to determine the nutrient intakes, markers of nutritional status, and physiological and psychological performance of military personnel during training and operations. This information is needed to critically evaluate the adequacy of rations provided to and consumed by soldiers exposed to multiple stressors. Findings of this research will enhance the development of rations that promote optimal nutrition and, accordingly, the performance of soldiers engaged in assault operations.

ACKNOWLEDGMENTS

Mention of a trademark or proprietary product does not constitute a guarantee of the product by the US Department of Agriculture and does not imply its approval to the exclusion of other products that may also be suitable. US Department of Agriculture, Agricultural Research, Northern Plains Area, is an equal opportunity/affirmative action employer and all agency services are available without discrimination.

REFERENCES

Baker-Fulco CJ. 1995. Overview of dietary intakes during military exercises. In: Marriott BM, ed. *Not Eating Enough*. Washington, DC: National Academy Press. Pp. 121–149.

Baker-Fulco CJ, Bathalon GP, Bovill ME, Lieberman HR. 2001. *Military Dietary Reference Intakes: Rationale for Tables Values*. Technical Note TN-00/10. Natick, MA: US Army Research Insitute of Environmental Medicine.

Baker-Fulco CJ, Kramer FM, Lesher LL, Merrill E, Johnson J, DeLany J. 2002. *Dietary Intakes of Female and Male Combat Support Hosptial Personnel Subsisting on Meal-Focused or Standard Versions of the Meal, Ready-to-Eat*. Technical Report T-01/23. Natick, MA: US Army Research Institute of Environmental Medicine.

Benton D, Cook R. 1991. The impact of selenium supplementation on mood. *Biol Psychiatry* 29(11):1092–1098.

Booth CK, Coad RA, Forbes-Ewan CH, Thomson GF, Niro PJ. 2003. The physiological and psychological effects of combat ration feeding during a 12-day training exercise in the tropics. *Mil Med* 168(1):63–70.

Brilla LR, Gunter KB. 1995. Effect of magnesium supplementation on exercise time to exhaustion. *Med Exerc Nutr Health* 4:230–233.

Brilla LR, Haley TF. 1992. Effect of magnesium supplementation on strength training in humans. *J Am Coll Nutr* 11(3):326–329.

Brownlie T 4th, Utermohlen V, Hinton PS, Giordano C, Haas JD. 2002. Marginal iron deficiency without anemia impairs aerobic adaptation among previously untrained women. *Am J Clin Nutr* 75(4):734–742.

Brun JF, Dieu-Cambrezy C, Charpiat A, Fons C, Fedou C, Micallef JP, Fussellier M, Bardet L, Orsetti A. 1995. Serum zinc in highly trained adolescent gymnasts. *Biol Trace Elem Res* 47(1–3):273–278.

Bruner AB, Joffe A, Duggan AK, Casella JF, Brandt J. 1996. Randomised study of cognitive effects of iron supplementation in non-anaemic iron-deficient adolescent girls. *Lancet* 348(9033):992–996.

Brutsaert TD, Hernandez-Cordero S, Rivera J, Viola T, Hughes G, Haas JD. 2003. Iron supplementation improves progressive fatigue resistance during dynamic knee extensor exercise in iron-depleted, nonanemic women. *Am J Clin Nutr* 77(2):441–448.

Delorme O, Bourdin H, Viel JF, Rigaud ML, Kantelip JP. 1992. Spectral analysis of electro-encephalography data in athletes with low erythrocyte magnesium. *Magnes Res* 5(4):261–264.

Dubray C, Rayssiguier Y. 1997. Magnesium, inflammation and pain. In: Theophanides TM, Anastassopoulou J, eds. *Magnesium: Current Status and New Developments:Theoretical, Biological, and Medical Aspects.* Dordrecht, Netherlands: Kluwer Academic. Pp. 303–311.

Finley JW, Penland JG. 1998. Adequacy or deprivation of dietary selenium in healthy men: Clinical and psychological findings. *J Trace Elem Exp Med* 11:11–27.

Friedl KE. 1995. When does energy deficit affect soldier physical performance? In: Marriott BM, ed. *Not Eating Enough.* Washington, DC: National Academy Press. Pp. 253–283.

Golf SW, Bohmer D, Nowacki PE. 1994. Is magnesium a limiting factor in competitive exercise? A summary of relevant scientific data. In: Golf S, Dralle D, Vecchiet L, eds. *Magnesium 1993.* London: John Libbey & Co. Pp. 209–219.

Groner JA, Holtzman NA, Charney E, Mellits ED. 1986. A randomized trial of oral iron on tests of short-term memory and attention span in young pregnant women. *J Adolesc Health Care* 7(1):44–48.

Hinton PS, Giordano C, Brownlie T, Haas JD. 2000. Iron supplementation improves endurance after training in iron-depleted, nonanemic women. *J Appl Physiol* 88(3):1103–1111.

Hirsch ES, Kramer FM. 1993. Situational influences on food intake. In: Marriott BM, ed. *Nutritional Needs in Hot Environments.* Washington, DC: National Academy Press. Pp. 215–243.

IOM (Institute of Medicine). 1997. *Dietary Reference Intakes for Calcium, Phosphorus, Magnesium, Vitamin D, and Fluorine.* Washington, DC: National Academy Press.

IOM. 2000a. *Dietary Reference Intakes: Applications in Dietary Assessment.* Washington, DC: National Academy Press.

IOM. 2000b. *Dietary Reference Intakes for Vitamin C, Vitamin E, Selenium, and Carotenoids.* Washington, DC: National Academy Press.

IOM. 2001. *Dietary Reference Intakes for Vitamin A, Vitamin K, Arsenic, Boron, Chromium, Copper, Iodine, Iron, Manganese, Molybdenum, Nickel, Silicon, Vanadium, and Zinc.* Washington, DC: National Academy Press.

Khaled S, Brun JF, Micallel JP, Bardet L, Cassanas G, Monnier JF, Orsetti A. 1997. Serum zinc and blood rheology in sportsmen (football players). *Clin Hemorheol Microcirc* 17(1):47–58.

Klevay LM, Buchet JP, Bunker VW, Clayton BE, Gibson RS, Medeiros DM, Moser-Veillon PB, Patterson KY, Taper LJ, Wolf WR. 1993. Copper in the western diet (Belgium, Canada, UK, and USA). In: Anke M, Meissner D, Mills CF, eds. *Trace Elements in Man and Animals.* TEMA 8. Gersdorf, Germany: Verlag Media Touristik. Pp. 207–210.

Kretsch MJ, Fong, AKH, Penland JG, Sutherland B, King JC. 2000. Cognitive effects of adaptation to a low zinc diet in healthy men. In: Roussel AM, Favier AE, Anderson RA, eds. *Trace Elements in Man and Animals: TEMA 10: Proceedings of the Tenth International Symposium on Trace Elements in Man and Animals.* New York: Kluwer Academic/Plenum Publishers. Pp. 999–1001.

Lukaski HC. 2005. Low dietary zinc decreases erythrocyte carbonic anhydrase activities and impairs cardiorespiratory function during exercise in men. *Am J Clin Nutr* 81(5):1045–1051.

Lukaski HC, Johnson PE. 2005. Dietary copper at the recommended intake decreases muscle cytochrome c oxidase activity and alters metabolic responses during exercise in men. *FASEB J* 19:A982.

Lukaski HC, Hoverson BS, Milne DB, Bolonchuk WW. 1989. Copper, zinc, and iron status of female swimmers. *Nutr Res* 9(5):493–502.

Lukaski HC, Hoverson BS, Gallagher SK, Bolonchuk WW. 1990. Physical training and copper, iron, and zinc status of swimmers. *Am J Clin Nutr* 51(6):1093–1099.

Mays MZ. 1993. Cognitive function in a sustained multi-stressor environment. In: Marriott BM, ed. *Review of the Results of Nutritional Intervention, Ranger Training Class 11/92 (Ranger II).* Washington, DC: National Academy Press. Pp. 199–214.

Mays MZ. 1995. Impact of underconsumption on cognitive performance. In: Marriott BM, ed. *Not Eating Enough.* Washington, DC: National Academy Press. Pp. 285–302.

Murray-Kolb LE, Whitfield KE, Beard JL. 2004. Iron status alters cognitive functioning in women during reproductive years. 2004 Experimental Biology Meeting Abstracts. *FASEB J* 18:Abstract #500.8. [Online]. Available at http://select.biosis.org/faseb [accessed April 13, 2005].

Pang Y, MacIntosh DL, Ryan PB. 2001. A longitudinal investigation of aggregate oral intake of copper. *J Nutr* 131(8):2171–2176.

Penland JG. 1988. Effects of trace element nutrition on sleep patterns in adult women. *FASEB J* 2(4):A434.

Penland JG. 1989. Relationship between essential trace element nutrition and self-reported mood states. *N Dak Acad Sci Proc* 43:68.

Penland JG. 1991. Cognitive performance effects of low zinc (Zn) intakes in healthy adult men. *FASEB J* 5(5):A938.

Penland JG, Finley JW. 1995. Dietary selenium and mood states in healthy young men. *N Dak Acad Sci Proc* 49:26.

Penland JG, Milne DB, Davis CD. 2000. Moderately high zinc intake impairs verbal memory of healthy postmenopausal women on a low copper diet. In: Roussel AM, Favier AE, Anderson RA, eds. *Trace Elements in Man and Animals*: *TEMA 10: Proceedings of the Tenth International Symposium on Trace Elements in Man and Animals.* New York: Kluwer Academic/Plenum Publishers. Pp. 1025–1030.

Rose MS, Buchbinder JC, Dugan TB, Szeto EG, Allegretto JD, Rose DW, Carlson DE, Sammonds KW, Schnakenberg DD. 1987. *Determination of Nutrient Intakes by a Modified Visual Estimation Method and Computerized Nutritional Analysis for Dietary Assessments.* Technical Report T6-88. Natick, MA: US Army Research Institute of Environmental Medicine.

Shils ME. 1997. Magnesium. In: O'Dell BL, Sunde RA, eds. *Handbook of Nutritionally Essential Mineral Elements.* New York: Marcel Dekker. Pp. 117–152.

Shippee RL. 1993. Nutritional status and immune function of Ranger trainees given increased caloric intake. Briefing for the National Academy of Sciences. In: Marriott BM, ed. *Review of the Results of Nutritional Intervention, Ranger Training Class 11/92 (Ranger II).* Washington, DC: National Academy Press. Pp. 86–104.

Tessier F, Hida H, Favier A, Marconnet P. 1995a. Muscle GSH-Px activity after prolonged exercise, training, and selenium supplementation. *Biol Trace Elem Res* 47(1–3):279–285.

Tessier F, Margaritis I, Richard MJ, Moynot C, Marconnet P. 1995b. Selenium and training effects on the glutathione system and aerobic performance. *Med Sci Sports Exerc* 27(3):390–396.

Tharion WJ, Baker-Fulco CJ, Bovill ME, Montain SM, DeLany JP, Champagne CM, Hoyt RW, Lieberman HR. 2004. Adequacy of Garrison feeding for Special Forces soldiers during training. *Mil Med* 169(6):483–490.

Tharion WJ, Baker-Fulco CJ, McGraw S, Johnson Wk, Niron P, Warber JP, Kramer FM, Allen R, Champagne CM, Falco C, Hoyt RW, DeLany JP, Lesher LL. 2000. *The Effects of 60 Days of Tray Ration Consumption in Marine Combat Engineers While Deployed on Great Inagua Island, Bahamas.* Technical Report T-00-16. Natick, MA: US Army Research Institute of Environmental Medicine.

Thomas CD, Friedl KE, Mays MZ, Mutter SH, Moore RJ, Jezior DA, Baker-Fulco CJ, Marchitelli LJ, Tulley RT, Askew EW. 1995. *Nutrient Intakes and Nutritional Status of Soldiers Consuming the Meal, Ready-to-Eat (MREXII) During a 30-Day Field Training Exercise.* Technical Report T95-6. Natick, MA: US Army Research Institute of Environmental Medicine.

Tobin BW, Beard J. 1997. Iron. In: Wolinsky I, Driskell JA, eds. *Sports Nutrition: Vitamins and Trace Elements.* Boca Raton, FL: CRC Press. Pp. 137–156.

Tucker DM, Sandstead HH. 1981. Spectral electroencephalographic correlates of iron status: Tired blood revisited. *Physiol Behav* 26(3):439–449.

Tucker DM, Sandstead HH. 1984. Neuropsychological function in experimental zinc deficiency in humans. In: Frederickson CJ, Howell GA, Kasarskis EJ, eds. *The Neurobiology of Zinc. Part B: Deficiency, Toxicity, and Pathology.* Vol. 11B. New York: Alan R. Liss. Pp. 139–152.

Tucker DM, Sandstead HH, Penland JG, Dawson SL. Milne DB. 1984. Iron status and brain function: Serum ferritin levels associated with asymmetries of cortical electrophysiology and cognitive performance. *Am J Clin Nutr* 39(1):105–113.

Tucker DM, Sandstead HH, Swenson RA, Sawler BG, Penland JG. 1982. Longitudinal study of brain function and depletion of iron stores in individual subjects. *Physiol Behav* 29(4):737–740.

US Departments of Army, Navy, and Air Force. 2001. *Nutrition Standards and Education.* AR 40-25/BUMEDINST 10110.6/AFI 44-141. Washington, DC: US Department of Defense Headquarters.

Vallee BL, Falchuk KH. 1993. The biochemical basis of zinc physiology. *Physiol Rev* 73(1):79–118.

Van Loan MD, Sutherland B, Lowe NM, Turnlund JR, King JC. 1999. The effects of zinc depletion on peak force and total work of knee and shoulder extensor and flexor muscles. *Int J Sport Nutr* 9(2):125–135.

Veverka DV, Anderson J, Auld GW, Coulter GR, Kennedy C, Chapman PL. 2003. Use of the stages of change model in improving nutrition and exercise habits in enlisted Air Force men. *Mil Med* 168(5):373–379.

Effect of Inadequate B Vitamin Intake and Extreme Physical Stress

Lynn B. Bailey and Kristina von Castel-Dunwoody, University of Florida

INTRODUCTION

The primary objective of this paper is to evaluate the potential effect of inadequate B vitamin intake in relation to the consumption of assault rations under extreme physical stress during intense military combat operations. The goal is to characterize the optimal B vitamin content for future rations that will be designed to maximize the physical and mental performance of soldiers engaged in intensely stressful combat operations. The specific questions that were posed by the Committee on Optimization of Nutrient Composition of Military Rations for Short-Term, High-Stress Situations are the following:

- What are the types and levels of B vitamins and choline that could be added to such rations to enhance performance and/or improve recovery during combat missions?
- Does exercise increase B vitamin use? Does decreased energy intake impact this? Will supplementation regardless of energy level meet B vitamin requirement during exercise?
- Do B vitamins and choline affect the bioavailability of other nutrients?

The current ration is hypocaloric in that it provides approximately 2,400 kcal for an expected energy expenditures of 4,000 to 4,500 kcal/day. The B vitamin content of the assault ration has not been analyzed chemically; however, the ration is designed to meet the nutrition standards of a restricted energy ration in which the vitamin content is proportionally reduced with the energy content. The estimated B vitamin content of the current assault ration is as follows: (1) thiamin, 0.6 mg; (2) riboflavin, 0.7 mg; (3) niacin, 8 mg NE; (4) vitamin B_6, 0.7 mg; (5) folic acid, 200 μg dietary folate equivalents (DFE); and (6) vitamin B_{12}, 1.2 μg [personal communication, S. Montain, USARIEM, July 16, 2004)]. These estimated quantities are approximately 50 percent of the Recommended Dietary Allowance (RDA) or Adequate Intake (AI) for young adult males (IOM, 1998); therefore, the current ration is both hypocaloric and deficient in B vitamin content (Table B-11). This paper presents examples of data supporting the conclusions

TABLE B-11 Dietary B Vitamins in a Ration Compared with the RDA or AI for Men Ages 19 to 30 Years

Vitamin	Estimated B Vitamin Content in Current Ration	RDA or AI
Thiamin	0.6 mg	1.2 mg
Riboflavin	0.7 mg	1.3 mg
Niacin	8 mg NE	16 mg NE
Vitamin B_6	0.7 mg	1.3 mg
Folic Acid	200 μg	400 μg DFE
Vitamin B_{12}	1.2 μg	2.4 μg
Biotin	—	30 μg[a]
Pantothenic Acid	—	5 mg[a]

NOTE: AI = Adequate Intake; DFE = dietary folate equivalents; NE = niacin equivalents; RDA = Recommended Dietary Allowance.
[a]Indicates the value is an AI rather than a RDA.
SOURCE: IOM (1998); personal communication, S. Montain, USARIEM, July 16, 2004.

that (1) inadequate B vitamin intake and caloric restriction impair physical and cognitive performance, and (2) extreme physical exertion coupled with caloric restriction significantly increases the requirement for B vitamins.

THE EFFECT OF INCREASED ENERGY DEMAND ON B VITAMIN USE

The B vitamins are required coenzymes for energy production in hundreds of metabolic reactions, including those required for glycolysis, the citric acid cycle, β-oxidation, amino acid metabolism, glycogenolysis, and gluconeogenesis (Bowman and Russel, 2001). Evidence suggests that when energy needs are increased by physical exertion, the B vitamin requirement increases to sustain energy production and maintain normal vitamin status.

Van der Beek and colleagues (1988) investigated the effect of low B vitamin intake on vitamin status and physical performance. These investigators conducted an eight-week, double-blind, controlled metabolic study in healthy young adult males (n = 24) described as moderately active. The study compared the effect of consumption of a diet low in thiamin, riboflavin, and vitamin B_6 with that of a deficient diet plus a supplement providing twice the Dutch RDA for these B vitamins. (2.5 mg, 4 mg, and 4 mg, respectively). The quantities of dietary B vitamins in the low vitamin group were similar to the quantities in the current military assault rations (i.e., 0.42 mg/day of thiamin; 0.53 mg/day of riboflavin; and 0.32 mg/day of vitamin B_6). The subjects consuming the low B vitamin diet were supplemented with twice the Dutch RDA for all vitamins except thiamin, riboflavin, and vitamin B_6 during the eight-week period of low vitamin intake. Unlike the combat ration, both experimental diets contained adequate calories (3,070 kcal/day).

Thiamin status was determined by measuring thiamin diphosphate concentration (TDP) and erythrocyte transketolase (ETK) activity as well as its in vitro stimulation by TDP (α-ETK or activation coefficient). Riboflavin status was assessed by means of flavin adenine dinucleotide (FAD) and erythrocyte glutathione reductase (EGR) activity as well as its in vitro stimulation by FAD (α-EGR). Vitamin B_6 status assessment was based on pyridoxal-5′-phosphate (PLP, the active form of the vitamin) concentration and erythrocyte glutamate oxaloacetate (EGOT) activity as well as its in vitro stimulation by PLP (α-EGOT). Within three to six weeks, deterioration of the vitamin status was indicated by decreased B vitamin coenzyme concentrations in blood, decreased erythrocyte enzyme activities, and elevation of stimulation tests of these enzymes, indicating an insufficient supply of coenzyme to maintain normal enzyme activity.

Physical performance was quantified by means of submaximal and maximal oxygen consumption (VO_2max). The onset of blood lactate accumulation (OBLA) was measured as well. To determine VO_2max and OBLA, the subjects performed incremental bicycle exercise tests. Both the aerobic power and maxi-

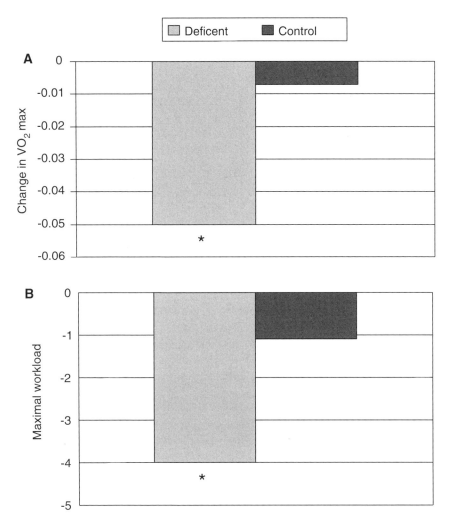

FIGURE B-21 Effect of combined low B vitamin intake on aerobic power (A) and work capacity (B). This effect is illustrated by the change of maximal performance from the baseline to 10 weeks during the study.
*Significantly different compared to control at $p < 0.01$.
SOURCE: van der Beek et al. (1988).

mal workload were significantly lower in the low vitamin group than in the control group (Figure B-21). The blood lactate concentration increase occurred at a lower intensity of physical exertion in the low vitamin group than in the control group. In summary, consumption of a diet adequate in calories but low in thiamin, riboflavin, and vitamin B_6 resulted in significantly impaired biochemical

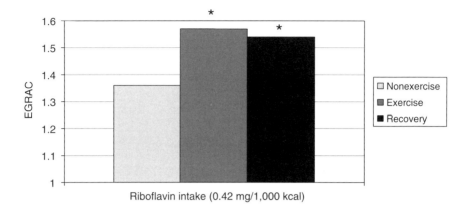

FIGURE B-22 Effect of exercise on riboflavin requirement in men.
NOTE: EGRAC = erythrocyte glutathione reductase activation coefficient.
*Significantly different compared to control (nonexercise) at $p < 0.05$.
SOURCE: Soares et al. (1993).

status, impaired aerobic power, decreased work capacity, and increased blood
lactate at a lower intensity of work.

Soares and colleagues (1993) evaluated the effect of exercise on the riboflavin
status of adult men whose baseline riboflavin status was inadequate. Energy balance was maintained throughout the study. Riboflavin status, based on increases
in the erythrocyte glutathione reductase activation coefficient (EGRAC), deteriorated significantly and the impaired status persisted during the subsequent
recovery period when the study participants exercised (Figure B-22). These data
indicate that riboflavin status further deteriorates during a short period of
increased physical activity in individuals whose riboflavin status is marginal.

As reviewed by Manore (2000), the results of a number of controlled metabolic studies in women indicate that exercise, dieting for weight loss, or a combination of both all increase riboflavin requirements. In one study by Belko and
colleagues (1983), young women consumed various amounts of riboflavin over a
10-week period, and their EGRAC values were determined. The EGRAC values
were above the cutoff of 1.25, indicating poor riboflavin status during the first
two weeks, when they consumed 0.14 mg of riboflavin/MJ (239 kcal). In
response to the consumption of 0.24 mg/MJ during the second two-week period,
the EGRAC values returned to normal. For the next three weeks, the riboflavin
intake was 0.24 mg/MJ, and the women started to exercise (20 to 50 minutes, six
days a week). The initiation of exercise increased the mean EGRAC values
above the cutoff. During the last three weeks, the women continued to exercise,
and their riboflavin intake increased to 0.33 mg/MJ. At this higher riboflavin

intake, the mean EGRAC values were normal, indicating that exercise led to an increase in the riboflavin requirement.

In two other metabolic studies, Belko and colleagues (1984, 1985) examined the effect of energy restriction and energy restriction plus physical exertion on riboflavin status. Overweight women consumed a metabolic diet that provided 1,195 to 1,266 kcal/day and various quantities of riboflavin (0.14 to 0.19 mg/MJ). The amount of riboflavin required to maintain good status was increased by energy restriction and increased even more by energy restriction plus exercise. It was concluded that a 0.38 mg/MJ level of riboflavin is required to keep EGRAC values in the normal range when female subjects dieted and exercised three to four hours week at 75 to 85 percent of the maximal heart rate.

The effect of exercise and energy restriction on riboflavin status was also evaluated by Winters and colleagues (1992), who fed older female subjects (50 to 67 years old) a metabolic diet that contained adequate calories to maintain weight and either 0.15 or 0.22 mg/MJ of riboflavin for five weeks. During the period when no exercise was performed, EGRAC values increased significantly. When subjects were exercising, 0.22 mg/MJ was required to maintain mean EGRAC values within the normal range. The conclusion from this investigation was that while energy restriction alone or exercise alone may increase riboflavin requirements above the RDA, calorie restriction plus exercise increases the requirement even more.

Manore and colleagues (1987) evaluated the effect of exercise on vitamin B_6 status. Plasma PLP concentrations increased significantly in response to exercise and returned to baseline within 60 minutes after exercise stopped (Figure B-23). The marked increase in plasma PLP in response to exercise increases the probability that the active coenzyme form of the vitamin (PLP) may be metabolized to the major excretory form (4-pyridoxic acid) and lost in the urine (Crozier et al., 1994). It has been proposed, therefore, that exercise may increase the turnover and loss of vitamin B_6 in active individuals.

In addition, Fogelholm and colleagues (1993) evaluated the effect of energy restriction coupled with exercise on vitamin B_6 status. A diet (1,673 kcal/day) consumed by elite male wrestlers over a three-week period resulted in a significant increase in vitamin B_6-dependent enzyme stimulation. Since no dietary intake data were obtained, there is a possibility that poor vitamin B_6 dietary intake may have also contributed to the impairment of vitamin B_6 status. In a different study, van Dale and colleagues (1990) compared the vitamin B_6 status in two groups of obese adult males who consumed low-calorie diets (716–931 kcal/day) for 14 weeks. In the group that consumed the weight-reduction diet coupled with exercise, plasma PLP concentration decreased from 54 to 40 mmol/L, but no such change occurred in the group who consumed the same diet but did not exercise. In addition, riboflavin status was also decreased in the diet-plus-exercise group.

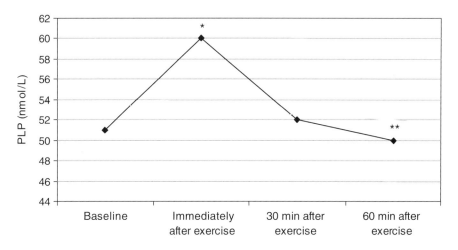

FIGURE B-23 Changes in a blood coenzyme form of vitamin B$_6$ (PLP) in response to very moderate exercise.
NOTE: PLP = pyridoxal 5′-phosphate.
*Sgnificant increase from baseline to immediately after exercise at $\alpha = 0.05$ level.
**Significant decrease from immediately after exercise to 60 minutes after exercise at $\alpha = 0.05$ level.
SOURCE: Manore et al. (1987).

EFFECT OF LOW B VITAMIN INTAKE ON MENTAL PERFORMANCE

The B vitamins are essential for normal neurological function. Deficiencies of vitamin B$_6$ and thiamin result in rapid neurological abnormalities (McCormick, 2001; Wood and Currie, 1995). The synthesis of key neurotransmittors, including serotonin, dopamine, norepinephrine, and γ-amniobutyric acid, is dependent on an adequate supply of vitamin B$_6$. Thiamin is required for normal neural cell function with different mechanisms of action proposed for normal nerve cell function (Bates, 2001). Folate is also required for the synthesis of a number of different neuroactive substances through its role as a methyl group donor (Bottiglieri, 1996). In addition, folate is a required coenzyme for homocysteine remethylation; low folate intake results in elevated homocysteine concentrations that have been associated with excitotic properties (Fava et al., 1997).

The effect of a low intake of thiamin (0.42 mg/day), riboflavin (0.53 mg/day), and vitamin B$_6$ (0.32 mg/day) on mental performance was evaluated in an eight-week double-blind controlled study in healthy young adult males (van der Beek et al., 1988). The mental performance test results indicated that subjects who consumed the low B vitamin diet made more errors (described as displaying a more risky behavior) and needed more time to complete tasks than subjects consuming the control diet, which contained twice the Dutch RDA (2.5 mg/d thiamin, 4 mg/day riboflavin and vitamin B_6) for these substances.

Low folate status has been associated with depression, cognitive dysfunction, psychosocial disorders, insomnia, irritability, impaired memory, and fatigue (Alpert et al., 2000; Bottiglieri et al., 1995). A meta-analysis of randomized controlled trials suggests that folate may have a potential role as a supplement to other treatments for depression (Taylor et al., 2004). Table B-12 includes a summary of studies that evaluated the association between folate status and mental performance.

TABLE B-12 Studies on Folate Levels and Mental Status

Authors	Subjects	Folate
Goodwin et al., 1983	Healthy noninstitutionalized, compared top 10% with bottom 5% and 10%	Lower concentration associated with lower test scores ($p < 0.01$) (Halstead-Reitan Categories Test)
Joosten et al., 1997	AD patients (A); Hospitalized control subjects (B); Healthy elderly (C)	Blood concentration significantly lower in A versus C ($p < 0.04$)
Kristensen et al., 1993	Patients with AD (A), other dementia (B), and mental disorders (C). Control subjects (D)	Blood concentration significantly lower in A versus D ($p < 0.05$)
Levitt and Karlinsky, 1992	AD patients and controls	Blood concentration significantly lower in subjects ($p > 0.05$)
Nilsson et al., 1996	Neuropsychiatric dementia patients (A); Neuropsychiatric patients no dementia (B); Control patients (C)	Blood concentration significantly lower in A versus B and C ($p < 0.001$)
Renvall et al., 1989	AD patients and normal individuals (A); Dementia patients and normal patients (B)	Blood concentration significantly lower in A ($p > 0.03$) and B ($p < 0.05$)
Riggs et al., 1996	Male volunteers	Lower concentration associated with lower test scores ($p = 0.003$) (Spatial copying test)

NOTE: AD = Alzheimer's disease.

RESPONSE TO SPECIFIC QUESTIONS RELATED TO REVISING THE B VITAMIN CONTENT OF THE PROPOSED MILITARY COMBAT RATION

A key question related to formulation of the proposed military ration is whether increasing the B vitamin content will enhance the performance of combat soldiers. The current combat ration is hypocaloric and estimated to have approximately 50 percent of the RDA for the B vitamins (personal communication, S. Montain, USARIEM, July 16, 2004). Data from the controlled studies reviewed above support the conclusion that increasing the B vitamin content in the current combat ration will likely enhance the physical and mental performance of soldiers. The studies consistently indicate that either exercise or energy restriction will increase the requirement of select B vitamins, and combining physical exertion with energy restriction will decrease B vitamin status and performance.

A second key question is whether the energy content of the combat ration should be maximized to reduce the energy debt. Based on findings from the controlled metabolic studies discussed above, energy restriction alone will result in impaired B vitamin status. There are no data that support the conclusion that supplemental B vitamins will compensate for all of the metabolic changes that occur due to energy restriction, but to maintain the B vitamin status, it is recommended that the B vitamins be added to the diet in excess of the RDA.

SUMMARY AND CONCLUSIONS

Energy restriction or moderate exercise increases the body's use of B vitamins to maintain metabolic pathways involved in energy production. A combination of energy restriction and moderate exercise increases B vitamin use to an even greater extent. In contrast to the short, intermittent periods of moderate exercise evaluated in the controlled studies, the intensity and duration of physical exertion during military combat operations are much greater and sustained for much longer periods. It is logical to assume that the effect of energy restriction and extreme physical exertion on B vitamin metabolism would be exacerbated during military combat. The recommended B vitamin content of the proposed new combat ration is twice the current RDA (Table B-13). For the B vitamins and choline not considered in this review, it is also recommended that the ration contain twice the RDA or AI (Table B-13).

REFERENCES

Alpert JE, Mischoulon D, Nierenberg AA, Fava M. 2000. Nutrition and depression: Focus on folate. *Nutrition* 16(7–8):544–546.
Bates CJ. 2001. Thiamin. In: Bowman BA, Russell RM, eds. *Present Knowledge in Nutrition*. Washington, DC: ILSI Press. Pp. 184–190.

TABLE B-13 Suggested B Vitamin Content for the Ration

Vitamin	RDA or AI Doubled for Daily Intake
Thiamin	2.4 mg
Riboflavin	2.6 mg
Niacin	32 mg NE
Vitamin B_6	2.6 mg
Folate	800 µg DFE (475 mg folic acid × 1.7)
Vitamin B_{12}	4.8 µg
Biotin	60 µg[a]
Pantothenic Acid	10 µg[a]
Choline	1,100 mg[a]

NOTE: AI = Adequate Intake; DFE = dietary folate equivalents; NE = niacin equivalents; RDA = Recommended Dietary Allowance.
[a]Indicates the value is an AI rather than a RDA.
SOURCE: IOM (1998).

Belko AZ, Meredith MP, Kalkwarf HJ, Obarzanek E, Weinberg S, Roach R, McKeon G, Roe DA. 1985. Effects of exercise on riboflavin requirements: Biological validation in weight reducing women. *Am J Clin Nutr* 41(2):270–277.

Belko AZ, Obarzanek E, Kalkwarf HJ, Rotter MA, Bogusz S, Miller D, Haas JD, Roe DA. 1983. Effects of exercise on riboflavin requirements of young women. *Am J Clin Nutr* 37(4):509–517.

Belko AZ, Obarzanek E, Roach R, Rotter M, Urban G, Weinberg S, Roe DA. 1984. Effects of aerobic exercise and weight loss on riboflavin requirements of moderately obese, marginally deficient young women. *Am J Clin Nutr* 40(3):553–561.

Bottiglieri T. 1996. Folate, vitamin B12, and neuropsychiatric disorders. *Nutr Rev* 54(12):382–390.

Bottiglieri T, Crellin R, Renolds EH. 1995. Folates and neuropsychiatry. In: Bailey LB, ed. *Folate in Health and Disease*. New York: Marcel Dekker. Pp. 435–462.

Bowman BA, Russel RM. 2001. *Present Knowledge in Nutrition*. 8th ed. Washington, DC: ILSI Press.

Crozier PG, Cordain L, Sampson DA. 1994. Exercise-induced changes in plasma vitamin B-6 concentrations do not vary with exercise intensity. *Am J Clin Nutr* 60(4):552–558.

Fava M, Borus JS, Alpert JE, Nierenberg AA, Rosenbaum JF, Bottiglieri T. 1997. Folate, vitamin B12, and homocysteine in major depressive disorder. *Am J Psychiatry* 154(3):426–428.

Fogelholm M, Ruokonen I, Laakso JT, Vuorimaa T, Himberg JJ. 1993. Lack of association between indices of vitamin B_1, B_2, and B_6 status and exercise-induced blood lactate in young adults. *Int J Sport Nutr* 3(2):165–176.

Goodwin JS, Goodwin JM, Garry PJ. 1983. Association between nutritional status and cognitive functioning in a healthy elderly population. *J Am Med Assoc* 249(21):2917–2921.

IOM (Institute of Medicine). 1998. *Dietary Reference Intakes for Thiamin, Riboflavin, Niacin, Vitmain B_6, Folate, Vitamin B_{12}, Pantothenic Acid, Biotin, and Choline*. Washington, DC: National Academy Press.

Joosten E, Lesaffre E, Riezler R, Ghekiere V, Dereymaeker L, Pelemans W, Dejaeger E. 1997. Is metabolic evidence for vitamin B-12 and folate deficiency more frequent in elderly patients with Alzheimer's disease? *J Gerontol A Biol Sci Med Sci* 52(2):M76–M79.

Kristensen MO, Gulmann NC, Christensen JE, Ostergaard K, Rasmussen K. 1993. Serum cobalamin and methylmalonic acid in Alzheimer dementia. *Acta Neurol Scand* 87(6):475–481.

Levitt AJ, Karlinsky H. 1992. Folate, vitamin B12 and cognitive impairment in patients with Alzheimer's disease. *Acta Psychiatr Scand* 86(4):301–305.

Manore MM. 2000. Effect of physical activity on thiamine, riboflavin, and vitamin B-6 requirements. *Am J Clin Nutr* 72(2 Suppl):598S–606S.

Manore MN, Leklem JE, Walter MC. 1987. Vitamin B-6 metabolism as affected by exercise in trained and untrained women fed diets differing in carbohydrate and vitamin B_6 content. *Am J Clin Nutr* 46(6):995–1004.

McCormick DB. 2001. Vitamin B-6. In: Bowman BA, Russel RM, eds. *Present Knowledge in Nutrition.* Washington, DC: ILSI Press. Pp. 207–213.

Nilsson K, Gustafson L, Faldt R, Andersson A, Brattstrom L, Lindgren A, Israelsson B, Hultberg B. 1996. Hyperhomocysteinaemia—A common finding in a psychogeriatric population. *Eur J Clin Invest* 26(10):853–859.

Renvall MJ, Spindler AA, Ramsdell JW, Paskvan M. 1989. Nutritional status of free-living Alzheimer's patients. *Am J Med Sci* 298(1):20–27.

Riggs KM, Spiro A 3rd, Tucker K, Rush D. 1996. Relations of vitamin B-12, vitamin B-6, folate, and homocysteine to cognitive performance in the Normative Aging Study. *Am J Clin Nutr* 63(3):306–314.

Soares MJ, Satyanarayana K, Bamji MS, Jacob CM, Ramana YV, Rao SS. 1993. The effect of exercise on the riboflavin status of adult men. *Br J Nutr* 69(2):541–551.

Taylor MJ, Carney SM, Goodwin GM, Geddes JR. 2004. Folate for depressive disorders: Systematic review and meta-analysis of randomized controlled trials. *J Psychopharmacol* 18(2):251–256.

van Dale D, Schrijver J, Saris WH. 1990. Changes in vitamin status in plasma during dieting and exercise. *Int J Vitam Nutr Res* 60(1):67–74.

van der Beek EJ, van Dokkum W, Schrijver J, Wedel M, Gaillard AW, Wesstra A, van de Weerd H, Hermus RJ. 1988. Thiamin, riboflavin, and vitamins B-6 and C: Impact of combined restricted intake on functional performance in man. *Am J Clin Nutr* 48(6):1451–1462.

Winters LR, Yoon JS, Kalkwarf HJ, Davies JC, Berkowitz MG, Haas J, Roe DA. 1992. Riboflavin requirements and exercise adaptation in older women. *Am J Clin Nutr* 56(3):526–532.

Wood B, Currie J. 1995. Presentation of acute Wernicke's encephalopathy and treatment with thiamine. *Metab Brain Dis* 10(1):57–72.

Optimization of the Nutrient Composition in Military Rations for Short-Term, High-Stress Situations: Sodium, Potassium, and Other Electrolytes

Susan Shirreffs, Loughborough University, UK

INTRODUCTION

The specific questions addressed in this manuscript are as follows:

1. What are the types and levels or ratios of electrolytes that could be added to such rations to enhance performance during combat missions? Specifically address the effects of environmental stress.
2. What are the interactions between electrolytes (e.g., sodium and potassium)?

Certain illnesses and medications influence electrolyte balance. In this manuscript, however, dietary electrolyte requirements have not been considered for individuals with illnesses that may cause repeated vomiting, prolonged diarrhea, heat illness, or collapse or for individuals with ongoing medical treatment.

One recent publication from the Institute of Medicine (IOM, 2004) provides an up-to-date review of sodium and potassium dietary requirements. The recommendations given within this publication have been used in this manuscript as a starting point for determining a healthy diet with specific requirements for short-term, high stress situations. Adequate Intakes (AIs) were set for both sodium and potassium because an Estimated Average Requirement, and thus a Recommended Dietary Allowance could not be established.

POTASSIUM

Potassium is the major cation in the intracellular fluid, and it is maintained at a concentration of approximately 145 mmol/L; the extracellular concentration is approximately 4 to 5 mmol/L. Potassium is required for normal cellular function, and relatively small changes in the extracellular potassium can greatly affect the extra- to intracellular ratio, thereby affecting neural transmission, muscle contraction, and vascular tone.

Severe potassium deficiency, characterized by hypokalemia and indicated by a serum potassium concentration of less than 3.5 mmol/L, has consequences that include cardiac arrhythmia, muscle weakness, and glucose intolerance. Moderate potassium deficiency is characterized by increased blood pressure, salt sensitivity, and risk of kidney stones and shows evidence of increased bone turnover.

In normal circumstances, 77 to 90 percent of dietary potassium is excreted in urine with the remaining excreted in feces and sweat (Holbrook et al., 1984).

The AI for potassium set by the Panel on Dietary Reference Intakes for Electrolytes and Water (IOM, 2004) is 4.7 g (120 mmol) per day. This recommendation, however, is based on potassium intake from food, excluding supplementation, and is therefore based on forms of potassium with bicarbonate precursors. The rationale for this AI is that it should help maintain lower blood pressure levels, reduce the effects of sodium chloride intake on blood pressure, reduce the risk of kidney stones, and, possibly, decrease bone loss. The Panel assigned no Tolerable Upper Intake Level (UL) because for healthy individuals with normal kidney function, any excess dietary potassium intake from foods is excreted in the urine, feces, and sweat. However, the National Health and Nutrition Examination Survey (NHANES III, 1988–1994) in the United States indicated that the median potassium intake by male adults was approximately 2.8 to 3.3 g (72 to 84 mmol) per day. Only 10 percent of men consumed potassium in a quantity equal to or greater than the AI.

SODIUM

Sodium is the major cation in extracellular fluid, and it is maintained at a concentration of approximately 140 mmol/L; the intracellular concentration is approximately 4 mmol/L. Along with the anion chloride, sodium maintains extracellular volume, and therefore, plasma volume and serum osmolality. It is also an important determinant of cell membrane potential and an active transporter of molecules across membranes.

In the absence of substantial sweating, individuals in sodium and water balance typically excrete 90 to 95 percent of their dietary sodium intake in their urine (Table B-14). The total obligatory sodium losses are very small, amounting to approximately 0.18 g (8 mmol) per day (Dahl, 1958).

On the basis of available data, the AI for sodium set by the Panel on Dietary Reference Intakes for Electrolytes and Water (IOM, 2004) is 1.5 g (65 mmol) per day. Based on the effects of higher sodium intake levels on blood pressure, the UL for sodium is 2.3 g (100 mmol) per day. However, while both the AI and UL were said to be appropriate for unacclimatized individuals exposed to high environmental temperatures or for people who are physically active, they were deemed inappropriate for highly active individuals or individuals who are exposed to prolonged heat and lose large amounts of sweat daily. Although the AI and UL parameters were not quantified, it is clear that the AI allows for an intake of approximately 1.3 g (57 mmol) above the maximum obligatory losses (Table B-14), meaning that this amount may be taken to accommodate increased sweat sodium loss.

Hyponatremia, which is defined as a serum sodium concentration of less than 135 mmol/L, does not generally occur with low sodium intakes (Kirkendall et al., 1976; Overlack et al., 1995), but rather is related to excessive sodium loss from the body or to excessive consumption of fluids low in sodium.

The National Health and Nutrition Examination Survey (NHANES III, 1988–1994) in the United States indicated that the median sodium intake by male adults ranged from 3.1 to 4.7 g (135 to 204 mmol) per day (IOM, 2004). This estimate, however, excludes any salt added at the table, so the intake levels

TABLE B-14 Obligatory Losses of Sodium

Source	g/day	mmol/day
Urine	0.005–0.035	0.2–1.5
Skin (nonsweating)	0.025	1.1
Feces	0.010–0.125	0.4–5.4
Total	0.040–0.185	1.7–8.0

SOURCE: Dahl (1958).

may be an underestimate for many individuals. Total dietary sodium intake was recently estimated to be 4.2 g (183 mmol) per day as shown in a study that quantified intake based on 24-hour urine collections (Zhou et al., 2003).

CHLORIDE

Sodium and chloride are commonly found together in foods as sodium chloride. For this reason, and because both are commonly in association in the body, the AI for chloride set by the Panel on Dietary Reference Intakes for Electrolytes and Water (IOM, 2004) is at a level equivalent, on a molar basis, to that of sodium and thus amounts to 2.3 g (65 mmol) per day.

SODIUM-WATER INTERACTION

A brief mention of water intake is warranted because of its links with body sodium balance and sodium's role in maintaining extracellular fluid volume. Water is the largest single constituent in the body in nonobese individuals. It acts as a solvent for biochemical reactions and as a medium of transport of other compounds, and it has a high specific heat to absorb metabolic heat, maintains vascular volume, supports the supply of nutrients, and removes waste. However, an individual's total water intake includes drinking water, water in other drinks, and water in foods. The AI for water was established at a sufficient level to prevent the acute deleterious effects of dehydration, including functional and metabolic abnormalities. For example, the AI for total water intake for young men is 3.7 liters per day (IOM, 2004); however, higher intakes will be required for individuals who are physically active or are exposed to hot environments. In very unusual circumstances, an excess consumption of fluids combined with a low sodium intake may lead to excess body water, resulting in hyponatremia.

THE EFFECTS OF ENVIRONMENTAL STRESS ON ELECTROLYTE REQUIREMENTS

An increased environmental temperature is more physiologically stressful to free living humans than is a cold environment. Exposure to a cold environment, provided that appropriate clothing is available and, perhaps, some form of exercise to generate heat is possible, presents no special consideration with regard to electrolyte requirements. They should be no different from requirements for a "normal" environment for that individual. However, the same is not true for a warm environment because of the sweating mechanism that is activated to regulate body temperature.

When sweating it stimulated, it can have a significant influence on electrolyte losses. Sodium is the main electrolyte present in sweat, but significant amounts of other electrolytes are present (Table B-15).

TABLE B-15 The Normal Concentration Range
of Some of the Main Electrolytes in Sweat

Electrolyte	Concentration (mmol/L)
Sodium	10–80
Chloride	10–60
Potassium	4–14
Calcium	0.3–2
Magnesium	0.2–1.5
Sulfate	0.1–0.2

SOURCE: Costill (1977); Lentner (1981); Maughan (1991); Pitts (1959); Schmidt and Thews (1989).

Clearly, the extent of any electrolyte loss incurred will also depend on the sweat rate. As summarized by IOM (2004) when an individual is at rest and not visibly sweating, the rate of water loss through the skin is approximately 0.020 L per hour. At the other extreme, an individual that experiences shorter periods of intense activity in a warm environment could have a maximum sweat rate of 3 L per hour (Sawka and Pandolf, 1990). Other data from the literature suggest sweat rates of 0.3 to 1.2 L per hour (Adolph, 1947) for residents of desert climates performing occupational activities, while persons performing low-intensity exercise but wearing protective clothing commonly have sweat rates of 1 to 2 L per hour (Levine et al., 1990). Finally, when calculated on a daily basis from water turnover studies, sweat water losses of 0.2 to 2 L per day have been reported for sedentary individuals in a temperate climate while volumes of 1 to 9 L per day have been reported for individuals undertaking manual work or exercise in varying climates (Leiper et al., 1996, 2001; Singh et al., 1989). These very different sweat rates clearly have the potential to induce electrolyte losses, thus affecting total body electrolyte loss. Taking 0.20 L per hour (4.8 L per day) as the lowest sweat rate and 9 L per day as the highest, the losses of the main electrolytes could range as shown in Table B-16.

Many other factors, however, influence sweat composition. These include the dietary electrolyte intake (Allsopp et al., 1998; Armstrong et al., 1985b), the heat acclimation status of an individual, and the individual's sweat rate at any time. However, as shown in Box B-2, while sodium levels are influenced by all three factors noted, divergent findings for potassium have been reported in the literature.

Many studies have attempted to quantify sodium and potassium loss through sweat and urine in a variety of settings, and some of these have been summarized in Table B-17. However, a key factor when considering dietary electrolyte intakes for groups of individuals is the vast differences individuals have in both sweat rate and sweat electrolyte losses when doing the same task, at the same time, in the same environment, and wearing the same clothing.

TABLE B-16 The Range of Losses for the Main Electrolytes Attributed to Sweat Rates Ranging from 4.8 L per Day to 9 L per Day

Electrolyte	Loss (mmol/day)[a]
Sodium	5–720
Chloride	5–540
Potassium	4–126

[a]See Table B-15 for the range of normal sweat electrolyte concentrations.

BOX B-2
The Influence of Diet, Heat Acclimation, and Sweat Rate on Sodium and Potassium Concentrations in Sweat

SODIUM
- ↑ dietary Na intake, ↑ sweat [Na]
- heat acclimation, ↓ sweat [Na]
- ↑ sweat rate, ↑ sweat [Na]

POTASSIUM
- ↑ dietary K intake, ? sweat [K]
- heat acclimation, ? sweat [K]
- ↑ sweat rate, ? sweat [K]

SODIUM AND POSTEXERCISE REHYDRATION

In situations when large sweat losses occur over a relatively short time, effective recovery from dehydration will not occur when replacing water loss until the sodium loss is replaced as well. Solid food consumed along with the water will replace the sodium, but if food is not consumed, sodium salts should be added to the water (Maughan et al., 1996; Ray et al., 1998; Shirreffs and Maughan, 1998).

SODIUM–POTASSIUM INTERACTIONS

Sodium and potassium are complementary to each other in a number of ways and their consumption has particular effects on urinary excretion of the alternate cation, salt sensitivity, and blood pressure. However, in the studies referred to in the final sections below, the subjects were not stressed to a level that would add to significant sweat electrolyte losses in addition to the urinary losses described.

TABLE B-17 Sweat (S) and Urinary (U) Loss of Potassium and Sodium

Condition	Intake and Loss	Reference
Potassium		
24 hr exposed to heat stress	97 mmol (D); 60 mmol (S); 116 mmol (U+S)	Malhotra et al., 1976
6 hr intermittent walking	32 mmol (S); 23–70 mmol (U+S)	Armstrong et al., 1985a
Projected 24 hr losses	62–240 mmol (U+S)	Armstrong et al., 1985b
4 days with exercise	25 mmol verses 80 mmol (D); 31 mmol versus 67 mmol (U); 12 mmol versus 11 mmol (S)	Costill et al., 1982
Sodium		
6 hr intermittent walking	72–244 mmol (U+S)	Armstrong et al., 1985a
Projected 24 hr losses	193–425 mmol (U+S)	Armstrong et al., 1985b
5 days heat acclimatization at 40 °C	348 vs. 174 vs. 66 mmol (D); 105 vs. 78 vs. 50 mmol (S); + 15 vs. + 29 vs. + 0.2 mmol (Balance)	Allsopp et al., 1998
5–9 L sweat per day	Sodium balance with 1.9–3.2 g (83–139 mmol)/day	Conn, 1949

NOTE: Where available, the dietary intake (D) of sodium or potassium is shown.

Dietary Intake and Sodium Excretion

With dietary sodium intakes of up to 3.2 g (140 mmol) per day, urinary potassium excretion generally remains lower than dietary potassium intake for at least 28 days (Sacks et al., 2001). However, with dietary sodium intakes greater that 6.9 g (300 mmol) per day, the urinary potassium excretion was greater than the dietary potassium intake over three days (Luft et al., 1982).

When potassium in the form of potassium bicarbonate or potassium chloride was supplemented in quantities greater than 4.7 g (120 mmol) per day, an increase in urinary sodium excretion was reported (van Buren et al., 1992). However, a potassium bicarbonate intake of either 2.7 or 4.7 g (70 to 120 mmol) per day was sufficient to reverse this increased loss when dietary sodium chloride intake was increased from 1.8 to 14.6 g (30 to 250 mmol) per day (Morris et al., 1999).

Salt Sensitivity

Salt sensitivity refers to the degree of blood pressure response to a change in dietary sodium intake. It is frequently classified by a dietary sodium chloride-induced increase in mean arterial blood pressure of 3 mm Hg or more. Studies have demonstrated that the expression of salt sensitivity is modulated by dietary potassium intake, and this is one of the main rationales given for encouraging a high potassium intake. Morris and colleagues (1999) reported a 50 to 80 percent decrease of the identified salt-sensitive individuals who had a sodium chloride intake of 14.6 g (250 mmol) per day while they increased their potassium bicarbonate intake from 1.2 g (30 mmol) to 2.7 g (70 mmol) per day. It has been postulated that these effects on salt sensitivity occur with the natriuretic (high level of sodium loss in urine) effects of the potassium, increasing renal tubule excretion of sodium chloride, which seems to be unaffected by the anion accompanying potassium (IOM, 2004).

Blood Pressure

The modulating effects of dietary potassium intake on blood pressure appear to be related to the sodium/potassium ratio, and the effects increase with higher sodium chloride intake (Morris and Sebastian, 1995; Whelton et al., 1997). Reductions in systolic blood pressure of 2.5 mm Hg and in diastolic blood pressure of 1.5 mm Hg have been reported when 2 g (50 mmol) of urinary potassium was excreted, indicative of higher potassium intakes (Intersalt Cooperative Research Group, 1988).

CONCLUSIONS

For the most part, appropriate electrolyte intake for combat rations would be similar to that for daily intake in a healthy, balanced diet. Sodium requirements may be the main exception because of environmental influences. Because adaptations to significant changes in dietary intake of sodium take a number of days to fully develop, there are compelling reasons to have sodium in a short-term ration be present in a least the same quantities as those in the preceding daily diet.

The types of stresses experienced and their effects on sweat production may influence dietary electrolyte requirements. After a period of heavy sweating, sodium should be consumed, if possible, with any large volume of water to minimize diuresis. It is possible that sodium requirements may well differ with prolonged low sweat rates in comparison with the high sweat rates seen during periods of intense activity.

In keeping with the conclusions of the Panel on Dietary Reference Intakes for Electrolytes and Water, "data are presently insufficient to set different potassium intake recommendations according to the level of sodium intake, and vice versa. Likewise, data are insufficient to set requirements based on the sodium/potassium ratio" (IOM, 2004, p. 230).

REFERENCES

Adolph EF. 1947. *Physiology of Man in the Desert.* New York: Intersciences.

Allsopp AJ, Sutherland R, Wood P, Wootton SA. 1998. The effect of sodium balance on sweat sodium secretion and plasma aldosterone concentration. *Eur J Appl Physiol* 78(6):516–521.

Armstrong LW, Costill DL, Fink WJ, Bassett D, Hargreaves M, Nishibata I, King DS. 1985a. Effects of dietary sodium on body and muscle potassium content during heat acclimation. *Eur J Appl Physiol* 54(4):391–397.

Armstrong LE, Hubbard RW, Szlyk PC, Matthew WT, Sils IV. 1985b. Voluntary dehydration and electrolyte losses during prolonged exercise in the heat. *Aviat Space Environ Med* 56(8): 765–770.

Costill D. 1977. Sweating: Its composition and effects on body fluids. *Ann N Y Acad Sci* 301: 160–174.

Costill DL, Cote R, Fink WJ. 1982. Dietary potassium and heavy exercise: Effects on muscle water and electrolytes. *Am J Clin Nutr* 36(2):266–275.

Conn JW. 1949. The mechanism of acclimatization to heat. *Adv Int Med* 3:373–393.

Dahl LK. 1958. Salt intake and salt need. *N Engl J Med* 258(23):1152–1157.

Holbrook JT, Patterson KY, Bodner JE, Douglas LW, Veillon C, Kelsay JL, Mertz W, Smith JC Jr. 1984. Sodium and potassium intake and balance in adults consuming self-selected diets. *Am J Clin Nutr* 40(4):786–793.

Intersalt Cooperative Research Group. 1988. Intersalt: An international study of electrolyte excretion and blood pressure. Results for 24 hour urinary sodium and potassium excretion. *Br Med J* 297(6644):319–328.

IOM (Institute of Medicine). 2004. *Dietary Reference Intakes for Water, Potassium, Sodium, Chloride and Sulfate.* Washington, DC: The National Academies Press.

Kirkendall AM, Connor WE, Abboud F, Rastogi SP, Anderson TA, Fry M. 1976. The effect of dietary sodium chloride on blood pressure, body fluids, electrolytes, renal function, and serum lipids of normotensive man. *J Lab Clin Med* 87(3):411–434.

Leiper JB, Carnie A, Maughan RJ. 1996. Water turnover rates in sedentary and exercising middle aged men. *Br J Sports Med* 30(1):24–26.

Leiper JB, Pitsiladis Y, Maughan RJ. 2001. Comparison of water turnover rates in men undertaking prolonged cycling exercise and sedentary men. *Int J Sports Med* 22(3):181–185.

Lentner C, ed. 1981. *Geigy Scientific Tables.* 8th ed. Basel: Ciba-Geigy Ltd.

Levine L, Quigley MD, Cadarette BS, Sawka MN, Pandolf KB. 1990. Physiologic strain associated with wearing toxic-environment protective systems during exercise in the heat. In: Das B, ed. *Advances in Industrial Ergonomics and Safety II.* London: Taylor & Francis. Pp. 897–904.

Luft FC, Weinberger MH, Grim CE. 1982. Sodium sensitivity and resistance in normotensive humans. *Am J Med* 72(5):726–736.

Malhotra MS, Sridharan K, Venkataswamy Y. 1976. Potassium losses in sweat under heat stress. *Aviat Space Environ Med* 47(5):503–504.

Maughan RJ. 1991. Fluid and electrolyte loss and replacement in exercise. *J Sports Sci* 9 (Special):117–142.

Maughan RJ, Leiper JB, Shirreffs SM. 1996. Resortation of fluid balance after exercise-induced dehydration: Effects of food and fluid intake. *Eur J Appl Physiol* 73:317–325.

Morris RC, Sebastian A. 1995. Potassium-responsive hypertension. In: Laragh JH, Brenner BM, eds. *Hypertension: Pathophysiology, Diagnosis, and Management.* 2nd ed. New York: Raven Press. Pp. 2715–2726.

Morris RC Jr, Schmidlin O, Tanaka M, Forman A, Frassetto L, Sebastian A. 1999. Differing effects of supplemental KCl and KHCO3: Pathophysiological and clinical implications. *Semin Nephrol* 19(5):487–493.

Overlack A, Ruppert M, Kolloch R, Kraft K, Stumpe KO. 1995. Age is a major determinant of the divergent blood pressure responses to varying salt intake in essential hypertension. *Am J Hypertens* 8(8):829–836.

Pitts RF. 1959. *The Physiological Basis of Diuretic Therapy.* Springfield, IL: C.C. Thomas.

Ray ML, Bryan MW, Ruden TM, Baier SM, Sharp RL, King DS. 1998. Effect of sodium in a rehydration beverage when consumed as a fluid or meal. *J Appl Physiol* 85(4):1329–1336.

Sacks FM, Svetkey LP, Vollmer WM, Appel LJ, Bray GA, Harsha D, Obarzanek E, Conlin PR, Miller ER 3rd, Simons-Morton DG, Karanja N, Lin PH. 2001. Effects on blood pressure of reduced dietary sodium and the Dietary Approaches to Stop Hypertension (DASH) diet. DASH-Sodium Collaborative Research Group. *N Engl J Med* 344(1):3–10.

Sawka M, Pandolf K. 1990. Effects of body water loss on physiological function and exercise performance. In: Gisolfi C, Lamb D, eds. *Perspectives In Exercise Science and Sports Medicine.* Vol. 3. Fluid homeostasis during exercise. Carmel, IN: Benchmark Press Inc. Pp. 1–38.

Schmidt RF, Thews G, eds. 1989. *Human Physiology.* 2nd ed. Berlin: Springer-Verlag.

Shirreffs SM, Maughan RJ. 1998. Volume repletion after exercise-induced volume depletion in humans: Replacement of water and sodium losses. *Am J Physiol* 274(5 Pt 2):F868–F875.

Singh J, Prentice AM, Diaz E, Coward WA, Ashford J, Sawyer M, Whitehead RG. 1989. Energy expenditure of Gambian women during peak agricultural activity measured by the doubly-labelled water method. *Br J Nutr* 62(2):315–329.

van Buren M, Rabelink TJ, van Rijn HJ, Koomans HA. 1992. Effects of acute NaCl, KCl and KHCO$_3$ loads on renal electrolyte excretion in humans. *Clin Sci (Lond)* 83(5):567–574.

Whelton PK, He J, Cutler JA, Brancati FL, Appel LJ, Follmann D, Klag MJ. 1997. Effects of oral potassium on blood pressure. Meta-analysis of randomized controlled clinical trials. *J Am Med Assoc* 277(20):1624–1632.

Zhou BF, Stamler J, Dennis B, Moag-Stahlberg A, Okuda N, Robertson C, Zhao L, Chan Q, Elliott P. 2003. Nutrient intakes of middle-aged men and women in China, Japan, United Kingdom, and United States in the late 1990s: The INTERMAP study. *J Hum Hypertens* 17(9):623–630.

Other Bioactive Food Components and Dietary Supplements

Rebecca B. Costello and George P. Chrousos, National Institutes of Health

INTRODUCTION

Evaluation of the potential beneficial effects of nutrition supplements or bioactive food components should consider an individual's baseline status and the many different stress states in response to discrete types of stressors. Also, we need to distinguish between acute, subacute, and chronic stressors and the type, amount, and duration of demands that each imposes on the individual. Another issue is the constitution of the individual, dictated by genetics, developmental intrauterine and early life history, and late postnatal and current environment.

Psychosocial or physical stressors or a combination of the two produce different kinds of adaptive responses and have different types of material requirements depending on both the size and duration of the stressor. During stress, be it psychosocial or physical, all four major neurotransmitter systems—noradrenergic, serotonergic, cholinergic, and γ-aminobutyric acid (GABA)ergic—are activated. This poses increased needs for precursor amino acid molecules as well as for the energy necessary for their synthesis, secretion, and electrochemical effects. Also, there is increased demand for the necessary coenzymes, some of which are essential vitamins that must be taken from the environment. When physical stress is present, one has to consider both the increased needs for the stress neurotransmitter synthesis, secretion, and effects, and the peripheral energy demands, the latter becoming of major importance. In this instance, the availability of nutrients and oxygen and the presence of healthy energy-producing machinery, including adequate numbers of healthy mitochondria and the ability to switch from aerobic to anaerobic metabolism, are crucial components of a successful adaptation.

This chapter reviews a number of bioactive food components and dietary supplements that have been tested or suggested for their performance-enhancing effects. Among these are the well-characterized and extensively studied amino acids tyrosine and tryptophan for their role in modulating neurotransmitter concentrations. Also reviewed are L-carnitine and coenzyme Q_{10} for their role in supporting mitochondrial energy metabolism, as well as several botanical ingredients, *Eleutherococcus senticosus* (Siberian ginseng), *Cordyceps sinensis*, and *Rhodiola*, for their adaptogenic qualities, and *Ginkgo biloba* for cognitive function and mitigation of acute mountain sickness.

NEUROTRANSMITTER PRECURSORS

Tyrosine and tryptophan, two of the large neutral amino acids (LNAA), when given in single, nonphysiologic doses or within special diets, have been shown to alter brain activity. Tyrosine is the precursor for the neurotransmitters dopamine, norepinephrine, and epinephrine. The working hypothesis is that tyrosine can mitigate the adverse effects of acute stress by modulating levels of norepinephrine. Tryptophan is the precursor for the neurotransmitter serotonin. Its role in regulating mood (particularly depression) and alertness but also pain sensitivity, aggression and food consumption may, under certain circumstances, support various aspects of performance. This topic has been well described in previous IOM reports (IOM, 1994, 1999) and in reviews by Lieberman (1994, 1999, 2003) and thus this chapter will concentrate on more recent research findings dealing with the roles of tyrosine and tryptophan in modulating performance.

TYROSINE

Animal studies have demonstrated that performance decline observed in highly stressed animals can be restored by supplementation with tyrosine (IOM, 1994). This has recently been confirmed (Yeghiayan et al., 2001); rats pretreated with L-tyrosine (200 to 400 mg/kg body weight) in a dose-dependent fashion improved performance in a forced-swim test following acute cold stress. Tyrosine also improved mood and performance concomitant with increases in hippocampal norepinephrine concentrations following cold exposure.

Human studies involved in supplementing with L-tyrosine have shown that the adverse effects of hypoxia and cold, lower body negative-pressure stress, and psychological stress can be reduced by tyrosine supplementation in dose ranges of 85 to 100 mg/kg body weight (IOM, 1994). Work by Neri and colleagues (1995) in a clinical study of a small number of US Marine research subjects, demonstrated that 75 mg/kg of L-tyrosine, compared to the results of a corn-starch control given in banana-flavored yogurt on two occasions to the soldiers after one night's sleep loss, ameliorated the usual performance decline on a set of psychomotor tasks over a 13-hour test session. A significant reduction in lapse probability on a high-event rate vigilance task was also demonstrated with improvements lasting approximately three hours. When two grams of L-tyrosine was administered in the form of a protein-rich drink for a period of five days, military cadets performed better on enhanced memory and tracking tests compared with those who ingested an isocaloric placebo drink (Deijen et al., 1999). Most recently in a study designed to test whether repeated ingestions of tyrosine during prolonged exercise would improve physical performance in competitive cyclists, Chinevere and colleagues (2002) administered L-tyrosine alone (25 mg/kg), tyrosine with a carbohydrate supplement, or a placebo in a double-blind controlled study and found a lack of effect on physical endurance parameters of oxygen uptake, heart rate, rate of perceived exertion (RPE) at any time during the 90-minute cycling session. Although an increase in the plasma to free-tyrosine:tryptophan ratio (a more sensitive marker of amino acid transport across the blood-brain barrier than plasma levels alone) was noted for those who consumed the tyrosine-containing supplements, it did not translate into an increase in performance. Thus, it appears that the benefits of tyrosine supplementation continue to be accrued for enhancements in cognitive function but not for physical performance.

L-Tyrosine is generally recognized as safe (GRAS) status in the United States. It is safe in doses up to 150 mg/kg/day for two weeks (IOM, 2002), although a number of issues remain to be addressed concerning routine supplementation with tyrosine. Yet to be demonstrated is tyrosine's effects across a wider range of stressors. There is a need to establish a dose-response function for tyrosine in humans and to estimate an upper level of intake. Documentation in human studies is still lacking regarding its efficacy in situations of chronic stress. The most effective method of supplementation for the soldiers (foods versus supplements) has yet to be determined.

TRYPTOPHAN

Tryptophan has been shown to have sedative-like effects on humans when administered in pure form and in sufficient quantity (IOM, 1994; Lieberman et al., 1986). It may also be useful as a mild sleep aid in military operations as it does not appear to impair some aspects of performance (IOM, 1994; Lieberman et al., 1986). Research on supplementation with L-tryptophan was halted in 1990 when products were removed from the market due to an outbreak of a rare condition called eosinophilia-myalgia syndrome (EMS). The exact etiology of this outbreak remains undefined. L-Tryptophan however is available in the United States in special dietary products for limited use under medical supervision, such as infant formulas. Consumption of increased levels of L-tryptophan when "balanced" with other amino acids in foods or as a fortificant has not been associated with EMS.

Dietary carbohydrates produce major, insulin-mediated decreases in the availability of LNAA, with lesser reductions in plasma tryptophan, which in effect raises the plasma tryptophan:LNAA ratio, facilitating tryptophan's entry into the brain. In contrast, intake of dietary protein has been shown to lower this ratio as they contribute less tryptophan to the circulation than do other LNAAs. Strüder and Weicker (2001) reviewed more than 20 human studies and concluded that nutritional manipulation of serotonin in the brain has variable effects on reducing fatigue and enhancing performance outcomes. This physiologic response has been recently reexamined by Wurtman et al. (2003) evaluating a high-carbohydrate versus a high-protein breakfast meal, as typically eaten by Americans, on the plasma tryptophan:LNAA ratio. It was found that the carbohydrate-rich and protein-rich breakfasts had significantly different effects on the plasma tryptophan:LNAA ratio (54 percent median difference) and tyrosine:LNAA ratio (28 percent median difference). In evaluating carbohydrate-rich and protein-poor diets in stress-prone individuals, Markus et al. (1998, 1999), have demonstrated that a carbohydrate-rich/protein-poor diet compared with a protein-rich/carbohydrate-poor diet increased the ratio of tryptophan:LNAA in the plasma and improved stress coping during high, uncontrollable laboratory stress in the high stress subjects only; thus suggesting a higher requirement for tryptophan and enhanced serotonergic functioning in the high-stress compared with low-stress subjects.

Following on these findings and further manipulating dietary constituents, Markus and colleagues (2000; 2002) designed clinical studies to evaluate mood and cognitive performance in high-stress-vulnerable subjects by using an enriched whey protein supplement high in tryptophan content (6 percent from α-lactalbumin) in a double-blind, placebo crossover study. Tryptophan 12.32 g/kg (in the form of α-lactabumin), when given in a chocolate beverage drink versus a sodium caseinate control beverage containing 9.51 g/kg of tryptophan twice daily, increased the plasma ratio of tryptophan:LNAA, enhanced plasma prolactin levels (a measure of enhanced brain serotonin function), and decreased cortisol levels (a measure of the reactivity of the stress response system) with improvements in cognitive performance in high-stress-vulnerable subjects only, as compared with low-stress subjects. Additional work in this area has been performed by Beulens and colleagues (2004) in healthy male subjects randomized to either an α-lactalbumin supplement plus carbohydrate or carbohydrate supplement only consumed after a breakfast consisting of 19 percent protein. Measurements were obtained at baseline, 30 minutes, and 90 minutes postingestion. The team demonstrated moderately increased levels (16 percent) of the plasma tryptophan:LNAA ratio with the α-lactalbumin supplement with no effect on appetite, food intake, macronutrient preference, or mood as compared with the carbohydrate-only supplemented group.

What is yet to be determined from these studies is the threshold level of tryptophan necessary in a protein-rich/carbohydrate-poor diet that will elicit the maximum response on the plasma tryptophan:LNAA ratio and subsequent levels of serotonin in the brain needed to effect changes in cognitive performance. A study by Teff and colleagues (1989) suggests that only an increase in tryptophan:LNAA ratio of 50 percent or more causes meaningful increases in brain serotonin; however, animal studies have shown effects at lower levels. What can be ascertained at present from this work is the relative safety of use from naturally occurring, enriched levels of tryptophan in food-based products. Improvements in cognitive function were evident together with immediate and short-term effects on plasma ratios of amino acids. Table B-18 summarizes the details of these studies.

METABOLIC COFACTORS

Carnitine

Carnitine is a conditionally essential nutrient because, under certain conditions, its requirements may exceed the body's capacity to synthesize it. Orally, L-carnitine is used for treating primary carnitine deficiency, secondary carnitine deficiency due to inborn errors of metabolism, and carnitine deficiency in people requiring hemodialysis. Aside from primary or secondary deficiency states, typical intake of carnitine from foods provides 50 to 100 mg/day in the United States. No evidence suggests a greater amount is needed to support normal metabolic functions. The role of carnitine is to chaperone the transport of medium- to long-chain fatty acids across mitochondrial membranes to facilitate their oxidation with subsequent energy production. By formation of acylcarnitines from acyl-CoA metabolic intermediates, carnitine may optimize the intracellular milieu for complete oxidation of glucose and fatty acids. Carnitine also has an important metabolic role in the exercising muscle. The hypothesis is that supplementation might enhance the oxidation of fatty acids during exercise, sparing the use of muscle glycogen, thereby delaying the onset of fatigue and culminating in enhanced physical performance. The data in this area are mixed and are not robust. For a number of reasons, carnitine supplementation would not be expected to enhance physical performance: whole-body carnitine homeostasis is highly regulated and compartmentalized; it exists in a large endogenous pool refractive to rapid change; exhibits low bioavailability (16 to 18 percent), with a rapid renal excretion; and it is regulated by a number of saturable transport

TABLE B-18 Results of Human Studies Utilizing Whole Foods on Tryptophan:LNAA Ratio

Reference	Subjects	Study Design	Preparation
Beulens et al., 2004	N = 18 healthy males, mean age 22 ± 4 y	DBRPC-CO	CHO only (10 g CHO, 0 protein) versus α-lactalbumin plus CHO (CHO 20 g, protein 12 g as α-lactalbumin enriched whey protein)
Markus et al., 1998	N = 48 healthy men and women; mean age 21.2 ± 0.4 years 24 high stress prone; 24 low stress prone	Open	CR/PP (62% CHO, 3.6% protein) versus PR/CP (26.3% CHO, 40.4% protein)
Markus et al., 1999	N= 43 healthy men and women; mean age 22.5 years 22 high stress prone and 21 low stress prone	Open	Same as above
Markus et al., 2000	N = 58 healthy mean and women; mean age 20.5 years. 29 high stress prone and 21 low stress prone	DBPC	α-lactalbumin enriched whey protein (12.32 g/kg tryptophan; ratio tryptophan:LNAA 8.7) versus Sodium caseinate control (9.51 g/kg tryptophan; ratio tryptophan:LNAA 4.7)

Dosing Schedule	Test Exposure	Effects
Drink supplement— one hour after breakfast containing CHO 50%, protein 15% and fat 35%.	2 test sessions, each separated by 2 weeks. Assessment of plasma amino acids, serum prolactin, insulin concentrations and mood (POMS) at baseline, 60 and 90 minutes.	Mean tryptophan: LNAA ratio increased (16%) from 0.084 ± 0.003 on α-lactalbumin diet to 0.097 ± 0.003 and decreased 17% from 0.087 ± 0.003 to 0.073 ± 0.002 after CHO only diet. Decrease in serum prolactin slightly smaller after α-lactalbumin than CHO alone. No significant differences in appetite, food intake, macronutrient preference, insulin levels or mood between diets. After α-lactalbumin, changes in tryptophan:LNAA ratio correlated significantly with changes in anger score ($r=-0.65$), and tension score ($r=0.59$).
Consumed as breakfast, snack and lunch; diet test periods were 4 weeks apart.	Mental arithmetic and memory scanning test during uncontrollable stress (POMS).	Mean tryptophan:LNAA ratio increased from 0.074 ± 0.01 on PR/CP to 0.105 ± 0.015 on CR/PP (42% increase). High stress subjects on CR/PP did not show stress-induced rise in depression (POMS). Mean reaction time was not significantly different between high stress and low stress subjects and increased for both groups on CR/PP diet.
Same as above	Mental arithmetic and memory scanning test and mood assessment (POMS) during controllable and uncontrollable stress.	Memory scanning after controllable stress improved in high stress subjects on CR/PP diet. Mean reaction time for high stress on PR/CP increased significantly after controllable stress from 700 to 900 minutes.
Active ingredients given in matching chocolate drink given before breakfast and before lunch. Diets were isoenergetic with equal amounts of CHO, fats, and protein.	Stress-inducing timed mental arithmetic task with industrial noise stress, and POMS. Salivary and plasma cortisol levels. Skin conductance. Heart rate.	Mean tryptophan:LNAA ratio increased from 0.071 ± 0.012 on casein diet to 0.104 ± 0.013 on α-lactalbumin diet (48%). High stress subjects had higher (40%) prolactin concentrations, decreased salivary and plasma cortisol levels and reduced depressive (POMS) feelings under stress on α-lactalbumin. Rise in the cortisol stress response was prevented in high stress but not in low stress on α-lactalbumin diet.

continued

TABLE B-18 Continued

Reference	Subjects	Study Design	Preparation
Markus et al., 2002	N = 52 healthy men and women 23 high stress prone and 29 low stress prone	DBPC	Same as above
Wurtman et al., 2003	N = 9 healthy, normal weight men women, mean age 24.2 ± 1.3 years	RC	CR (69.9 g CHO, 5.2 g protein) versus PR (15.4 g CHO, 46.8 g protein)

NOTE: CHO = carbohydrate; CP = carbohydrate poor; CR = carbohydrate rich; CR/PP = carbohydrate rich/ protein poor; DBPC = double-bind placebo controlled; DBRPC-CO = double-blind randomized placebo controlled crossover; LNAA = large neutral amino acids; POMS = Profile of Mood States; PP = protein poor; PR = protein rich; PR/CP = protein rich/carbohydrate poor; RC = randomized control.

mechanisms. Studies suggest that muscle function is sensitive to carnitine supplementation when muscle carnitine content is < 25 to 50 percent of normal but insensitive to changes in muscle carnitine content around normal levels (Brass, 2004). Exercise studies in healthy subjects have failed to consistently define an effect of supplementation on more than one metabolic parameter of interest. Many of the studies suffer from small sample sizes, lack of appropriate control groups, and short duration. In general, L-carnitine appears to be well tolerated, and no serious toxicity has been demonstrated when given in oral doses up to several grams (Goa and Brogden, 1987). The D-isomer is not biologically active and D-isomer formulations can compete with the L-isomer. At this time, it appears that L-carnitine does not have a significant role in enhancing physical performance in the short term, but additional research is needed to ascertain the benefits of L-carnitine in certain states that alter the requirements for L-carnitine, such as physical or psychological stress. These studies would benefit from well-designed, adequately powered clinical trials with robust clinical performance endpoints.

Also of interest is L-carnitine's emerging role in immunomodulation, as

Dosing Schedule	Test Exposure	Effects
Same as above	Computerized stress-inducing timed mental task	Mean tryptophan: LNAA ratio increased from 0.073± 0.012 on casein diet to 0.104 ± 0.013 on α-lactalbumin diet (43%). Mean reaction time for high stress on α-lactalbumin was significantly lower (758 ± 137 ms) compared to casein control (800 ± 173 minutes).
2 breakfasts, 3–7 days apart	Timed collection of plasma for assessment of tryptophan:LNAA ratio at baseline, 40, 80, 120, and 240 min	Tryptophan:LNAA and tyrosine/LNAA ratios on CR diet at 40, 80, 120, 240 were not different from baseline. Tryptophan:LNAA and tyrosine/LNAA ratios on PR diet at 40, 80, 120, 240 minutes were statistically significant from baseline. Median difference for tryptophan:LNAA was 54% (range 36–88%) and for tyrosine:LNAA was 28 % (range 10–64%).

demonstrated in both animal and human studies. In rodent studies, carnitine (50 to 100 mg/kg body weight) was shown to reduce lipopolysaccharide (LPS)-induced cytokine production with improved survival during cachexia and septic shock (Ruggiero et al., 1993; Winter et al., 1995). Carnitine was also shown to reduce the ex vivo release of tumor necrosis factor alpha (TNF-α) by *S. aureus*-stimulated human polymorphonuclear white blood cells (Fattorossi et al., 1993). Carnitine administration in patients undergoing surgery (8 g intravenously) or in patients with HIV+ (6 g/day for two weeks) can significantly decrease serum TNF-α levels (De Simone et al., 1993; Delogu et al., 1993). Recently, Alesci and colleagues (2004) have suggested that the immunomodulatory properties of L-carnitine may be mediated by its interaction with the glucocorticoid receptor. Similar to dexamethasone, which is a synthetic glucocorticoid, carnitine at milli-molar concentrations triggered nuclear translocation of human glucocorticoid-receptor alpha (GRα), stimulated GRα-mediated transactivation of known glucocorticoid-responsive promoters, suppressed in a GRα-dependent fashion; and stimulated release of proinflammatory cytokines from human monocytes. These proposed modulatory actions of L-carnitine on the glucocorticoid receptor may be of interest to the military as related to the stressful training undertaken by soldiers in the Army Ranger program. As noted previously by Kramer et al. (1997) and Martinez-Lopez et al. (1993), infection rates in Rangers were notably elevated in association with derangements in indices of immune function. High levels of glucocorticoids during chronic stress suppress most aspects of the immune response (Dhabhar and McEwen, 1997) and the ability to fight infection and mount an antibody response (Dhabhar, 2002). The net effect is a suppression of proinflammatory cytokines by glucocorticoids, with an increase in anti-inflammatory cytokines leading to overall immunosuppression (IOM, 2004). New mechanistic data on L-carnitine may warrant research studies in situations of high stress and compromised nutritional status.

Coenzyme Q_{10}

Coenzyme Q_{10} (CoQ_{10}) is a member of the family of compounds known as ubiquinones. All animals, including humans, can synthesize ubiquinones, and no CoQ_{10} deficiency syndromes have been reported in humans; therefore, a varied diet provides sufficient CoQ_{10} for healthy individuals. Oral supplementation with CoQ_{10} increases the plasma and lipoprotein concentrations of CoQ_{10} in humans (Crane, 2001; Mohr et al., 1992). What is not clear is whether supplementation increases CoQ_{10} concentrations in other tissues of individuals with normal endogenous CoQ_{10} synthesis. Several placebo-controlled clinical trials in either trained or untrained men have demonstrated a lack of effect of CoQ_{10} on parameters of physical performance. These parameters include VO_2max and exercise time to exhaustion (Braun et al., 1991; Malm et al., 1997; Porter et al., 1995; Weston et al., 1997), blood lactate levels, and rate of perceived exertion (Porter et al., 1995) in response to cycle ergometer testing. Doses ranging from 100 to 150 mg of CoQ_{10}, with intervention periods lasting from three to eight weeks in duration, have been reported. Two studies in trained men found significantly greater improvements in measures of anaerobic (Malm et al., 1997) and aerobic exercise performance (Laaksonen et al., 1995) with a placebo as compared with CoQ_{10}. While supplementation with CoQ_{10} appears safe in doses as high as 1,200 mg/day up to 16 months (Shults et al., 2002) its role for enhancing performance cannot be supported with existing data.

PERFORMANCE-ENHANCING BOTANICALS

Panax ginseng

Among the botanicals considered as adaptogens, agents taken as a general tonic to increase resistance to environmental stress, *Panax ginseng* (Asian ginseng) is the most studied in terms of enhancing performance. Its ergogenic effects have been characterized in terms of physical performance (exercise outcomes, physiological changes, metabolic measures, and assessment of hormone levels) as well as in terms of cognitive performance (psychomotor measures, reaction time, mood, cognition, memory, and accuracy of repetitive tests) [see review by Bucci et al. (2004)]. Conclusions drawn from a recent systematic review of the literature note that the evidence is contradictory for benefits to physical performance but may be suggestive of benefit for psychomotor performance and cognitive behavior (Vogler et al., 1999). The majority of the studies found at least one significant change in mental functions with Asian ginseng, but responses were not uniform across studies. While the use of ginseng is associated with a feeling of general well-being, in addition, reaction times to auditory or visual cues improved and fatigue and errors in cognitive tasks reduced. Short-term use (four weeks or less) of ginseng does not result in benefits to mental or physical performance, but long-term use (over 12 weeks) in situations of compromised performance suggests some benefit in mood, reaction times, neuromuscular control, mental functions, and work capacity (Bucci et al., 2004). As with other clinical studies evaluating dietary supplements, ginseng studies also suffer from small sample sizes, short duration of use, and poorly characterized products. Also, it appears that ginseng with its delayed onset of action would not be an appropriate supplement for military use in acute situations.

Ginkgo biloba

Ginkgo biloba extract is one of the most prescribed phytomedicines in Germany and France. Physicians prescribe it for dementia, vertigo, anxiety, headaches, tinnitus, peripheral vascular occlusive disease, and other problems. There are also indications that it is an effective antioxidant with free-radical scavenging activity (Christen, 2004). In recent years, ginkgo has been a top selling dietary supplement in the United States. Ginkgo preparations are derived from the dried, green leaf of *Ginkgo biloba*. L. *Ginkgo biloba* extracts (GBEs), contain several constituents including flavonoids, terpenoids, and organic acids. GBE is standardized to contain 24 percent flavonoids and 6 percent terpenes. Although many of ginkgo's individual constituents have intrinsic pharmacological effects, there is some evidence that the constituents work synergistically to produce more potent pharmacological effects than any individual constituent.

Evidence suggests that chronic administration of standardized extracts of *Ginkgo biloba* can ameliorate cognitive decline associated with aging (Ernst and Pittler, 1999; Oken et al., 1998). However, relatively few studies of ginkgo's effect on cognitive measures in healthy adults are available. A systematic review (Canter and Ernst, 2002) identified nine placebo-controlled, double-blind studies utilizing standardized extracts of *Ginkgo biloba*, the longest trial lasting 30 days. The authors concluded that there were no consistent positive effects of ginkgo on objective measures of cognitive function in healthy populations. Two studies published since the 2002 review provide additional data suggesting beneficial effects for ginkgo on measures of cognitive function. Kennedy and colleagues (2002), building on a series of previous investigations (Kennedy et al., 2000, 2001), evaluated the acute cognitive effects of herbal extracts. They conducted a randomized placebo-controlled double-blind crossover study to compare the effects of single doses of GBE, ginseng, and a combination product on aspects of mood (Bond-Lader visual analogue scale) and cognitive performance (Cognitive Drug Research computerized assessment battery, CDR) and several subtraction mental arithmetic tasks (Kennedy et al., 2002). Fifteen female and five male healthy young subjects (mean age 21.2) received 360 mg of GBE (GK501), 400 mg of ginseng (G115), 960 mg of a product combining the two extracts (Ginkoba M/E), and a matching placebo on four separate occasions. Each test session was separated by a seven-day washout period. Measurements were obtained at baseline 1, 2.5, 4, and 6 h after dosing. All three treatments were associated with improved secondary memory performance defined as accuracy of immediate and delayed word recall, picture, and word recognition tasks on the CDR battery. Ginseng showed some improvement in the speed of performing memory tasks (speed of performance of spatial and numeric working memory and picture and word recognition tasks) at four hours postdose. Additionally, ginseng showed improvements in the accuracy of attentional tasks (accuracy of performing choice reaction time and digit vigilance tasks) at 2.5 h postdose. GBE and the GBE/ginseng combination improved performance on both the serial threes and serial sevens subtraction tests at six hours postdose. In another study conducted in 60 healthy adults aged 50 to 65 years, Cieza and colleagues (2003) demonstrated positive effects of 240 mg of GBE (EGb761) three times daily over a four-week period. Primary outcome measures included the subject's judgment of their own mental health, their general health and their quality of life determined on the basis of three difference visual analog scales. Secondary outcomes (15 tests and procedures) were chosen to represent neurobiologically based functions. Results of finger tapping test-maximal tempo indicated favorable effects of GBE on mental function action and reaction times.

Perhaps of greater interest in the military theater, GBE has also been studied for the prevention and mitigation of acute mountain sickness or high-altitude illness. The Lake Louise Consensus Group defined acute mountain sickness (AMS) as the presence of headache in an unacclimatized person who has recently arrived at an altitude above 2,500 meters plus the presence of other symptoms such as: gastrointestinal symptoms (anorexia, nausea, or vomiting), insomnia, dizziness, and lassitude or fatigue (Roach et al., 1993). If left untreated the condition may progress to life threatening pulmonary or cerebral edema. Whether or not AMS occurs is determined by the rate of ascent, the altitude reached, the altitude at which an affected person sleeps, and individual physiology. Physical fitness does not appear to be protective against AMS (Hackett and Roach, 2001). Safe and effective drugs, such as acetazolamide, are available to treat AMS.

Four randomized double-blind placebo-controlled studies (Chow et al., 2002;

Gertsch et al., 2002, 2004; Roncin et al., 1996) and one nonrandomized but double-blind placebo-controlled study (Leadbetter et al., 2001) totaling 781 participants have been reported utilizing GBE for AMS with mixed results. The dosage of GBE ranged from 160 to 240 mg (brands not always identified) daily with pretreatment ranging from one to thirty days prior to ascent. In the studies by Chow et al. (2002) and Gertsch et al. (2004) the comparator drug was acetazolamide, given as 250 mg twice daily, which demonstrated superiority in prevention of acute symptoms as coded using the Lake Louise Scoring system and showed that ginkgo offered no additional benefit in reduction of symptoms compared to placebo. While the study by Gertsch et al. (2004) enrolled 614 healthy western trekkers, mean age 36.6 years old, and predominately male, a number of shortcomings of the study were identified. These included short duration of dosing prior to ascent (3 to 4 doses), administration of the intervention to participants at a high baseline altitude (as opposed to starting the intervention at sea level before ascent), coupled with a 20 percent drop-out rate (although analysis was by intention-to-treat). In the study by Chow et al. (2002), both men and women were enrolled (age range 25 to 65, mean 36.5 years) and were dosed five days prior to ascent, and were driven from a level of 4,000 feet to a final altitude of 12,470 feet over a two-hour period. An earlier study by Gertsch and colleagues (2002) demonstrated that pretreatment of 180 mg of GBE (GK501) one day prior to ascent from sea level to 4,205 meters over three hours by air showed that ginkgo lowered the incidence of AMS but not significantly as compared to placebo. The two studies with positive outcomes for GBE (Leadbetter et al., 2001; Roncin et al., 1996) provided either 160 or 240 mg of GBE daily with pretreatment ranging from 5 to 30 days prior to ascent. The study by Roncin and colleagues (1996) tested EGb761 for the prevention of AMS and also studied vasomotor changes (cold gradient) of the extremities using plethysmorgraphy during a 30-day Himalayan expedition. These investigators found that none of the subjects randomized to EGb761 developed acute mountain sickness versus 40.9 percent of subjects in the placebo group as determined by responses to an Environmental Symptoms Questionnaire (ESQ)–cerebral factor (Sampson et al., 1983). A small percentage (13.6 percent) of subjects on EGb761 compared with subjects on placebo (81.8 percent) developed AMS as determined by the ESQ–respiratory factor. Evaluation of a "cold gradient" was measured by plethysmography and a specific questionnaire. Subjects randomized to EGb 761 showed a mean improvement of the cold gradient of 22.8 percent compared to the placebo group that deteriorated by 104 percent across 20 days of study. There was a marked increase in hand blood flow in the subjects on ginkgo compared to placebo. Also of possible importance to field maneuvers, diuresis of the EGb 761 group was decreased to a much lesser extent than in the placebo group suggesting a tendency for poorly adapted subjects to accumulate excess fluid, which could predispose them to an increased risk of developing altitude edema. The mechanism of action for the effects of GBE cannot be attributed to a single action or to a single molecule in the extract. Research suggests that ginkgo could act in several different ways to prevent AMS. It may block the enzyme inducible nitric oxide synthase, which produces nitric oxide, act as an antioxidant oxygen radical scavenger, or may block platelet-activating factors (Christen, 2004).

In the studies reviewed above, ginkgo was well tolerated and without side effects and is likely safe when used orally and appropriately. Ginkgo may be contraindicated in individuals with epilepsy or in individuals who are prone to seizures, individuals with diabetes or those taking prescription anticoagulants.

New data on GBE for the prevention of AMS from controlled trials coupled with data from basic and mechanistic studies provides justification for additional investigation of this product. Lastly, if GBE were to be incorporated into food-based products and depending on the intended use of the product, potential regulatory issues (unlike vitamin and mineral nutrients) would need to be addressed prior to distribution.

OTHER ADAPTOGENIC HERBS

Preliminary data exist for a number of other adaptogenic herbs to include *Cordyceps sinensis*, *Eleutherococcus senticosus*, and *Rhodiola*. *Cordyceps sinensis* gained the interest of Americans in 1994 following the unprecedented record-breaking running performances by Chinese athletes (Steinkraus and Whitfield, 1994). In China, *Cordyceps sinensis* is an herbal pharmaceutical under investigation for treatment of immune deficiencies, cardiovascular diseases, diabetes, cancer, and inflammatory diseases (Zhu et al., 1998a, b). Five small, controlled, human studies measuring parameters of physical performance (such as VO_2max, ventilatory threshold, respiratory exchange ratio, anaerobic threshold, and exercise time) using the same *Cordyceps sinensis* product (3 g/day) for 4 to 12 weeks suggest that *Cordyceps sinensis* may be associated with some improvements in untrained persons, but these improvements could not be routinely expected for trained persons (Bucci et al., 2004).

Rhodiola species, also known as goldenroot, roseroot, and Arctic ginseng, have been well studied and characterized by Russian and Scandinavian researchers. The Soviet Ministry of Health has approved a *Rhodiola* extract liquid (in 40 percent ethanol) for use as a stimulant to relieve fatigue, improve memory, improve attention span and work productivity in healthy persons (Brown et al., 2002; Germano et al., 1999; Kelly, 2001). Sweden and Denmark also have approved *Rhodiola* extracts (SHR-5) as antifatigue stimulants and adaptogens (Brown et al., 2002; Shevtsov et al., 2003). In one randomized double-blind placebo controlled trial in 121 military cadets on night duty, 185 mg of *Rhodiola rosea* SHR-5 extract acutely improved an antifatigue index for mental work while fatigued, and it decreased errors on ring attention and numbers tests (Shevtsov et al., 2003). In summary, standardized extracts used in clinical trials show potential for improving some aspects of mental (electroencephalogram, memory, reduction of errors performing tasks, shooting accuracy, and hearing) and physical (increased work, increased run time to exhaustion, heart rate record post-exercise, and less fatigue) performance in athletes and sedentary subjects (Bucci et al., 2004). A combination formula containing 1,000 mg of *Cordyceps sinensis* and 300 mg of *Rhodiola* was recently tested with a two week treatment in 17 competitive amateur cyclists in a randomized, placebo-controlled, double-blind study design. The formula failed to elicit positive changes for peak exercise variables (VO_2max, time to exhaustion, peak workload, or peak heart rate) as well as for subpeak exercise variables (power output ventilatory threshold, respiratory compensation or VO_2) (Earnest et al., 2004). The authors note that a longer period of supplementation may have provided a more efficacious response, but this awaits further study.

SUMMARY

This chapter has focused on a number of bioactive food and dietary supplement components that have been evaluated for their performance enhancing qualities. The data presented suggest that if amino acid precursors are to be further tested, their incorporation into a food matrix is preferable over that of a dietary supplement. While research on L-carnitine for enhancing physical performance has not been promising, the role for L-carnitine and its interactions with the glucocorticoid receptor, and particularly for its potential effects on immunomodulation, warrant further exploration. The use of botanicals most likely would not provide short-term or immediate enhancement to performance, except possibly for standardized extracts of *Rhodiola* and *Ginkgo biloba*, which warrant more rigorous study.

In the design of future studies, important considerations are the increased precursor, coenzyme, and energy demands during stress that would be met differently by the human population, possibly distributed in the form of a bell-shaped curve, with individuals ranging from coping poorly to coping extremely well. Individuals to benefit the most from necessary supplements would most likely be in the "coping poorly" category, as was shown in the studies by Markus et al. (1998, 1999, 2000). Of course, persons with discrete defects in stress coping, constituting a separate group of individuals with their own transposed bell-shaped curve, could also benefit from needed supplements if their defects could be corrected in the presence of excess bioactive food components. The possibility that only a subgroup of the population would benefit from bioactive food components, and only when they are challenged by stress, makes the design of clinical studies of these agents difficult, because it presupposes controlling two continuous variables—degree of coping capacity and amount of stress impose—both of which depend on myriad factors. The former is a product of genetics, developmental history, and environment, while the latter depends on the diverse types of stressors applied with different strengths for different times.

REFERENCES

Alesci S, De Martino MU, Kino T, Ilias I. 2004. L-Carnitine is a modulator of the glucocorticoid receptor alpha. *Ann N Y Acad Sci* 1024:147–152.

Beulens JW, Bindels JG, de Graaf C, Alles MS, Wouters-Wesseling W. 2004. Alpha-lactalbumin combined with a regular diet increases plasma Trp-LNAA ratio. *Physiol Behav* 81(4):585–593.

Brass EP. 2004. Carnitine and sports medicine: Use or abuse? *Ann N Y Acad Sci* 1033:67–78.

Braun B, Clarkson PM, Freedson PS, Kohl RL. 1991. Effects of coenzyme Q_{10} supplementation on exercise performance, VO_2max, and lipid peroxidation in trained cyclists. *Int J Sport Nutr* 1(4):353–365.

Brown RP, Gerbarg PL, Ramazanov Z. 2002. *Rhodiola rosea*: A phytomedicinal overview. [Online] HerbalGram. American Botanical Council. 56:40–52. Available at: http://www.herbalgram.org/herbalgram/articleview.asp?a=2333 [accessed April 1, 2005].

Bucci LR, Turpin AA, Beer C, Feliciano J. 2004. Ginseng. In: Wolinsky I, Driskell JA, eds. *Nutritional Ergogenic Aids*. Boca Raton, FL: CRC Press. Pp. 379–410.

Canter PH, Ernst E. 2002. *Ginkgo biloba*: A smart drug? A systematic review of controlled trials of the cognitive effects of ginkgo biloba extracts in healthy people. *Psychopharmacol Bull* 36(3):108–123.

Chinevere TD, Sawyer RD, Creer AR, Conlee RK, Parcell AC. 2002. Effects of L-tyrosine and carbohydrate ingestion on endurance exercise performance. *J Appl Physiol* 93(5):1590–1597.

Chow TK, Browne VA, Heileson HL, Wallace DR, Anholm JD. 2002. Comparison of *Ginkgo biloba* versus acetazolamide in the prevention of acute mountain sickness. *Med Sci Sports Exerc* 34(Suppl 1):S246.

Christen Y. 2004. *Ginkgo biloba*: From traditional medicine to molecular biology. In: Packer L, Ong CN, Halliwell B, eds. *Herbal and Traditional Medicine. Molecular Aspects of Health*. New York: Marcel Dekker. Pp. 145–164.

Cieza A, Maier P, Poppel E. 2003. Effects of *Ginkgo biloba* on mental functioning in healthy volunteers. *Arch Med Res* 34(5):373–381.

Crane FL. 2001. Biochemical functions of coenzyme Q10. *J Am Coll Nutr* 20(6):591–598.

De Simone C, Tzantzoglou S, Famularo G, Moretti S, Paoletti F, Vullo V, Delia S. 1993. High dose L-carnitine improves immunologic and metabolic parameters in AIDS patients. *Immunopharmacol Immunotoxicol* 15(1):1–12.

Deijen JB, Wientjes CJ, Vullinghs HF, Cloin PA, Langefeld JJ. 1999. Tyrosine improves cognitive performance and reduces blood pressure in cadets after one week of a combat training course. *Brain Res Bull* 48(2):203–209.

Delogu G, De Simone C, Famularo G, Fegiz A, Paoletti F, Jirillo E. 1993. Anaesthetics modulate turnover necrosis factor alpha: Effects of L-carnitine supplementation in surgical patients. Preliminary results. *Med Inflamm* 2:S33–S36.

Dhabhar FS. 2002. Stress-induced augmentation of immune function—The role of stress hormones, leukocyte trafficking, and cytokines. *Brain Behav Immun* 16(6):785–798.

Dhabhar FS, McEwen BS. 1997. Acute stress enhances while chronic stress supresses cell-mediated immunity in vivo: A potential role for leukocyte trafficking. *Brain Behav Immun* 11(4):286–306.

Earnest CP, Morss GM, Wyatt F, Jordan AN, Colson S, Church TS, Fitzgerald Y, Autrey L, Jurca R, Lucia A. 2004. Effects of a commercial herbal-based formula on exercise performance in cyclists. *Med Sci Sports Exerc* 36(3):504–509.

Ernst E, Pittler MH. 1999. *Ginkgo biloba* for dementia: A systematic review of double-blind placebo controlled trials. *Clin Drug Invest* 17(4):301–308.

Fattorossi A, Biselli R, Casciaro A, Tzantzoglou S, De Simone C. 1993. Regulation of normal human polymorphonuclear leucocytes by arnitine. *Med Inflamm* 2:S37–S41.

Germano C, Ramazanov Z, Del Mar Bernal Suarez M. 1999. *Rhodiola rosea* and human performance. In: Appell B, ed. *Arctic Root (*Rhodiola rosea*) The Powerful New Ginseng Alternative.* New York: Kensington Publishing. P. 112.

Gertsch JH, Basnyat B, Johnson EW, Onopa J, Holck PS. 2004. Randomised, double blind, placebo controlled comparison of *Ginkgo biloba* and acetazolamide for prevention of acute mountain sickness among Himalayan trekkers: The prevention of high altitude illness trial (PHAIT). *Br Med J* 328(7443):797–801.

Gertsch JH, Seto TB, Mor J, Onopa J. 2002. *Ginkgo biloba* for the prevention of severe acute mountain sickness (AMS) starting one day before rapid ascent. *High Alt Med Biol* 3(1):29–37.

Goa KL, Brogden RN. 1987. l-Carnitine. A preliminary review of its pharmacokinetics, and its therapeutic use in ischaemic cardiac disease and primary and secondary carnitine deficiencies in relationship to its role in fatty acid metabolism. *Drugs* 34(1):1–24.

Hackett PH, Roach RC. 2001. High-altitude illness. *N Eng J Med* 345(2):107–114.

IOM (Institute of Medicine). 1994. *Food Components to Enhance Performance.* Washington, DC: National Academy Press.

IOM. 1999. *The Role of Protein and Amino Acids in Sustaining and Enhancing Performance.* Washington, DC: National Academy Press.

IOM. 2002. *Dietary Reference Intakes: Energy, Carbohydrate, Fiber, Fat, Fatty Acids, Cholesterol, Protein, and Amino Acids.* Washington DC: The National Academies Press.

IOM. 2004. *Monitoring Metabolic Status. Predicting Decrements in Physiological and Cognitive Performance.* Washington, DC: The National Academies Press.

Kelly GS. 2001. *Rhodiola rosea*: A possible plant adaptogen. *Altern Med Rev* 6(3):293–302.

Kennedy DO, Scholey AB, Wesnes KA. 2000. The dose-dependent cognitive effects of acute administration of *Ginkgo biloba* to healthy young volunteers. *Psychopharmacology (Berl)* 151(4):416–423.

Kennedy DO, Scholey AB, Wesnes KA. 2001. Differential, dose dependent changes in cognitive performance following acute administration of a *Ginkgo biloba/Panax ginseng* combination to healthy young volunteers. *Nutr Neurosci* 4(5):399–412.

Kennedy DO, Scholey AB, Wesnes KA. 2002. Modulation of cognition and mood following administration of single doses of *Ginkgo biloba*, ginseng, and a ginkgo/ginseng combination to healthy young adults. *Physiol Behav* 75(5):739–751.

Kramer TR, Moore RJ, Shippee RL, Friedl KE, Martinez-Lopez L, Chan MM, Askew EW. 1997. Effects of food restriction in military training on T-lymphocyte responses. *Int J Sports Med* 18(Suppl 1):S84–S90.

Laaksonen R, Fogelholm M, Himberg JJ, Kaakso J, Salorinne Y. 1995. Ubiquinone supplemetation and exercise capacity in trained young and older men. *Eur J Appl Physiol Occup Physiol* 72(1-2):95–100.

Leadbetter G, Maakestad K, Olson S, Hackett P. 2001. *Ginkgo biloba* reduces the incidence and severity of acute mountain sickness. *High Altitude Med Biol* 2(1):110.

Lieberman HR. 1994. Tyrosine and stress: Human and animal studies. In: Marriott BM, ed. *Food Components to Enhance Performance.* Washington, DC: National Academy Press. Pp. 277–299.

Lieberman HR. 1999. Amino acid and protein requirements: Cognitive performance, stress, and brain function. In: *The Role of Protein and Amino Acids in Sustaining and Enhancing Performance.* Washington, DC: National Academy Press. Pp. 289–307.

Lieberman HR. 2003. Nutrition, brain function and cognitive performance. *Appetite* 40(3):245–254.

Lieberman HR, Spring BJ, Garfield GS. 1986. The behavioral effects of food constituents: Strategies used in studies of amino acids, protein, carbohydrate and caffeine. *Nutr Rev* 44(Suppl):61–70.

Malm C, Svensson M, Ekblom B, Sjodin B. 1997. Effects of ubiquinone-10 supplementation and high intensity training on physical performance in humans. *Acta Physiol Scand* 161(3):379–384.

Markus CR, Olivier B, de Haan EH. 2002. Whey protein rich in alpha-lactalbumin increases the ratio of plasma tryptophan to the sum of the other large neutral amino acids and improves cognitive performance in stress-vulnerable subjects. *Am J Clin Nutr* 75(6):1051–1056.

Markus CR, Olivier B, Panhuysen GE, Van Der Gugten J, Alles MS, Tuiten A, Westenberg HG, Fekkes D, Koppeschaar HF, de Haan EE. 2000. The bovine protein alpha-lactalbumin increases the plasma ratio of tryptophan to the other large neutral amino acids, and in vulnerable subjects raises brain serotonin activity, reduces cortisol concentration, and improves mood under stress. *Am J Clin Nutr* 71(6):1536–1544.

Markus CR, Panhuysen G, Jonkman LM, Bachman M. 1999. Carbohydrate intake improves cognitive performance of stress-prone individuals under controllable laboratory stress. *Br J Nutr* 82(6):457–467.

Markus CR, Panhuysen G, Tuiten A, Koppeschaar H, Fekkes D, Peters ML. 1998. Does carbohydrate-rich, protein-poor food prevent a deterioration of mood and cognitive performance of stress-prone subjects when subjected to a stressful task? *Appetite* 31(1):49–65.

Martinez-Lopez LE, Friedl KE, Moore RJ, Kramer TR. 1993. A longitudinal study of infections and injuries of Ranger students. *Mil Med* 158(7):433–437.

Mohr D, Bowry VW, Stocker R. 1992. Dietary supplementation with coenzyme Q_{10} results in increased levels of ubiquinol-10 within circulating lipoproteins and increased resistance of human low-density lipoprotein to the initiation of lipid peroxidation. *Biochim Biophys Acta* 1126(3):247–254.

Neri DF, Wiegmann D, Stanny RR, Shappell SA, McCardie A, McKay DL. 1995. The effects of tyrosine on cognitive performance during extended wakefulness. *Aviat Space Environ Med* 66(4):313–319.

Oken BS, Storzbach DM, Kaye JA. 1998. The efficacy of *Ginkgo biloba* on cognitive function in Alzheimer disease. *Arch Neurol* 55(11):1409–1415.

Porter DA, Costill DL, Zachwieja JJ, Krzeminski K, Fink WJ, Wagner E, Folkers K. 1995. The effect of oral coenzyme Q_{10} on the exercise tolerance of middle-aged, untrained men. *Int J Sports Med* 16(7):421–427.

Roach RC, Bartsch P, Oelz O, Hackett PH. 1993. Lake Louise AMS Scoring Consensus Committee. The Lake Louise acute mountain sickness scoring system. In: Sutton JR, Houston CS, Coates G, eds. *Hypoxia and Molecular Medicine*. Proceedings of the 8th International Hypoxia Smposium held at Lake, Louise, Canada, February 9–13, 1993. Burlington, VT: Queen City Printers. Pp. 272–274.

Roncin JP, Schwartz F, D'Arbigny P. 1996. EGb 761 in control of acute mountain sickness and vascular reactivity to cold exposure. *Aviat Space Environ Med* 67(5):445–452.

Ruggiero V, D'Urso CM, Albertoni C, Campo S, Foresta P, Arrigoni-Martelli E. 1993. LPS-induces serum TNF production and lethality in mice: Effect of L-carnitine and some acyl-derivatives. *Med Inflamm* 2:S43–S50.

Sampson JB, Cymerman A, Burse RL, Mahr JT, Rock PB. 1983. Procedures for the measurement of acute mountain sickness. *Aviat Space Environ Med* 54(12 Pt 1):1063–1073.

Shevtsov VA, Zholus BI, Shervarly VI, Vol'skij VB, Korovin YP, Khristich MP, Roslyakova NA, Wikman G. 2003. A randomized trial of two different doses of a SHR-5 *Rhodiola rosea* extract versus placebo and control of capacity for mental work. *Phytomedicine* 10(2–3):95–105.

Shults CW, Oakes D, Kieburtz K, Beal MF, Haas R, Plumb S, Juncos JL, Nutt J, Shoulson I, Carter J, Kompoliti K, Perlmutter JS, Reich S, Stern M, Watts RL, Kurlan R, Molho E, Harrison M, Lew M. 2002. Effects of coenzyme Q_{10} in early Parkinson disease: Evidence of slowing of the functional decline. *Arch Neurol* 59(10):1541–1550.

Steinkraus DC, Whitfield JB. 1994. Chinese caterpillar fungus and world record runners. *Am Entomologist* 40:235–239.

Strüder HK, Weicker H. 2001. Physiology and pathophysiology of the serotonergic system and its implications on mental and physical performance. Part II. *Int J Sports Med* 22(7):482–497.

Teff KL, Young SN, Marchand L, Botez MI. 1989. Acute effect of protein or carbohydrate breakfasts on human cerebrospinal fluid monoamine precursor and metabolite levels. *J Neurochem* 52(1):235–241.

Vogler BK, Pittler MH, Ernst E. 1999. The efficacy of ginseng. A systematic review of randomised clinical trials. *Eur J Clin Pharmacol* 55(8):567–575.

Weston SB, Zhou S, Weatherby RP, Robson SJ. 1997. Does exogenous coenzyme Q_{10} affect aerobic capacity in endurance athletes? *Int J Sport Nutr* 7(3):197–206.

Winter BK, Fiskum G, Gallo LL. 1995. Effects of L-carnitine on serum triglyceride and cytokine levels in rat models of cachexia and septic shock. *Br J Cancer* 72(5):1173–1179.

Wurtman RJ, Wurtman JJ, Regan MM, McDermott JM, Tsay RH, Breu JJ. 2003. Effects of normal meals rich in carbohydrates or proteins on plasma tryptophan and tyrosine ratios. *Am J Clin Nutr* 77(1):128–132.

Yeghiayan SK, Luo S, Shukitt-Hale B, Lieberman HR. 2001. Tyrosine improves behavioral and neurochemical deficits caused by cold exposure. *Physiol Behav* 72(3):311–316.

Zhu JS, Halpern GM, Jones K. 1998a. The scientific rediscovery of a precious ancient Chinese herbal regimen: *Cordyceps sinensis*: Part II. *J Altern Complement Med* 4(4):429–457.

Zhu JS, Halpern GM, Jones K. 1998b. The scientific rediscovery of an ancient Chinese herbal medicine: *Cordyceps sinensis*: Part I. *J Altern Complement Med* 4(3):289–303.

Effect of Physical Activity and Other Stressors on Appetite: Overcoming Underconsumption of Military Operational Rations, Revisited

R. James Stubbs and Stephen Whybrow, Rowett Research Institute
Neil King and John E. Blundell, Leeds University
Marinos Elia, Southhampton General Hospital

INTRODUCTION

The ready availability of a huge variety of energy-dense, palatable food is considered partly responsible for the current trends in obesity and attendant diseases in Western society. Although intuitively, it would seem that widescale underconsumption should not be a problem, underconsumption of military operational rations has been a subject of some concern to the United States. In 1995, the Committee on Military Nutrition Research (CMNR) produced a report entitled *Not Eating Enough* (IOM, 1995), a comprehensive report covering the causes and consequences of underconsumption in field operations, the strategies, and need for research to increase intake of military rations in combat (IOM, 1995). The majority of data sourced for this report is related to experimental, comprehensive field studies during military exercises and with garrisoned soldiers. These environments clearly differ from each other and from combat itself. The report acknowledged a lack of data from combat or near-combat situations regarding ration intake, acceptability, appetite and feeding behavior. Understandably, most data are anecdotal; however, the report noted that the nagging hunger of energy restriction differs from the appetite-suppressed state that is characteristic of illness, trauma or emotional disturbances. They observed that "Based on the discomforts associated with the field situation—the anxiety, fatigue, aches and pains, and assorted other problems—decline of appetite is likely to be a prominent factor in explaining underconsumption of military operational rations. Field training or combat anorexia thus may be the result of a generalized stress response" (IOM, 1995).

The purpose of this paper is to consider appetite control in relation to the high energy expenditure and additional stressors in a combat operation. Apparently, during combat operations, the expected daily energy expenditure is 4,000 to 4,500 kcal, achieved through intermittent periods of high energy expenditure (> 50 percent VO_2max) mixed with longer periods of low intensity movement sustained for about 20 h per day. The daily ration must fit within 0.12 cubic feet and weigh 3 pounds or less. The soldiers rely on this ration for three to seven days followed by one to three days of recovery when they will have access to more nutritionally complete meals (i.e., ad libitum food availability served in field kitchen setting). During combat these troops will therefore experience a 1,600 to 2,100 kcal/day energy deficit. This work focuses on these conditions and time window(s). Specifically, the following questions were addressed:

- Is the energy deficit that soldiers experience in combat due to the relationship between high levels of physical activity, appetite, and energy intake during periods of high energy requirements?
- How do the additional stresses of combat impinge on appetite and what do we know of the mechanisms?
- What types of nutritional ingredients or packaging can be added to maintain appetite and hence, presumably, physiological and cognitive performance?

RELATIONSHIP BETWEEN HIGH LEVELS OF PHYSICAL ACTIVITY, APPETITE, AND ENERGY INTAKE

Extremes of Intake and Expenditure

Extremes of energy intake have been recorded during overfeeding studies (Diaz et al., 1992; Norgan and Durnin, 1980; Ravussin et al., 1985), ceremonial overfeeding (Pasquet et al., 1992), prolonged underfeeding studies (Keys et al., 1950), as well as from energy intake records derived from recovering famine, prisoners of war, and concentration camp victims during World War II. These cases represent states of acclimation to extreme environmental conditions, rather than voluntarily energy intake. Compensatory responses subsequent to such induced extremes of energy balance can be spectacular, especially in relation to energy deficits. During rehabilitation from severe malnutrition, famine and concentration camp victims (with body weights below 55 kg) were recorded as spontaneously ingesting 6,900 to 7,900 kcal/day that ceased as body mass and composition were restored.

TABLE B-19 Effect of Extreme Endurance On Energy Balance In Humans

Study	Nature of the Event	Subjects	Energy Intake (MJ/day)	Energy Expenditure (MJ/day)
Eden and Abernethy, 1994	1,005 km running, 9 days	1 male	25.0	NA
Forbes-Ewan et al., 1989	Military jungle training, 7 days	4	16.9	19.9
Gabel et al., 1995	3,280 km cycling, 10 days	2	29.8	NA
Hoyt et al., 1991	Military mountain training, 11 days	23 males	13.1	20.6
Jones et al., 1993	Military arctic training	10	11.0	18.0
Keys et al., 1950	Ad libitum energy intake post weight loss (25% loss of body weight at first week)	12 males	42.6	NA
Sjodin et al., 1994	Cross-country skiing, 7 days	4 males; 4 females	25.7–36.0; 15.7–20.4	25.4–34.9; 15.1–20.2
Stroud (unpublished results)	Sahara multimarathon, 7 days	4	14.6	22.0–32.5
Stroud, 1987	South Pole expedition, 70 days	3 males	21.0	25–29
Stroud et al., 1993	North Pole expedition, 48 days	2	19.2	28.1–32.4
Stroud et al., 1997	Trans-antarctic expedition:			
	Days 0–50;	2 males;	19.9;	29.1–35.5;
	Days 51–95;	2 males;	22.2;	18.8–23.1;
	Maximum: days 21–30	2 males	22.2;	46.6–48.7
Westerterp et al., 1986	Tour de France, 20 days	4	24.7	33.7

NOTE: NA = not available.
SOURCE: Adapted from Stroud (1998).

In healthy subjects, such high levels of energy intake have only been recorded under conditions of extreme physical activity such as the Tour de France (Saris, 1989) or military and polar expeditions (Stroud et al., 1993). In the case of the Tour de France, not all the energy intake is voluntary because the participants receive intravenous nutrition during sleep. These examples illustrate the extremes to which energy intake can adapt to intense physiological demands imposed by very high levels of physical activity (Saris, 1989) or severe malnutrition. The primary stressor in these situations is the physical stress of the event. Under these relatively acute conditions in which every attempt is made to meet energy requirements, subjects are nonetheless typically characterized by a marked negative daily energy balance (Table B-19). This is not surprising because this level of expenditure represents the maximal sustainable level of human endurance. In these situations, it is not easy to eat enough to meet elevated expenditures.

The overconsumption characteristic of Western society (with the exception of binging disorders) is not rampant but episodic. Attempting to persuade individuals to continually overeat, even to 150 percent of their maintenance requirements, is actually quite difficult when imposed as an acute change. This has implications for underconsumption in both endurance and military contexts.

Human populations have been known to subsist for quite prolonged periods on extreme ranges of diet composition despite our general tendency to consume 12 to 20 percent of our energy from protein, 35 to 40 percent from fat, and most of the rest from carbohydrate (Mela, 1995). For example, the Inuit have been reported as subsisting for months on high-fat, high-protein diets almost entirely comprising of animal matter and virtually devoid of all carbohydrate (Mowat, 1975). This produces markedly ill effects during lean months when the energy to protein ratio of the diet falls too low. Similarly, the traditional Japanese diet has been reported as constituting some 8 percent of energy intake from dietary fat, in extreme cases. It appears clear from these accounts that human populations are capable of adapting (through their physiological plasticity) to meet their physiological requirements from a wide range of macronutrient ratios in the diet. As indicated by Phinney and collegues (1983a, b) in the case of virtually carbohydrate free diets (< 20 g/day), the period of adaptation can take some days, therefore abrupt, extreme changes in the composition of rations should perhaps be avoided.

The Impact of Altered Energy Expenditure on Energy Intake

When studying the relationship between energy expenditure and energy intake, it is useful to consider how high and low levels of energy expenditure influence intake, and vice versa (Stubbs et al., 2003). The main focus of the present discussion is the relationship between appetite and energy expenditure during high levels of energy turnover. The general population is remarkably sedentary as indicated by cross-sectional surveys of levels of activity among adults and children and the fact that average levels of physical fitness are remarkably low in the population at large (Activity and Health Research, 1992). Black et al. (1996) have estimated from tracer studies that the established limits of total daily energy expenditure ranges from 1.2 to 4.5 times the basic metabolic rate (BMR) over periods of two weeks or more. Intense, sustained activity tends to be a little lower for most people at approximately 2.3 to 2.9 times the BMR, which is similar to combat levels of energy expenditure. For the general, "rather sedentary" population the average daily energy expenditures are in the range of 1.4 to 1.8 times the BMR (Black et al., 1996).

Acute increases in physical activity is believed to promote weight loss (Garrow and Summerbell, 1995). However, this is unlikely to happen over a prolonged period (e.g., Sum et al., 1994). Over time, energy intake will begin to track energy expenditure. The exact manner in which changes in levels of physical activity influence feeding behavior over periods long enough to affect energy balance is not clearly understood. There is a large body of literature on the effect of training programs on body weight and composition in athletes (Barr and Costill, 1992; McGowan et al., 1986; van Baak, 1999; van Etten et al., 1997; Westerterp, 1998). Likewise a number of studies have examined the effects of training programs on weight loss in obese subjects (Saris, 1993; Schoeller et al., 1997). Fewer studies have examined the relationship between changes in energy expenditure and feeding behavior in nonobese subjects who do not have a pre-conceived goal associated with weight reduction or a training program. A review of the effects of exercise regimes on appetite and/or energy intake shows that in short-to medium-term intervention studies (often no longer than two to five days), 19 percent reported an increase in energy intake after exercise; 65 percent showed no change, and 16 percent showed a decrease (Blundell and King, 1999; King et al., 1997). Longer-term studies that measure body composition suggest some fat mass is lost, but lean body mass tends to be preserved in response to exercise regimes, depending on the absolute level of energy balance (Ballor and Poehlman, 1994; Sum et al., 1994). These studies suggest that in the short- to medium-term (1 day to 20 days) energy intake does not accurately track changes in energy expenditure. This raises the critical question: What is the time course over which humans begin to compensate for energy imbalances induced by systematic manipulations of energy intake or of energy expenditure? This is a difficult question to answer because the majority of studies do not track energy intake and energy expenditure on a day-by-day basis. The most precise means of objectively measuring energy expenditure in free-living humans is the doubly labeled water method, which tends to give average estimates of daily energy expenditure over periods of 10 to 20 days (Schoeller and van Santen, 1982). Daily energy expenditure can also be estimated using heart rate monitoring (Ceesay et al., 1989; Spurr et al., 1988), but this technique is widely regarded as having relatively low precision and accuracy, especially with sedentary people (Murgatroyd et al., 1993). However, in studies that employ within-subject comparisons and for which most changes in energy expenditure occur through the same exercise activities that were used to individually calibrate the heart rate monitors, this approach is most efficacious. Stubbs and colleagues (2004b) assessed the effect of no exercise (Nex:control) and high-exercise level (Hex; 4 MJ [955 kcal]/day) and two dietary manipulations, (a high-fat diet [HF]; 50 percent of energy, 167 kcal/100 g) and a low- and high-fat diet [LF]; 20 percent of energy, 71 kcal/100g) on compensatory changes in energy intake and energy expenditure over seven-day periods. Eight lean men were each studied four times, in a 2×2 randomized design. Energy intake was directly quantified by weight of food consumed. Energy expenditure was assessed by heart rate monitoring. Body weight was measured daily. Mean daily energy expenditures were 4,200 and 2,750 kcal/day ($p < 0.001$) on the pooled Hex and Nex treatments, respectively. Energy intake was higher on HF diets (3,200 kcal/day) compared to the LF diets (2,150 kcal/day). Regression analysis showed that these energy imbalances induced significant compensatory changes in energy balances over time of 70 to 96 kcal/day (p < 0.05). These were caused by changes in both energy intake and energy expenditure in the opposite direction to the small changes in energy balance (Figure B-24). These changes were significant and small, but persistent, amounting to approximately 48 and 84 kcal/day for energy intake and energy expenditure, respectively. Under these relatively acute conditions it would take two to four weeks for a person to adjust to the altered level of energy turnover (Stubbs et al., 2004b). However, it is likely that compensation could be accelerated using, for example, sports drinks.

There is evidence that it takes considerable time for energy intake to adjust to elevations of energy expenditure in ad libitum feeding subjects. One direct intervention also supports this view (Figure B-25). Sum et al. (1994) studied the effects of five-month basic military training on body weight, body fat, and lean body mass in 42 Singapore males, classified as being normal weight (BMI 25 to 29.9 kg/m^2), obese (BMI 30 to 34.9 kg/m^2), and very obese (BMI > 35 kg/m^2). Two key features of this study are that training was incremental, allowing subjects to gradually become fitter, and food intake was ad libitum. Over the 5 months of training, fat-free mass (FFM) did not change, but subjects lost substantial amounts of weight and body fat. Subjects who were initially fatter lost more weight and fat. This suggests that responses of intake to exercise-induced changes in energy expenditure may depend on how much fat one has. In other words, it is likely that fat mass is acting as an energy buffer, and intake rises markedly when lean-body mass is threatened by the exercise induced energy deficit. The importance of changes in lean-body mass and appetite control has been discussed by Stubbs and Elia (2001). If responses of intake to exercise-induced changes in energy expenditure depend on body fat level and compensation is due to small changes in both intake and expenditure, then crosstalk between energy expenditure and intake is initially too weak; that is, soldiers would not spontaneously adjust intake to energy requirements during short missions of three to seven days. Most likely, soldiers will need to consciously overcome this lack of spontaneous appetite response by eating more than they feel is sufficient. It appears that substantial fat loss is possible before intake begins to track a sustained elevation of energy expenditure. Friedl (1995) has considered the implications of the baseline nutritional status for physical performance during energy deficit in modern soldiers. Because modern soldiers tend to be larger and better nourished than in earlier studies, they appear to withstand the insults of an energy deficit with less decrement in performance. However, under conditions close to combat (the Ranger I study), ". . . soldiers who began training with very low body fat (< 10 percent) were less likely to succeed than were slightly fatter soldiers (Moore et al., 1992)" (Friedl, 1995). These data indicate that soldiers who are slightly fatter withstand the rigors of extreme field training better than those who are very lean; they also point to the importance of ensuring soldiers are fed (or overfed) for the coming mission. The Ranger I and II studies provide further

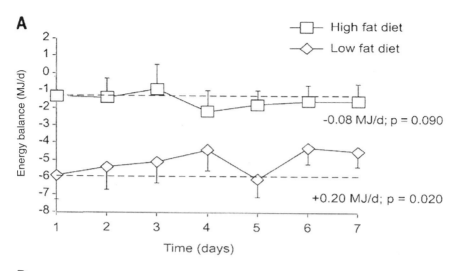

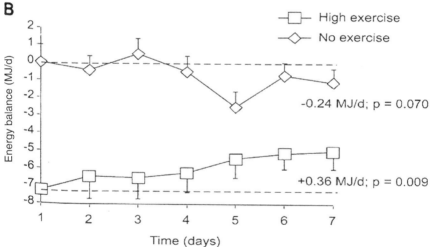

FIGURE B-24 Effect of no-exercise, (Nex) and high exercise level [(Hex); (approximately 4 MJ/day)] and two dietary manipulations [a high-fat diet (HF: 50 percent of energy, 700 kJ/100 g) and low-fat diet (LF: 20 percent of energy, 300 kJ/100 g)] on compensatory changes in energy intake (EI) and energy expenditure (EE) over 7 day periods. Eight lean men were each studied four times, in a 2×2 randomised design. EI was directly quantified by weight of food consumed. EE was assessed by heart rate monitoring. Top panel gives plots over time for the HF and LF diet conditions. The bottom panel plots energy balance across days for the Hex and Nex conditions.
SOURCE: Stubbs et al. (2004b). *Am J Physiol Regul Integr Comp Physiol* used with permission.

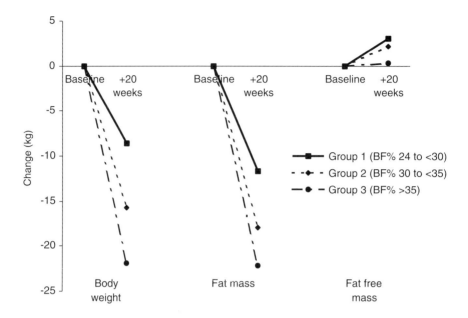

FIGURE B-25 The impact of five-month basic military training on body weight, body fat, and fat-free mass in 42 obese Singapore males.
NOTE: BF = body fat.
SOURCE: Data adapted from Sum et al. (1994).

insights into the time course over which appetite can be suppressed. While energy intake does not accurately track energy expenditure in the short to medium term, over periods of weeks and months, appetite increases again. Friedl (1995) notes that the Ranger students would all have consumed more if food was available and observes that "at least at the extreme level of deprivation of Ranger students (in the studies concerned), there was a strong hunger drive even in the face of multiple stressors" (Friedl, 1995). The same is true of the concentration camp and prisoners of war accounts.

The implications of these data for field training and combat conditions are that (1) when energy expenditure is acutely and significantly elevated, energy intake is slow to respond, and a negative energy balance ensues; (2) the degree of energy deficit will, if continued, compromise physical and cognitive function; (3) use of foods and beverages that are conducive to overconsumption may help limit the extent of the negative energy balance; and (4) if the energy deficit becomes severe over a longer period, appetite will again drive feeding behavior despite multiple stressors (Keys et al., 1950).

THE IMPORTANCE OF THE RECOVERY PERIOD TO INCREASED FOOD INTAKE

During acute, high levels of energy expenditure, both appetite and energy intake characteristically fail to track elevated energy expenditure (Stubbs et al., 2004a). What is remarkable about these situations is the extent of negative energy balance subjects appear able to sustain, at least in the short to medium term. One factor that is likely to account for the slow response of food intake to increased energy demands is the priority the body has given to the control of water balance. Hypohydration decreases appetite and leads to anorexia (Engell, 1995). Soldiers can lose 3 to 5 percent of body weight during deployment because of the effects of dehydration (IOM, 1995) which may reduce appetite and food intake during combat. In addition, individuals who overfeed tend to be relatively sedentary and relaxed at the time, which obviously is not the case in combat. High levels of activity that redistribute blood flow to the muscles and away from the splanchnic circulation reduce the rate of gastric emptying (Leiper et al., 2001; Mudambo et al., 1997). In addition, there is evidence that dehydration further delays gastric emptying and increases gastrointestinal distress if a person is physically active (running) (Rehrer et al., 1990). Training while consuming carbohydrate-rich beverages may lead to some adaptation in terms of increased or maintained rates of gastric emptying during exercise (Carrio et al., 1989; Rehrer et al., 1992). However, to eat more, one needs to increase to flow of blood to the gut to increase gut motility and digestion of the additional food. It is anecdotally universal that people do not exercise on a full stomach. In summary, the demands of exercise are in conflict with the demands of food intake (e.g., a relaxed meal and increased gut motility). This conflict makes it difficult for a soldier to increase the consumption and digestion of food. It is likely that as with athletes, consumption of readily digested (low-bulk and low-protein) foods and already digested (beverages) nutrients may help bypass this problem. In summary, the decreased blood flow to the gut during conditions of continuous moderate to intense activity, will decrease gut motility and increase indigestion when food is consumed. A limited capacity to increase food intake, coupled with the effects of hypohydration on appetite, results in energy intake that does not effectively track energy expenditure. To rapidly restore energy balance, a sedentary period may be most effective, not just to decrease energy expenditure, but also to facilitate higher levels of energy intake such as refeeding between missions. It is no coincidence that during the Guru-Walla overfeeding ritual, the subjects remain entirely sedentary during a period when they consumed some 6,000 to 7,000 kcal/day (Pasquet et al., 1992). The little evidence available relating to abrupt decreases in energy expenditure caused by training cessation or injury suggests that reduced activity leads to acute decreases in energy expenditure, that then leads to reduced activity marked by gain in body weight. Figure B-26 indicates that reduced energy expenditure from inactivity is very weakly linked, through

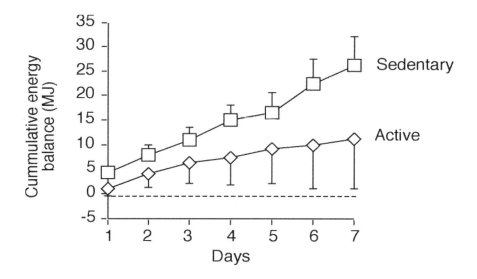

FIGURE B-26 Mean (standard error of means) cumulative energy balance (MJ) for six men who were continually resident in a whole-body indirect calorimeter for 7 days on either a sedentary or active treatment. On the sedentary treatment, daily energy expenditure was held at $1.4 \times BMR$ (the low end of the sedentary range), and on the active treatment daily energy expenditure was held at $1.8 \times BMR$. Subjects were fed ad libitum throughout on a medium-fat diet of constant measurable composition.
NOTE: BMR = basal metabolic rate.
SOURCE: Stubbs et al. (2004a) *Am J Physiol Regul Integr Comp Physiol* used with permission.

physiological signals, to energy intake and has little effect in reducing intake (Stubbs et al., 2004a). A period of rest may promote greater levels of energy intake by providing opportunities and a physiological capacity for overconsumption. Thus, refeeding soldiers during recovery periods should be considered; it may be somewhat harder to supplement them during acute elevations of activity. In addition to these problems for appetite control, the soldiers are subjected to a variable range of stressors that do not generally occur during attend athletic and endurance events. This raises the question: Is all of the negative energy balance observed under combat conditions entirely due to the relationship between increased exercise and appetite?

EFFECTS OF ADDITIONAL COMBAT STRESSORS ON APPETITE

Stresses Associated with Combat

Hypohydration

A major stress of deployment and combat is hypohydration. This is not necessarily related to levels of energy expenditure. Soldiers appear particularly susceptible to hypohydration during deployment, in hot environments, and where they are required to wear protective clothing (IOM, 1995). The CMNR considered that a weight loss of > 3 percent and < 10 percent was principally due to an inadequate fluid intake, which would likely reduce performance (IOM, 1995). Engell (1995) has reviewed the evidence that shows inadequate water intake restricts ad libitum food intake. The converse does not appear to be true. Figure B-27 shows the effects of changes in the composition of the diet on ad libitum daily energy intake in 78 subjects self-recording their own food intake (Stubbs et al., 2000). Large variations in water intake, presumably in well-hydrated people, have little effect on energy intake. Given the likelihood of hypohydration and its effects on energy intake, it is critical that attempts are made to avoid this stress and its knock on effects for appetite and performance.

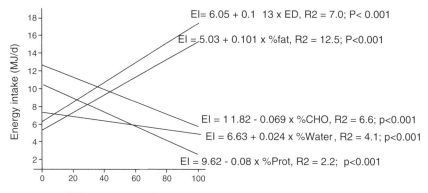

FIGURE B-27 Relationship between energy density (ED) of the diet (expressed as a daily percentage of the maximum daily ED of each subject's diet) and energy intake (EI) in 76 subjects self-recording their food intake by weighed dietary record over 7 consecutive days. Subjects with energy intakes < 1.2 × BMR who did not lose weight during the seven days were previously excluded.
NOTE: BMR = basal metabolic rate.
SOURCE: Stubbs et al. (2000).

Sleep Deprivation

Another stress of combat is sleep deprivation. In rats sleep deprivation appears to cause an increase in locomotor behaviour, and increase in food intake, and increase in the activity of the hypothalamic-pituitary-adrenal axis (increased plasma thyroxine, norepinephrine) and increased heat loss (Rechtschaffen et al., 2002), leading to considerable loss of function and even death. These problems may relate to altered thermoregulation. In rats sleep deprivation causes mal-nutrition (despite the increased energy intake), which is secondary to increased energy expenditure (Everson and Wehr, 1993). Horne (1985) has noted that the extreme problems of thermoregulation, induced by sleep deprivation in rodents, do not appear to apply to humans. Many studies relevant to military situations also include periods of intense activity (e.g., Oektedalen et al., 1982; Opstad and Aakvaag, 1981; Opstad et al., 1984) and it is difficult to separate the effects of a negative energy balance induced by sleep deprivation or by exercise. Akerstedt et al. (1980) exposed twelve healthy males to 48 h of sleep deprivation under conditions where time isolation and activity and feeding were strictly controlled. They found that under these otherwise unstressed conditions adrenocortical and gonadal steroid hormones were lower or unchanged, indicating a lack of emer-gency stress response, due to sleep deprivation. Redwine et al. (2000) have found that mild sleep deprivation affects IL (interleukin)-6 levels, suggesting sleep deprivation may influence the integrity of immune functioning. The cognitive effects of sleep deprivation are documented elsewhere (Foo et al., 1994; Fu and Ma, 2000). It seems that sleep deprivation induces a negative energy balance (due to increased activity that causes the lack of sleep) and obviously, fatigue. In rats at least, these changes are alleviated better with supplements of energy than of protein (Everson and Wehr, 1993). There is no clear evidence that sleep deprivation decreases appetite and energy intake; on the contrary, in rats it appears to increase energy intake. However, in both rats and humans, under the disparate conditions of the studies conducted, intake does not appear to match elevated energy requirements associated with sleep deprivation. It is not clear why this is so, particularly when the limited indications are that supplemental energy intakes may alleviate some of the stress of sleep deprivation.

Anxiety

There is no doubt that the combat environment induces the most extraordi-nary levels of anxiety. The modernization of warfare methods increases stress, anxiety and emotional trauma, which have an acute effect at decreasing appetite. These levels of stress are rarely quantified, but they have been documented in the diaries and records of numerous soldiers throughout humankind's continuing and ongoing conduct of various wars. In several classical accounts, especially those associated with the D-Day landings when there was a period of prebattle anticipation, the inability to eat or even hold food down was not uncommon (see accounts at http://www.bbc.co.uk/dna/ww2/C54665). Some of these disturbances remain after the war is over as combat-stress disorder and posttraumatic stress disorder, as documented by a growing literature (Hyams et al., 1996; Pearn, 2000; Pereira, 2002; Witztum et al., 1996).

Stress-Related Mechanisms of Appetite Suppression

Stress-related mechanisms of appetite suppression are multiple, redundant, and poorly understood in humans. In rats, hypohydration-induced anorexia appears to involve corticotrophin releasing factor and neurotensin in the lateral hypothalamus (Watts, 1999). Brain stem mechanisms are also involved (Flynn et al., 1995). Sleep deprivation will clearly affect the peptide families controlling biorhythms, which may disrupt diurnal patterns of feeding. Anxiety-based responses will be mediated through the hypothalamic-pituitary-adrenal axis and inflammation/physical trauma will be mediated by the immune-inflammatory system (Newsholme and Leach, 1992). Most evidence is derived from animal models except for the growing body of psychological evidence relating to human stress. Because of the wide range of components of these responses, there is no simple stress-associated mechanism that can be alleviated by a simple nutritional or pharmacological manipulation to improve appetite. While the interactions of these different components are unknown, it is reasonable to conclude that together, they will decrease appetite under combat situations. The intuitive solution would be to minimize the perception of satiety. It is important to supplement rations with energy because as a negative energy balance proceeds, performance will deteriorate and appetite will increase, even under stressed conditions [see Keys et al. (1950) for consideration of responses to undernutrition in war].

When and When Not to Bypass Satiety

When considering strategies to bypass the decreased appetite associated with combat, one can gain insights by analogy with clinical conditions. In the clinical setting under conditions of severe stress, such as surgery and shock, the patient experiences a period of catabolism, during which inter alia plasma glucagon, coticosteriods, and catecholamines are elevated. These are all hormones that induce an acute negative nitrogen balance and raise plasma glucose, providing metabolic fuels to deal with the stress at hand (Newsholme and Leach, 1992). Under these conditions, appetite is also characteristically suppressed and there is some debate as to whether supplementation should occur ever be provided through enteral or parenteral nutrition. This is important because a number of the stresses to which soldiers are exposed on the battlefield (beyond the obvious injuries and risks) may well be similar, in extent, to those experienced during shock, trauma, or other illness in the clinical setting. Under these conditions people are intolerant of food in the following three ways: (1) appetite suppression; (2) increased gastric stasis (decreased gastric emptying) caused by intense exercise, acute systemic injury, or postoperative stress; and (3) intolerance to specific nutrients during stress (Newsholme and Leach, 1992).

The following examples illustrate how the use of bioactive substances to improve clinical outcomes can produce unpredictable serious side-effects, including death. The first example involves injections of pharmacological doses of growth hormone (GH) in critically ill patients. It was thought that GH might be beneficial by limiting the marked nitrogen loss that frequently occurs in such patients (equivalent to overcoming a metabolic block in net protein synthesis). Growth hormone is known to stimulate protein synthesis and had previously been shown to improve nitrogen balance in a wide range of clinical conditions. However, in a large multicenter trial involving patients admitted to intensive care units, pharmacological doses of GH doubled (from about 20 percent to 40 percent) mortality as compared with the placebo group. Although the mechanisms responsible for the increased mortality are still uncertain, several suggestions have been made (Takala et al., 1999).

A second example shows how outcomes in the critically ill can be improved through the control of delivered nutrients. The importance of strict glucose homeostasis in critically ill patients was demonstrated by a large study involving about 1,500 patients who were randomized to receive insulin to control their plasma glucose concentrations strictly between 4.4 and 6.1 mmol/L, or to receive standard therapy in which a circulating concentration of 10.0 to 11.1 mmol/L was considered acceptable. In the strictly controlled group there was a four-fold reduction in mortality and a two-fold reduction in the number of transfusions and the incidence of critical care polyneuropathy (van den Berghe et al., 2001). Thus, the use of bioactive ingredients and nutrients to bypass suppressed appetite must be considered with caution under conditions of acute and unpredictable stress. The nature and extent of the stress will be important in determining tolerance to the supplement.

It is known that during military training and combat, the rate, extent, and composition of weight loss influence physical performance and cognitive function (Freidl, 1995). We know from these studies that protein is largely adequate and mineral and vitamin short-term deficits are well tolerated under field conditions (Baker-Fulco, 1995). The main purpose of supplementation is to overcome suppressed appetite and meet, as closely as possible, energy and fluid requirements. The timing of energy supplementation is likely to have a large impact on tolerability and, indirectly, on performance. Most evidence about stress and tolerability of rations is derived from noncombat conditions in which the most acute stressors are largely absent. It is perhaps necessary to ascertain under combat or similar conditions how different stressors will influence appetite and physiological and cognitive function. From a research perspective, the authors suggest it is important to: (1) quantify the likely nature and extent of the stress under combat or similar conditions; (2) test strategies to optimize energy intake before, after, or during combat (with focus on timing and composition of the supplement); and (3) quantify the tolerability and performance response. From the perspectives of both appetite and performance, timing and composition are the two critical features of the ration that determine the benefits of supplementation. Timing is important because it will determine the most efficacious and feasible strategy of supplementation. Composition of foods influences the amount that can be ingested (Stubbs, 1998; Stubbs et al., 1995, 2001).

NUTRITIONAL INGREDIENTS OR PACKAGING TO MAINTAIN APPETITE

Diet Composition and Appetite

A number of reviews have considered the means and mechanisms by which dietary macronutrients, macronutrient substitutes, and associated nutritional parameters, such as dietary energy density influence appetite and energy balance in humans (Stubbs, 1998; Stubbs et al., 2000). As they exist in the diet, macronutrients differ in their metabolisable energy coefficients (Elia and Livesey, 1992). Average values for alcohol, protein, carbohydrate, and fat are 7, 4, 4, and 9 kcal/g. Fat and alcohol are more energy dense (energy per wet weight of food eaten) than protein and carbohydrate (Elia and Livesey, 1992).

Not all of the different macronutrients affect satiety to the same degree. There is a hierarchy in the satiating efficiency of the macronutrients such that, under a variety conditions per unit of energy ingested, protein suppresses appetite to a greater extent than carbohydrate, which has a greater effect than fat (Stubbs, 1995; Figure B-28). Caloric compensation can be defined as a unit decrease in energy intake for each unit of energy given as a particular nutrient. Protein produces supercaloric compensation, carbohydrate caloric compensation and fat ingestion leads to subcaloric compensation (Figure B-27). Thus, high-protein diets are particularly satiating and limit energy intake. Because of this, foods conducive to a high-energy intake tend to be low in protein. When ingested at the same level of energy density, protein is still the most satiating macronutrient (Johnstone et al., 1996; Stubbs et al., 1996). Under these conditions differences between carbohydrate and fat are less clear cut. Carbohydrate tends to exert a more acute effect on satiety than does fat (Johnstone et al., 1996; Stubbs et al., 1996).

Dietary energy density tends to act as a constraint on feeding behavior (Stubbs et al., 2000). A diet that has too low-an energy density will induce an energy deficit determined by the rate at which low-energy-dense foods can be digested and absorbed. There is evidence that food intake will increase in the longer term to offset this deficit. With high energy density diet, overconsumption tends to occur because the amount of food a person eats tends to be conditioned and weak against excess energy intake (Stubbs et al., 2000).

Because of its contribution to energy density, fat is often seen as the nutrient that will induce the greatest energy intake. It is possible to produce maltodextrin supplements that produce equally large elevations of energy intake (Stubbs et al., 1997, 2001). Very active subjects can also benefit from water that is stored with glycogen in a 3:1 ratio. Given that hydration is critical to troops in combat, the ability to carry water locked in glycogen may help alleviate hypohydration-induced anorexia.

Certain types of protein, carbohydrates, and fat may exert different effects on appetite (Stubbs et al., 1999) but this is a relatively new area. Current evidence suggests that sweet, wet, carbohydrate solutions induce lower caloric compensation (i.e., facilitate supplementation) than the same carbohydrates given as solid foods (diMeglio and Mattes, 2000; Stubbs et al., 2001). Women soldiers consume more when given ready access to commercial snack foods (Rose, 1989). This raises an

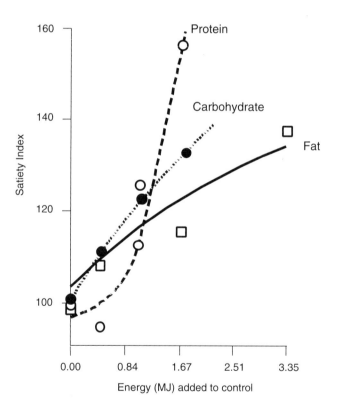

FIGURE B-28 Effect of increasing the energy content of macronutrient loads on Satiety Index subjectively expressed over 3.25 h.
SOURCE: Weststrate (1992).

important research issue of whether energy-dense dry foods (rich in fats and sugars) will elevate energy intake more than lower energy-dense beverages (rich in carbohydrates). In this context the hydration status of the subject is likely to be critical. Another question is raised about the effects of consumption of foods that require minimal digestion and place minimal stress on the gut, like athletes do (see above).

According to our data, large amounts of water intake in well-hydrated subjects will displace little or no energy from the diet (Figure B-27; Stubbs et al., 2001). Energy-containing beverages appear to have a supplemental effect. Stratton et al. (2003) showed that using a continuously infusing naso-gastric drip, it is possible to increment daily energy intake by approximately 1,000 kcal/day in ad libitum, free-living, well-hydrated subjects. These observations support the CMNR suggestions (IOM, 1995) that increased snacking and beverage intake may help elevate energy intake in the field.

Possible Strategies to Elevate Energy Intake and Performance in Combat

Timing

We know that loss of weight, especially as water and/or lean tissue, can be detrimental to performance in combat. Given that even in a 60-day Ranger study (Moore et al., 1992) during which subjects were in an energy deficit, approximately 1,200 kcal/day subjects who had < 10 percent body fat performed less well than slightly fatter subjects, soldiers with even relatively small amounts of extra body fat may have certain performance advantages in combat. This will be more so if the stressors are such that neither opportunity nor motivational appetite facilitate food intake. It would be valuable to compare the effects of overfeeding subjects before combat or during resting periods with the effects of supplemention during combat. One way to optimize nutritional status and hence performance in combat is to focus on supplementation during those recovery periods. A major research question is: When could energy be supplemented to achieve the best results?

Ingredients

During deployment it may be advantageous to supplement troops with carbohydrate-rich beverages to avoid hypohydration. In addition, the extra water stored with glycogen will act as a small internal water reservoir. It is our opinion that the most effective way to supplement a person that has free-living, ad libitum feeding is to trickle readily assimilated energy by using small snacks and beverages; such design also provides greater flexibility than a pack of three Meals, Ready-to-Eat (MREs). The use of flavor enhancers has had remarkable effects on soft drink sales and intakes. It is likely that soft drinks will readily replace the fluid and carbohydrate requirement for performance if the problems of portability can be overcome (see below).

Given the high satiety value of protein and, to a lesser extent, fiber's negative association with energy density, these components of foods are not conducive to high energy intakes. Similarly, very high-fat food items on their own might also be avoided because there is evidence that fat loads can enhance satiety at the level of the gut (Welch et al., 1988), an effect to be avoided in combat. On the other hand, except when in cold environments (Stroud et al., 1993), satiety with low food consumption is desirable to minimize gastrointestinal disturbances. Mixtures of fats and carbohydrates are particularly conducive to overconsumption as indicated by the fact that most commercial snacks are of this composition (Holland et al., 1991).

Portion Size

Previous authors have suggested that maximizing portion size will help elevate energy intake in the field setting (Rolls, 1995). In combat, however, a greater number of smaller portions will facilitate snacking and maintain energy levels. In terms of the pattern of daily intake, it is pertinent to note that meal size actually increases through the day. On average, breakfast is smaller than lunch, which is smaller than dinner (de Castro, 2000). In our experience, when offered three meals equal in size and energy content for breakfast, lunch, and dinner, subjects complain that breakfast is too large and dinner is too small. This may contribute to underconsumption of MREs because troops are unlikely to save half of one ration until later.

Packaging

A good deal of work has already been done on the way variety, packaging, and social and situational influences may help enhance intake during field training and combat (see IOM, 1995). In particular, some of the modeling approaches and marketing techniques used in commerce (Thompson, 1995) may be of considerable value in raising expectation and acceptability of rations. Companies use a variety of messages to repeatedly maintain consumer interest in their products, and it has already been shown that troops consume more if military rations are packed in a manner that resembles commercial products (Kalick, 1992; Kramer et al., 1989). There may be value in adding food-based aromas to foods to enhance their appeal given the influence of aromas in taste perceptions. After Desert Storm, many commanders expressed their belief in the importance of hot cooked food with an appealing aroma as being vital to morale (see IOM, 1995). While this luxury may not be available in combat, it should be a priority between missions.

Given the problems of hydration and food portability, the new packaging developments are of critical importance. The new packaging provides a remarkable system whereby a variety of water sources, including a filtration of one's own urine, can safely be ingested. A range of super-soluble, low-weight supplements could be mixed with water, thus replacing fluid, electrolytes, and glucose under conditions during which other rations cannot be consumed.

It may be valuable, in addition, to develop tools whereby soldiers can monitor their own fluid and fuel status (in that order). Dehydration can be assessed with urine sticks, and this may provide rapid feedback to soldiers who may not be experiencing the usual urges to eat and drink.

RESEARCH

Given the extreme energy deficit encountered in combat, nutritional supplementation should be the primary focus of rations for soldiers in short-term, high-intensity operations. We have provisionally recommended that research be focused on (1) better understanding of the nature and extent of stressors experienced in combat; (2) determining the optimum timing for nutritional supplementation (including between missions), bearing in mind that supplementation during unpredictable stress may not be advantageous; and (3) finding the most effective means of bypassing suppressed appetite to maintain hydration and optimize energy intake for performance in combat. More data derived from combat or similar situations on the nature of stress, types of intervention, and outcome would be valuable but difficult to obtain. Assessing how initial body composition relates to performance during extreme field training (e.g., Ranger I study) would help to derive guides for feeding before combat.

CONCLUSIONS

Three basic questions regarding the relationship of stress and appetite have been considered. First, in considering the relationship between energy intake and expenditure, it is apparent that appetite poorly tracks acute and extreme elevations of exercise-induced energy expenditure. This might be partly due to the fact that hypohydration itself induces anorexia. Behavior should be geared first to fluid ingestion and then to energy balance. In addition, intense exercise influences gastrointestinal physiology and blood flow and decreases gastric emptying. Hypohydration makes these effects more acute. Under conditions in which increased gastric emptying is needed (i.e, greater food intake), in addition to indigestion, a conflict between the demands of eating and those of exercising will occur. In the short- to medium-term, eating can limit exercise, but exercise can continue without necessarily consuming more thus intake will fail to track expenditure. The best approach to this low energy intake under these circumstances is to consume readily digestible energy and carbohydrate-rich beverages.

Second, the additional stressors of combat may exert further suppressive effects on appetite and have been considered; however, the nature and extent of these stressors is highly unpredictable. The general rule in the clinical setting is that during periods of extreme metabolic instability, do not feed. It is critical to quantify the nature and effects of combat-related stresses and the way they affect both appetite and performance.

Third, other factors such as timing, type of ingredients, and packaging have been considered. When combat is likely to involve extreme stressors, it may be more advantageous to supplement soldiers before deployment and postmission and to maintain fluid and energy (carbohydrate) intakes during acute phases of combat. We suggest that research priorities in this area should focus on quantifying the nature and extent of stressors experienced in combat and their effects on physical and cognitive performance; in addition, assessing the effects of timing, and determining the composition of supplements to improve performance in combat should be a priority.

REFERENCES

Activity and Health Research. 1992. *Allied Dunbar National Fitness Survey*. London: Health Education Authority and Sports Council.

Akerstedt T, Palmblad J, de la Torre B, Marana R, Gillberg M. 1980. Adrenocortical and gonadal steroids during sleep deprivation. *Sleep* 3(1):23–30.

Baker-Fulco C. 1995. Overview of dietary intakes during military exercises. In: Marriott BM, ed. *Not Eating Enough*. Washington, DC: National Academy Press. Pp. 121–149.

Ballor DL, Poehlman ET. 1994. Exercise-training enhances fat-free mass preservation during diet-induced weight loss: A meta-analytical finding. *Int J Obes Relat Metab Disord* 18(1):35–40.

Barr SI, Costill DL. 1992. Effect of increased training volume on nutrient intake of male collegiate swimmers. *Int J Sports Med* 13(1):47–51.

Black AE, Coward WA, Cole TJ, Prentice AM. 1996. Human energy expenditure in affluent societies: An analysis of 574 doubly-labelled water measurements. *Eur J Clin Nutr* 50(2):72–92.

Blundell JE, King NA. 1999. Physical activity and regulation of food intake: Current evidence. *Med Sci Sports Exerc* 31(11 Suppl):S573–S583.

Carrio I, Estorch M, Serra-Grima R, Ginjaume M, Notivol R, Calabuig R, Vilardell F. 1989. Gastric emptying in marathon runners. *Gut* 30(2):152–155.

Ceesay SM, Prentice AM, Day KC, Murgatroyd PR, Goldberg GR, Scott W, Spurr GB. 1989. The use of heart rate monitoring in the estimation of energy expenditure: A validation study using indirect whole-body calorimetry. *Br J Nutr* 61(2):175–186.

de Castro JM. 2000. Eating behavior: Lessons from the real world of humans. *Nutrition* 16(10):800–813.

Diaz EO, Prentice AM, Goldberg GR, Murgatroyd PR, Coward WA. 1992. Metabolic response to experimental overfeeding in lean and overweight healthy volunteers. *Am J Clin Nutr* 56(4):641–655.

DiMeglio DP, Mattes RD. 2000. Liquid versus solid carbohydrate: Effects on food intake and body weight. *Int J Obes Relat Metab Disord* 24(6):794–800.

Eden BD, Abernethy PJ. 1994. Nutritional intake during an ultraendurance running race. *Int J Sport Nutr* 4(2):166–174.

Elia M, Livesey G. 1992. Energy expenditure and fuel selection in biological systems: The theory and practice of calculations based on indirect calorimetry and tracer methods. *World Rev Nutr Diet* 70:68–131.

Engell D. 1995. Effects of beverage consumption and hypdration status on caloric intake. In: Marriott BM, ed. *Not Eating Enough*. Washington, DC: National Academy Press. Pp. 217–237.

Everson CA, Wehr TA. 1993. Nutritional and metabolic adaptations to prolonged sleep deprivation in the rat. *Am J Physiol* 264(2 Pt 2):R376–R387.

Flynn FW, Curtis KS, Verbalis JG, Stricker EM. 1995. Dehydration anorexia in decerebrate rats. *Behav Neurosci* 109(5):1009–1012.

Foo SC, How J, Siew MG, Wong TM, Vijayan A, Kanapathy R. 1994. Effects of sleep deprivation on naval seamen: II. Short recovery sleep on performance. *Ann Acad Med Singapore* 23(5):676–679.

Forbes-Ewan CH, Morrissey BL, Gregg GC, Waters DR. 1989. Use of doubly labeled water technique in soldiers training for jungle warfare. *J Appl Physiol* 67(1):14–18.

Friedl KE. 1995. When does energy deficit affect soldier physical performance. In: Marriott BM, ed. *Not Eating Enough*. Washington, DC: National Academy Press. Pp. 253–283.

Fu ZJ, Ma RS. 2000. Effects of sleep deprivation on human performance. *Space Med Med Eng (Beijing)* 13(4):240–243.

Gabel KA, Aldous A, Edgington C. 1995. Dietary intake of two elite male cyclists during 10-day, 2,050-mile ride. *Int J Sport Nutr* 5(1):56–61.

Garrow JS, Summerbell CD. 1995. Meta-analysis: Effect of exercise, with or without dieting, on the body composition of overweight subjects. *Eur J Clin Nutr* 49(1):1–10.

Holland B, Welch AA, Unwin ID, Buss DH, Paul AA, Southgate DAT. 1991. *McCance and Widdowson's The Composition of Foods*. 5th ed. Cambridge: The Royal Society of Chemistry.

Horne JA. 1985. Sleep function, with particular reference to sleep deprivation. *Ann Clin Res* 17(5):199–208.

Hoyt RW, Jones TE, Stein TP, McAninch GW, Lieberman HR, Askew EW, Cymerman A. 1991. Doubly labeled water measurement of human energy expenditure during strenuous exercise. *J Appl Physiol* 71(1):16–22.

Hyams KC, Wignall FS, Roswell R. 1996. War syndromes and their evaluation: From the US Civil War to the Persian Gulf War. *Ann Intern Med* 125(5):398–405.

IOM (Institute of Medicine). 1995. *Not Eating Enough*. Washington, DC: National Academy Press.

Johnstone AM, Stubbs RJ, Harbron CG. 1996. Effect of overfeeding macronutrients on day-to-day food intake in man. *Eur J Clin Nutr* 50(7):418–430.

Jones PJ, Jacobs I, Morris A, Ducharme MB. 1993. Adequacy of food rations in soldiers during an arctic exercise measured by doubly labeled water. *J Appl Physiol* 75(4):1790–1797.

Kalick JB. 1992. *The Effect of Consumer Oriented Packaging Designs on Acceptance and Consumption of Military Rations*. Technical Report TR-92-034. Natick, MA: US Army Natick Research, Development and Engineering Centre.

Keys A, Brozek J, Henschel A, Mickelsen O, Taylor HL. 1950. *The Biology of Human Starvation*. Minneapolis, MN: The University of Minnesota Press.

King NA, Tremblay A, Blundell JE. 1997. Effects of exercise on appetite control: Implications for energy balance. *Med Sci Sports Exerc* 29(8):1076–1089.

Kramer FM, Edinberg J, Luther S, Engell D. 1989. The impact of food packaging on food consumption and palatability. Paper presented to the Association for the Advancement of Behaviour Therapy, Washington, DC.

Leiper JB, Prentice AS, Wrightson C, Maughan RJ. 2001. Gastric emptying of a carbohydrate-electrolyte drink during a soccer match. *Med Sci Sports Exerc* 33(11):1932–1938.

McGowan CR, Epstein LH, Kupfer DJ, Bulik CM, Robertson RJ. 1986. The effect of exercise on non-restricted caloric intake in male joggers. *Appetite* 7(1):97–105.

Mela DJ. 1995. Understanding fat preference and consumption: Applications of behavioural sciences to a nutritional problem. *Proc Nutr Soc* 54(2):453–464.

Moore RJ, Friedl KE, Kramer TR, Martinez-Lopez LE, Hoyt RW, Tulley RE, DeLany JP, Askew EW, Vogel JA. 1992. *Changes in Soldier Nutritional Status & Immune Function During the Ranger Training Course.* Technical Report No. T13-92. Natick, MA: US Army Medical Research & Development Command.

Mowat F. 1975. *People of the Deer.* Toronto: Seal Books.

Mudambo KS, Leese GP, Rennie MJ. 1997. Gastric emptying in soldiers during and after field exercise in the heat measured with the [^{13}C]acetate breath test method. *Eur J Appl Physiol Occup Physiol* 75(?):109–114.

Murgatroyd PR, Shetty PS, Prentice AM. 1993. Techniques for the measurement of human energy expenditure: A practical guide. *Int J Obes Relat Metab Disord* 17(10):549–568.

Newsholme EA, Leach AR. 1992. *Biochemistry for the Medical Sciences.* Chichester, England: John Wiley and Sons Ltd.

Norgan NG, Durnin JV. 1980. The effect of 6 weeks of overfeeding on the body weight, body composition, and energy metabolism of young men. *Am J Clin Nutr* 33(5):978–988.

Oektedalen O, Flaten O, Opstad PK, Myren J. 1982. hPP and gastrin response to a liquid meal and oral glucose during prolonged severe exercise, caloric deficit, and sleep deprivation. *Scand J Gastroenterol* 17(5):619–624.

Opstad PK, Aakvaag A. 1981. The effect of a high calory diet on hormonal changes in young men during prolonged physical strain and sleep deprivation. *Eur J Appl Physiol Occup Physiol* 46(1):31–39.

Opstad PK, Falch D, Oktedalen O, Fonnum F, Wergeland R. 1984. The thyroid function in young men during prolonged exercise and the effect of energy and leep deprivation. *Clin Endocrinol* 20(6):657-669.

Pasquet P, Brigant L, Froment A, Koppert GA, Bard D, de Garine I, Apfelbaum M. 1992. Massive overfeeding and energy balance in men: The Guru Walla model. *Am J Clin Nutr* 56(3):483–490.

Pearn J. 2000. Traumatic stress disorders: A classification with implications for prevention and management. *Mil Med* 165(6):434–440.

Pereira A. 2002. Combat trauma and the diagnosis of post-traumatic stress disorder in female and male veterans. *Mil Med* 167(1):23–27.

Phinney SD, Bistrian BR, Evans WJ, Gervino E, Blackburn GL. 1983a. The human metabolic response to chronic ketosis without caloric restriction: Preservation of submaximal exercise capability with reduced carbohydrate oxidation. *Metabolism* 32(8):769–776.

Phinney SD, Bistrian BR, Wolfe RR, Blackburn GL. 1983b. The human metabolic response to chronic ketosis without caloric restriction: Physical and biochemical adaptation. *Metabolism* 32(8):757–768.

Ravussin E, Schutz Y, Acheson KJ, Dusmet M, Bourquin L, Jequier E. 1985. Short-term, mixed-diet overfeeding in man: No evidence for "luxuskonsumption." *Am J Physiol* 249(5 Pt 1):E470–E477.

Rechtschaffen A, Bergmann BM, Everson CA, Kushida CA, Gilliland MA. 2002. Sleep deprivation in the rat: X. Integration and discussion of the findings. 1989. *Sleep* 25(1):68–87.

Redwine L, Hauger RL, Gillin JC, Irwin M. 2000. Effects of sleep and sleep deprivation on interleukin-6, growth hormone, cortisol, and melatonin levels in humans. *J Clin Endocrinol Metab* 85(10):3597–3603.

Rehrer NJ, Beckers EJ, Brouns F, ten Hoor F, Saris WH. 1990. Effects of dehydration on gastric emptying and gastrointestinal distress while running. *Med Sci Sports Exerc* 22(6):790–795.

Rehrer NJ, Wagenmakers AJ, Beckers EJ, Halliday D, Leiper JB, Brouns F, Maughan RJ, Westerterp K, Saris WH. 1992. Gastric emptying, absorption, and carbohydrate oxidation during prolonged exercise. *J Appl Physiol* 72(2):468–475.

Rolls B. 1995. Effects of food quality, quantity, and variety on food intake. In: Marriott BM, ed. *Not Eating Enough.* Washington, DC: National Academy Press. Pp. 203–215.

Rose MS. 1989. *Between-Meal Food Intake for Reservists Training in the Field.* Technical Report T15-89. Natick, MA: US Army Research Institute of Environmental Medicine.

Saris WH. 1989. Physiological aspects of exercise in weight cycling. *Am J Clin Nutr* 49(5 Suppl):1099–1104.

Saris WH. 1993. The role of exercise in the dietary treatment of obesity. *Int J Obes Relat Metab Disord* 17 (Suppl 1):S17–S21.

Schoeller DA, van Santen E. 1982. Measurement of energy expenditure in humans by doubly labeled water method. *J Appl Physiol* 53(4):955–959.

Schoeller DA, Shay K, Kushner RF. 1997. How much physical activity is needed to minimize weight gain in previously obese women? *Am J Clin Nutr* 66(3):551–556.

Sjodin AM, Andersson AB, Hogberg JM, Westerterp KR. 1994. Energy balance in cross-country skiers: A study using doubly labeled water. *Med Sci Sports Exerc* 26(6):720–724.

Spurr GB, Prentice AM, Murgatroyd PR, Goldberg GR, Reina JC, Christman NT. 1988. Energy expenditure from minute-by-minute heart-rate recording: Comparison with indirect calorimetry. *Am J Clin Nutr* 48(3):552–559.

Stratton RJ, Stubbs RJ, Elia M. 2003. Short-term continuous enteral tube feeding schedules did not suppress appetite and food intake in healthy men in a placebo-controlled trial. *J Nutr* 133(8):2570–2576.

Stroud M. 1998. The nutritional demands of very prolonged exercise in man. *Proc Nutr Soc* 57(1):55–61.

Stroud MA. 1987. Nutrition and energy balance on the 'Footsteps of Scott' expedition 1984–86. *Hum Nutr Appl Nutr* 41(6):426–433.

Stroud MA, Coward WA, Sawyer MB. 1993. Measurements of energy expenditure using isotope-labelled water ($^2H_2{}^{18}O$) during and Arctic expedition. *Eur J Apl Physiol* 67(4):375–379.

Stroud MA, Ritz P, Coward WA, Sawyer MB, Constantin-Teodosiu D, Greenhaff PL, Macdonald IA. 1997. Energy expenditure using isotope-labelled water ($^2H_2{}^{18}O$), exercise performance, skeletal muscle enzyme activities and plasma biochemical parameters in humans during 95 days of endurance exercise with inadequate energy intake. *Eur J Appl Physiol Occup Physiol* 76(3):243–252.

Stubbs J, Ferres S, Horgan G. 2000. Energy density of foods: Effects on energy intake. *Crit Rev Food Sci Nutr* 40(6):481–515.

Stubbs RJ. 1995. Macronutrient effects on appetite. *Int J Obes Relat Metab Disord* 19(Suppl 5):S11–S19.

Stubbs RJ. 1998. Nutrition Society Medal Lecture. Appetite, feeding behaviour and energy balance in human subjects. *Proc Nutr Soc* 57(3):341–356.

Stubbs RJ, Elia M. 2001. Macronutrients and appetite control with implications for the nutritional management of the malnourished. *Clin Nutr* 20(Suppl 1):129–139.

Stubbs RJ, Hughes DA, Johnstone AM, Horgan GW, King N, Blundell JE. 2004a. A decrease in physical activity affects appetite, energy, and nutrient balance in lean men feeding ad libitum. *Am J Clin Nutr* 79(1):62–69.

Stubbs RJ, Hughes DA, Johnstone AM, Horgan GW, King N, Elia M, Blundell JE. 2003. Interactions between energy intake and expenditure in the development and treatment of obesity. In: Mederios-Neto G, Halpern A, Bouchard C, eds. *Progress in Obesity Research: 9. Proceedings of the 9th International Congress on Obesity.* United Kingdom: John Libbey Eurotext.

Stubbs RJ, Hughes DA, Johnstone AM, Whybrow S, Horgan GW, King N, Blundell J. 2004b. Rate and extent of compensatory changes in energy intake and expenditure in response to altered exercise and diet composition in humans. *Am J Physiol Regul Integr Comp Physiol* 286(2):R350–R358.

Stubbs RJ, Mazlan N, Whybrow S. 2001. Carbohydrates, appetite and feeding behavior in humans. *J Nutr* 131(10):2775S–2781S.

Stubbs RJ, Prentice AM, James WP. 1997. Carbohydrates and energy balance. *Ann N Y Acad Sci* 819:44–69.

Stubbs RJ, Raben AR, Westerterp-Plantenga MS. 1999. Macronutrient metabolism and appetite. In: Westerterp-Plantenga S, Steffens AB, Tremblay A, eds. *Regulation of Food Intake and Energy Expenditure*. Milan: Edra Press. Pp. 59–84.

Stubbs RJ, Ritz P, Coward WA, Prentice AM. 1995. Covert manipulation of the ratio of dietary fat to carbohydrate and energy density: Effect on food intake and energy balance in free-living men eating ad libitum. *Am J Clin Nutr* 62(2):330–337.

Stubbs RJ, van Wyk MC, Johnstone AM, Harbron CG. 1996. Breakfasts high in protein, fat or carbohydrate: Effect on within-day appetite and energy balance. *Eur J Clin Nutr* 50(7):409–417.

Sum CF, Wang KW, Choo DC, Tan CE, Fok AC, Tan EH. 1994. The effect of a 5-month supervised program of physical activity on anthropometric indices, fat-free mass, and resting energy expenditure in obese male military recruits. *Metabolism* 43(9):1148–1152.

Takala J, Ruokonen E, Webster NR, Nielsen MS, Zandstra DF, Vundelinckx G, Hinds CJ. 1999. Increased mortality associated with growth hormone treatment in critically ill adults. *N Engl J Med* 341(11):785–792.

Thompson EG. 1995. Industry approaches to food research. In: Marriott BM, ed. *Not Eating Enough*. Washington, DC: National Academy Press. Pp. 239–250.

van Baak MA. 1999. Physical activity and energy balance. *Public Health Nutr* 2(3A):335–339.

van den Berghe G, Wooters P, Weekers F, Verwaest C, Bruyninckx F, Schetz M, Vlasserlaers D, Ferdinande P, Lauwers P, Bouillon R. 2001. Intensive insulin therapy in critically ill patients. *N Engl J Med* 345(19):1359–1367.

van Etten LM, Westerterp KR, Verstappen FT, Boon BJ, Saris WH. 1997. Effect of an 18-wk weight-training program on energy expenditure and physical activity. *J Appl Physiol* 82(1): 298–304.

Watts AG. 1999. Dehydration-associated anorexia: Development and rapid reversal. *Physiol Behav* 65(4–5):871–878.

Welch IM, Sepple CP, Read NW. 1988. Comparisons of the effects on satiety and eating behaviour of infusion of lipid into the different regions of the small intestine. *Gut* 29(3):306–311.

Westerterp KR. 1998. Alterations in energy balance with exercise. *Am J Clin Nutr* 68(4):970S–974S.

Westerterp KR, Saris WH, van Es M, ten Hoor F. 1986. Use of the doubly labeled water technique in humans during heavy sustained exercise. *J Appl Physiol* 61(6):2162–2167.

Weststrate JA. 1992. Effects of nutrients on the regulation of food intake. Unilever Research, Vlaardingen, the Netherlands.

Witztum E, Levy A, Solomon Z. 1996. Therapeutic response to combat stress reaction during Israel's wars. *Isr J Psychiatry Relat Sci* 33(2):77–78.

Optimization of Immune Function in Military Personnel

Simin Nikbin Meydani and Faria Eksir, Tufts University

INTRODUCTION

Although moderate amount of exercise could result in improving the immune function, it has been shown that strenuous physical activity can suppress the immune response (Hoffman-Goetz and Pedersen, 1994). Studies have reported that during combat as well as during times of rigorous training, soldiers are exposed to many types of stress factors that can affect different components of the immune system (Moore et al., 1992). Lack of sleep, low energy food ration, and psychological stress are among those factors that contribute to a low immune response. The fact that during military work, soldiers are often exposed to long durations of strenuous physical activity, makes the danger even more serious. The duration of physical stress as well as the low energy intake that is associated with military life can cause severe alterations in the immune response and increase risk of infection among soldiers. Many studies have been conducted on the effects of individual stress factors on the immune function. A few studies have shown that the combined effect of the stress factors can be even more damaging to the immune response than the effect of each individual factor (Booth et al., 2003; Kramer et al., 1997).

Immunological studies conducted on military personnel have reported several unfavorable consequences resulting from stresses associated with military life. A major concern has to do with the low-calorie food ration provided for soldiers in combat. Studies have well documented the impact of dietary intake on physical performance and on the immune response (Booth, 2003; Montain and Young, 2003). Undernutrition and/or malnutrition, especially during stressful times, can result in suppression of the immune response, which can lead to increased susceptibility to infection (particularly respiratory infection) and diarrheal diseases often experienced by combat personnel. In fact, it has been documented that during combat, diseases account for more inactive days than either combat wounds or nonbattle injury cases among military personnel. The question would be: What measures can be taken to ameliorate the situation for our military personnel? Clearly, reducing the level of stress would be an effective course. However, given the nature of the job, in all likelihood, that is also the most unattainable option. A more feasible choice would be to conduct vaccinations against various possible diseases, a practice that already has been taken up by the military sectors. Still, available vaccinations only protect against certain diseases and do not provide protection against new pathogens to which the soldiers would likely be exposed. In addition, the vaccines are less effective in immuno-suppressed individuals. An effective and more promising means of protecting the immune function during combat would be through an optimal nutrition plan, which is the focus of this paper. The specific questions that this paper addresses are the following:

- What links are known to exist between nutritional factors and the optimization of the immune system? Specifically which nutritional factors would help reduce occurrence of infections or enhance disease resistance?
- Are there consequences on immune function from a short-term hypocaloric diet?
- Are there nutrients that might improve resistance to infection despite a hypocaloric diet?

NUTRITIONAL STRATEGIES TO IMPROVE
THE IMMUNE RESPONSE

Most nutrient deficiencies result in the impairment of the host defense system and increase susceptibility to infectious diseases (Chandra and Sarchielli, 1993; Keusch et al., 1983). Additionally, recent studies have shown that malnutrition, such as deficiency of selenium and vitamin E, plays a major role in increasing the pathogenicity of microbes and surfacing of unusual viral infections (Beck and Levander, 1998). This is quite important in the case of soldiers at combat in foreign lands, because they frequently encounter pathogens that they have not previously been exposed to. A strong host defense system is critical in the ability of the body to fight off novel pathogens and develop an immune response for future attacks. Supplying the soldiers with adequate nutrients could reduce the risk of a suppressed immune response. Furthermore, providing more than adequate levels of some nutrients can strengthen the immune function and protect against infection and disease.

Using animal models, a number of studies have demonstrated the role of micronutrients (vitamins and trace minerals) in enhancing the immune function. However, studies of micronutrients and immune function in human subjects have been limited and very few have looked at the effect of nutrients on disease and susceptibility to infection. Recently, however, a few studies have examined the relationship between nutritional deficit and/or supplementation and disease in the elderly population.

It should be noted that in spite of the chronological age difference between the elderly population and the military personnel (mostly consisting of a young population), there are similarities in their immune systems. In both groups, the elderly and the military personnel in combat, immunosuppression is evident and characterized by a decrease in cell-mediated immunity and changes in the ability of lymphocytes to proliferate. Notably, the elderly, as a consequence of immunological changes, have a higher susceptibility to, and a greater morbidity and mortality from, infectious diseases, particularly respiratory infections and diarrheal diseases, which are some of the major concerns for soldiers in combat as well. Thus, in the absence of data for military combat personnel, results from a recent clinical trial on vitamin E and respiratory infections will be reviewed as an example of how nutrient intervention could be used to optimize the immune response and reduce risk of infection in an immunocompromised individual.

VITAMIN E AND INFECTIOUS DISEASES

The immunostimulatory effect of vitamin E has been shown to be associated with resistance to infections. Most of the animal studies that investigated the effects of vitamin E on infectious diseases reported a protective effect despite the variations in the dose and duration of the supplementation, infectious organisms involved, and route of administration as reviewed by Meydani et al. (2001).

Vitamin E supplementation in old mice resulted in significantly lower viral titer and preserved antioxidant nutrient status following influenza virus infection (Hayek et al., 1997). This protective effect of vitamin E against influenza infection seems to be partly due to enhancement of Th1 (T helper 1) response, increased IL (interleukin)-2 and IFN-γ production (Han et al., 2000).

VITAMIN E AND RESPIRATORY INFECTIONS IN THE ELDERLY

Only a limited number of studies have investigated the effect of vitamin E on resistance against infections in humans. The subjects in these studies were mainly elderly persons. Infections, particularly respiratory infections (RI), are common in the elderly, resulting in decreased daily activity, prolonged recovery times, increased health care service use, and more frequent complications that may lead to death (Alvarez et al., 1988; Crossley and Peterson, 1996; Farber et al., 1984; Garibaldi et al., 1981; Gugliotti, 1987; Hasley et al., 1993; Jackson et al., 1992; Mehr et al., 1992; Nicolle et al., 1984; Plewa, 1990; Schneider, 1983). Contributing to the increased incidence of infection with age is the well-described decline in immune response (Siskind, 1980). For example, there are higher morbidity and mortality from cancer, pneumonia, and postoperative complications in those who have a diminished delayed-type hypersensitivity (DTH) skin test response (Christou et al., 1989; Cohn et al., 1983; Wayne et al., 1990).

Nutritional status is an important determinant of immune function (Chandra, 1990; Keusch et al., 1983), and nutritional supplementation has been shown to enhance older subjects' immune response (Chandra, 1992; Meydani and Blumberg, 1989). In our earlier placebo-controlled, double-blind trials in elderly persons, vitamin E supplementation improved immune response, including DTH and response to vaccines (Meydani et al., 1990, 1997). In this study we also reported a nonsignificant (p < 0.09) 30 percent lower incidence of self-reported infections among the groups supplemented with vitamin E (60, 200, or 800 mg/day for 235 days) compared with the placebo group (Meydani et al., 1997). Because infection was not the primary outcome, the study did not have enough power to detect significant differences in the incidence of infections. To overcome these limitations, we conducted a large double-blind, placebo-controlled trial to determine the effect of one-year supplementation with vitamin E on objectively recorded respiratory illnesses in elderly nursing home residents (Meydani et al., 2004).

In this randomized, double-blind study, 617 people older than 65 and residing at 33 nursing homes in the Boston area who met the study's eligibility criteria received either a placebo or 200 IU of vitamin E (dl-α-tocopherol) daily for one year. All participants received a capsule containing half the recommended daily allowance of essential vitamins and minerals. The main outcomes of the study were incidence of respiratory tract infections, number of persons and number of days with RIs (upper and lower), and number of new antibiotic prescriptions for RIs among all randomized participants and those who completed the study (Meydani et al., 2004).

Supplementation with vitamin E had no significant effect on the incidence or duration of all RIs taken together, or on upper or lower respiratory tract infections measured separately. However, fewer vitamin E-supplemented subjects acquired one or more RIs (65 percent versus 74 percent, RR = 0.87, CI = 0.73–0.99, p = 0.035), or upper RIs (50 percent versus 62 percent, RR = 0.81, CI = 0.65–0.96, p = 0.015). Further analysis on the foremost RI, the common cold, indicated that the vitamin E group had a lower incidence of common colds (0.66 versus 0.83 per subject-year, RR = 0.80, CI = 0.64–0.98, p = 0.046) and fewer subjects in the vitamin E group acquired one or more common colds (46 percent versus 57 percent, RR = 0.79, CI = 0.63–0.96, p = 0.016) (Meydani et al., 2004). The vitamin E-treated group also had fewer days with common cold per person-year compared with those in the placebo group, but the difference did not reach statistical significance (22 percent less, p = 0.11).

In conclusion, the results of this clinical trial show that vitamin E supplementation significantly reduces the risk of acquiring upper respiratory infections, particularly the common cold.

CONCLUSIONS

Several investigations have demonstrated that vitamin E significantly enhances immune functions in humans, especially in the elderly. Animal studies as well as recently completed clinical trials strongly suggest that this effect of vitamin E is associated with reduced risk of acquiring infections, particularly upper respiratory infections in the elderly. Given that, similar to the elderly, military personnel in combat are immunosuppressed, these studies strongly suggest that they might also benefit from consuming additional level of vitamin E. Studies by Lee and Wan (2000), in which they demonstrated vitamin E to be effective in improving the immune response of young adults, further supports this recommendation. Thus, studies to demonstrate efficacy of increasing the vitamin E level in military combat ration are warranted.

ACKNOWLEDGMENTS

The work of the authors was supported by NIA, National Institute of Health Grant 1 R01-AG13975, and US Department of Agriculture agreement 58-1950-9-001, and National Institute of Health Grant 2R01 AG009140-10A1 and a gift for preparation of supplement from Roche, Inc.

REFERENCES

Alvarez S, Shell CG, Woolley TW, Berk SL, Smith JK. 1988. Nosocomial infections in long-term facilities. *J Gerontol* 43(1):M9–M17.

Beck MA, Levander OA. 1998. Dietary oxidative stress and the potentiation of viral infection. *Annu Rev Nutr* 18:93–116.

Booth CK. 2003. Combat rations and military performance. Do soldiers on active service eat enough? *Asia Pac J Clin Nutr* 12(Suppl):S2.

Booth CK, Coad RA, Forbes-Ewan CH, Thomson GF, Niro PJ. 2003. The physiological and psychological effects of combat ration feeding during a 12-day training exercise in the tropics. *Mil Med* 168(1):63–70.

Chandra RK. 1990. Nutrition is an important determinant of immunity in old age. In: Prinsley DM, Sandstead HH, eds. *Nutrition and Aging. Proceedings of the 1988 International Conference on Nutrition and Aging, held in Galveston, Texas, October 5-7, 1988*. New York: Alan R. Liss, Inc. Pp. 321–334.

Chandra RK. 1992. Effect of vitamin and trace-element supplementation on immune responses and infection in elderly subjects. *Lancet* 340(8828):1124–1127.

Chandra RK, Sarchielli P. 1993. Nutritional status and immune responses. *Clin Lab Med* 13(2):455–461.

Christou NV, Tellado-Rodriguez J, Chartrand L, Giannas B, Kapadia B, Meakins J, Rode H, Gordon J. 1989. Estimating mortality risk in preoperative patients using immunologic, nutritional, and acute-phase response variables. *Ann Surg* 210(1):69–77.

Cohn JR, Hohl CA, Buckley CE 3rd. 1983. The relationship between cutaneous cellular immune responsiveness and mortality in a nursing home population. *J Am Geriatr Soc* 31(12):808–809.

Crossley KB, Peterson PK. 1996. Infections in the elderly. *Clin Infect Dis* 22(2):209–215.

Farber BF, Brennen C, Puntereri AJ, Brody JP. 1984. A prospective study of nosocomial infections in a chronic care facility. *J Am Geriatr Soc* 32(7):499–502.

Garibaldi RA, Brodine S, Matsumiya S. 1981. Infections among patients in nursing homes: Policies, prevalence, problems. *N Engl J Med* 305(13):731–735.

Gugliotti R. 1987. The incidence of nosocomial infections in a skilled nursing facility. *Conn Med* 51(5):287–290.

Han SN, Wu D, Ha WK, Beharka A, Smith DE, Bender BS, Meydani SN. 2000. Vitamin E supplementation increases T helper 1 cytokine production in old mice infected with influenza virus. *Immunology* 100(4):487–493.

Hasley PB, Brancati FL, Rogers J, Hanusa BH, Kapoor WN. 1993. Measuring functional change in community-acquired pneumonia. A preliminary study using the Sickness Impact Profile. *Med Care* 31(7):649–657.

Hayek MG, Taylor SF, Bender BS, Han SN, Meydani M, Smith DE, Eghtesada S, Meydani SN. 1997. Vitamin E supplementation decreases lung virus titers in mice infected with influenza. *J Infect Dis* 176(1):273–276.

Hoffman-Goetz L, Pedersen BK. 1994. Exercise and the immune system: A model of the stress response? *Immunol Today* 15(8):382–387.

Jackson MM, Fierer J, Barrett-Connor E, Fraser D, Klauber MR, Hatch R, Burkhart B, Jones M. 1992. Intensive surveillance for infections in a three-year study of nursing home patients. *Am J Epidemiol* 135(6):685–696.

Keusch GT, Wilson CS, Waksal SD. 1983. Nutrition, host defenses, and the lymphoid system. *Adv Host Def Mech* 2:275–306.

Kramer TR, Moore RJ, Shippee RL, Friedl KE, Martinez-Lopez L, Chan MM, Askew EW. 1997. Effects of food restriction in military training on T-lymphocyte responses. *Int J Sports Med* 18(Suppl 1):S84–S90.

Lee CY, Man-Fan Wan J. 2000. Vitamin E supplementation improves cell-mediated immunity and oxidative stress of Asian men and women. *J Nutr* 130(12):2932–2937.

Mehr DR, Foxman B, Colombo P. 1992. Risk factors for mortality from lower respiratory infections in nursing home patients. *J Fam Pract* 34(5):585–591.

Meydani SN, Blumberg JB. 1989. Nutrition and the immune function in the elderly. In: Munro H, Danforth A, eds. *Human Nutrition: A Comprehensive Treatise.* Vol. VII. New York: Plenum Press. Pp. 61–87.

Meydani SN, Barklund MP, Liu S, Meydani M, Miller RA, Cannon JG, Morrow FD, Rocklin R, Blumberg JB. 1990. Vitamin E supplementation enhances cell-mediated immunity in healthy elderly subjects. *Am J Clin Nutr* 52(3):557–563.

Meydani SN, Fawzi WW, Han SN. 2001. The effect of vitamin deficiencies (E and A) and supplementation on infection and immune response. In: Suskind RM, Tontisirin K, eds. *Nutrition, Immunity, and Infection in Infants and Children.* Vol. 45. Philadelphia, PA: Lippincott Williams & Wilkins. Pp. 213–241.

Meydani SN, Leka LS, Fine BC, Dallal GE, Keusch GT, Singh MF, Hamer DH. 2004. Vitamin E and respiratory tract infections in elderly nursing home residents: A randomized controlled trial. *J Am Med Assoc* 292(7):828–836.

Meydani SN, Meydani M, Blumberg JB, Leka LS, Siber G, Loszewski R, Thompson C, Pedrosa MC, Diamond RD, Stollar BD. 1997. Vitamin E supplementation and in vivo immune response in healthy elderly subjects. A randomized controlled trial. *J Am Med Assoc* 277(17):1380–1386.

Montain SJ, Young AJ. 2003. Diet and physical performance. *Appetite* 40(3):255–267.

Moore RJ, Friedl KE, Kramer TR, Martinez-Lopez LE, Hoyt RW, Tulley RE, DeLany JP, Askew EW, Vogel JA. 1992. *Changes in Soldier Nutritional Status & Immune Function During the Ranger Training Course.* Technical Report No. T13-92. Natick, MA: US Army Medical Research & Development Command.

Nicolle LE, McIntyre M, Zacharias H, MacDonell JA. 1984. Twelve-month surveillance of infections in institutionalized elderly men. *J Am Geriatr Soc* 32(7):513–519.

Plewa MC. 1990. Altered host response and special infections in the elderly. *Emerg Med Clin North Am* 8(2):193–206.

Schneider EL. 1983. Infectious diseases in the elderly. *Ann Intern Med* 98(3):395–400.

Siskind GW. 1980. Immunological aspects of aging: An overview. In: Schimke RT, ed. *Biological Mechanism in Aging.* Bethesda, MD: US Department of Health and Human Services. Pp. 455–467.

Wayne SJ, Rhyne RL, Garry PJ, Goodwin JS. 1990. Cell-mediated immunity as a predictor of morbidity and mortality in subjects over 60. *J Gerontol* 45(2):M45–M48.

Optimization of Nutrient Composition for Assault Rations: Interaction of Stress with Immune Function

Ronenn Roubenoff, Millenium Pharmaceuticals

INTRODUCTION

Both military missions and military training cause major stress to the body on a number of levels: dehydration, whole-body inflammation and immune modulation, muscle catabolism, oxidative stress, and increased energy requirements are the most readily demonstrable effects of these activities. During high-tempo, stressful combat missions, it is expected that soldiers will not be able to carry adequate calories and nutrients to meet the heightened requirements of their environment and activity. Therefore, the goal of a model military ration must be to reduce the effects of these stresses in the sure foreknowledge that they cannot be avoided or fully countered under combat or rigorous training conditions. The goal of this discussion is to answer the following questions:

- What theoretical constructs should be considered in evaluating the interplay of stress, diet, exercise, and immune function in determining functional capacity?
- What dietary factors can affect muscle injury and immune function?
- What biomarkers could be used to assess the effects of dietary interventions?
- What more do we need to know to enhance the benefits of military rations?

The body's stress response is multifaceted, with endocrine, immune, and neuropsychiatric systems participating in a complex interaction that remains poorly understood (Marsland et al., 2002; Stowell et al., 2001; Webster et al., 2002). The stress response invokes cellular, humoral, and neurological responses (see Figure B-29). The ability of nutritional elements to modulate these responses varies by both nutrient and system (Venkatraman and Pendergast, 2002). Although, as athletes and coaches have known for years, poor nutrition can increase the risk of injury and be detrimental to performance, the expectaction that nutrition can markedly improve performance may be unrealistic (Venkatraman and Pendergast, 2002). Nutritionists face a challenge to improve the immune system responses to the multiple stresses in a combat situation through changing the nutritional composition of the combat ration. Nevertheless some aspects of the stress response are most amenable to dietary manipulations and include:

- Modulating the immune function with signal-transducing fatty acids, prostaglandins, leukotrienes, and cytokines.
- Decreasing of total energy deficit caused by low-caloric intake.
- Reducing oxidative stress by way of antioxidant intake.
- Limiting muscle damage exacerbation caused by inadequate energy and protein intake.
- Modulating emotional response to stress by offering hedonic foods (e.g., chocolate, caffeine).

An important consideration in devising optimal meal content for supporting intensive physical activity (Rasmussen et al., 2000; Tipton et al., 2001). Several researchers have suggested that there is an "open window" of immune suppression after an exercise bout, and its severity correlates with the intensity and duration of exercise (Figure B-30) (Lakier Smith, 2003; Nieman, 2003). This concept has not been fully explored and limited data support it; however, if it is correct, then dietary intake during the open window should be considered as a potential route of delivery of immune-supportive nutrients (see below). Further investigation of this possibility is warranted.

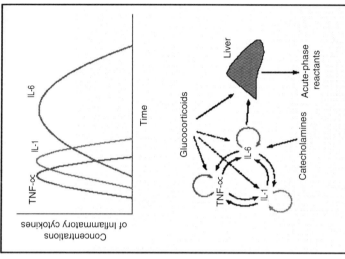

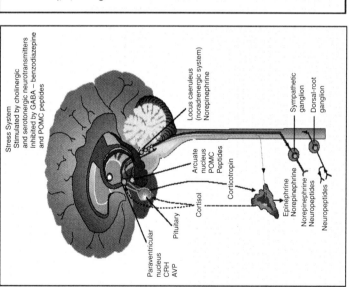

FIGURE B-29 Selected elements of the stress response: left panel, central nervous system; right panel, cytokine secretion.

NOTE: AVP = arginine vasopressin; CRH = corticotrophin-releasing hormone; GABA = γ-aminobutyric acid; IL = interleukin; POMC = pro-opiomelanocortin; TNF = tumor necrosis factor.

SOURCE: Chrousos (1995), used with permission. Copyright © 1995 Massachusetts Medical Society. All Rights Reserved.

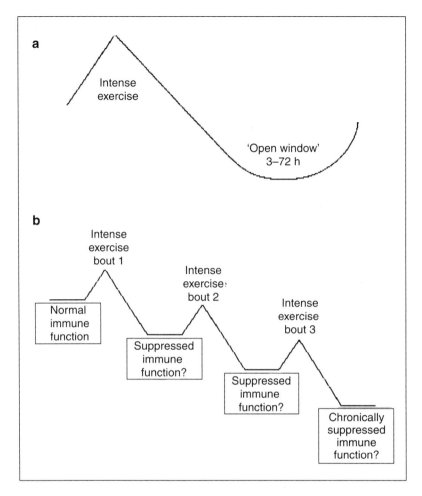

FIGURE B-30 (a) "Open Window" theory of the (b) cumulative effects of intense exercise on immune function.
SOURCE: Lakier Smith (2003).

DIETARY FACTORS THAT AFFECT MUSCLE INJURY AND IMMUNE FUNCTION

The physical stress of combat and high-intensity training causes (1) damage to skeletal muscle, (2) a systemic inflammatory response, and (3) alterations in immune function (Zoico and Roubenoff, 2002). A variety of nutrients may, to some extent, affect aspects of these responses to stress. For example, fatty acids, such as omega-3 fatty acids, that suppress inflammation may reduce inflammation at the site of injury, although this benefit to soldiers under combat situations remain to be proven (Sethi, 2002). Similarly, amino acids such as arginine and glutamine may be important for combat situations and should be considered for enrichment in soldiers' diets (Nieman, 2001; Nieves and Langkamp-Henken, 2002). In addition, high-intensity physical activity (and perhaps mental stress as well) increase insulin resistance, which could be exacerbated by diets high in simple sugars. Finally, antioxidant nutrients—both vitamins (such as vitamins E and C) and nonvitamin antioxidants (such as catechins found in tea), as well as anthocyanins found in blueberries and other highly colored fruits—can have protective effects on both muscle and systemic inflammatory responses (Nieman, 2001; Nieves and Langkamp-Henken, 2002).

POTENTIAL BIOMARKERS OF DIETARY INTERVENTIONS

A key factor limiting the ability to evaluate the effectiveness of nutritional and pharmacological interventions in combat situations is the limited number of biomarkers of response that are currently known. It is crucial to be able to evaluate the effects of such interventions by using simple blood or functional tests that can be implemented in the field. In the future, it should be feasible to assess any soldier's level of stress during combat or training in relation to his baseline and, ideally, alter his dietary intake or prescribe medications that could mitigate downstream injury.

At this time, the best candidates for such biomarkers include indicators of inflammation such as C-reactive protein, cytokines such as interleukin-1 and -6, tumor necrosis factor-α, and their antagonists or receptors (Bosch et al., 2003; Lakier Smith, 2003; Zoico and Roubenoff, 2002). However, these biomarkers will need to be validated in real-life situations and then converted into portable, environmentally stable, easily interpretable tests for field use.

FUTURE DIRECTIONS

The study of how military rations can maintain troops' fitness for combat is in its infancy. Further studies are needed to evaluate the results of various diets on immune function and on other effects of exercise and stress. Although studies of some individual nutrients have been undertaken, more are needed with more sophisticated outcome measures, evaluation of biomarkers, and application to real-life situations. However, the real work must come in evaluating combinations of nutrients in true diets. This will obviously take a great deal of time and effort to achieve, but the benefits to troop functionality and ability to recover from intense exertion are potentially great. As the cost and time needed to train soldiers for the modern battlefield increase, dietary interventions offer a cost-effective and exciting way to maximize the troops' effectiveness in the field.

REFERENCES

Bosch JA, de Geus EJ, Veerman EC, Hoogstraten J, Nieuw Amerongen AV. 2003. Innate secretory immunity in response to laboratory stressors that evoke distinct patterns of cardiac autonomic activity. *Psychosom Med* 65(2):245–258.

Chrousos GP. 1995. The hypothalamic-pituitary-adrenal axis and immune-mediated inflammation. *N Engl J Med* 332(20):1351–1362.

Lakier Smith L. 2003. Overtraining, excessive exercise, and altered immunity: Is this a T helper-1 versus T helper-2 lymphocyte response? *Sports Med* 33(5):347–364.

Marsland AL, Bachen EA, Cohen S, Rabin B, Manuck SB. 2002. Stress, immune reactivity and susceptibility to infectious disease. *Physiol Behav* 77(4-5):711–716.

Nieman DC. 2001. Exercise immunology: Nutritional countermeasures. *Can J Appl Physiol* 26(Suppl):S45–S55.

Nieman DC. 2003. Current perspective on exercise immunology. *Curr Sports Med Rep* 2(5):239–242.

Nieves C Jr, Langkamp-Henken B. 2002. Arginine and immunity: A unique perspective. *Biomed Pharmacother* 56(10):471–482.

Rasmussen BB, Tipton KD, Miller SL, Wolf SE, Wolfe RR. 2000. An oral essential amino acid-carbohydrate supplement enhances muscle protein anabolism after resistance exercise. *J Appl Physiol* 88(2):386–392.

Sethi S. 2002. Inhibition of leukocyte-endothelial interactions by oxidized omega-3 fatty acids: A novel mechanism for the anti-inflammatory effects of omega-3 fatty acids in fish oil. *Redox Rep* 7(6):369–378.

Stowell JR, Kiecolt-Glaser JK, Glaser R. 2001. Perceived stress and cellular immunity: When coping counts. *J Behav Med* 24(4):323–339.

Tipton KD, Rasmussen BB, Miller SL, Wolf SE, Owens-Stovall SK, Petrini BE, Wolfe RR. 2001. Timing of amino acid-carbohydrate ingestion alters anabolic response of muscle to resistance exercise. *Am J Physiol Endocrinol Metabol* 281(2):E197–E206.

Venkatraman JT, Pendergast DR. 2002. Effect of dietary intake on immune function in athletes. *Sports Med* 32(5):323-337.

Webster JI, Tonelli L, Sternberg EM. 2002. Neuroendocrine regulation of immunity. *Ann Rev Immunol* 20:125–163.

Zoico E, Roubenoff R. 2002. The role of cytokines in regulating protein metabolism and muscle function. *Nutr Rev* 60(2):39–51.

The Potential Impact of Probiotics and Prebiotics on Gastrointestinal and Immune Health of Combat Soldiers

Mary Ellen Sanders, Food Culture Technologies
Joshua Korzenik, Harvard Medical School

INTRODUCTION

This paper evaluates the health benefits associated with pro- and prebiotics and their potential utility as a component of combat rations. Combat rations are intended for short-term (three to seven days) use by soldiers during high-intensity, stressful, repetitive combat missions. Desired benefits from this ration, which may potentially be derived from pro- or prebiotics, include prevention of diarrhea;

prevention of infections; reduction of infection-caused morbidity; enhancement of the immune system function; and prevention of kidney stones.

A group of experts assembled by the Food and Agriculture Organization/ World Health Organization (FAO/WHO) defined probiotics as "live micro-organisms which, when administered in adequate amounts, confer a health benefit on the host" (FAO/WHO, 2002). To meet this definition, probiotics must remain alive. Some immune modulatory effects have been documented for killed cells or bacterial cell components, but this is beyond the scope of this paper. Probiotics are not synonymous with our native, beneficial microbiota, although they are often derived from this source. Prebiotics are food ingredients that provide selective stimulation of the growth or activity of beneficial native bacteria (Gibson and Roberfroid, 1995). They are generally complex carbohydrates, such as fructo-oligosaccharides (FOS) and inulin, which are synthesized from food components or isolated from plant materials.

Some technological issues must be considered for the incorporation of pro- and prebiotics in combat rations for healthy soldiers. For example, the effects for probiotics are strain specific and microorganisms must remain viable in the chosen delivery vehicle. Also, probiotics would be considered a food ingredient, and therefore, any particular strain or combination of strains chosen must have documented safety and efficacy. Furthermore, the dose chosen must be documented to elicit the desired physiological effects. Likewise, prebiotics must be chosen based on documentation of efficacy and used at doses which elicit specific microbiota responses and do not cause any gastrointestinal side effects.

Although a body of supportive data exist that document the role of certain prebiotics and strains of probiotics in enhancing gastrointestinal health, pro- and prebiotics have not been tested specifically on healthy, hypocaloric young adults under stress. Furthermore, data documenting physiological benefits of pro- and prebiotics after short-term (three to seven days) administration are rare. To take advantage of pro- or prebiotic-induced benefits, a more effective strategy may be to supplement the soldier's diet in the weeks or months before and during the period of combat ration. The use of these compounds for longer time may allow these physiologic effects to be harnessed in a way that would be beneficial during the period of combat stress. In addition, pro- or prebiotic use should be considered as a possible nutritional supplement for soldiers taking antibiotics, and as enteral nutrition during surgical procedures or when exposure to pathogens is likely. Demonstrated actions of pro- and prebiotics are potentially highly relevant to the design of combat rations. However, existing research, while promising, does not convincingly support their inclusion in combat rations administered for a short term. More research is needed to understand how best to take advantage of the utility of these supplements.

Ensuring optimal nutritional status is the primary goal of combat rations. Advances in nutritional science suggest that adequate nutrition means much more than providing macronutrients and preventing nutrient deficiency diseases. A host of food components have been shown to play roles both in reducing the risk of acute and chronic illnesses and optimizing physiological performance. Pro- and prebiotics are being studied as agents that can play a role in enhancing human health via infection prevention and immune enhancement. The rationale for including these components in combat rations stems from data demonstrating the physiologic effects these substances caused which could potentially benefit intestinal immunity, prevent enteric infections, decrease recovery time from enteric infections and improve bowel habits. Other theoretical, but unproven, benefits of pro- and prebiotics that could be of use include optimizing intestinal function by maximizing nutrient utilization and improving stamina. Unfortunately many of the randomized, controlled studies on probiotics are in pediatric populations or in adults having specific health concerns and these data cannot be directly extrapolated to a healthier population.

This review will consider the human studies that may be applicable to improving the nutritional status of combat troops and explore technological issues associated with inclusion of probiotics or prebiotics in combat rations.

The specific questions that are addressed in this paper are:

- What are the current applications for pro- and prebiotics in preventing or protection from infections/disease?
- What are the types and levels of pro- and prebiotics that could be added to such rations of presumably healthy soldiers to optimize their immune system, which may best sustain physical and cognitive performance and prevent possible adverse health consequences with a hypocaloric diet?

EFFECTS OF PROBIOTICS AND PREBIOTICS

A huge and diverse range of bacterial species colonize the human body. Internally, the microbiota extend from mouth to anus, and, for women, into the vaginal tract. Externally they reside on the skin surface. Many lines of research have demonstrated the significant role of the microbiota in human physiology. The microbiota are involved in the development of the immune system, prevention of infection from pathogenic or opportunistic microbes, and maintenance of intestinal barrier function. Recently, the role of commensal microbes in adiposity was established (Backhed et al., 2004). Conventional mice were found to have higher percent body fat, greater feed consumption and higher oxygen utilization than their germ-free counterparts. For a variety of reasons, normal native bacteria may not always perform these functions optimally. The use of pro- and prebiotics to alter native microbiota and thus improve these functions has been studied.

The effects of the components of the gut microbiota may range from potentially pathogenic to health promoting. Lactic acid producing genera such as *Bifidobacterium* or *Lactobacillus* have a long-established association with health. These bacteria can be increased either by feeding appropriate strains as a probiotic or appropriate prebiotic substrates which selectively stimulate the growth or function of beneficial microbiota.

Research into the physiological benefits of probiotics use in the normal population is extensive. Published effects include regulation of immune function and prevention of infection (Bengmark, 2003; Gill, 2003); possible reduction of the risk of relapse in inflammatory bowel conditions (Gionchetti et al., 2003; Ishikawa et al., 2003; Tamboli et al., 2003); reduction of duration of infectious diarrhea in infants (Van Niel et al., 2002); reduction of the onset of atopic dermatitis in high-risk infants (Kalliomaki et al., 2001, 2003); and control of symptoms associated with lactose intolerance (de Vrese et al., 2001). Less dramatic, albeit statistically significant, results have shown the ability of certain probiotic bacteria to decrease the incidence of dental caries (Nase et al., 2001), antibiotic use (Hatakka et al., 2001), respiratory infections (Hatakka et al., 2001), and antibiotic-associated diarrhea (Cremonini et al., 2002). There is emerging research in the areas of probiotics reducing the risk of oxalate kidney stone formation (Duncan et al., 2002; Sidhu et al., 2001); and decreasing stomach colonization by *Helicobacter pylori* (Cruchet et al., 2003; Linsalata et al., 2004).

The proposed benefits of prebiotics are focused on their effects on the colon and include: (1) increasing colonic bifidobacteria (Buddington et al., 1996); (2) increasing intestinal levels of lactate and short chain fatty acids, especially acetate, butyrate, and propionate (Campbell et al., 1997); (3) decreasing fecal pH (Campbell et al., 1997); (4) altering activities of certain fecal enzymes (Gudiel-Urbano and Goni, 2002); (5) reducing constipation (Kleessen et al., 1997); and (6) increasing mineral absorption (Roberfroid et al., 2002). Most of these effects have been most convincingly demonstrated with prebiotics such as inulin or oligofructose. The effects of prebiotics on reducing the incidence of infectious enteric disease or on immune function has not been well documented.

The relevance of many of these studies to short-term use (three to seven days) of pre- or probiotics in healthy (albeit stressed and hypocaloric) soldiers is questionable because most of these studies focus on longer term administration to subgroups of at-risk individuals such as preterm infants, infants and children with infectious diarrhea, individuals with chronic illnesses, or the elderly. However, it has been noted that a high incidence of noninfectious diarrhea occurs in deployed soldiers. In this case, some value to short-term administration of prebiotics may be realized via prebiotic-mediated osmotic effects. There is some evidence that may be applicable to support a role of pro- or prebiotics in combat rations although benefits may require longer term administration than three to seven days.

STRAIN-DEPENDENCY AND DOSE-DEPENDENCY OF PROBIOTIC AND PREBIOTICS EFFECTS

The benefits reported for probiotics should be considered specific to the strain or strains used and the levels of viable microbes consumed. Although few studies have evaluated strain-dependent clinical effects (due to the high cost of conducting human studies), numerous in vitro and animal studies have demonstrated that different strains of the same probiotic species can have different or opposing effects. For example, in mouse models of inflammation, different strains have been shown to stimulate expression of different classes of cytokines, which may result in anti- or pro-inflammatory effects (personal communication, B. Pot, Institut Pasteur de Lille, France). In time, however, it may be possible to generalize that certain effects are associated with specific species or even genera of bacteria but the limited body of results from controlled human studies precludes this conclusion at present. Consequently, the target for intervention and the probiotic component must be carefully selected.

Few controlled studies have evaluated the effecst of pro- or prebiotic dose in humans. Doses achieving statistically significant results in a sample of clinical targets are listed in Table B-20. One meta-analysis of studies on *Lactobacillus* and infectious diarrhea in infants demonstrated a direct correlation between dose and effect (see Figure B-31, Van Niel et al., 2002). Using the endpoint of fecal recovery of an orally administered probiotic, Saxelin and coworkers (1991) demonstrated that there was no recovery of *L. rhamnosus* GG in feces at feeding levels of 10^6–10^8 colony forming units (cfu)/day. However, at 10^9 cfu/day, two of seven volunteers showed *L. rhamnosus* GG in feces. At 10^{10} cells/day all were colonized. Generally speaking, studies using higher doses of probiotics are likely to have positive effects. Therefore, using the highest dose possible, considering

TABLE B-20 Daily Doses Used in Different Studies Documenting Clinical Effects

Clinical Effect	References	Dose (cfu/day)
↓Day care center antibiotic use/infections/ dental caries	Hatakka, et al. 2001; Nase et al. 2001	10^8
↓Incidence of antibiotic associated diarrhea	Vanderhoof et al., 1999	1–2×10^{10}
↑Fecal lactobacilli (*L. rhamnosus* GG)	Saxelin et al., 1991	10^9
↑Fecal *L. reuteri*	Valeur et al., 2004	10^{8-9}
↓Incidence atopic eczema	Kalliomaki et al., 2001	10^{10}
↑Lactose digestion	de Vrese et al., 2001	$10^{10}*$
↓IBS abdominal pain	Niedzielin et al., 2001	2×10^{10}
↓Duration of infant diarrhea	Majamaa et al., 1995	10^{11}
↑Remission of pouchitis	Mimura et al., 2004	10^{12}

NOTE: cfu = colony-forming units; IBS = irritable bowel syndrome.
*Dose in this case more closely tied to quantity of lactose ingested than in daily amount. In general, symptom relief caused by the lactose present in one serving of milk or yogurt can be significantly reduced by consumption of 10^{10} cfu live cultures.

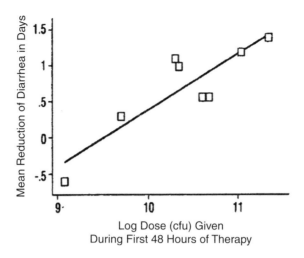

FIGURE B-31 Relationship between *Lactobacillus* dose and reduction of diarrhea in children.
NOTE: cfu = colony-forming units.
SOURCE: Van Niel et al. (2002), used with permission of *Pedatrics*.

the product format and cost constraints, is a reasonable approach to formulation. In general, it is important to be mindful of the strain(s) and dose(s) used in studies of clinical documentation and not generalize these results to other strains and doses.

PHYSIOLOGICAL EFFECTS OF PROBIOTICS AND PREBIOTICS

Effects on Fecal Microbiota

One of the most thoroughly documented effects of pro- and prebiotics is their ability to influence fecal microbiota. Limitations of this work, however, stem from assumptions about the composition of an "ideal" microbiota, methodologies for quantification of the diverse microbial communities in feces, and ability to use composition of fecal microbiota as an indicator of microbiota upstream in the intestinal tract. Nonetheless, prebiotics and probiotics comprised of lactobacilli and bifidobacteria have been shown to increase levels of those bacteria in the feces (Bouhnik et al., 1999). Although effects have been shown to be dose-dependent, it should be noted that in the case of subjects with already high bifidobacteria counts, prebiotic feeding has little to no measurable effect. In

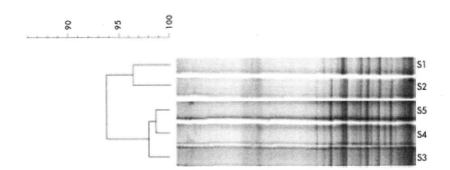

FIGURE B-32 Temporal temperature gradient gel electrophoresis of 16S rDNA amplicons of the dominant fecal flora in a healthy control subject sampled over a two-year period. S1, fecal sample collected in 1997; S2-S5, samples collected in 1999 on days 1, 23, 58, and 78, respectively. The dendrogram gives a statistically optimal representation of similarities between temporal temperature gradient gel electrophoresis profiles. SOURCE: Seksik et al. (2003), used with permission from the BMJ Publishing Group.

some cases, changes in enzymatic (Buddington et al., 1996), physical, or biochemical (Campbell et al., 1997) parameters of the feces also have been documented.

Significantly altering the intestinal microbiota is a difficult task. Normal gut microbiota have their own intrinsic stability, which is poorly understood (see Figure B-32). In addition, the body has its own defenses against bacteria that must be traversed before they reach the colon. Both gastric acidity and bile act as barriers to the survival of transiting bacteria. Once they reach the colon, probiotic bacteria enter a complex environment with more than 450 different species and as many as 10^{12} cfu per gram of stool. An effective probiotic will increase the number of the particular species being added but usually has little effect on other species. Prebiotics are more consistently delivered as they are largely unaltered by their transit through the gastrointestinal tract until they reach the colon, where they serve as a substrate for particular bacteria. In addition to increasing the numbers of certain bacteria, many prebiotics have a potentially broader effect on the colonic microbiota by altering the pH and making the colonic environment less hospitable for certain species, decreasing their concentration.

Effects on the Gut Barrier

Elements of the intestinal barrier which protect the host from a potential microbial threat include the mucous layer or biofilm adjacent to the epithelial lining, other secreted products [such as immunoglobulin A (IgA)], the epithelial cell layer itself and circulating immune cells. Probiotics have been demonstrated to influence each of these components. Research using cell culture systems, animal models, and humans suggests that probiotics may have a role, along with commensal bacteria, in maintaining intestinal barrier integrity. A recent paper (Resta-Lenert and Barrett, 2003) examined the ability of live and killed *L. acidophilus* ATCC4356 and *Steptococcus thermophilus* ATCC19258 to interfere with the infection of human intestinal epithelial cell lines (HT29 and Caco-2) by enteroinvasive *Escherichia coli* (EIEC). The live probiotic blend interfered with EIEC adhesion and invasion, protected against physiological disruption caused by EIEC, and increased transepithelial resistance (a marker for improved epithelial barrier function). Antibiotic killed blend did not significantly effect EIEC adhesion or protect against physiological disruption. This model suggests that *L. acidophilus* and *S. thermophilus* could protect the cell lines from EIEC and enhance barrier function. A variety of other mechanisms demonstrated by probiotics may be important for an anti-infective capacity, including enhancement of mucus secretion, competitive binding of mucosal cells, displacement of pathogenic microbes, production of bacteriocins (compounds with bacterial antibiotic activity) and reduction of bacterial translocation from the gut lumen (Eijsink et al., 2002; Garcia-Lafuente et al., 2001; Mack et al., 2003; Resta-Lenert and Barrett, 2003).

Effects on Immune System

Probiotic bacteria have been demonstrated to bolster the immune defense against potential bacterial threats. Studies have indicated that certain probiotics can modulate nonspecific and specific aspects of immune responses. According to Gill (1999), these findings suggest that probiotics "could be used as valuable dietary adjuncts for optimizing immunocompetence" in population groups with less than optimal immune systems.

Probiotics appear to alter the activity of phagocytic cells and natural killer (NK) cells, both important against infections and integral to the non-specific immune network. In humans, increases in peripheral blood phagocytic activity and/or NK cell function with *L. acidophilus* La1 (Schiffrin et al., 1997); *Bifidobacterium lactis* Bb12 (Schiffrin et al., 1997); *L. rhamnosus* HN001 (Gill et al., 2001b; Sheih et al., 2001); *B. lactis* HN019 (Arunachalam et al., 2000; Chiang et al., 2000; Gill et al., 2001b); and *L. casei* Shirota (Nagao et al., 2000) have been observed.

The components of the specific immune response, humoral- (mediated by antibodies) and cell-mediated (mediated by T-lymphocytes), have also been shown to be affected by probiotics in animal models and, to a lesser extent, in healthy human subjects. *Lactobacillus rhamnosus* GG stimulated antibody response during rotavirus infection (Kaila et al., 1992; Majamaa et al., 1995). Increased antibody response to vaccines has been observed with a mixture of *L. acidophilus* La1 and *B. lactis* BB12 (Link-Amster et al., 1994) and *L. rhamnosus* GG (Isolauri et al., 1995). In humans, cell-mediated responses to probiotics include

B. lactis HN019-induced (Gill et al., 2001b) and *L. brevis*-induced production of interferon α (Kishi et al., 1996). Also, *B. lactis* HN019 has been shown to increase proportions of total, helper (CD4+) and activated (CD25+) T-lymphocytes in the blood of elderly persons (Gill et al., 2001c). Effects seem to be most clearly demonstrable in human subjects with compromised immune function (Gill et al., 2001a; Nagao et al., 2000). Dendritic cell function, pivotal cells for T-cell immune response, is stimulated by lactobacilli; interferon γ production is increased in these cells (Halpern et al., 1991); and systemic and mucosal IgA production is increased as well (Kaila et al., 1992)—these effects were also demonstrated by *Bifidobacterium bifidum* and *B. breve* (Roller et al., 2004; Yasui et al., 1999). These effects may be clinically important in the viral immune response, as demonstrated by increasing IgA production to rotaviruses in children with rotavirus diarrhea (Majamaa et al., 1995). In addition, numerous studies have also demonstrated a probiotic effect at limiting aberrant, excessive intestinal inflammation seen in inflammatory bowel disease through modulating the T-cell-driven process (Pavan et al., 2003; Rachmilewitz et al., 2004).

Effects on Protection from Pathogenic Infections

A simple study provides some insight into the potential of certain probiotics to interfere with intestinal pathogens. Shu and colleagues (2000) documented the ability of *B. lactis* HN019 to protect conventionally colonized mice from lethality caused by *Salmonella typhimurium* (see Figure B-33). In addition to their improved survival, a higher post-challenge food intake and weight gain and a reduced pathogen translocation to spleen and liver was observed. These results were correlated with improved immune parameters. Similar results were observed using a synbiotic (i.e., a mixture of prebiotic and probiotic) product (Asahara et al., 2001). Using a Shiga toxin-producing *E. coli* (STEC) model of infection in mice, *B. breve* strain Yakult also decreased mortality (Asahara et al., 2004). Interestingly, neither *B. bifidum* ATCC 15696 nor *B. catenulatum* ATCC 27539 had the ability to reduce STEC-induced mortality in this model, perhaps due to the fact that the *B. breve* strain produced a high quantity of acetic acid in the feces, but the *B. bifidum* or *B. cantenulatum* strains did not.

The clinical relevance of these effects is less certain. A 4 to 7 day (until discharged from the hospital) treatment of preterm infants with *L. rhamnosus* GG failed to prevent urinary tract infections, necrotizing enterocolitis, or sepsis (Dani et al., 2002). This same strain failed to prevent urinary tract infections in women with a history of previous infections (Kontiokari et al., 2001). A mixture of five probiotics failed to eradicate *H. pylori* infection, although some suppression was demonstrated. In another study, *L. plantarum* 299V was administered in a juice drink for one week before and after elective surgery. No differences in gastric colonization (assessed by nasogastric aspirates); bacterial translocation (assessed by culture of a mesenteric lymph node and serosal scraping at laparotomy);

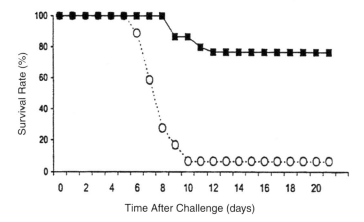

FIGURE B-33 Survival rate of conventionally colonized mice fed *B. lactis* DR10 or no supplement following a single challenge with *Salmonella typhimurium* (○, control mice; ■, mice fed *B. lactis*).
SOURCE: Shu et al. (2000).

or septic complications were observed as compared with the control group (McNaught et al., 2002). A second study with similar endpoints was conducted on patients undergoing elective abdominal surgery. Two weeks before their surgery, 72 patients were given either a placebo or a synbiotic preparation containing *L. acidophilus* La5, *B. lactis* Bb12, *S. thermophilus*, *L. bulgaricus,* and oligofructose. The resulting lack of differences in bacterial translocation, systemic inflammation, or septic complications questions the benefit of this synbiotic intervention (Anderson et al., 2004).

The results of studies using probiotics and/or prebiotics to prevent travelers' diarrhea or minimize its symptoms are mixed. One study followed British soldiers deployed to Belize. Soldiers were given one of three preparations (*L. fermentum* KLD, *L. acidophilus* LA, or placebo). Although the probiotic was administered at a high dose (2×10^{11}/day), no improvement in the incidence of diarrhea was observed after three weeks administration (Katelaris et al., 1995). FOS (10 g/day) was not shown to improve symptoms in a randomized, double-blind, placebo-controlled study of 244 healthy subjects traveling to different destinations and, in fact, increased flatulence (Cummings et al., 2001). Studies using probiotics to prevent travelers diarrhea have generated both positive and negative results (de dios Pozo-Olano et al., 1978; Oksanen et al., 1990).

Effects on Decreasing Duration of Enteric Infections

Pro- and prebiotics have been investigated as a means of decreasing symptoms from enteric infections. Of potentially direct relevance to the population of interest in combat nutrition is a study that demonstrated a benefit in acute amebiasis. In a study of 57 adults, using *Saccharomyces boulardii* as an adjunct to antibiotic therapy in the treatment of acute amebiasis decreased the duration of clinical symptoms and cyst passage (Mansour-Ghanaei et al., 2003).

Supplementation with prebiotics may be of benefit in decreasing symptoms from diarrhea as well, perhaps by mechanisms that may not only alter gut microbiota but also enhance fluid reabsorbtion through the colon. This may be accomplished by the conversion of complex carbohydrates to short chain fatty acids by bacteria and subsequent use by a short chain fatty acid-sodium transporter in colonocytes. Ramakrishna and coworkers (2000) supplemented oral rehydration solution with amylase-resistant starch in a study of adults and adolescents with cholera. They found that fecal weight and duration of diarrhea were reduced by the addition of this prebiotic.

Probiotics have been studied extensively with the aim of decreasing duration of symptoms in children with acute illness. A meta-analysis of 18 studies of coadministration of probiotics with oral rehydration demonstrated a shorter duration of the disease (Huang et al., 2002). Supplementation of infant cereal with a prebiotic in two randomized controlled trials did not demonstrate any difference in infant diarrhea, frequency of use of medical resources or response to immunizations. However, these trials were done in infants who also were being breastfed, and breast milk contains significant amounts of complex carbohydrates with prebiotic properties (Duggan et al., 2003).

A fermented milk product containing a probiotic strain of *L. casei* DN-114001 did not prevent gastrointestinal or respiratory infection in an elderly population (Turchet et al., 2003), but it did reduce the duration of infections.

The infection rate observed in brain injury patients was lower (50 percent compared with 100 percent) and the length of hospitalization was shorter (10 compared with 22 days) in a group receiving a probiotic- and glutamine-supplemented enteral diet than in a control group receiving the unsupplemented enteral diet (Falcao de Arruda and de Aguilar-Nascimento, 2004). This study, however, evaluated only 10 patients per group.

The effects of probiotics on the prevention and treatment of symptoms associated with consumption of antibiotics have been evaluated in several studies. The majority of these studies were conducted with a yeast, *Saccharomyces boulardii*, which has been shown to have a specific ability to decrease recurrence of *Clostridium difficile* infection (Surawicz, 2003). A study of a probiotic and prebiotic treatment was effective in reducing antibiotic associated diarrhea (AAD) in children (La Rosa et al., 2003). The probiotic used in this study was listed as a "Lactobacillus sporogenes." This is not a recognized species of *Lacto-*

bacillus, but is more likely a species of *Bacillus* (Sanders et al., 2001). A meta-analysis concluded that *S. boulardii* and lactobacilli have the potential to reduce frequency of AAD incidence; however, benefits from probiotic treatment remain to be proven (D'Souza et al., 2002). This conclusion was challenged (Beckly and Lewis, 2002), and several reports documenting probiotic administration having no effect on AAD have been published (Lewis et al., 1998; Takanow et al., 1990; Thomas et al., 2001). Furthermore, the biological basis for conducting a meta-analysis on studies using such different probiotic preparations as a yeast and bacterium is questionable.

Effects on Colitis

Inflammation can lead to a breakdown of the gut barrier, leaving the host more susceptible to the translocation of infectious agents and autoimmune responses. The manner in which the immune components manage to discriminate (and respond) between foreign microbes and the diverse microbe population of the intestinal tract (approximately 2 kg) is gradually being deciphered. Tolerance towards the intestinal microbe population may derive from the reaction of commensal microbiota with immune components and consequently from prevention of innate immune responses. For example, an important class of transmembrane proteins, various toll-like receptors (TLRs), react specifically with bacteria (both commensal and pathogenic) and their components (Rakoff-Nahoum et al., 2004).

Rodent (Pavan et al., 2003; Rachmilewitz et al., 2004) and human (Gionchetti et al., 2003) models of gut inflammation have been used to assess the ability of different probiotic bacteria or blends of bacteria to downregulate the inflammatory response. For example, a rat model was used to demonstrate the effects of *L. farciminis*, a producer of nitric oxide, on colitis. In colitic rats, *L. farciminis* treatment reduced several markers of inflammation (macroscopic damage scores, myeloperoxidase and nitric oxide synthase activities) as compared with controls. Hemoglobin, used as a nitric oxide scavenger, negated the anti-inflammatory effect if infused colonically, suggesting the role of nitric oxide in mediating this anti-inflammatory effect. Oral administration of nitric oxide-producing *L. farciminis* improved 2,4,6-trinitrobenzene sulfonic acid-induced colitis in rats. Nitric oxide is a smooth muscle dilator produced in situ by intestinal bacteria. However, no evidence has been published about its ability to provide relief from intestinal cramping.

In humans, the most compelling data come from studies conducted on subjects with pouchitis (inflammation of the internal mucosa of a pouch, part of the small intestine created as a neo-rectum in postcolectomy patients having had ulcerative colitis). Administration of high levels (9×10^{11} viable lyophilized bacteria/day) of a commercial probiotic product, VSL#3 (comprising eight different species of *Streptococcus*, *Lactobacillus,* and *Bifidobacterium*) extended remission (Gionchetti et al., 2003). None of the 20 patients receiving the placebo maintained remission, while 17 of 20 patients receiving active treatment maintained remission for at least nine months.

While these studies are important in showing the distinct and dramatic effects of probiotics on gut inflammation, these results may not be directly relevant to formulation of combat rations because they were conducted with ill subjects.

EFFECTS ON DEVELOPMENT OF KIDNEY STONES

The gut microbiota have been hypothesized to play a role in oxalate accumulation in the urine. The absence of *Oxalobacter formigenes* from fecal microbiota has been shown to be a risk factor in the development of kidney stones (Mittal et al., 2003). Manipulation of the gut microbiota has been proposed to reduce the risk of kidney stones. No studies in humans have documented that probiotic administration reduces the incidence of kidney stones. However, animal and human studies have documented that *O. formigenes* can establish itself in the gut and reduce the urinary oxalate concentration (Duncan et al., 2002; Sidhu et al., 2001).

EFFECTS ON ALLERGIC RESPONSES

Although the best studies on allergy are with infants and the prevention of atopic dermatitis, one study does show the ability of viable yogurt bacteria to reduce the symptoms associated with allergies in healthy college students. Trapp and colleagues (1993) studied the effects of the long-term consumption (12 months) of 200 g yogurt daily compared with pasteurized yogurt or no yogurt on self-reported symptoms and immune parameters in young (n = 42) and senior (n = 56) adults. This study was a follow-up to a previous study showing that consumption of yogurt for four months led to a 4 fold increase in γ-interferon in adults (Halpern et al., 1991). In this study, 200 g of daily yogurt (Y), pasteurized yogurt (PY), or no yogurt (NY) was consumed by the two age groups. The number of subjects in each of the six resulting groups was not disclosed in the paper. The paper also did not clarify the microbiological content of the yogurt, so it is likely that the yogurt ("similar to commercially available low-fat yogurt") only contained *L. bulgaricus* and *S. thermophilus* at levels $> 10^8$ cfu/gram. Health questionnaires that were completed weekly provided data on the incidence of a variety of gastrointestinal, respiratory, and skin symptoms. Blood samples yielded results on blood cell count and chemistry (including blood lipids and γ-glutamyl transpeptidase [GTT]). Interferon, immunoglobulin E (IgE), and antibody titers to a pneumococcal vaccine were also assessed. The young-adult Y group recorded a significantly lower frequency of allergies and itching as compared with both the PY and NY groups. The senior Y group recorded a significant decrease in allergies over time. Interestingly, the senior NY group recorded a steady increase in total cholesterol and LDL (6.4 percent increase), which did not occur in the Y or PY groups. Gamma-glutamyl transpeptidase, a liver enzyme associated with fat and/or alcohol or drug metabolism, decreased only in the Y or PY groups. In general the groups consuming yogurt rated their overall health as better than that in the NY group. Total serum IgE was lower for senior subjects in the Y or PY groups. No other statistically significant differences were seen among groups.

PRACTICAL CONSIDERATIONS FOR USE

Several issues should be considered before the use of a pro- or prebiotic in any product, including combat rations.

Probiotic Strain Selection and Prebiotic Selection

There are many probiotic strains commercially available that have been studied for efficacy in humans. Despite the wealth of information available on probiotics, it can be difficult to determine the best strains for a particular situation, such as for healthy soldiers under short-term, high-stress combat situations. Strains such as *B. lactis* HN019, *B. lactis* BB12, *L. rhamnosus* GG, and *L. plantarum* 299V have a solid basis of scientific support and might be good strains to consider initially. It may be prudent to restrict probiotic strains to species of lactobacilli or bifidobacteria to minimize any safety risk. The best candidate prebiotics for this application would be fructooligosaccharides, including inulin, or galactooligosaccharides. Careful review of scientific documentation for commercial strains of probiotics and prebiotics under consideration with attention to the desired effect must be the basis for strain selection for combat rations.

Safety and Efficacy

The use of pro- and prebiotics in the human diet is not new. Many species of probiotics have been tested for tolerance in humans and have been sold in the supplement and food market for years. However, many other species have not been tested or may carry unnecessary risk. Generally, the pathogenic potential of probiotic species of lactobacilli and bifidobacteria is considered to be quite low (Boriello et al., 2003). If the product developed is in the "drug" category, then the concept of risk versus benefit should be considered. Lactobacilli and bifidobacteria have a very low pathogenic potential, a conclusion supported by several international groups (Borriello et al., 2003; FAO/WHO, 2002). However, probiotics of other genera (e.g., *Enterococcus*, *Escherichia*) should be carefully screened for characteristics that may present risks of antibiotic transfer or infectivity.

Prebiotics must be used at levels that provide selective stimulation of the growth or activity of beneficial native bacteria but at the same time do not result in unpleasant side effects. The level used must be determined for the specific prebiotic under consideration. Side effects can be minimized through a gradual increase in dose.

Strains of probiotics and types of prebiotics should be chosen using science-based evidence for efficacy in humans, ideally in the subjects of interest. Unfortunately, there are no published reports on the efficacy of any prebiotics or probiotic strains to be used for combat troops.

The dose of a pro- or prebiotic is an important consideration, and it should be based on studies showing a physiological effect and lack of significant safety risks. Generally, the higher the level of probiotics, the greater effect observed. With prebiotics, however, if the dose is too high, there is a risk of adverse gastrointestinal effects (diarrhea, gas) or loss of specificity of the effect. Most research studies have used a dose of 5 to 12 g/day, which is a reasonable target.

Stability

For probiotics, stability of the microorganisms is critical for effectiveness but its maintenance can present challenges. For example, viability depends on many factors, including temperature, moisture, atmosphere, pH, and the surrounding matrix. Typically, cell counts can be maintained for one year at room temperature in a freeze-dried state in unopened packages. However, when they are added to food, their stability might be altered and should be tested in the food matrix. For prebiotics, however, stability as supplements or in food matrices is not a concern.

SUMMARY

Existing data are insufficient to make definite strong recommendations for inclusion of pro- or prebiotics as part of a combat ration provided to soldiers for three to seven days. Adequate studies both on this specific population and on the duration of consumption have not been performed. While immune and intestinal benefits have been demonstrated in a variety of settings and populations, some assumptions are required to extrapolate these results to this particular application. Nevertheless, a strong potential exists in using pro- or prebiotics to prevent or decrease symptoms from enteric illnesses. To take advantage of these benefits, we recommend that pro- and prebiotics be evaluated for administration to individuals in the weeks or months before and during the period of combat ration use. The use of these compounds for a longer period may result in beneficial effects during the period of combat stress.

Stability challenges of keeping probiotics alive under the conditions of storage may preclude their incorporation into soldiers' rations, even if efficacy data strongly supported their inclusion. However, this is not a limitation of prebiotics. Although there are limits to the evidence supporting the efficacy of prebiotics in this specific application, it should be recognized that a basal level of prebiotics (approximately 5 g/day) is consumed as part of the normal American diet. Even this low level is likely not present in the soldiers' rations. Therefore, supplementing the rations with this minimal level may provide some support for intestinal function that could be beneficial with essentially no risk. Nourishment of the gut with fiber in the form of these prebiotics could be very worthwhile.

Research priorities that would help advance this field and allow for the possible practical application of pro- and prebiotics to combat rations belong to two broad categories: questions regarding the human microbial biome and more specific issues concerning pro- and prebiotics in the combat population: (1) defining the complete complement or biome (populations and activities) of normal intestinal microbes; (2) understanding the stability of normal intestinal microbiota to resist perturbations and infection; (3) detailing the response of that complement of microbes to diet, stress, drugs, and daily lifestyle fluctuations; and (4) understanding the mechanisms of communication between microbial and host cells.

Before prebiotics or probiotics can be applied to the military population and conditions, specific studies need to be developed to address (1) preventing gastrointestinal illness in soldiers in field conditions; (2) decreasing morbidity and enhancing recovery from a variety of noncombat related illnesses; and (3) using pro- and prebiotics in other areas of interest to this population, such as increase in nutrient utilization; effects on stamina and fatigue; and using of bioengineered probiotics for the delivery of other compounds such as those that may be important for dealing with fatigue resistance or wound healing. Furthermore, to assess the potential benefits for soldiers, more information is needed about noncombat morbidity and risk factors for soldiers to develop infections or other health problems.

In summary, pro- and prebiotics may provide a very low risk intervention for supporting gastrointestinal and immune function. They are quite compatible in dairy-based formats (drinkable yogurt, for example) or as nutritional supplements. Key questions on the extent of these ingredients' effects on healthy populations, their mechanisms of action, and the parameters for their optimal use remain to be researched. With current knowledge, it is reasonable to recommend a basal level of prebiotic supplementation of combat rations. However, additional research on soldier populations should be conducted before the inclusion of probiotics in combat rations can be recommended.

ACKNOWLEDGMENTS

Thanks to Dominique Brassart, Lorenzo Morelli, and Glenn Gibson for their perspectives on this topic.

REFERENCES

Anderson AD, McNaught CE, Jain PK, MacFie J. 2004. Randomised clinical trial of synbiotic therapy in elective surgical patients. *Gut* 53(2):241–245.

Arunachalam K, Gill HS, Chandra RK. 2000. Enhancement of natural immune function by dietary consumption of *Bifidobacterium lactis* (Hn019). *Eur J Clin Nutr* 54(3):263–267.

Asahara T, Nomoto K, Shimizu K, Watanuki M, Tanaka R. 2001. Increased resistance of mice to Salmonella enterica serovar typhimurium infection by synbiotic administration of Bifidobacteria and transgalactosylated oligosaccharides. *J Appl Microbiol* 91(6):985–996.

Asahara T, Shimizu K, Nomoto K, Hamabata T, Ozawa A, Takeda Y. 2004. Probiotic bifidobacteria protect mice from lethal infection with Shiga toxin-producing *Escherichia coli* O157:H7. *Infect Immun* 72(4):2240–2247.

Backhed F, Ding H, Wang T, Hooper LV, Koh GY, Nagy A, Semenkovich CF, Gordon JI. 2004. The gut microbiota as an environmental factor that regulates fat storage. *Proc Natl Acad Sci USA* 101(44):15718–15723.

Beckly J, Lewis S. 2002. The case for probiotics ramains unproven. *Br Med J* 325(7350):902.

Bengmark S. 2003. Use of some pre-, pro- and synbiotics in critically ill patients. *Best Pract Res Clin Gastroenterol* 17(5):833–848.

Borriello SP, Hammes WP, Holzapfel W, Marteau P, Schrezenmeir J, Vaara M, Valtonen V. 2003. Safety of probiotics that contain lactobacilli or bifidobacteria. *Clin Infect Dis* 36(6):775–780.

Bouhnik Y, Vahedi K, Achour L, Attar A, Salfati J, Pochart P, Marteau P, Flourie B, Bornet F, Rambaud JC. 1999. Short-chain fructo-oligosaccharide administration dose-dependently increases fecal bifidobacteria in healthy humans. *J Nutr* 129(1):113–116.

Buddington RK, Williams CH, Chen SC, Witherly SA. 1996. Dietary supplement of neosugar alters the fecal flora and decreases activities of aome reductive enzymes in human subjects. *Am J Clin Nutr* 63(5):709–716.

Campbell JM, Fahey GC Jr, Wolf BW. 1997. Selected indigestible oligosaccharides affect large bowel mass, cecal and fecal short-chain fatty acids, pH and microflora in rats. *J Nutr* 127(1):130–136.

Chiang BL, Sheih YH, Wang LH, Liao CK, Gill HS. 2000. Enhancing immunity by dietary consumption of a probiotic lactic acid bacterium (*Bifidobacterium lactis* HN019): Optimization and definition of cellular immune responses. *Eur J Clin Nutr* 54(11):849–855.

Cremonini F, Di Caro S, Covino M, Armuzzi A, Gabrielli M, Santarelli L, Nista EC, Cammarota G, Gasbarrini G, Gasbarrini A. 2002. Effect of different probiotic preparations on anti-helicobacter pylori therapy-related side effects: A parallel group, triple blind, placebo-controlled study. *Am J Gastroenterol* 97(11):2744–2749.

Cruchet S, Obregon MC, Salazar G, Diaz E, Gotteland M. 2003. Effect of the ingestion of a dietary product containing *Lactobacillus johnsonii* La1 on *Helicobacter pylori* colonization in children. *Nutrition* 19(9):716-721.

Cummings JH, Christie S, Cole TJ. 2001. A study of fructo oligosaccharides in the prevention of travellers' diarrhoea. *Aliment Pharmacol Ther* 15(8):1139–1145.

Dani C, Biadaioli R, Bertini G, Martelli E, Rubaltelli FF. 2002. Probiotics feeding in prevention of urinary tract infection, bacterial sepsis and necrotizing enterocolitis in preterm infants. A prospective double-blind study. *Biol Neonate* 82(2):103–108.

de dios Pozo-Olano J, Warram JH Jr, Gomez RG, Cavazos MG. 1978. Effect of a lactobacilli preparation on traveler's diarrhea. A randomized, double blind clinical trial. *Gastroenterology* 74(5 Pt 1):829–830.

de Vrese M, Stegelmann A, Richter B, Fenselau S, Laue C, Schrezenmeir J. 2001. Probiotics— Compensation for lactase insufficiency. *Am J Clin Nutr* 73(2 Suppl):421S–429S.

D'Souza AL, Rajkumar C, Cooke J, Bulpitt CJ. 2002. Probiotics in prevention of antibiotic associated diarrhoea: Meta-analysis. *Br Med J* 324(7350):1361–1364.

Duggan C, Penny ME, Hibberd P, Gil A, Huapaya A, Cooper A, Coletta F, Emenhiser C, Kleinman RE. 2003. Oligofructose-supplemented infant cereal: 2 randomized, blinded, community-based trials in peruvian infants. *Am J Clin Nutr* 77(4):937–942.

Duncan SH, Richardson AJ, Kaul P, Holmes RP, Allison MJ, Stewart CS. 2002. *Oxalobacter formigenes* and its potential role in human health. *Appl Environ Microbiol* 68(8):3841–3847.

Eijsink VG, Axelsson L, Diep DB, Havarstein LS, Holo H, Nes IF. 2002. Production of class II bacteriocins by lactic acid bacteria. An example of biological warfare and communication. *Antonie Van Leeuwenhoek* 81(1–4):639–654.

Falcao de Arruda IS, de Aguilar-Nascimento JE. 2004. Benefits of early enteral nutrition with glutamine and probiotics in brain injury patients. *Clin Sci* 106(3):287–292.

FAO/WHO (Food and Agriculture Organization/World Health Organization). 2002. *Guidelines for the Evaluation of Probiotics in Food*. Geneva, Switzerland: FAO/WHO.

Garcia-Lafuente A, Antolin M, Guarner F, Crespo E, Malagelada JR. 2001. Modulation of colonic barrier function by the composition of the commensal flora in the rat. *Gut* 48(4):503–507.

Gibson GR, Roberfroid MB. 1995. Dietary modulation of the human colonic microbiota: Introducing the concept of prebiotics. *J Nutr* 125(6):1401–1412.

Gill HS. 1999. Potential of using dietary lactic acid bacteria for enhancement of immunity. *Dialogue* 32:6–11. New Zealand Dairy Advisory Bureau.

Gill HS. 2003. Probiotics to enhance anti-infective defences in the gastrointestinal tract. *Best Pract Res Clin Gastroenterol* 17(5):755–773.

Gill HS, Darragh AJ, Cross ML. 2001a. Optimizing immunity and gut function in the elderly. *J Nutr Health Aging* 5(2):80–91.

Gill HS, Rutherfurd KJ, Cross ML. 2001b. Dietary probiotic supplementation enhances natural killer cell activity in the elderly: An investigation of age-related immunological changes. *J Clin Immunol* 21(4):264–271.

Gill HS, Rutherfurd KJ, Cross ML, Gopal PK. 2001c. Enhancement of immunity in the elderly by dietary supplementation with the probiotic *Bifidobacterium lactis* HN019. *Am J Clin Nutr* 74(6):833–839.

Gionchetti P, Rizzello F, Helwig U, Venturi A, Lammers KM, Brigidi P, Vitali B, Poggioli G, Miglioli M, Campieri M. 2003. Prophylaxis of pouchitis onset with probiotic therapy: A double-blind, placebo-controlled trial. *Gastroenterology* 124(5):1202–1209.

Gudiel-Urbano M, Goni I. 2002. Effect of short-chain fructooligosaccharides and cellulose on cecal enzyme activities in rats. *Ann Nutr Metab* 46(6):254–258.

Halpern GM, Vruwink KG, Van de Water J, Keen CL, Gershwin ME. 1991. Influence of long-term yoghurt consumption in young adults. *Int J Immunotherapy* 7(4):205–210.

Hatakka K, Savilahti E, Ponka A, Meurman JH, Poussa T, Nase L, Saxelin M, Korpela R. 2001. Effect of long term consumption of probiotic milk on infections in children attending day care centres: Double blind, randomised trial. *Br Med J* 322(7298):1327–1329.

Huang JS, Bousvaros A, Lee JW, Diaz A, Davidson EJ. 2002. Efficacy of probiotic use in acute diarrhea in children: A meta-analysis. *Dig Dis Sci* 47(11):2625–2634.

Ishikawa H, Akedo I, Umesaki Y, Tanaka R, Imaoka A, Otani T. 2003. Randomized controlled trial of the effect of bifidobacteria-fermented milk on ulcerative colitis. *J Am Coll Nutr* 22(1): 56–63.

Isolauri E, Joensuu J, Suomalainen H, Luomala M, Vesikari T. 1995. Improved immunogenicity of oral D x RRV reassortant rotavirus vaccine by *Lactobacillus casei* GG. *Vaccine* 13(3):310–312.

Kaila M, Isolauri E, Soppi E, Virtanen E, Laine S, Arvilommi H. 1992. Enhancement of the circulating antibody secreting cell response in human diarrhea by a human *Lactobacillus* strain. *Pediatr Res* 32(2):141–144.

Kalliomaki M, Salminen S, Arvilommi H, Kero P, Koskinen P, Isolauri E. 2001. Probiotics in primary prevention of atopic disease: A randomised placebo-controlled trial. *Lancet* 357(9262):1076–1079.

Kalliomaki M, Salminen S, Poussa T, Arvilommi H, Isolauri E. 2003. Probiotics and prevention of atopic disease: 4-year follow-up of a randomised placebo-controlled trial. *Lancet* 361(9372):1869–1871.

Katelaris PH, Salam I, Farthing MJ. 1995. Lactobacilli to prevent traveler's diarrhea? *N Engl J Med* 333(20):1360–1361.

Kishi A, Uno K, Matsubara Y, Okuda C, Kishida T. 1996. Effect of the oral administration of *Lactobacillus brevis* subsp. *coagulans* on interferon-alpha producing capacity in humans. *J Am Coll Nutr* 15(4):408–412.

Kleessen B, Sykura B, Zunft HJ, Blaut M. 1997. Effects of inulin and lactose on fecal microflora, microbial activity, and bowel habit in elderly constipated persons. *Am J Clin Nutr* 65(5):1397–1402.

Kontiokari T, Sundqvist K, Nuutinen M, Pokka T, Koskela M, Uhari M. 2001. Randomised trial of cranberry-lingonberry juice and Lactobacillus GG drink for the prevention of urinary tract infections in women. *Br Med J* 322(7302):1571–1575.

La Rosa M, Bottaro G, Gulino N, Gambuzza F, Di Forti F, Ini G, Tornambe E. 2003. Prevention of antibiotic-associated diarrhea with *Lactobacillus spororgens* and furcto-oligosaccharides in children. A multicentric double-blind vs placebo study. *Minerva Pediatr* 55(5):447–452.

Lewis SJ, Potts LF, Barry RE. 1998. The lack of therapeutic effect of *Saccharomyces boulardii* in the prevention of antibiotic-related diarrhoea in elderly patients. *J Infect* 36(2):171–174.

Link-Amster H, Rochat F, Saudan KY, Mignot O, Aeschlimann JM. 1994. Modulation of a specific humoral immune response and changes in intestinal flora mediated through fermented milk intake. *FEMS Immunol Med Microbiol* 10(1):55–63.

Linsalata M, Russo F, Berloco P, Caruso ML, Matteo GD, Cifone MG, Simone CD, Ierardi E, Di Leo A. 2004. The influence of *Lactobacillus brevis* on ornithine decarboxylase activity and polyamine profiles in *Helicobacter pylori*-infected gastric mucosa. *Helicobacter* 9(2):165–172.

Mack DR, Ahrne S, Hyde L, Wei S, Hollingsworth MA. 2003. Extracellular MUC3 mucin secretion follows adherence of *Lactobacillus* strains to intestinal epithelial cells in vitro. *Gut* 52(6):827–833.

Majamaa H, Isolauri E, Saxelin M, Vesikari T. 1995. Lactic acid bacteria in the treatment of acute rotavirus gastroenteritis. *J Ped Gastroenterol Nutr* 20(3):333–338.

Mansour-Ghanaei F, Dehbashi N, Yazdanparast K, Shafaghi A. 2003. Efficacy of *Saccharomyces boulardii* with antibiotics in acute amoebiasis. *World J Gastroenterol* 9(8):1832–1833.

McNaught CE, Woodcock NP, MacFie J, Mitchell CJ. 2002. A prospective randomised study of the probiotic *Lactobacillus plantarum* 299V on indices of gut barrier function in elective surgical patients. *Gut* 51(6):827–831.

Mimura T, Rizzello F, Helwig U, Poggioli G, Schreiber S, Talbot IC, Nicholls RJ, Gionchetti P, Campieri M, Kamm MA. 2004. Once daily high dose probiotic therapy (VSL#3) for maintaining remission in recurrent or refractory pouchitis. *Gut* 53(1):108–114.

Mittal RD, Kumar R, Mittal B, Prasad R, Bhandari M. 2003. Stone composition, metabolic profile and the presence of the gut-inhabiting bacterium *Oxalobacter formigenes* as risk factors for renal stone formation. *Med Princ Pract* 12(4):208–213.

Nagao F, Nakayama M, Muto T, Okumura K. 2000. Effects of a fermented milk drink containing *Lactobacillus casei* strain Shirota on the immune system in healthy human subjects. *Biosci Biotechnol Biochem* 64(12):2706–2708.

Nase L, Hatakka K, Savilahti E, Saxelin M, Ponka A, Poussa T, Korpela R, Meurman JH. 2001. Effect of long-term consumption of a probiotic bacterium, *Lactobacillus rhamnosus* GG, in milk on dental caries and caries risk in children. *Caries Res* 35(6):412–420.

Niedzielin K, Kordecki H, Birkenfeld B. 2001. A controlled, double-blind, randomized study on the efficacy of *Lactobacillus plantarum* 299V in patients with irritable bowel syndrome. *Eur J Gastroenterol Hepatol* 13(10):1143–1147.

Oksanen PJ, Salminen S, Saxelin M, Hamalainen P, Ihantola-Vormisto A, Muurasniemi-Isoviita L, Nikkari S, Oksanen T, Porsti I, Salminen E. 1990. Prevention of travellers' diarrhoea by Lacto-bacillus GG. *Ann Med* 22(1):53–56.

Pavan S, Desreumaux P, Mercenier A. 2003. Use of mouse models to evaluate the persistence, safety, and immune modulation capacities of lactic acid bacteria. *Clin Diagn Lab Immunol* 10(4):696–701.

Rachmilewitz D, Katakura K, Karmeli F, Hayashi T, Reinus C, Rudensky B, Akira S, Takeda K, Lee J, Takabayashi K, Raz E. 2004. Toll-like receptor 9 signaling mediates the anti-inflammatory effects of probiotics in murine experimental colitis. *Gastroenterology* 126(2):520–528.

Rakoff-Nahoum S, Paglino J, Eslami-Varzaneh F, Edberg S, Medzhitov R. 2004. Recognition of commensal microflora by toll-like receptors is required for intestinal homeostasis. *Cell* 118(2):229–241.

Ramakrishna BS, Venkataraman S, Srinivasan P, Dash P, Young GP, Binder HJ. 2000. Amylase-resistant starch plus oral rehydration solution for cholera. *N Engl J Med* 342(5):308–313.

Resta-Lenert S, Barrett KE. 2003. Live probiotics protect intestinal epithelial cells from the effects of infection with enteroinvasive *Escherichia coli* (EIEC). *Gut* 52(7):988–997.

Roberfroid MB, Cumps J, Devogelaer JP. 2002. Dietary chicory inulin increases whole-body bone mineral density in growing male rats. *J Nutr* 132(12):3599–3602.

Roller M, Rechkemmer G, Watzl B. 2004. Prebiotic inulin enriched with oligofructose in combina-tion with the probiotics *Lactobacillus rhamnosus* and *Bifidobacterium lactis* modulates intestinal immune functions in rats. *J Nutr* 134(1):153–156.

Sanders ME, Morelli L, Bush S. 2001. *Lactobacillus sporogenes* is not a *Lactobacillus* probiotic. *ASM News* 67(8):385–386.

Saxelin M, Elo S, Salminen S, Vapaatalo H. 1991. Dose response colonization of faeces after oral administration of *Lactobacillus casei* strain GG. *Microbial Ecol Health Dis* 4:209–214.

Schiffrin EJ, Brassart D, Servin AL, Rochat F, Donnet-Hughes A. 1997. Immune modulation of blood leukocytes in humans by lactic acid bacteria: Criteria for strain selection. *Am J Clin Nutr* 66(2):515S–520S.

Seksik P, Rigottier-Gois L, Gramet G, Sutren M, Pochart P, Marteau P, Jian R, Dore J. 2003. Alterations of the dominant faecal bacterial groups in patients with Crohn's disease of the colon. *Gut* 52(2):237–242.

Sheih YH, Chiang BL, Wang LH, Liao CK, Gill HS. 2001. Systemic immunity-enhancing effects in healthy subjects following dietary consumption of the lactic acid bacterium *Lactobacillus rhamnosus* HN001. *J Am Coll Nutr* 20(2 Suppl):149–156.

Shu Q, Lin H, Rutherfurd KJ, Fenwick SG, Prasad J, Gopal PK, Gill HS. 2000. Dietary Bifidobacterium lactis (HN019) enhances resistance to oral *Salmonella typhimurium* infection in mice. *Microbiol Immunol* 44(4):213–222.

Sidhu H, Allison MJ, Chow JM, Clark A, Peck AB. 2001. Rapid reversal of hyperoxaluria in a rat model after probiotic administration of *Oxalobacter formigenes*. *J Urol* 166(4):1487–1491.

Surawicz CM. 2003. Probiotics, antibiotic-associated diarrhoea and *Clostridium* difficile diarrhoea in humans. *Best Pract Res Clin Gastroenterol* 17(5):775–783.

Takanow RM, Ross MB, Eretel IN, Dickinson DG, McCormick LS Garfinkel JF. 1990. A double-blind, placebo-controlled study of the efficacy of lactinex in the prophylaxis of amoxicillin-induced diarrhea. *DECP Ann Pharmacother* 224:(38)2–4.

Tamboli CP, Caucheteux C, Cortot A, Colombel JF, Desreumaux P. 2003. Probiotics in inflamma-tory bowel disease: A critical review. *Best Pract Res Clin Gastroenterol* 17(5):805–820.

Thomas MR, Litin SC, Osmon DR, Corr AP, Weaver AL, Lohse CM. 2001. Lack of effect of *Lactobacillus* GG on antibiotic-associated diarrhea: A randomized, placebo-controlled trial. *Mayo Clin Proc* 76(9):883–889.

Trapp DL, Chang CC, Halpern GM, Keen CL, Gershwin ME. 1993. The influence of chronic yogurt consumption on populations of young and elderly adults. *Int J Immunotherapy* IX:53–64.

Turchet P, Laurenzano M, Auboiron S, Antoine JM. 2003. Effect of fermented milk containing the probiotic *Lactobacillus casei* DN-114 001 on winter infections in free-living elderly subjects: A randomised, controlled pilot study. *J Nutr Health Aging* 7(2):75–77.

Valeur N, Engel P, Carbajal N, Connolly E, Ladefoged K. 2004. Colonization and immunomodulation by *Lactobacillus reuteri* ATCC 55730 in the human gastrointestinal tract. *Appl Environ Microbiol* 70(2):1176–1181.

Van Niel CW, Feudtner C, Garrison MM, Christakis DA. 2002. Lactobacillus therapy for acute infectious diarrhea in children: A meta-analysis. *Pediatrics* 109(4):678–684.

Vanderhoof JA, Whitney DB, Antonson DL, Hanner TL, Lupo JV, Young RJ. 1999. *Lactobacillus* GG in the prevention of antibiotic-associated diarrhea in children. *J Pediatr* 135(5):564–568.

Yasui H, Shida K, Matsuzaki T, Yokokura T. 1999. Immunomodulatory function of lactic acid bacteria. *Antonie Van Leeuwenhoek* 76(1–4):383–389.

Developing a Low Residue Diet

Joanne L. Slavin, University of Minnesota

LOW-RESIDUE DIETS

A low-residue (low-fiber) diet[1] is for people who need to care for their intestinal tracts. This diet limits the amount of food waste that moves through the large intestine, which should help control diarrhea and abdominal cramping. Low-residue diets are also recommended for diverticulitis, after some types of intestinal surgery such as colostomy or ileostomy, and in the acute phases of certain inflammatory bowel conditions such as ulcerative colitis or Crohn's disease. Diet therapy texts suggest that patients on a low-residue diet avoid foods made with seeds, nuts, or raw or dried fruit; with whole grains; and with raw fruits and vegetables. In addition, they should remove fruit and vegetable skins before cooking, limit dairy consumption to two cups per day, limit fats because they increase stool bulk, and avoid tough, fibrous meats with gristle.

Low-residue diets have been around for a long time, but there is little research in support for their use or effectiveness. Kember and coworkers (1995), in a blind prospective trial of low-residue diet versus normal diet in preparation for barium enema, found no difference in fecal residue between the groups. They recommended that patients just consume their usual diet, rather than the low-residue one before the procedure.

---

[1] In general, a low-residue diet is synonymous with a low-fiber diet.

WHAT IS NORMAL LAXATION?

The term "laxation" describes a wide range of gastrointestinal effects, including stool weight, transit time, bloating and distention, flatus, and constipation, and diarrhea. Digestive problems are one of the most common medical complaints, with 40.5 percent of individuals reporting one or more adverse digestive symptoms in a recent survey (Sandler et al., 2000). Many of these complaints are associated with the consumption of high-fiber foods, such as beans, cabbage, and onions, or with malabsorption of carbohydrates such as lactose. Diarrhea is a potentially life-threatening condition, and although it is associated with a high intake of nondigestible carbohydrates, it is more likely related to the consumption of bacteria-contaminated food, viral infection, irritable bowel syndrome, Crohn's disease, or colonic tumors (Schiller, 2004). Commonly accepted criteria for clinical diarrhea are (1) elevated stool output (> 250 g/day); (2) watery, difficult-to-control bowel movements; and (3) elevated frequency of bowel movements (> 3/day) (McRorie et al., 2000).

In general, stools are about 75 percent water although this is highly variable and increases greatly with diarrhea. Of the remaining stool, about 33 percent is dead bacteria, 33 percent is undigested carbohydrate, and the remaining 33 percent is protein, fat, mucus, dead cells, and inorganic material. Consumption of highly digestible foods and a limited intake of dietary fiber, dairy products, and other poorly digested material will produce a small stool. Although dairy products are typically listed as foods to avoid on a low-residue diet, presumably because of their lactose content, clinical studies that document dairy foods producing more residue are lacking.

Other factors that affect stool size are often noted in studies, but are not well supported by research trials. Stress associated with exams or competition can speed intestinal transit. Exercise is known to speed intestinal transit as well (Oettle, 1991), although data on this topic are conflicting (Bingham and Cummings, 1989). Bingham and Cummings (1989) found that on a controlled dietary intake, transit time increased in nine subjects and decreased in five after participating in a nine-week exercise program. The exercise program did not change other measures of bowel function, stool weight, or fecal frequency. Patients often relate the importance of that morning cup of coffee or smoking on regular bowel habit. Drugs, both laxatives designed to speed transit and others, alter bowel function and fecal composition (Lembo and Camilleri, 2003). Even on rigidly controlled diets of the same composition, subjects had a large variation in daily stool weights. Tucker and colleagues (1981) examined the predictors of stool weight when completely controlled diets were fed to normal volunteers. They found that personality was a better predictor of stool weight than was dietary fiber intake, with outgoing subjects more likely to produce higher stool weights.

DEFINING DIETARY FIBER

Consumption of high-fiber, carbohydrate-based diets protects against life-threatening illnesses such as heart disease, diabetes, obesity, and cancer. Since the mid-1970s, attention has focused on dietary fiber as the active component in this protection. Dietary fiber is generally divided into soluble and insoluble fiber to reflect differences in physiological effects. These descriptors, however, have serious limitations because the effects of dietary fiber in whole foods are often greater than that found with isolated fiber fractions.

The Panel on Dietary Reference Intakes for Macronutrients reviewed the research on dietary fiber and disease prevention to decide whether to set a recommended intake level for dietary fiber. Before their report, there was no Recommended Dietary Allowance (RDA) for dietary fiber. The panel also found in its deliberations that there was no official definition of dietary fiber. Thus, an Institute of Medicine Panel on the Definition of Dietary Fiber was formed to review the existing literature on dietary fiber and to determine its best scientific definition (IOM, 2001). Dietary fiber consists of nondigestible carbohydrates and lignin that are intrinsic and intact in plants. Functional Fiber consists of isolated nondigestible carbohydrates that have beneficial physiological effects in humans. Total fiber is the sum of dietary fiber and functional fiber.

The DRI committee used the updated definitions from the Panel on the Definition of Dietary Fiber for dietary, functional, and total fiber in their report (IOM, 2002). Additionally, they set an Adequate Intake (AI) for total fiber from foods at 38 g and 25 g/day for young men and women, respectively, based on intake levels observed to protect against coronary heart disease (CHD). Adequate Intake is the recommended average daily intake level based on observed or experimentally determined approximations or estimates of nutrient intake by a group (or groups) of apparently healthy people; AI is used when an RDA cannot be determined. The committee concluded that a recommended intake level for total fiber based on the prevention of CHD should be sufficient to reduce constipation in most normal people given an adequacy of hydration of the large bowel. There was insufficient evidence to set a Tolerable Upper Intake Level (UL) for dietary fiber and functional fiber. The usual intake of dietary fiber in the United States is only about 14 grams per day (Martlett et al., 2002). Thus, there is a large fiber gap to fill between usual intake of dietary fiber and recommended intakes.

DEFINING AND MEASURING THE
PHYSIOLOGICAL EFFECTS OF FIBER

The physiological effects of fibers differ and scientists have attempted to categorize fibers according to function, methods of extraction, or solubility. In an attempt to assign physiological effects to chemical types of fiber, scientists classified fibers into soluble and insoluble fiber. Unfortunately, scientific support that soluble fibers can lower serum cholesterol while insoluble fibers can increase stool size is inconsistent at best. A meta-analysis testing the effects of pectin, oat bran, guar gum, and psyllium on blood lipid concentrations found that 2 to 10 g/day of viscous fiber (e.g., oat bran and psyllium) was associated with small, but significant, decreases in total and low-density lipoprotein cholesterol concentrations (Brown et al., 1999). Oat bran lowers serum lipids, but wheat bran does not (Anderson et al., 1991). Resistant starch, generally a soluble fiber, does not affect serum lipids (Jenkins et al., 1998). Thus, not all soluble fibers are hypocholesterolemic agents, and other traits, such as viscosity of fiber, play a role and must be considered.

The insoluble fiber association with laxation also is inconsistent. Fecal weight increases 5.4 g per gram of wheat bran fiber (mostly insoluble), 4.7 g per gram of fruits and vegetables (soluble and insoluble), 3.5 g per gram of isolated cellulose (insoluble), and 1.2 g per gram of isolated pectin (soluble) consumed (Table B-21) (Cummings, 1993). When subjects were fed 15, 30, or 42 g/day of dietary fiber from a mixed diet, there was a significant increase in stool weight on all diets. Most of the increased stool weight was from undigested dietary fiber, although the mid-range of fiber intake was also associated with an increase in bacterial mass (Kurasawa et al., 2000).

Many fiber sources (e.g., oat bran and psyllium) are mostly soluble but still increase stool weight. Not all insoluble fibers (e.g., isolated cellulose) are particularly good at relieving constipation. The disparities between the amounts of soluble and insoluble fiber measured chemically and the magnitude of their physiological effects led the Institute of Medicine Panel on the Definition of Dietary Fiber to recommend that with fiber, the terms "soluble" and "insoluble" gradually be eliminated and replaced by specific beneficial physiological effects of a fiber, perhaps viscosity (the ability of a liquid to resist flow under shear-

TABLE B-21 Average Increase in Fecal Weight Per Gram of Fiber Consumed

Source	Increased Fecal Weight (g/g fiber fed)
Wheat	5.4
Fruits and vegetables	4.7
Gums and mucilages	3.7
Cellulose	3.5
Oats	3.4
Corn	3.3
Legumes	2.2
Pectin	1.2

SOURCE: Cummings (1993), reprinted with permission from CRC Press, Boca Raton, Florida.

stress) and fermentability (ability of a carbohydrate to be converted to alcohol, acids, or other compounds (IOM, 2001).

Perhaps less invasive measures of bowel function could be used to evaluate functional fibers. Bowel movement frequency would not require stool collection and appears to be linked to higher fiber intakes (Sanjoaquin et al., 2004). Another approach would be to model systems for bowel function attributes. A fecal bulking index has been described for rats (Monro, 2004). Other animal models or model systems could be devised standardized, and included in regulations. Noninvasive methods are available to estimate fiber fermentation in humans (Symonds et al., 2004).

SUMMARY

Many of the diseases of public health significance—obesity, cardiovascular disease, type 2 diabetes—as well as the less prevalent, but no less significant, diseases—colonic diverticulosis, constipation, and inflammatory bowel conditions such as ulcerative colitis or Crohn's disease—can be prevented or treated by increasing the consumption of a variety of foods containing various fibers. Promotion of such a food plan by the dietetics professional and implementation by the adult population should increase fiber intakes across the life cycle (Martlett et al., 2002). Since the assault rations are meant for short-term use (three to seven days for up to a month), the prevention of chronic diseases is not a factor considered when recommending dietary fiber.

More relevant to the case of soldiers in military operations are the dietary fiber effects on the prevention of constipation and diarrhea and the maintenance of proper gastrointestinal function. Also, decreasing stool weight and volume would be an advantage for soldiers deployed to these missions. To decrease stool weight, less dietary fiber is advised. The lower limit of dietary fiber intake for small stool size, yet normal bowel function, is difficult to define. With functional fibers, many possibilities are available, shorter or longer chain length, different chemical composition, increasing or decreasing fiber fermentation, and increasing or decreasing fiber viscosity. The choice of fiber will also depend on the delivery system. For example, soluble fibers (such as oligosaccharides and arabinogalactan) are easier to use in liquid systems, and others are easier to use in food, such as grain fibers. In general, shorter chain nondigestible carbohydrates may be less well tolerated physiologically, but they are easy to incorporate into liquids. A mixture of isolated fibers might be better tolerated than any one fiber source.

REFERENCES

Anderson JW, Gilinsky NH, Deakins DA, Smith SF, O'Neal DS, Dillon DW, Oeltgen PR. 1991. Lipid responses of hypercholesterolemic men to oat-bran and wheat-bran intake. *Am J Clin Nutr* 54(4):678–683.

Bingham SA, Cummings JH. 1989. Effect of exercise and physical fitness on large intestinal function. *Gastroenterology* 97(6):1389–1399.

Brown L, Rosner B, Willett WW, Sacks FM. 1999. Cholesterol-lowering effects of dietary fiber: A meta-analysis. *Am J Clin Nutr* 69(1):30–42.

Cummings JH. 1993. The effect of dietary fiber on fecal weight and composition. In: Spiller GA, ed. *CRC Handbook of Dietary Fiber in Human Nutrition.* 2nd ed. Boca Raton, FL: CRC Press. Pp. 263–349.

Jenkins DJ, Vuksan V, Kendall CW, Wursch P, Jeffcoat R, Waring S, Mehling CC, Vidgen E, Augustin LS, Wong E. 1998. Physiological effects of resistant starches on fecal bulk, short chain fatty acids, blood lipids and glycemic index. *J Am Coll Nutr* 17:609–616.

IOM (Institute of Medicine). 2001. *Dietary Reference Intakes: Proposed Definition of Dietary Fiber.* Washington, DC: National Academy Press.

IOM. 2002. *Dietary Reference Intakes: Energy, Carbohydrates, Fiber, Fat, Fatty Acids, Cholesterol, Protein and Amino Acids.* Washington, DC: The National Academies Press.

Kember PG, McBride KD, Tweed CS, Collins MC. 1995. A blinded prospective trial of low-residue versus normal diet in preparation for barium enema. *Br J Radiol* 68(806):128–129.

Kurasawa S, Haack VS, Marlett JA. 2000. Plant residue and bacteria as bases for increased stool weight accompanying consumption of higher dietary fiber diets. *J Am Coll Nutr* 19(4):426–433.

Lembo A, Camilleri M. 2003. Current concepts: Chronic constipation. *N Engl J Med* 349(14):1360–1368.

Martlett JA, McBurney MI, Slavin JL. 2002. Position of the American Dietetic Association: Health implications of dietary fiber. *J Am Diet Assoc* 102(7):993–1000.

McRorie J, Zorich N, Riccardi K, Bishop L, Filloon T, Wason S, Giannella R. 2000. Effects of olestra and sorbitol consumption on objective measures of diarrhea: Impact of stool viscosity on common gastrointestinal symptoms. *Regul Toxicol Pharmacol* 31(1):59–67.

Munro JA. 2004. Adequate intake values for dietary fibre based on faecal bulking indexes of 66 foods. *Eur J Clin Nutr* 58(1):32–39.

Oettle GJ. 1991. Effect of moderate exercise on bowel habit. *Gut* 32(8):941–944.

Sandler RS, Stewart WF, Liberman JN, Ricci JA, Zorich NL. 2000. Abdominal pain, bloating, and diarrhea in the United States: Prevalence and impact. *Dig Dis Sci* 45(6):1166–1171.

Sanjoaquin MA, Appleby PN, Spencer EA, Key TJ. 2004. Nutrition and lifestyle in relation to bowel movement frequency: A cross-sectional study of 20630 men and women in EPIC-Oxford. *Public Health Nutr* 7(1):77–83.

Schiller LR. 2004. Chronic diarrhea. *Gastroenterology* 127(1):287–293.

Symonds EL, Kritas S, Omari TI, Butler RN. 2004. A combined $^{13}CO_2/H_2$ breath test can be used to assess starch digestion and fermentation in humans. *J Nutr* 134(5):1193–1196.

Tucker DM, Sandstead HH, Logan GM Jr, Klevay LM, Mahalko J, Johnson LK, Inman L, Inglett GE. 1981. Dietary fiber and personality factors as determinants of stool output. *Gastroenterology* 81(5):879–883.

Diet and Kidney Stones: Optimizing Military Field Rations

Linda K. Massey, Washington State University

INTRODUCTION

More than 90 percent of kidney stones in the adult US population are made of calcium oxalate, calcium phosphate, urate salts, or a combination of these.

The risk of developing any of these types of stones varies with urinary composition, which can be improved by appropriate dietary choices. The components of urinary composition affecting stone formation include volume, oxalate, calcium, citrate, magnesium, phosphate, and pH. The relationship of these compounds to saturation levels of the salt forms (e.g., calcium oxalate, calcium phosphate) has been summarized by Tiselius (1997). In addition, sodium and potassium concentrations affect the salt form of urate, which in turn affects solubility (Moe et al., 2002). Urate salts can often form the core for calcium stone formation, enhance calcium stone growth, and form stones directly (Coe, 1978).

Two mechanisms have been proposed for stone formation and growth. In the classic paradigm, stones grow slowly with layers of calcium oxalate or calcium phosphate building on a core, frequently urate. When sectioned, these stones have the concentric layers that can also be seen in the candy known as a "jawbreaker." Recently, another model has been proposed to explain rapidly forming stones. In accordance with hydraulic models, urine flows more slowly along the outside of the urethral lumen. When urines are supersaturated with potential stone-forming salts, which frequently happens when urine production is limited, stones may form rapidly (within hours) in concentrated urines. In this model, aggregation of small crystals into large conglomerates occurs. These stones frequently have the appearance of a raspberry. Even if not expelled, they may bind to the epithelium, forming the core for a new stone.

Many "normal" urines contain small calcium oxalate crystals, but the crystals do not form stones. Inhibitory proteins may keep these crystals from aggregating or accumulating as additional layers on a stone attached to the epithelium. Variations in these proteins cannot yet be measured clinically.

This paper addresses the types and levels of nutritional factors that could be added to assault rations of a presumably healthy soldier to lower the risk of kidney stones formation. These factors should be included in a ration which may also best sustain physical and cognitive performance and prevent possible adverse health consequences of soldiers under stress and consuming a hypocaloric diet.

RISK OF URINARY STONE FORMATION UNDER COMBAT MISSIONS

Combat conditions that affect urinary composition associated with stone risk include extreme physical activity, impaired caloric intake, increased sweating, and dehydration. First, urinary volume decreases. The causes include increased sweat loss accompanying physical exertion, protective clothing retaining body heat, and inadequate fluid intake. In the only study on physical exercise and stone risk, Sakhaee and colleagues (1987) found that moderate physical exercise, six hours on a bicycle ergometer at 70 to 75 percent of maximum oxygen consumption, increased stone risk by decreasing urinary volume from 847 to 290 mL. Even though total renal excretion of stone-forming constituents decreased, the reduction in volume resulted in higher saturation of calcium oxalate and uric acid. In addition, the pH dropped from 6.35 to 5.79. A decreased pH will increase urinary calcium.

The pH will also drop if energy intake is not sufficient to meet increased energy use. Reddy and colleagues (2002) reported that two weeks' consumption of a high-protein, low-carbohydrate weight reduction diet (1,930 versus 2,314 kcal usual energy) decreased urinary pH from 6.1 to 5.5 and increased urinary calcium from 160 to 258 mg/day. During this study, hydration was maintained as participants maintained urinary outputs of 2.4 L/day for all study phases, but even with the relatively modest hypocaloric status in this study, stone risk indices increased.

Studies have shown that diet can be modified in nonmilitary situations to reduce the risk of supersaturated urines. Interventions include maintaining adequate water intake and hydration. A clinical trial by Borghi and colleagues (1996) reported that stone recurrence was reduced significantly by even modest increases in urinary volume. Hydration is considered adequate if urine production is 2 L/day (Borghi et al., 1999).

Restriction of several dietary components may also be effective in reducing stone risk. Avoiding high-oxalate foods is the highest priority.The foods highest in oxalate per serving are listed in Table B-22. For example, soy food consumption can increase urinary oxalate significantly (Massey et al., 2002). To complicate the issue, soy protein concentrates contain high but variable amounts of oxalate depending on cultivar, growing conditions, and processing methods, so each soy product would have to be checked for oxalate content. Caffeine increased urinary calcium for several hours after its consumption (Massey and Sutton, 2004), but there is no adaptation to the hypercalciuric effects of caffeine as there is with mental stimulatory effects. Reduction of caffeine may not be possible because soldiers need to be mentally alert under combat conditions. Urinary pH is affected by protein intake as well, in particular by the sulfur content of the proteins (Frassetto et al., 1998; Massey, 2003). Both animal and

TABLE B-22 Foods Highest in Oxalate, Recommended to Avoid

Food
Parsley
Rhubarb
Spinach
Beets, both roots and leaves
Legumes, including beans, soy, and peanuts
Tea, green or black, regular not herbal
Chocolate
Tree nuts, almonds, walnuts, pecans
Concentrated brans, especially wheat

TABLE B-23 Potential Acid as Sulfate from Sulfur-Containing Amino Acids

Food	Potential Acid as Sulfate (mEq per 100 g of protein)
Oatmeal	82
Egg	80
Walnuts	74
Pork	73
Wheat	69
White Rice	68
Barley	68
Tuna	65
Chicken	65
Corn	61
Beef	59
Milk	59
Cheddar	46
Soy	40
Peanuts	40
Millet	31
Almonds	23
Potato	23

SOURCE: Massey (2003).

plant protein sources have the potential to increase sulfuric acid excretion, thereby decreasing pH (Table B-23). Substitution of plant protein for an equivalent amount of beef resulted in no change in risk as shown in a metabolic study (Massey and Kynast-Gales, 2001). High-purine foods should be restricted, but these are not commonly found in field rations (e.g., gravies and meat extracts; organ meats: kidneys, liver, sweetbreads; anchovies; herring, sardines). In addition, dietary purine catabolism to uric acid only contributes about one-third of the daily uric acid excretion.

Dietary components to be enhanced include potassium, citrate, and magnesium. Potassium reduces urinary calcium excretion (Lemann et al., 1991), and potassium urate is more soluble than sodium urate and, therefore, presents a lower risk of stone formation (Maalouf et al., 2004).

Higher urinary potassium is associated with decreased stone growth after shockwave lithotripsy (Pierratos et al., 2000). Finally food potassium is associated with basic compounds that counteract the acidic effects of protein (Sebastian et al., 1994). Good sources of potassium include milk legumes and most fruits and vegetables. Citrate is also beneficial because citrate competes with oxalate for binding calcium, but calcium citrate is more soluble. Citrus fruits and juices are good sources of citrate, and citrate salts are used in some combat foods.

Finally, higher urinary magnesium from increased magnesium intakes is beneficial because magnesium competes with calcium to bind oxalate, and magnesium oxalate is 100 times more soluble than calcium oxalate. Whole grains and green vegetables are good sources of magnesium. Because food intake may be less than optimal, consider using a potassium–magnesium–citrate supplement. Ettinger and colleagues (1997) showed that 60 mEq/day of citrate as the combined potassium–magnesium salt reduced stone recurrence by 85 percent in a three-year clinical trial.

Two nutrients should be controlled to amounts appropriate for combat situations: calcium and salt (sodium chloride). Calcium intakes of 1,000 mg/day are appropriate for individuals with normal calciuria, while 600 mg/day is appropriate for individuals with diagnosed hypercalciuria. Because populations contain with individuals with both of these conditions, an intake of 800 mg/day is recommended. This level of calcium will reduce minimize the risk of hypercalciuria and will reduce urinary oxalate by binding dietary oxalate in the gut lumen (Massey and Kynast-Gales, 1998). Salt intake in excess of amounts needed to replace sweat losses increases urinary calcium losses by 1 mmol of calcium (40 mg) for each 100 mmol of salt (5,844 mg) excreted. Individuals typically show a range of responses, from virtually none to more than twice the average amounts of calcium excreted (Massey and Whiting, 1996). The need of the soldier for adequate salt to replace sweat losses is more important than reducing risk of kidney stones.

Ten milligrams per day of urinary oxalate comes from endogenous synthesis (Holmes, 2000), and ascorbate is one precursor. Massey and colleagues (2005) recently reported that 40 percent of both stone formers and nonstone formers increased urinary oxalate after taking 2 g/day supplements of ascorbate. Supplementation amounts as low as 500 mg/day have been reported to increase urinary oxalate significantly (Massey, 2000). Therefore, supplementation of any amount of vitamin C above the RDA (e.g., men 19–30 years is 75 mg/day) should be avoided. The hyperoxaluric effect of ascorbate was seen primarily within two to six hours after supplementation, and urinary oxalate levels declined to non-supplementation levels within three days.

SUMMARY

A combination of factors during combat situations might increase the risk of stone formation during combat situations. For instance, the increased sweat volumes that occur during high-intensity physical activity combined with a fluid restriction may result in dehydration, a risk factor for stone formation. Furthermore, changes in pH that may occur as a result of diet changes (decrease in pH due to inadequate caloric intake to meet energy expenditure) might also alter saturation levels of certain salts and result also in an increased risk of stone formation.

Provision of adequate amounts of water is critical when soldiers are deployed to high-intensity combat missions, where high sweat volumes can induce dehydration. Adequate hydration is the most important factor to reduce the risk of stone formation but it is difficult to maintain in field combat conditions. Adequate caloric intake to meet energy needs would be beneficial to maintain the urinary pH at normal levels; this, however, is also unlikely to occur.

A more practical approach to lessening concerns of stone formation might be the simultaneous modification of some nutrients and dietary components along with food fortification with potassium–magnesium–citrate salts that may reduce the risk of urinary crystallization (Pak et al., 2003). For example, food developers should avoid the inclusion of foods high in oxalate in the ration, such as soy protein sources. Calcium intakes of 800 mg/day are appropriate for individuals when genetic predisposition to hypercalciuria is not known. In addition, supplementation of any amount of vitamin C above the RDA for adult men (75 mg/day) should also be avoided.

REFERENCES

Borghi L, Meschi T, Amato F, Briganti A, Novarini A, Giannini A. 1996. Urinary volume, water and recurrences in idiopathic calcium nephrolithiasis: A 5-year randomized prospective study. *J Urol* 155(3):839–843.

Borghi L, Meschi T, Schianchi T, Briganti A, Guerra A, Allegri F, Novarini A. 1999. Urine volume: Stone risk factor and preventive measure. *Nephron* 81(Suppl 1):31–37.

Coe FL. 1978. Hyperuricosuric calcium oxalate nephrolithiasis. *Kidney Int* 13(5):418–426.

Ettinger B, Pak CY, Citron JT, Thomas C, Adams-Huet B, Vangessel A. 1997. Potassium-magnesium citrate is an effective prophylaxis against recurrent calcium oxalate nephrolithiasis. *J Urol* 158(6):2069–2073.

Frassetto LA, Todd KM, Morris RC Jr, Sebastian A. 1998. Estimation of net endogenous noncarbonic acid production in humans from diet potassium and protein contents. *Am J Clin Nutr* 68(3):576–583.

Holmes RP. 2000. Oxalate synthesis in humans: Assumptions, problems, and unresolved issues. *Mol Urol* 4(4):329–332.

Lemann J Jr, Pleuss JA, Gray RW, Hoffmann RG. 1991. Potassium administration reduces and potassium deprivation increases urinary calcium excretion in healthy adults. *Kidney Int* 39(5):973–983.

Maalouf NM, Cameron MA, Moe OW, Sakhaee K. 2004. Novel insights into the pathogenesis of uric acid nephrolithiasis. *Curr Opin Nephrol Hypertens* 13(2):181–189.

Massey LK. 2000. Effects of ascorbate supplements on urinary oxalate and risk of kidney stones. *J Am Diet Assoc* 100(5):516.

Massey LK. 2003. Dietary animal and plant protein and human bone health: A whole foods approach. *J Nutr* 133(3):862S–865S.

Massey LK, Kynast-Gales SA. 1998. Substituting milk for apple juice does not increase kidney stone risk in most normocalciuric adults who form calcium oxalate stones. *J Am Diet Assoc* 98(3):303–308.

Massey LK, Kynast-Gales SA. 2001. Diets with either beef or plant proteins reduce risk of calcium oxalate precipitation in patients with a history of calcium kidney stones. *J Am Diet Assoc* 101(3):326–331.

Massey LK, Sutton RA. 2004. Acute caffeine effects on urine composition and calcium kidney stone risk in calcium stone formers. *J Urol* 172(2):555–558.

Massey LK, Whiting SJ. 1996. Dietary salt, urinary calcium, and bone loss. *J Bone Miner Res* 11(6):731–736.

Massey LK, Grentz LM, Horner HT, Palmer RG. 2002. Soybean and soyfood consumption increase oxalate excretion. *Top Clin Nutr* 17(2):49–59.

Massey LK, Kynast-Gales SA, Liebman M. 2005. Ascorbate increases human oxaluria and kidney stone risk. *J Nutr* 135: (in press)

Moe OW, Abate N, Sakhaee K. 2002. Pathophysiology of uric acid nephrolithiasis. *Endocrinol Metab Clin North Am* 31(4):895–914.

Pak CY, Heller HJ, Pearle MS, Odvina CV, Poindexter JR, Peterson RD. 2003. Prevention of stone formation and bone loss in absorptive hypercalciuria by combined dietary and pharmacological interventions. *J Urol* 169(2):465–469.

Pierratos A, Dharamsi N, Carr LK, Ibanez D, Jewett MA, Honey RJ. 2000. Higher urinary potassium is associated with decreased stone growth after shock wave lithotripsy. *J Urol* 164(5):1486–1489.

Reddy ST, Wang CY, Sakhaee K, Brinkley L, Pak CY. 2002. Effect of low-carbohydrate high-protein diets on acid-base balance, stone-forming propensity, and calcium metabolism. *Am J Kidney Dis* 40(2):265–274.

Sakhaee K, Nigam S, Snell P, Hsu MC, Pak CY. 1987. Assessment of the pathogenetic role of physical exercise in renal stone formation. *J Clin Endocrinol Metab* 65(5):974–979.

Sebastian A, Harris ST, Ottaway JH, Todd KM, Morris RC Jr. 1994. Improved mineral balance and skeletal metabolism in postmenopausal women treated with potassium bicarbonate. *N Engl J Med* 330(25):1776–1781.

Tiselius HG. 1997. Risk formulas in calcium oxalate urolithiasis. *World J Urol* 15(3):176–185.

Assault Rations:
Organoleptic, Satiability, and Engineering Challenges

Dennis H. Passe, Scout Consulting, LLC

INTRODUCTION

The sensory and engineering challenges of developing an assault ration are complex but surmountable. The fundamentals that should be addressed are (1) the basics of sensory palatability (both the positive and negative) and the interactions that can occur between physical stress/exercise levels and hedonic (pleasure) levels; (2) the current statistical design methods for optimizing formulas and production processes; (3) the basics of packaging engineering; and (4) the psychological and behavioral aspects of the soldiers. Although most of the basics are reasonably well understood, an essential, but challenging, aspect to develop the best possible assault ration is to integrate these areas of understanding with a team approach.

The following sections focus primarily on beverages, but much of the material applies to solid foods as well. The following questions are addressed in this section:

- What are the challenges of developing nutritionally enhanced food products, especially beverages, for a special group of people, specifically people under physical, cognitive, and environmental stress?
- What are nutrients that have been added to food products with the purpose of enhancing the immune function, hydration status, or gastrointestinal processes; performance; or other physiological or cognitive functions?
- What are specific metabolic concerns, for example, interactions with other nutrients, bioavailability, and absorption?
- What are the issues to consider when such a nutritionally enhanced food product is developed, in terms of sensory, palatability, and storage/stability?
- What strategies have worked to maximize the consumption of such food product (or beverages) by soldiers under stress? What strategies have not worked?

THE IMPORTANCE OF PALATABILITY

Flavor and Fluid Intake

Flavor is an important palatability element in encouraging voluntary fluid intake. The preponderance of research shows that a flavored beverage is consumed in greater quantities than water (Table B-24).

TABLE B-24 Percentage of Increase in Voluntary Fluid Intake of a Flavored Drink Versus Water. Values in parentheses indicate a decrease in Voluntary Fluid Intake

Increase (%)	Reference
10–79	Szylyk et al., 1989
13–19	Minehan et al., 2002
24	Passe et al., 2004
31	Spioch and Nowara, 1980
32	Rivera-Brown et al., 1999
36	Clapp et al., 1999
41–83	Hubbard et al., 1984
42	Maughan et al., 1997
45–90	Wilk and Bar-Or, 1996
54–59 (5–6)	Wilmore et al., 1998
99–143	Rolls et al., 1980
110–115	Passe et al., 2000
233–318	Passe et al., 2000
247	Sohar et al., 1962

In early observations of military personnel, Rothstein and colleagues (1947) indicated that providing some flavoring resulted in enhanced palatability. In subsequent controlled field (Engell and Hirsch, 1991; Minehan et al., 2002; Sohar et al., 1962; Spioch and Nowara, 1980) and laboratory studies (Clapp et al., 1999; Hubbard et al., 1984; Maughan et al., 1997; Passe et al., 2004; Szlyk et al., 1987, 1989) with adults under varying degrees of physical stress, beverage palatability and voluntary fluid intake increased when a flavored drink was offered. Conversely, the least popular drinks were those containing carbonation (Sohar et al., 1962).

In addition, providing a choice of flavors can further enhance fluid intake. In a study of the effects of flavor variety, Rolls and colleagues (1980) reported that the addition of one flavor increased voluntary fluid intake by 99 percent in comparison with water intake. Adding three flavors increased voluntary fluid intake over water (control) by 143 percent.

Exercise and Palatability

In experiments taking a more systematic look at flavor palatability and voluntary fluid intake, Passe and colleagues (2000) investigated the effects of high- versus low-palatability beverages on intake during exercise. After athletes first screened beverages for palatability, both the most and least acceptable flavors for each subject and water were subsequently made available ad libitum during three hours of aerobic exercise. During screening, the most acceptable flavor scored higher than water ($p < 0.01$), which scored higher than the least acceptable flavor ($p < 0.01$) (Figure B-34). During exercise, however, the palatability of the least acceptable flavor increased and exceeded that of water ($p < 0.01$) (Figure B-35). Furthermore, in a replication experiment with the same flavors and a similar aerobic exercise protocol, but using a two-choice procedure, the flavored sports beverage, whether originally identified as most acceptable or least acceptable, was consumed in significantly greater quantities than water, even after only 15 minutes of exercise (Figures B-36 and B-37).

These findings highlight the importance of flavor in contributing to voluntary fluid intake when exercising. They also suggest that a powerful association exists between flavor palatability of a sports beverage and exercise status. That is, a beverage with low palatability during at-rest conditions can dramatically increase in palatability during exercise (Figure B-38) (Passe et al., 2000). This association is consistent with the findings of Horio and Kawamura (1998) who reported that a shift in the hedonic value of a beverage can occur as a function of exercise.

While the effect of flavor (and beverage temperature; see section below) may be a key driver of voluntary fluid intake during exercise, there appears to be a relationship between exercise and hedonic experience. That is, when considering the addition of flavors to a beverage, the hedonic experience of the flavor being

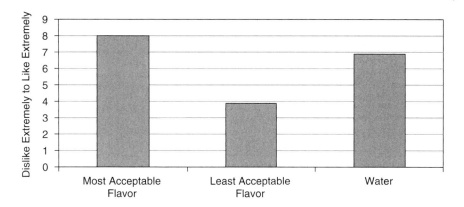

FIGURE B-34 Overall acceptance (liking) for most acceptable flavor, least acceptable flavor, and water during sedentary (at rest) conditions.
NOTE: All differences are significant at $p < 0.001$.
SOURCE: Data obtained from Passe et al. (2000).

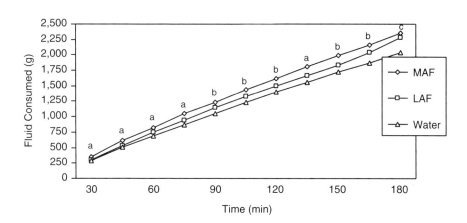

FIGURE B-35 Cumulative amount consumed (grams) of most acceptable flavor, least acceptable flavor, and water during three hours of exercise. Single-choice procedure.
NOTE: MAF = most acceptable flavor; LAF = least acceptable flavor. a = MAF > (LAF, Water), LAF = Water; b = MAF > Water, LAF = (MAF, Water); c = (MAF = LAF) > Water. a, b, c, significantly different $p < 0.05$.
SOURCE: Passe et al. (2000), used with permission from Elsevier.

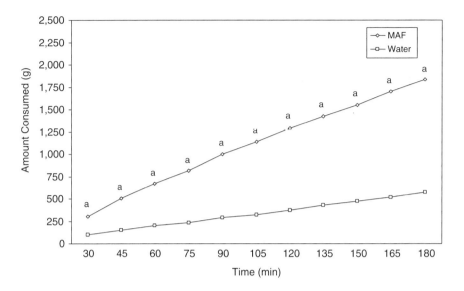

FIGURE B-36 Cumulative amount consumed of most acceptable flavor and water during three hours of exercise. Two-choice procedure.
NOTE: MAF = most acceptable flavor. Most acceptable flavor compared to water, $p < 0.05$.
SOURCE: Adapted from Passe et al. (2000), used with permission from Elsevier.

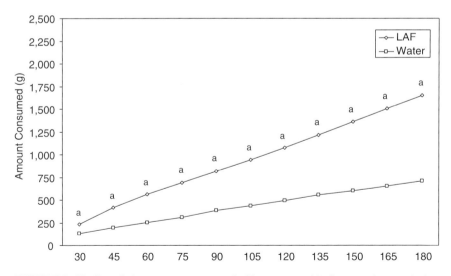

FIGURE B-37 Cumulative amount consumed of least acceptable flavor and water during three hours of exercise. Two-choice procedure.
NOTE: LAF = least acceptable flavor. Least acceptable flavor compared to water, $p < 0.05$.
SOURCE: Adapted from Passe et al. (2000), used with permission from Elsevier.

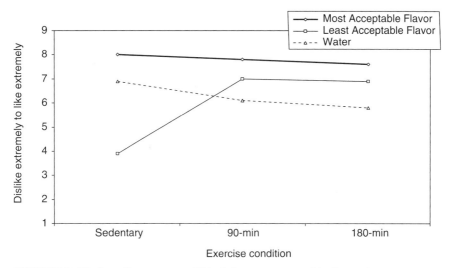

FIGURE B-38 Overall acceptance (liking) for most acceptable flavor, least acceptable flavor, and water during sedentary (at rest) conditions and after 90 minutes and 180 minutes of exercise. Overall acceptance scale 1–9: 1 (dislike extremely) through 9 (like extremely).
NOTE: Acceptability of least preferred flavor increased significantly from sedentary to exercise conditions. All drink comparisons at least $p < 0.05$.
SOURCE: Passe et al. (2000), used with permission from Elsevier.

tasted should be tested during or after exercise and rated for acceptability. Lluch and colleagues (1998) demonstrated in females that the appeal of a low-fat meal increased after exercise relative to the same meal consumed after rest, but not for males (King and Blundell, 1995; King et al., 1996). Lluch and colleagues (1998) also observed that the increase in the hedonic value of foods following exercise occurred predominantly for the high-carbohydrate (low-fat) items in the menu, consistent with the need for carbohydrate-related glycogen use during exercise.

To date, there have been few, if any, published reports of systematic investigations of flavor components that could increase or decrease the palatability of beverages during physical stress or exercise. In a series of experiments, Passe (2001) investigated the dose–response relationships between key flavor components (sweetness, saltiness, tartness, flavor strength) and palatability measured immediately following exercise. Healthy adults exercised for 30 minutes, after which they had ad libitum access to a beverage that they then evaluated for palatability and perceived intensity as a function of the key flavor components. Results indicated critical breakpoints for all of these sensory attributes (Figures B-39 through B-42). Together these studies suggest, at least for major flavor components in a sports beverage, that there are optima that must be achieved to fully enhance beverage flavor quality and that deviation from these optima, with either higher or lower concentrations, can reduce palatability.

The results from the sodium palatability study are consistent with those of Wemple and colleagues (1997), who investigated the effects of 25 and 50 mmol/L of sodium in flavored, six-percent carbohydrate drinks on voluntary fluid intake following dehydration. Fluid intake was significantly enhanced for the 25 mmol/L beverage over water but not for the 50 mmol/L beverage. Similarly, Leshem and colleagues (1999) have reported an increase in salt preference in soup following exercise. In this study subjects (21 male students, 24 years old) engaged in "routine exercise" for one hour after which they were allowed to self-adjust the salt level in tomato soup. Relative to baseline measurements and a control group that did not exercise, subjects increased the level of salt in the soup by about 50 percent (from 1.3 to 2 percent NaCl). A similar study investigated the effects of carbonation on beverage palatability in exercising subjects. In this case, the acceptability of a sports beverage drops precipitously with carbonation (Figure B-43) (Passe et al., 1997).

Negative Sensory Characteristics

In addition to increasing the benefits that the correct combination of beverage characteristics can have on hedonic experiences and voluntary fluid intake, it is also important to understand how negative characteristics can adversely affect palatability during physical stress or exercise. Failure to eliminate or reduce unacceptable beverage characteristics may produce unwanted reactions—this has been observed when water is tainted by off-flavors (Rothstein et al., 1947; Szlyk et al., 1987, 1989), when the beverage type is mismatched for the exercise occasion (Sohar et al., 1962), or when the temperature is too warm (Armstrong et al., 1985; Boulze et al., 1983; Hubbard et al., 1984; Sandick et al., 1984; Szlyk et al., 1987, 1989).

In a study investigating the potential acceptability of various beverage characteristics (Passe, 2001), adult subjects consumed, ad libitum, a variety of beverages (lemon-lime flavored 6 percent carbohydrate electrolyte sports beverage, apple juice, mixed-vegetable juice, bottled water, and a cola) after 30 minutes of aerobic activity. At the end of the study, subjects were asked to complete a questionnaire which probed how "annoyed" they would be by certain beverage characteristics if they occurred in a beverage. The most salient negative beverage characteristics for this group were related to feelings of nausea or bloating, objectionable mouthfeel, perceived viscosity, objectionable flavor, and excessive sweetness (Table B-25). The negative characteristics identified as being least important were low saltiness, low sweetness, low tartness, and high artificial color appearance. A replicate study was subsequently conducted with results that closely paralleled those of the first study (Table B-25).

Consistent with the above results, Pelchat and Rozin (1982) observed in a

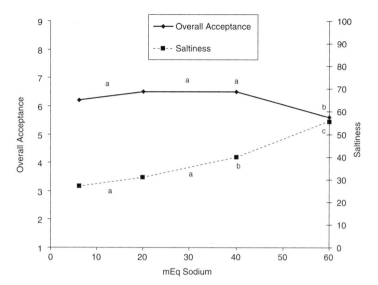

FIGURE B-39 Overall acceptance (liking) and perceived beverage saltiness after 30 minutes of exercise.
NOTE: For each curve, values not sharing a letter (a, b, c) in common are significantly different ($p \leq 0.05$). Overall acceptance scale 1–9: 1 (dislike extremely) through 9 (like extremely). Saltiness scale 0–100: 0 (not salty) through 100 (very salty).
SOURCE: Passe (2001).

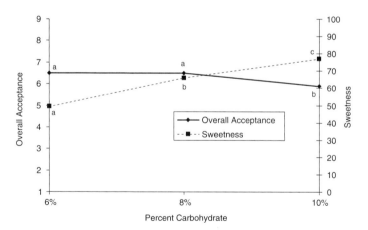

FIGURE B-40 Overall acceptance (liking) and perceived beverage sweetness after 30 minutes of exercise.
NOTE: For each curve, values not sharing a letter in common are significantly different ($p \leq 0.05$). Overall acceptance scale 1–9: 1 (dislike extremely) through 9 (like extremely). Sweetness scale 0–100: 0 (not sweet) through 100 (very sweet).
SOURCE: Passe (2001).

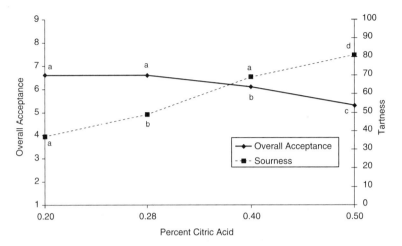

FIGURE B-41 Overall acceptance (liking) and perceived beverage sourness/tartness after 30 minutes of exercise.

NOTE: For each curve, values not sharing a letter in common are significantly different ($p \leq 0.05$). Overall acceptance scale 1–9: 1 (dislike extremely) through 9 (like extremely). Sourness scale 0–100: 0 (not tart) through 100 (very tart).

SOURCE: Passe (2001).

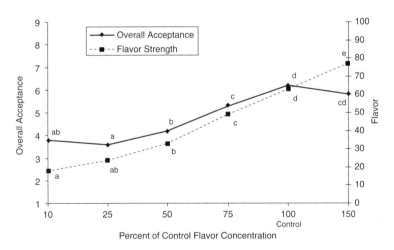

FIGURE B-42 Overall acceptance (liking) and perceived beverage flavor strength after 30 minutes of exercise.

NOTE: For each curve, values not sharing a letter in common are significantly different ($p \leq 0.05$). Overall acceptance scale 1–9: 1 (dislike extremely) through 9 (like extremely). Flavor scale 0–100: 0 (weak flavor) through 100 (strong flavor).

SOURCE: Passe (2001).

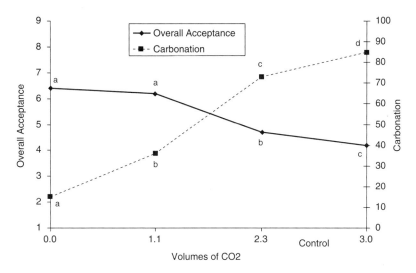

FIGURE B-43 Overall acceptance (liking) and perceived beverage carbonation after 30 minutes of exercise.
NOTE: For each curve, values not sharing a letter in common are significantly different ($p \leq 0.05$). Overall acceptance scale 1–9: 1 (dislike extremely) through 9 (like extremely). Carbonation scale 0–100: 0 (weak carbonation) through 100 (strong carbonation). CO2 = carbon dioxide.
SOURCE: Passe et al. (2000), used with permission from Elsevier.

survey study that nausea following ingestion of a food was the most potent correlate of acquired dislike of the taste of food. The effects of postingestion gastrointestinal distress can be powerful and are a central theme in the area of conditioned taste-aversion learning. The reader is referred to Garcia and colleagues (1974) and Rozin and Kalat (1971) for discussion.

BEVERAGE TEMPERATURE

One of the most effective ways to improve the palatability of a beverage to heat-stressed or exercising subjects is to chill it (Armstrong et al., 1985; Boulze et al., 1983; Hubbard et al., 1984; Passe, 2001; Rothstein et al., 1947; Sandick et al., 1984; Sohar et al., 1962; Szlyk et al., 1987, 1989). Research over the years has consistently shown that cooling a drink enhances its palatability and increases voluntary fluid intake (Table B-26).

In addition, there appears to be a perception-changing effect of beverage temperature in relation to flavor on voluntary fluid intake. Hubbard and colleagues (1984) reported a 50 percent increase in water consumption when water

TABLE B-25 Level of Annoyance[a] with Various Potential Beverage Flaws

Annoyance Question	Study 1	Study 2
Beverage causes nausea	93	91
Beverage leaves mouth sticky and dry	80	78
Beverage is too thick and syrupy	79	76
Beverage is too sweet	77	76
Beverage has off flavor	76	77
Beverage leaves you feeling bloated	72	70
Beverage does not quench thirst	68	65
Beverage is too salty	64	74
Aftertaste is too strong	62	60
Flavor is too strong	57	57
Beverage has artificial flavor	55	56
Beverage is too tart	45	50
Aroma is too strong	43	39
Flavor is too weak	42	46
Beverage is not tart enough	37	37
Beverage appears artificially colored	33	34
Beverage is not sweet enough	25	30
Beverage is not salty enough	20	17

[a]Scale is 100-point analogue line scale, anchored on the left by "not annoyed" and anchored on the right by "very annoyed."
SOURCE: Passe (2001).

TABLE B-26 Percentage of Increase in Voluntary Fluid Intake of a Chilled Drink over One at "Ambient" Temperature

Increase Intake (%)	Reference
23; 79	Sandick et al., 1984
87	Hubbard et al., 1984
88	Szlyk et al., 1989
127	Armstrong et al., 1985
393; 114	Boulze et al., 1983

was chilled, a 40 percent increase when it was flavored, and an 80-percent increase when it was both chilled and flavored.

In the case of sweetened beverages, temperature may exert an effect on palatability by modifying perceived sweetness intensity. Calvino (1986) generated psychophysical sweetness intensity curves at beverage temperatures (7°C, 37°C, and 50°C). Solutions at 37°C (99 °F) and 50°C (122 °F) were perceived as being sweeter than at 7°C (45°F). This study also confirm what others had reported before, that is, that this temperature effect diminishes with higher sucrose concentrations and becomes negligible at higher concentrations of approximately 0.4–0.5 M sucrose. In addition, the slopes of the sweetness functions at the higher temperatures were lower than at 7°C (45°F); that is, the sweetness function was steeper at 7°C (45°F) than at the warmer temperatures, which suggests an improved ability to discriminate sweetness differences with lower temperatures.

EXERCISE AND SALT APPETITE

Following exercise-induced dehydration, sodium in a rehydration beverage is important because it restores and maintains body fluid levels. Therefore, the influence of exercise on the preference for foods or high salt concentrations (salt appetite) is of special interest for soldiers under stress due to the loss of sodium during exercise. To date, however, there are only a few reports directly investigating the effect of exercise on salt appetite or salt preference in humans (Horio and Kawamura, 1998; Leshem et al., 1999; Takamata et al., 1994; Wald and Leshem, 2003).

Takamata and colleagues (1994) investigated the effect of exercise-induced water and sodium depletion on the palatability of various aqueous solutions of sodium chloride. Over a 23-hour rehydration period, the unpleasant taste of the higher salt solutions became less so. The perceived intensity of 0.3 M sodium chloride increased after exercise and remained elevated throughout most of the rehydration period.

In a study investigating the effect of exercise on preference for salt with a group of male university students who exercised versus a control group, Leshem and colleagues (1999) compared the acceptability of salt in soup between the two groups. The preferred concentration of salt in soup increased by 50 percent, relative to the concentration preferred by the control group, immediately after exercise (p < 0.02). Furthermore, on the morning after, the exercising group still preferred a higher level of salt in soup than the controls did (p < 0.05). A comparison of groups on the intake of salty snacks failed to find any significant differences; however, Leshem and colleagues (1999) concluded that there is not yet evidence demonstrating that increased salt preference results in an increase in intake. This is an area of research requiring additional attention.

Horio and Kawamura (1998), unlike Leshem and colleagues (1999) and Takamata and coworkers (1994), did not observe an increase in preference for salty taste following exercise in 58 university-student volunteers. Results indicated that the hedonic rating of the salt solutions and detection thresholds did not change following exercise. While Horio and Kawamura (1998) and Takamata and colleagues (1994) both investigated saltiness preference in aqueous solutions using sip-and-spit techniques, a potentially important methodological difference existed in that the exercise for the former was of 30 minute duration and was of moderate intensity compared with a six-hour exercise protocol designed to deplete the subjects of body water and sodium for the latter. It is possible that the exercise-induced sodium depletion (3.29 mEq/kg) contributed to the increased palatability ratings observed in Takamata and colleagues (1994). Support for such a mechanism has been suggested by Wald and Leshem (2003), who reported that following exercise, greater postingestive flavor conditioning of preference for a novel beverage (via pairing with salt capsules) occurred under conditions of greater sweating. The increase in physiological well-being from the sodium supplementation may be facilitating the acquisition of the flavor preference.

Wemple and colleagues (1997) investigated the effects of two levels of sodium chloride (25 mmol/L and 50 mmol/L) in a flavored, 6 percent sucrose beverage versus artificially sweetened and flavored water (no added sodium) in exercise subjects who lost three percent of their body weights through dehydration, after which they were allowed to rehydrate freely for three hours. The beverage with the added 25 mmol/L of sodium chloride was preferred. In support of these findings, Kanarek and colleagues (1995) have reported that preference for salted popcorn is greater for women who exercise more than three hours per week than for those who exercise less.

In summary, the role of sodium in a rehydration beverage is important because of its necessary role in restoring and maintaining body fluid levels following exercise-induced dehydration. Substantial amounts can be lost in sweat and must be replaced to maintain physiological functions. Although preliminary evidence suggests that the desire for saltiness may increase with exercise; getting sufficient quantities of sodium in a properly formulated rehydration beverage may be a sensory and palatability challenge. The research presented above suggests that a relatively low level of sodium, 25 mmol/L, may enhance beverage palatability. Research in the area of sodium palatability in sports beverages is in its infancy, and additional research is necessary to achieve acceptable palatability with higher levels of sodium.

PRODUCT DEVELOPMENT CHALLENGES

The challenges of developing an assault ration for a target population expending large amounts of energy are analogous to those faced by the developers of medicinal foods for patient populations also requiring high caloric intake. The most efficient way to achieve high caloric density is through fat, recognizing that we must also meet other nutritional goals.

The product, whether a solid or fluid, must also look and taste like "real" food—a hurdle that requires at least some basic understanding of our target population's food preferences. Our final product could be a solid food or a liquid or a combination of both. In addition it is helpful to identify palatability gold standards that we wish to achieve for a particular product. In this sense, obtaining the services of a chef during this phase can be helpful (e.g., to intensify the flavor profile of a high-energy beef stroganoff).

Cost is also important to consider in the early phases of our planning. Even though we may initially approach a project with a "no-cost-constraint" philosophy, experience tells us that we very quickly lose decision-making efficiency if we have to back track and reengineer our decisions later on the basis of cost. Perhaps the most efficient mode is to solve the energy density, palatability, and cost equations simultaneously. Once the type of product and the target are identified there are other requirements that must be established and will affect the nature of the final product. A key element of product development success is simultaneously improving the formula-component levels. For example, the following text outlines a simple approach (currently used by the food industry) to develop a shelf-stable, low-calorie electrolyte drink for high-stress environments to reduce the risk of hyponatremia:

- The product formula can be addressed by a response surface design incorporating the following key ingredients: water, iodine or another microstabilizer, electrolyte blend, sweetener, flavor.
- Cost is included in the model, so cost options must be identified as well.
- Sensory testing of the design points and subsequent statistical modeling will identify the best palatability.
- Microbiological stability should be checked through standard screening.
- The validity of the final product should be established by field testing.

SENSORY STORAGE TESTING

Sensory storage testing, while sometimes an afterthought, is critical to product survival. Such testing establishes that sensory quality is maintained at acceptable levels throughout the time when the product is available for use. Microbiological testing is typically done in parallel but is not covered in detail in this discussion.

There are two basic approaches to establishing shelf life. The first identifies whether the product is acceptable at a specified date. This is a simple approach that only requires two tests: initial and final. If we are fairly confident of the product's ability to maintain its sensory integrity, we use this kind of test as confirmatory of sensory integrity.

The second approach identifies when the product shifts in quality, if any shift occurs. This approach requires periodic testing between the initial and the final tests for time (above). To save time and cost, a feature that can and should be incorporated into the testing protocol is to include an accelerated portion of the test that mimics long-term storage studies by using elevated temperatures or other intentional challenges to the food. Most product development teams elect to conduct some variation of this second approach.

PROCESS AND PACKAGING ENGINEERING CHALLENGES

The first process engineering challenge is to determine whether the product can, in fact, be produced. Microbiological stability, production reliability (operating within production standards) and efficiency (cost effectiveness) are central for processing and packaging the product.

Processing usually damages flavor to some degree. Achieving the target flavor and texture profile while maintaining microbiological stability is usually a matter of trade-offs. Heat, pressure, shear, and the presence of preservatives usually conspire to degrade the final sensory experience. The process engineer's challenge is to get to the best compromise.

Packaging engineering takes up where process engineering leaves off. The key challenges here will be to create the most efficacious moisture, oxygen, microbial, and, possibly, ultraviolet barriers. If the product is inherently microbiologically stable (perhaps due to low water activity and low pH), the packaging options are simpler and less costly. However, if the product characteristics require a formula and process that leave it more vulnerable either in a sensory or microbiological way, the packaging can compensate by an enhanced barrier support. Hermetically sealing a product will provide protection against microbe ingress to a product that has been rendered safe but not stable. Oxygen-impermeable barriers will enhance sensory shelf life. Although more complex and more expensive, these approaches sometimes help to achieve the best value relative to achieving our food-target goal.

SPECIAL NUTRITIONAL ISSUES

Over the three to seven days that an assault ration will be used, the nutritional focus is likely to be on the macronutrient profile. Specifically, dietary components that help regulate the body's insulin response and maintain the correct glucose levels are crucial. As insulin lowers blood sugar levels and selectively drives amino acids into muscle tissue, tryptophan, normally competing with the branch-chain amino acids to cross the blood–brain barrier, can more freely cross into the brain. The increased tryptophan levels may facilitate an increase in serotonin levels, which can affect performance, cognitive function, alertness, mood, and appetite. Consequently, to maintain hormone and glucose balance, an assault ration may be improved from some augmented valine, leucine, and isoleucine levels in combination with some fiber, amylase-resistant starch, fat, and sufficient carbohydrate.

Important micronutrients to include are an electrolyte blend to encourage voluntary fluid intake. Although the science may be limited with respect to the benefits of antioxidants in performance, their inclusion may help protect healthy tissue from inflammation during muscle breakdown and repair.

SUMMARY

Flavor and temperature are the two most important sensory attributes at our disposal to optimize beverage quality. A high level of acceptability can be achieved by simultaneously improving the flavor, texture, and appearance profile and reducing any negative sensory and postingestive effects.

The most efficient and cost effective approach to improve complex formulas and processes is the use of advanced response surface statistical designs. These methods are, fortunately, intuitive and easily implemented.

In addition, storage testing is critical to ensure the field success of product quality. If possible, accelerated-temperature designs to facilitate an early read on potential problems should be conducted.

Finally, decisions should be made by an integrated team of experienced professionals that include experts on physiology, nutrition, product development, food processing, and sensory qualities of food.

ACKNOWLEDGMENTS

I gratefully acknowledge the valuable insights and suggestions from Steve Ink, Ph.D., Director of Agricultural Technology, Northern Illinois University, DeKalb; John Konieczka, JBK Consulting, LLC; Paula Manoski, Quality R&D Partners; Bob Murray, Ph.D., Gatorade Sports Science Institute.

REFERENCES

Armstrong LE, Hubbard RW, Szlyk PC, Matthew WT, Sils IV. 1985. Voluntary dehydration and electrolyte losses during prolonged exercise in the heat. *Aviat Space Environ Med* 56(8):765–770.

Boulze D, Montastruc P, Cabanac M. 1983. Water intake, pleasure and water temperature in humans. *Physiol Behav* 30(1):97–102.

Calvino AM. 1986. Perception of sweetness: The effects of concentration and temperature. *Physiol Behav* 36(6):1021–1028.

Clapp AJ, Bishop PA, Walker JL. 1999. Fluid replacement preferences in heat-exposed workers. *Am Ind Hyg Assoc J* 60(6):747–751.

Engell D, Hirsch E. 1991. Environmental and sensory modulation of fluid intake in humans. In: Ramsey DJ, Booth D, eds. *Thirst: Physiological and Psychological Aspects.* Berlin: Springer-Verlag. Pp. 382–402.

Garcia J, Hankins WG, Rusiniak KW. 1974. Behavioral regulation of the milieu interne in man and rat. *Science* 185(4154):824–831.

Horio T, Kawamura Y. 1998. Influence of physical exercise on human preferences for various taste solutions. *Chem Senses* 23(4):417–421.

Hubbard RW, Sandick BL, Matthew WT, Francesconi RP, Sampson JB, Durkot MJ, Maller O, Engell DB. 1984. Voluntary dehydration and alliesthesia for water. *J Appl Physiol* 57(3):868–873.

Kanarek RB, Ryu M, Przypek J. 1995. Preferences for foods with varying levels of salt and fat differ as a function of dietary restraint and exercise but not menstrual cycle. *Physiol Behav* 57(5):821–826.

King NA, Blundell JE. 1995. High-fat foods overcome the energy expenditure induced by high-intensity cycling or running. *Eur J Clin Nutr* 49(2):114–123.

King NA, Snell L, Smith RD, Blundell JE. 1996. Effects of short-term exercise on appetite responses in unrestrained females. *Eur J Clin Nutr* 50(10):663–667.

Leshem M, Abutbul A, Eilon R. 1999. Exercise increases the preference for salt in humans. *Appetite* 32(2):251–260.

Lluch A, King NA, Blundell JE. 1998. Exercise in dietary restrained women: No effect on energy intake but change in hedonic ratings. *Eur J Clin Nutr* 52(4):300–307.

Maughan RJ, Leiper JB, Shirreffs SM. 1997. Factors influencing the restoration of fluid and electrolyte balance after exercise in the heat. *Br J Sports Med* 31(3):175–182.

Minehan MR, Riley MD, Burke LM. 2002. Effect of flavor and awareness of kilojoule content of drinks on preference and fluid balance in team sports. *Int J Sport Nutr Exerc Metab* 12(1):81–92.

Passe DH. 2001. Physiological and psychological determinants of fluid intake. In: Maughan RJ, Murray R, eds. *Sports Drinks. Basic Science and Practical Aspects.* Boca Raton, FL: CRC Press. Pp. 45–87.

Passe DH, Horn M, Murray R. 1997. The effects of beverage carbonation on sensory responses and voluntary fluid intake following exercise. *Int J Sport Nutr* 7(4):286–297.

Passe DH, Horn M, Murray R. 2000. Impact of beverage acceptability on fluid intake during exercise. *Appetite* 35(3):219–229.

Passe DH, Horn M, Stofan J, Murray R. 2004. Palatability and voluntary intake of sports beverages, diluted orange juice, and water during exercise. *Int J Sport Nutr Exerc Metab* 14(3):272–284.

Pelchat ML, Rozin P. 1982. The special role of nausea in the acquisition of food dislikes by humans. *Appetite* 3(4):341–351.

Rivera-Brown AM, Gutierrez R, Gutierrez JC, Frontera WR, Bar-Or O. 1999. Drink composition, voluntary drinking, and fluid balance in exercising, trained, heat-acclimatized boys. *J Appl Physiol* 86(1):78–84.

Rolls BJ, Wood RJ, Rolls ET. 1980. Thirst: The initiation, maintenance, and termination of drinking. In: Sprague JM, Epstein AN, eds. *Progress in Psychobiology and Physiological Psychology.* New York: Academic Press. Vol. 9. Pp. 263–321.

Rothstein A, Adolph EF, Wills JH. 1947. Voluntary dehydration. In: Adolph EF, ed. *Physiology of Man in the Desert.* New York: Interscience Publishers. Pp. 254–270.

Rozin P, Kalat JW. 1971. Specific hungers and poison avoidance as adaptive specializations of learning. *Psychol Rev* 78(6):459–486.

Sandick BL, Engell DB, Maller O. 1984. Perception of drinking water temperature and effects for humans after exercise. *Physiol Behav* 32(5):851–855.

Sohar E, Kaly J, Adar R. 1962 The prevention of voluntary dehydration. In: *Symposium on Environmental Physiology and Psychology in Arid Conditions.* Proceedings of the Lucknow Symposium. Paris: United Nations Educational Scientific and Cultural Organization. Pp. 129–135.

Spioch FM, Nowara M. 1980. Voluntary dehydration in men working in heat. *Int Arch Occup Environ Health* 46(3):233–239.

Szlyk PC, Hubbard RW, Matthew WT, Armstrong LE, Kerstein MD. 1987. Mechanisms of voluntary dehydration among troops in the field. *Mil Med* 152(8):405–407.

Szlyk PC, Sils IV, Francesconi RP, Hubbard RW, Armstrong LE. 1989. Effects of water temperature and flavoring on voluntary dehydration in men. *Physiol Behav* 45(3):639–647.

Takamata A, Mack GW, Gillen CM, Nadel ER. 1994. Sodium appetite, thirst, and body fluid regulation in humans during rehydration without sodium replacement. *Am J Physiol* 266(5 Pt 2):R1493–R1502.

Wald N, Leshem M. 2003. Salt conditions a flavor preference or aversion after exercise depending on NaCl dose and sweat loss. *Appetite* 40(3):277–284.

Wemple RD, Morocco TS, Mack GW. 1997. Influence of sodium replacement on fluid ingestion following exercise-induced dehydration. *Int J Sport Nutr* 7(2):104–116.

Wilk B, Bar-Or O. 1996. Effect of drink flavor and NaCL on voluntary drinking and hydration in boys exercising in the heat. *J Appl Physiol* 80(4):1112–1117.

Wilmore JH, Morton AR, Gilbey HJ, Wood RJ. 1998. Role of taste preference on fluid intake during and after 90 min of running at 60% of VO₂max in the heat. *Med Sci Sports Exerc* 30(4):587–395.

Foods for People under Stress: Special Considerations

Steven M. Wood, Abbott Laboratories

INTRODUCTION

Developing foods for people under stress requires the examination of several critical issues. First, a product concept should be developed based on scientific evidence that includes identification of stress-induced changes and the rationale for using specific nutrients to modulate the identifiable changes. Second, food technology parameters, including physical stability, standardization of ingredients, and product sterility, need to be ensured. Third, to establish efficacy and bioavailability of nutrients, testing of the foods should be conducted in the intended population. Last, in the retail environment, regulatory issues and pathways that include product forms, claims, and labeling should be addressed. This section addresses the rationale for using specific nutrients, illustrated by examples in which supplemental nutrition has been studied and found to modulate physiological processes or physical condition (efficacy) in people under stress. In addition, the progression of a series of studies in trauma stress, military training, and senior populations is presented. These studies identified significant immunologic benefits of a novel nutritional formula shown to modulate stress-induced immune dysregulation.

The following are specific questions that this review attempts to answer:

- What are the challenges of developing nutritionally enhanced food products for a special group of people, specifically people under physical, cognitive, and environmental stress? Stress under military operations can be from exercise, extreme environmental temperature, dehydration, heat exhaustion, threat to personal safety, sleep deprivation, and other operational demands.
- Are there nutrients that could be added to these foods to minimize oxidative stress and therefore deterioration of performance?
- Are there other nutrients that could be added to these foods to optimize the immune system, nutrient absorption, hydration, or other physiological functions?
- What are nutrient specific metabolic concerns; for example, interaction with other nutrients, bioavailability, and absorption or others?

- Will nutrient addition affect the organoleptic qualities of a food as to make it less appealing? If so, how would you improve the palatability in order to maximize the consumption of the food product?
- If these nutrients where to be added to a food, what are the issues to consider in terms of packaging and shelf-life considerations?

EXAMPLE OF ACUTE STRESS AND NUTRITIONAL MODULATION

Acute stress, such as trauma, can cause increased nutritional requirements; furthermore, nutrients may be supplied to modulate stress-induced changes such as inflammation and lung function. Acute respiratory distress syndrome (ARDS) was described by Ashbaugh and coworkers (1967), who reported respiratory failure in association with sepsis, trauma, and drug overdoses. This respiratory syndrome, characterized by pulmonary infiltration, poor lung compliance, hypoxemia, and poor gas exchange, can cause significant mortality (Bigatello and Zapol, 1996). Although many factors are associated with the development of ARDS, adverse lung function changes can be attributed primarily to inflammatory cells concentrated within the lung (Fulkerson et al., 1996; Goodman et al., 1996). These specialized cells secrete mediators that typically help control pathogens; however, uncontrolled levels of mediators may ultimately damage healthy tissues.

Dietary lipids or fats have many functions within the body, and specific fatty acids can modulate inflammation. Metabolism of omega-3 fatty acids such as eicosapentaenoic acid (EPA) and γ-linolenic acid (GLA) can alter the arachidonic acid pathway, ultimately affecting potent neutrophil chemotactic factors and proinflammatory mediators such as prostanoids and leukotrienes. EPA shifts production of cellular metabolites to those that are less pro-inflammatory (thromboxane A3 and prostaglandin I3), while GLA inhibits arachidonic acid precursors. GLA can also be converted to dihomo-γ-linoleic acid (DGLA), a precursor of prostaglandin E1 that has anti-inflammatory properties (Fan and Chapkin, 1998). Animal and human studies have documented that feeding a specialized nutritional formula containing EPA and GLA, along with antioxidants, can rapidly change the phospholipid fatty acid composition of inflammatory cell membranes. This alteration can have the following benefits: (1) reduction of the synthesis of proinflammatory eicosanoids; (2) attenuation of endotoxin-induced increases in pulmonary neutrophil recruitment; (3) reduction of microvascular protein permeability; (4) reduction of time on a ventilator as well as days in the intensive care unit; and (5) increase in cardiopulmonary hemodynamics and respiratory gas exchange (Gadek et al., 1999; Mancuso et al., 1997a, 1997b; Murray et al., 1995, 2000; Palombo et al., 1996, 1997, 1999). These data demonstrate the potential of nutritional modulation to significantly reduce the consequences of acute stress on respiratory function.

MILITARY TRAINING-INDUCED STRESS AND
NUTRITIONAL INTERVENTION STUDIES

The inability to successfully adapt to stress as measured by immune function has been observed in military and nonmilitary groups (Bernton et al., 1995; Bonneau et al., 1990; Gray et al., 1997, 1999, 2001; Herbert and Cohen, 1993; Kasl et al., 1979; Kiecolt-Glaser et al., 2003; Kramer et al., 1997; Lee et al., 1992; Marsland et al., 1997; Martinez-Lopez et al., 1993; Segerstrom and Miller, 2004). Several studies have found an increased risk of infectious diseases (e.g., respiratory diseases and cellulitis) or decline in immunity and immune function as a result of military training-induced stress (Bernton et al., 1995; Gray et al., 1997, 1999, 2001; Kasl et al., 1979; Kramer et al., 1997; Lee et al., 1992; Martinez-Lopez et al., 1993). Immune function appears to be a sensitive indicator of health and stress. One in vivo immune marker that predicts susceptibility of infection and mortality is delayed-type skin hypersensitivity (DTH). Christou and coworkers (1995) studied hospitalized patients and found those who responded to a DTH test were less likely to become infected; furthermore, those who were already infected and nonresponsive had a significant elevation in mortality. Bernton and coworkers (1995) found that as Ranger Training progressed, there was a decline in total DTH induration (i.e., immune reaction causing reddening and hardening of skin tissue) diameter with a concomitant increase in the number of subjects not responding (anergy) to any antigens (see Figure B-44). Thus, it appears that training-induced stress reduces immune responsiveness and places soldiers at increased risk of infection.

Our laboratory, in collaboration with other colleagues, has studied stress-induced immune cell changes and antioxidant status changes that occur during military training. In prospective, randomized, double-blind control studies, we determined whether these factors could be attenuated by nutritional intervention (Chao et al., 1999; Pfeiffer et al., 1999; Shippee et al., 1995). Subjects from three military training courses were studied: Special Forces Selection and Assessment School (SFAS), 21 days in duration; Ranger Training (RT), 62 days in duration; and Marine Mountain Warfare Training (MMWT), 28 days in duration. These studies provided uniform stress factors and measurements of nutritional intake to evaluate immune modulation through nutritional supplementation.

Studies focusing on single nutrient deficiencies or nutrient supplementation, and their influence on immune function have provided valuable insights; however, multinutrient, rather than single nutrient, deficiencies typically occur. To meet the increased requirements of stress or lack of intake, the best approach would be to provide a multinutrient combination. Furthermore, there may also be intake or metabolic differences among soldiers and a multinutrient formula may be required to meet all of the nutrient requirements of a diverse group. A strategy (described below) was developed to identify specific nutrients and to supply adequate nutrition for optimal immune function. The implementation of this strategy led to the testing of a multinutrient formula that provided immunological

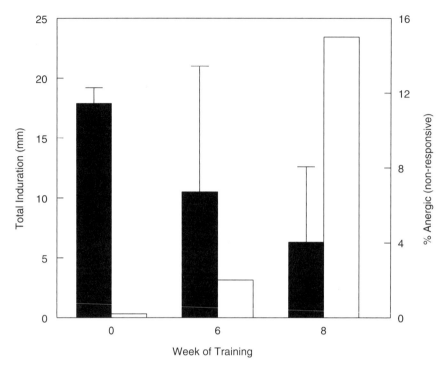

FIGURE B-44 Delayed-type skin hypersensitivity of soldiers participating in Ranger Training. Solid bars represent the mean total induration in milliliters ± standard error of the means) while the open bars are the percentage of soldiers that do not respond (anergic) to any antigen tested at the baseline and at six and eight weeks of Ranger Training. SOURCE: Data obtained from Bernton et al. (1995).

support to soldiers. The immune responsiveness to senior citizens was also tested (see next section).

The goal of the first study was to determine whether supplemental glutamine (15 g/day, a nutrient shown to decline with stress but important for immune function) could alter plasma amino acid profiles and immune function during the 21-day SFAS course (Shippee et al., 1995). SFAS assesses a soldier's physical, emotional, and mental stamina to predict success in Special Forces training. Soldiers consumed primarily Meals, Ready-to-Eat (MREs) and were given a drink containing glutamine (experimental) or glycine (control) twice, daily. Plasma glutamine and immune function were measured at baseline and at end of training. There was no difference in plasma glutamine levels between the control and experimental groups; both groups experienced an increase in plasma glutamine levels. There was a 20 percent decline in lymphocyte proliferation to phytohemagglutinin (PHA) from baseline to the end of stressful training in both groups, and 40 percent of the soldiers were anergic to the DTH test at the end of the study (Shippee et al., 1995). Weight loss was approximately six pounds per soldier during the course, and all nutrient intakes exceeded the military-recommended dietary allowances, except for folic acid (approximately 80 percent). It appeared that there was little immune benefit from glutamine supplementation.

Two additional studies were conducted with soldiers completing MMWT and SFAS courses to evaluate the effects of the antioxidants, vitamin E, vitamin C, β-carotene, and selenium either individually or in combination. Soldiers exposed to moderate altitude and cold weather training during MMWT had elevated levels of markers of oxidative stress (i.e., breath pentane, lipid peroxides, and urinary 8-hydroxydeoxyguanosine). The rise in breath pentane, a measure of oxidative stress, was only attenuated in the soldiers consuming the combination of antioxidants. There were no differences among the control group and the groups consuming individual antioxidants supplements (Figure B-45, Chao et al., 1999). Soldiers completing SFAS courses were then studied.

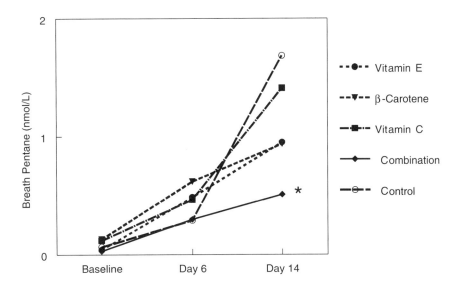

FIGURE B-45 Breath pentane concentrations (nmol/L) of marines in Marine Mountain Warfare Training consuming supplements [vitamin E (440 α-tocopherol equivalents); β-carotene (2,000 retinol equivalents); vitamin C (500 mg of ascorbic acid); and a combination of other supplements including 100 μg of selenium and 30 mg of zinc (the control was a supplement of 1,000 mg of oyster shell calcium)]. Baseline samples were collected immediately before field training, day 6 (during field training), and day 14 immediately after the end of field training.
NOTE: *Siginifcantly different from control ($p < 0.05$) at day 14.
SOURCE: Data obtained from Chao et al. (1999).

MRE diets were supplemented with a drink containing a similar level of the antioxidant combination described above (400 IU of vitamin E, 500 mg of vitamin C, 16 mg of β-carotene, 100 μg of selenium) or with an isonitrogenous–isoenergetic control drink. There were differences in serum vitamin E and vitamin C concentrations between the groups at the end of SFAS courses (p < 0.05). Even though markers of oxidative stress (plasma total radical antioxidant parameter, and lipid peroxide) pointed to substantial oxidative stress occurring during training, no differences in these markers were found between the two groups. At the end of the course, immune function declined in the control group, as seen previously in the glutamine study [lymphocyte proliferation from PHA stimulation (21 percent decline) and DTH (39 percent anergic decline)], while antioxidant supplementation attenuated the decline of lymphocyte proliferation to PHA stimulation (6 percent decline) and DTH (24 percent anergic decline). Weight loss (approximately six pounds) was similar between groups and comparable to the previous glutamine study.

It appears that a combination of antioxidants provided some benefit; therefore, a multinutrient formula was tested. The strategy, discussed in the following section, was to provide a novel nutritional immune formulation that contained energy (54 percent of kilocalories as carbohydrates, including a fermentable carbohydrate [fructooligosacchrarides] and 30 percent as fats, including structured lipids to provide a novel energy substrate as well as improved absorption of fat-soluble nutrients), protein (14 percent of kilocalories), antioxidants, and a mix of vitamins, minerals, and amino acids to sustain immune function for people under stress.

Nutritional Components for a Novel Immune Formula

Nutrition has been linked to cellular pathways essential for effective immune function (Beisel et al., 1981; Scrimshaw and SanGiovanni, 1997), and administration of selected supplemental nutrition may attenuate stress-induced immune changes. Several reviews have summarized the effects of individual nutrient deficiencies and their influence on immune function (Beisel et al., 1981; Corman, 1985; Santos et al., 1983). For example, zinc deficiency reduced effective immune function, while supplemental zinc improved effective immune function (Fraker et al., 2000). Plasma zinc levels decline in soldiers participating in intensive military training (Singh et al., 1989) as a result of elevated urinary excretion, although the decline is not classified as an "overt" nutrient deficiency (Miyamura et al., 1987). Because of the demands of increased metabolism or minor nutrient deficiencies, soldiers may benefit from selected supplemental nutrition resulting in optimal immune function, thereby improving soldiers' readiness.

During training, soldiers experience oxidative stress (Chao et al., 1999; Pfeiffer et al., 1999). As a result, free radical accumulation can result in tissue injury, delayed wound healing, and increased susceptibility to infectious diseases (Sandstead et al., 1982). Immune cells modulate free radical oxidation by using concentrated antioxidants (Moser, 1987). Antioxidants play a role in the proper functioning of immune cells (i.e., neutrophils) and help prevent oxidative stress and immune function decline (Greenman et al., 1988; Kanter et al., 1993; Prasad, 1980). Exercise and muscle stress rely on both fats and carbohydrates as fuel sources to meet energy demands. However, lipids have the advantage over carbohydrates in energy density. A factor contributing to muscle fatigue is muscle glycogen depletion and carbohydrate oxidation; therefore, researchers have attempted to maintain muscle glycogen through the delivery of lipids, e.g. medium-chain triacylglycerols (MCT). MCTs diffuse across enterocytes quickly and are absorbed through mitochondria independently of transport mechanisms and are oxidized as rapidly as glucose (Decombaz et al., 1983; Johnson et al., 1990), but few MCTs are available to the muscle because they are first absorbed through the portal vein and metabolized in the liver. Ingestion of large amounts of MCTs can also cause gastrointestinal (GI) discomfort. Studies have not detected any benefit in muscle performance resulting from supplemental MCTs as compared with supplemental carbohydrate during exercise (Horowitz et al., 2000; Jeukendrup et al., 1998). Other studies, however, have shown significant benefits in muscle performance when MCTs are consumed with carbohydrates (Jeukendrup et al., 1995; Van Zyl et al., 1996). For example, Van Zyl and coworkers (1996) compared cycling performance (two-hour ride at 60 percent of VO_2max followed by a simulated 40-kilometer race) of subjects consuming a 10-percent glucose polymer solution, an isocaloric 4.3-percent MCT emulsion, or a mixture of carbohydrate and MCT. The mixture of carbohydrate and MCT provided the best performance ($p < 0.05$) (see Figure B-46, Van Zyl et al., 1996).

A novel approach would be to include structured lipids in the formulation. Structured lipids have been shown to attenuate the hypermetabolic and protein catabolic responses of trauma and stress (DeMichele et al., 1988; Kenler et al., 1996; Mok et al., 1984; Selleck et al., 1994). Random re-esterification of MCT with long-chain fatty acids yields structured triacylglycerols or structured lipids that retain desirable characteristics of both types of fatty acids (DeMichele and Bistrian, 2001). Feeding fish oil–derived structured triacylglycerol containing MCT and long-chain fatty acids to patients undergoing surgery resulted in 50 percent fewer GI complications and infections in this susceptible population (Kenler et al., 1996).

Stress also influences GI health. Structured triacylglycerols (structured lipids) have been shown to increase the absorption of both lipids and fat-soluble nutrients important for immune function in models of GI injury (Tso et al., 1999, 2001). Furthermore, there was a two- to three-fold increase in decanoic acid and EPA in the lymphatic system (Figure B-47, Tso et al., 1999). Thus, structured lipid fatty acids, even those of medium-chain length, are absorbed through the lymphatic system and delivered to the blood stream, and are available as an energy source for active muscles. Similarly, researchers have determined that

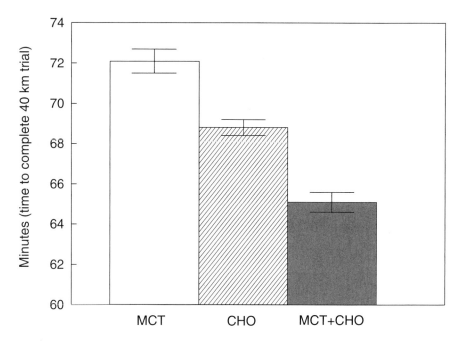

FIGURE B-46 Time needed to complete a 40 km simulated time-trial (performance). Subjects ingested either medium-chain triacylglyceride (MCT), carbohydrate (CHO), or MCT plus CHO.
NOTE: All groups are significantly diffferet from each other (p < 0.05).
SOURCE: Van Zyl et al. (1996), used with permission.

some nutrients (e.g., vitamin E) are absorbed better when given with structured lipids in normal and malabsorptive states (Tso et al., 2001). Therefore, dietary structured lipids may influence soldiers' physical readiness by providing a unique energy source to meet increased physical demands. By aiding in the absorption of fat-soluble nutrients necessary for optimal immune responses, they may also influence immune function (Calder et al., 2002).

In addition to alterations in absorption, nutrients can influence the immune cells in the GI tract. For example, fermentable carbohydrates are substrates for bifidobacteria and other beneficial bacteria (Barrangou et al., 2003). Mounting evidence suggests that fermentable carbohydrates are also beneficial to the immune system and general GI health (Pierre et al., 1999; Schley and Field, 2002).

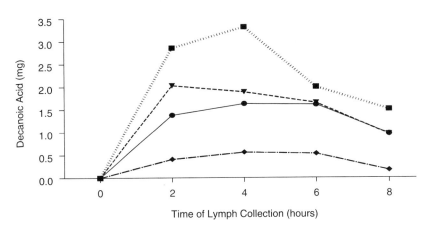

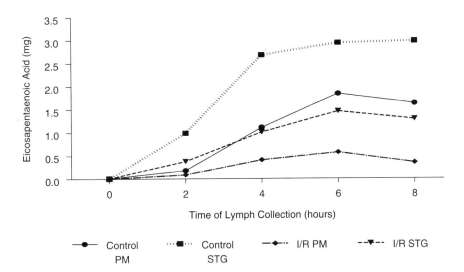

FIGURE B-47 Lymphatic output in Sprague-Dawley rats following an overnight fast. The intestinal lymph duct was cannulated and lymph was analyzed for decanoic acid (10:0 from medium chain triacylglycerols) and eicosapentaenoic acid 20:5 (long-chain ω-3 fatty acid) from intragastrically infusing a physical mix (PM) or structured lipid (STG) in normal (Control) and GI injured (Ischemia/Reperfusion–I/R) models. Measurements were made before lipid infusion (time 0) and at two, four, six, and eight hours after lipid feeding. Mean fasting lymph flow increased as a result of lipid infusion (peaking after three hours and reaching a steady output by the eighth hour) and was similar for all groups.
SOURCE: Tso et al. (1999), used with permission.

Testing the Novel Nutritional Immune Formula (NNIF) During Military Training

Soldiers participating in SFAS courses experienced similar weight loss (approximately six pounds per soldier) in both the control and NNIF groups even though more energy was offered along with the typical MRE diet due to the addition of either the control or NNIF supplements. Even with weight loss, however, a significant difference was observed between the control and NNIF groups with respect to DTH (41 percent versus 22 percent anergic; in addition, a trend towards increased whole blood lymphocyte proliferation to concanvalin A (–6 percent versus 17 percent for control and NNIF groups, respectively) was observed (Wood et al., in press). Furthermore, the consumption of NNIF attenuated stress-induced immune cell changes and reduced the number of soldiers reporting to the medical clinic with upper respiratory tract infections (16 percent versus 12 percent for control and NNIF groups, respectively, p = 0.08) (Wood et al., in press). Thus, among the formulas tested, NNIF was the most effective in supporting the immune function of soldiers during stressful military training.

SIMILARITIES BETWEEN MILITARY STRESS-INDUCED IMMUNE CHANGES AND THOSE OCCURRING IN SENIOR POPULATIONS

Stress-induced changes observed in military training include a reduction in lymphocyte proliferation, DTH responsiveness, and vaccine responses (data not shown), an increased oxidative stress as well as several cellular changes that ultimately may increase the soldiers' risk of infection. Similar results have been observed in senior populations. Factors that influence immune function, such as inadequate intake; GI changes that decrease nutrient absorption and nutrient metabolism; and the increased nutritional needs for optimal immune function, may be similar in both the military and aging populations. Therefore, the same multinutrient formula was tested in two studies of senior citizens (one study in a free- and assisted-living setting, and the other in an institutional setting). The first study evaluated whether senior citizens consuming NNIF for six months, before and during influenza season, experienced fewer days with symptoms of upper respiratory tract infections and improved response to influenza vaccine, compared with a control group consuming an isonitrogenous or isoenergetic formula. Significantly fewer days of upper respiratory tract infection symptoms (8.7 ± 3.8 versus 4.9 ± 3.2 [mean ± standard error of the mean for the control versus NNIF groups, respectively]) were observed for the NNIF group (see Figure B-48). Improved response to the influenza vaccine as measured by antibody responses; increased percentage of subjects with a four-fold increase in antibody production (an indication of response to the influenza vaccine); and increased lymphocyte proliferation to influenza antigens were also observed (Langkamp-Henken et al., 2004a) in the group consuming NNIF.

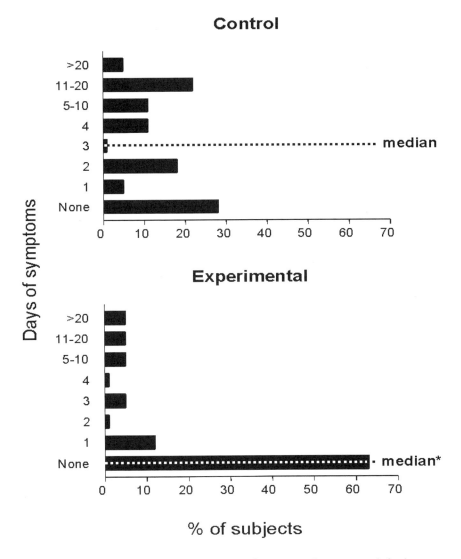

FIGURE B-48 Median days with symptoms of upper respiratory tract infections per subject were three (range 0–69) in the control group and zero (range 0–49, p < 0.05) in the experimental (NNIF) group. In the control group, 13 of 18 subjects recorded a total of 156 days of symptoms, while in the experimental group, 6 of 16 subjects recorded a total of 78 days of symptoms.

NOTE: NNIF = novel nutritional immune formulation.

SOURCE: Adapted from Langkamp-Henken et al. (2004a).

In the second study, institutionalized senior citizens consuming NNIF for three months experienced differences in immune function (response to influenza vaccines, lymphocyte subsets and activity, and cytokine production following stimulation with mitogens or influenza antigens) (Langkamp-Henken et al., 2004b).These findings were consistent with those noted in the previous studies of NNIF fed to soldiers undergoing training stress as well as to senior citizens in a free- and assisted-living setting.

SUMMARY AND CONCLUSIONS

Stress from military training and combat causes a reduction in immune function, placing soldiers at an increased risk of infection. The development of foods for people under stress, such as soldiers, requires the identification of stress-induced changes and specific nutrients to modulate these changes. The ability to identify gaps between healthy and stressed populations seems to be a critical point in developing such foods. Examples of nutritional manipulation of stress-induced changes were presented using immune function as a tool to evaluate susceptibility to infection. The similarities between stress-induced changes in soldiers in training courses and those observed in senior citizens in various settings provided an opportunity to evaluate the results of the same nutritional formula in two high-risk groups. A multinutrient formulation containing vitamins, antioxidants, minerals, structured lipids, fermentable carbohydrates, taurine, carnitine, and protein attenuated the stress-induced immune changes of soldiers in training. The same formula improved the immune system of senior citizens and led to increased responsiveness to influenza vaccine, fewer days of symptoms of upper respiratory tract infections, and less senescent immune cell profiles.

In summary, the multinutrient formulation attenuated lymphocyte proliferation decline and DTH anergy caused by stressful military training, and similarly, in senior citizens, reduced the number of days of symptoms of upper respiratory tract infections, improved responsiveness to influenza vaccine, and was associated with cellular changes indicating enhanced immunity. Thus, use of the NNIF could affect soldiers' immune function, recovery, and readiness that ultimately could influence overall performance.

ACKNOWLEDGMENT

The author thanks COL Ron Shippee, PhD, Jeff Kennedy, MD, Joann Arsenault, MS, RD, E. Wayne Askew, PhD, Don Roberts, PhD, Scott Montain, PhD, Tim Kramer, PhD, Bobbi Langkamp-Henken, PhD, Brad Bender, MD, Kelli Herrlinger-Garcia, BS, Stephen DeMichele, PhD, John McEwen, BS, Mike Simpson, BS, John Cramblit, BS, Debra Thomas, MS, Joseph Schaller, PhD, Peter Ruey, PhD, Deb Ataya, PhD, and Geraldine Baggs, PhD, who contributed significantly to the studies described. Furthermore, this work could not have been possible without the dedicated commitment of staff, command, soldiers, and personnel from US Army Research Institute of Environmental Medicine, Naval Health Research Center, US Army Special Operations, Marine Mountain Warfare Training Center, University of Utah, University of Florida, and Ross Products Division of Abbott Laboratories.

REFERENCES

Ashbaugh DG, Bigelow DB, Petty TL, Levine BE. 1967. Acute respiratory distress in adults. *Lancet* 2(7511):319–323.

Barrangou R, Altermann E, Hutkins R, Cano R, Klaenhammer TR. 2003. Functional and comparative genomic analyses of an operon involved in fructooligosaccharide utilization by *Lactobacillus acidophilus*. *Proc Natl Acad Sci U S A* 100(15):8957–8962.

Beisel WR, Edelman R, Nauss K, Suskind RM. 1981. Single-nutrient effects on immunologic functions. Report of a workshop sponsored by the Department of Food and Nutrition and its nutrition advisory group of the American Medical Association. *J Am Med Assoc* 245(1):53–58.

Bernton E, Hoover D, Galloway R, Popp K. 1995. Adaptation to chronic stress in military trainees. Adrenal androgens, testosterone, glucocorticoids, IGF-1, and immune function. *Ann N Y Acad Sci* 774:217–231.

Bigatello LM, Zapol WM. 1996. New approaches to acute lung injury. *Br J Anaesth* 77(1):99–109.

Bonneau RH, Kiecolt-Glaser JK, Glaser R. 1990. Stress-induced modulation of the immune response. *Ann N Y Acad Sci* 594:253–269.

Calder PC, Yaqoob P, Thies F, Wallace FA, Miles EA. 2002. Fatty acids and lymphocyte functions. *Br J Nutr* 87(Suppl 1):S31–S48.

Chao WH, Askew EW, Roberts DE, Wood SM, Perkins JB. 1999. Oxidative stress in humans during work at moderate altitude. *J Nutr* 129(11):2009–2012.

Christou NV, Meakins JL, Gordon J, Yee J, Hassan-Zahraee M, Nohr CW, Shizgal HM, MacLean LD. 1995. The delayed hypersensitivity response and host resistance in surgical patients. 20 years later. *Ann Surg* 222(4):534–546.

Corman LC. 1985. Effects of specific nutrients on the immune response. Selected clinical applications. *Med Clin North Am* 69(4):759–791.

Decombaz J, Arnaud MJ, Milon H, Moesch H, Philippossian G, Thelin AL, Howald H. 1983. Energy metabolism of medium-chain triglycerides versus carbohydrates during exercise. *Eur J Appl Physiol Occup Physiol* 52(1):9–14.

DeMichele SJ, Bistrian BR. 2001. Structured triacylglycerols in clinical nutrtion. In: Mansbach II CM, Tso P, Kuksis A, eds. *Intestinal Lipid Metabolism*. New York: Kluwer Acedemic/Plenum. Pp. 403–419.

DeMichele SJ, Karlstad MD, Babayan VK, Istfan N, Blackburn GL, Bistrian BR. 1988. Enhanced skeletal muscle and liver protein synthesis with structured lipid in enterally fed burned rats. *Metabolism* 37(8):787–795.

Fan YY, Chapkin RS. 1998. Importance of dietary g-linolenic acid in human health and nutrition. *J Nutr* 128(9):1411–1414.

Fraker PJ, King LE, Laakko T, Vollmer TL. 2000. The dynamic link between the integrity of the immune system and zinc status. *J Nutr* 130(5S Suppl):1399S–1406S.

Fulkerson WJ, MacIntyre N, Stamler J, Crapo JD. 1996. Pathogenesis and treatment of the adult respiratory distress syndrome. *Arch Intern Med* 156(1):29–38.

Gadek JE, DeMichele SJ, Karlstad MD, Pacht ER, Donahoe M, Albertson TE, Van Hoozen C, Wennberg AK, Nelson JL, Noursalehi M. 1999. Effect of enteral feeding with eicosapentaenoic acid, gamma-linolenic acid, and antioxidants in patients with acute respiratory distress syndrome. Enteral Nutrition in ARDS Study Group. *Crit Care Med* 27(8):1409–1420.

Goodman RB, Strieter RM, Martin DP, Steinberg KP, Milberg JA, Maunder RJ, Kunkel SL, Walz A, Hudson LD, Martin TR. 1996. Inflammatory cytokines in patients with persistence of the acute respiratory distress syndrome. *Am J Respir Crit Care Med* 154(3 Pt 1):602–611.

Gray GC, Blankenship TL, Gackstetter G. 2001. History of respiratory illness at the US Naval Academy. *Mil Med* 166(7):581–586.

Gray GC, Callahan JD, Hawksworth AW, Fisher CA, Gaydos JC. 1999. Respiratory diseases among US military personnel: Countering emerging threats. *Emerg Infect Dis* 5(3):379–385.

Gray GC, Duffy LB, Paver RJ, Putnam SD, Reynolds RJ, Cassell GH. 1997. Mycoplasma pneumoniae: A frequent cause of pneumonia among US Marines in southern California. *Mil Med* 162(8):524–526.

Greenman E, Phillipich MJ, Meyer CJ, Charamella LJ, Dimitrov NV. 1988. The effect of selenium on phagocytosis in humans. *Anticancer Res* 8(4):825–828.

Herbert TB, Cohen S. 1993. Stress and immunity in humans: A meta-analytic review. *Psychosom Med* 55(4):364–379.

Horowitz JF, Mora-Rodriguez R, Byerley LO, Coyle EF. 2000. Preexercise medium-chain triglyceride ingestion does not alter muscle glycogen use during exercise. *J Appl Physiol* 88(1):219–225.

Jeukendrup AE, Saris WH, Schrauwen P, Brouns F, Wagenmakers AJ. 1995. Metabolic availability of medium-chain triglycerides coingested with carbohydrates during prolonged exercise. *J Appl Physiol* 79(3):756–762.

Jeukendrup AE, Thielen JJ, Wagenmakers AJ, Brouns F, Saris WH. 1998. Effect of medium-chain triacylglycerol and carbohydrate ingestion during exercise on substrate utilization and subsequent cycling performance. *Am J Clin Nutr* 67(3):397–404.

Johnson RC, Young SK, Cotter R, Lin L, Rowe WB. 1990. Medium-chain-triglyceride lipid emulsion: Metabolism and tissue distribution. *Am J Clin Nutr* 52(3):502–508.

Kanter MM, Nolte LA, Holloszy JO. 1993. Effects of an antioxidant vitamin mixture on lipid peroxidation at rest and postexercise. *J Appl Physiol* 74(2):965–969.

Kasl SV, Evans AS, Niederman JC. 1979. Psychosocial risk factors in the developmental of infectious mononucleosis. *Psychosom Med* 41(6):445–466.

Kenler AS, Swails WS, Driscoll DF, DeMichele SJ, Daley B, Babineau TJ, Peterson MB, Bistrian BR. 1996. Early enteral feeding in postsurgical cancer patients. Fish oil structured lipid-based polymeric formula versus a standard polymeric formula. *Ann Surg* 223(3):316–333.

Kiecolt-Glaser JK, Preacher KJ, MacCallum RC, Atkinson C, Malarkey WB, Glaser R. 2003. Chronic stress and age-related increases in the proinflammatory cytokine IL-6. *Proc Natl Acad Sci U S A* 100(15):9090–9095.

Kramer TR, Moore RJ, Shippee RL, Friedl KE, Martinez-Lopez L, Chan MM, Askew EW. 1997. Effects of food restriction in military training on T-lymphocyte responses. *Int J Sports Med* 18(Suppl 1):S84–S90.

Langkamp-Henken B, Bender BS, Gardner EM, Herrlinger-Garcia KA, Kelley MJ, Murasko DM, Schaler JP, Stechmiller JK, Thomas DJ, Wood SM. 2004a. Nutritional formula enhanced immune function and reduced days of symptoms of upperrespiratory tract infection in seniors. *J Am Geriatr Soc* 52(1):3–12.

Langkamp-Henken B, Wood SM, Herrlinger-Garcia KA, Stechmiller JK, Thomas DJ, Bender BS, Schaller JP, Gardner EM, Murasko DM. 2004b. Nutritional formula improved immune profiles in a nursing home population. *FASEB J* 18(4):A9.

Lee DJ, Meehan RT, Robinson C, Mabry TR, Smith ML. 1992. Immune responsiveness and risk of illness in US Air Force Academy cadets during basic cadet training. *Aviat Space Environ Med* 63(6):517–523.

Mancuso P, Whelan J, DeMichele SJ, Snider CC, Guszcza JA, Claycombe KJ, Smith GT, Gregory TJ, Karlstad MD. 1997a. Effects of eicosapentaenoic and gamma-linolenic acid on lung permeability and alveolar macrophage eicosanoid synthesis in endotoxic rats. *Crit Care Med* 25(3):523–532.

Mancuso P, Whelan J, DeMichele SJ, Snider CC, Guszcza JA, Karlstad MD. 1997b. Dietary fish oil and fish and borage oil suppress intrapulmonary proinflammatory eicosanoid biosynthesis and attenuate pulmonary neutrophil accumulation in endotoxic rats. *Crit Care Med* 25(7):1198–1206.

Marsland AL, Herbert TB, Muldoon MF, Bachen EA, Patterson S, Cohen S, Rabin B, Manuck SB. 1997. Lymphocyte subset redistribution during acute laboratory stress in young adults: Mediating effects of hemoconcentration. *Health Psychol* 16(4):341–348.

Martinez-Lopez LE, Friedl KE, Moore RJ, Kramer TR. 1993. A longitudinal study of infections and injuries of Ranger students. *Mil Med* 158(7):433–437.

Miyamura JB, McNutt SW, Lichton IJ, Wenkam NS. 1987. Altered zinc status of soldiers under field conditions. *J Am Diet Assoc* 87(5):595–597.

Mok KT, Maiz A, Yamazaki K, Sobrado J, Babayan VK, Moldawer LL, Bistrian BR, Blackburn GL. 1984. Structured medium-chain and long-chain triglyceride emulsions are superior to physical mixtures in sparing body protein in the burned rat. *Metabolism* 33(10):910–915.

Moser U. 1987. Uptake of ascorbic acid by leukocytes. *Ann N Y Acad Sci* 498:200–215.

Murray MJ, Kanazi G, Moukabary K, Tazelaar HD, DeMichele SJ. 2000. Effects of eicosapentaenoic and gamma-linolenic acids (dietary lipids) on pulmonary surfactant composition and function during porcine endotoxemia. *Chest* 117(6):1720–1727.

Murray MJ, Kumar M, Gregory TJ, Banks PL, Tazelaar HD, DeMichele SJ. 1995. Select dietary fatty acids attenuate cardiopulmonary dysfunction during acute lung injury in pigs. *Am J Physiol* 269(6 Pt 2):H2090–H2099.

Palombo JD, DeMichele SJ, Boyce PJ, Lydon EE, Liu JW, Huang YS, Forse RA, Mizgerd JP, Bistrian BR. 1999. Effect of short-term enteral feeding with eicosapentaenoic and gamma-linolenic acids on alveolar macrophage eicosanoid synthesis and bactericidal function in rats. *Crit Care Med* 27(9):1908–1915.

Palombo JD, DeMichele SJ, Lydon E, Bistrian BR. 1997. Cyclic vs continuous enteral feeding with omega-3 and gamma-linolenic fatty acids: Effects on modulation of phospholipid fatty acids in rat lung and liver immune cells. *J Parenter Enteral Nutr* 21(3):123–132.

Palombo JD, DeMichele SJ, Lydon EE, Gregory TJ, Banks PL, Forse RA, Bistrian BR. 1996. Rapid modulation of lung and liver macrophage phospholipid fatty acids in endotoxemic rats by continuous enteral feeding with n-3 and gamma-linolenic fatty acids. *Am J Clin Nutr* 63(2):208–219.

Pfeiffer JM, Askew EW, Roberts DE, Wood SM, Benson JE, Johnson SC, Freedman MS. 1999. Effect of antioxidant supplementation on urine and blood markers of oxidative stress during extended moderate-altitude training. *Wilderness Environ Med* 10(2):66–74.

Pierre F, Perrin P, Bassonga E, Bornet F, Meflah K, Menanteau J. 1999. T cell status influences colon tumor occurrence in min mice fed short chain fructo-oligosaccharides as a diet supplement. *Carcinogenesis* 20(10):1953–1956.

Prasad JS. 1980. Effect of vitamin E supplementation on leukocyte function. *Am J Clin Nutr* 33(3):606–608.

Sandstead HH, Henriksen LK, Greger JL, Prasad AS, Good RA. 1982. Zinc nutriture in the elderly in relation to taste acuity, immune response, and wound healing. *Am J Clin Nutr* 36(5 Suppl):1046–1059.

Santos JI, Arredondo JL, Vitale JJ. 1983. Nutrition, infection and immunity. *Pediatr Ann* 12(3):182–194.

Schley PD, Field CJ. 2002. The immune-enhancing effects of dietary fibres and prebiotics. *Br J Nutr* 87(Suppl 2):S221–S230.

Scrimshaw NS, SanGiovanni JP. 1997. Synergism of nutrition, infection, and immunity: An overview. *Am J Clin Nutr* 66(2):464S–477S.

Segerstrom SC, Miller GE. 2004. Psychological stress and the human immune system: A meta-analytic study of 30 years of inquiry. *Psychol Bull* 130(4):601–630.

Selleck KJ, Wan JM, Gollaher CJ, Babayan VK, Bistrian BR. 1994. Effect of low and high amounts of a structured lipid containing fish oil on protein metabolism in enterally fed burned rats. *Am J Clin Nutr* 60(2):216–222.

Shippee RL, Wood S, Anderson P, Kramer TR, Neita M, Wolcott K. 1995. Effects of glutamine supplementation on immunological responses of soldiers during the Special Forces Assessment and Selection Course. *FASEB J* 9:A731.

Singh A, Day BA, DeBolt JE, Trostmann UH, Bernier LL, Deuster PA. 1989. Magnesium, zinc, and copper status of US Navy SEAL trainees. *Am J Clin Nutr* 49(4):695–700.

Tso P, Lee T, DeMichele SJ. 1999. Lymphatic absorption of structured triglycerides vs. physical mix in a rat model of fat malabsorption. *Am J Physiol* 277(40):G333–G340.

Tso P, Lee T, DeMichele SJ. 2001. Randomized structured triglycerides increase lymphatic absorption of tocopherol and retinol compared with the equivalent physical mixture in a rat model of fat malabsorption. *J Nutr* 131(8):2157–2163.

Van Zyl CG, Lambert EV, Hawley JA, Noakes TD, Dennis SC. 1996. Effects of medium-chain triglyceride ingestion on fuel metabolism and cycling performance. *J Appl Physiol* 80(6):2217–2225.

Wood SM, Kennedy JS, Arsenault J, Thomas DL, Buck RH, Shippee RL, DeMichele SJ, Winship TR, Schaller JP, Montain S, Cordle CT. In press. Novel nutritional immune formula maintains host defense mechanisms. *Mil Med.*

Food Intake Regulation: Liquid versus Solid

Richard D. Mattes, Purdue University

INTRODUCTION

Hunger is the term for sensations that prompt food seeking and ingestion. Satiation and satiety represent sensations that determine meal size and the intermeal interval, respectively. While hunger is on the opposite end of an ingestive behavior scale from satiation/satiety, the sensations do not stem from the presence or absence of a common set of cues. Different mechanisms regulate them, reflecting the fact that the sensations are multidimensional. For example, there is clearly a physiological basis for hunger, but there are cognitive and sensory components as well. One may eat to a high level of satiation, yet the availability of a palatable food can prompt sufficient hunger to eat more. Alternatively, stress may reduce interest in eating when sensations commonly associated with low satiation (e.g., weakness) are present. Thus, regulation of energy balance involves a complex interaction between these sensations and lifestyle.

In the context of soldiers in combat operations, where energy expenditure may surpass energy intake by 50 percent, there is particular concern about an energy deficit that may result in muscle loss and impaired performance. Such a deficit results from an inappropriate dominance of satiation/satiety cues relative to hunger. It may also be attributable to a low priority for appetitive sensations and intake (i.e., the appetitive system may still be functional just ignored or minimized). The body of scientific literature comprises work addressing the predominant health concern in the general population, that is, energy surfeit. Whether the factors that promote positive energy balance in the general population can be applied in the combat environment in which intake is less than desired, is an empirical question that warrants further consideration and testing.

Features of a diet that may contribute to its low satiety value include a high fat content, a low fiber level, a low calcium concentration and an increased proportion of energy derived from beverages. The latter will be the focus of this presentation. Evidence will be presented that energy-yielding beverages have weak satiety properties and elicit incomplete dietary compensation. The properties of beverages that account for these effects will be outlined followed by a consideration of possible mechanisms. The following are a set of more specific questions that this paper attempts to address:

- What are the rheological factors regulating food intake that could maximize the consumption of a food given to soldiers under physical, cognitive, and environmental stress?
- What products may enhance appetite and be added to maximize the consumption of a food product for soldiers under stress?
- What form (liquid versus solid and gels versus bars) could be given to a presumably healthy soldier to enhance appetite?

EFFECTS OF BEVERAGE CONSUMPTION ON FOOD INTAKE

Beverage Consumption and Appetite

Most studies of appetitive sensations (e.g., hunger, desire to eat, fullness, prospective consumption) support the view that fluids or semisolids are less satiating than solid foods (Haber et al., 1977; Hulshof et al., 1993; Raben et al., 1994; Tournier and Louis-Sylvestre, 1991). Indeed, an independent inverse influence of viscosity on hunger has been demonstrated (Mattes and Rothacker, 2001). There have been studies that failed to observe solid versus fluid differences in intake (Jordan and Spiegel, 1977; Kissileff et al., 1980; Levitz, 1975; Rolls et al., 1990), but their interpretation may be hampered by the use of foods that differed along many dimensions and testing under nonnormal eating conditions (e.g., delivery of load by pump or testing in a laboratory). For example, a number of these observations are based on studies conducted with soup (Hulshof et al., 1993; Jordan and Spiegel, 1977; Kissileff, 1985; Kissileff et al., 1980; Levitz, 1975; Raben et al., 1994; Rolls et al., 1990, 1999; Tournier and Louis-Sylvestre, 1991). Soup does appear to be an exception in the fluid–solid influence on appetite; although an explanation remains elusive, it likely involves a strong cognitive component (Mattes, 2005).

Beverage Consumption and Dietary Compensation

Dietary surveys indicate that the addition of a beverage to a meal leads to increased total energy intake at the meal by an amount roughly equal to the contribution of the beverage (de Castro, 1993). Similar findings have been reported over days for soda and alcohol (Colditz et al., 1991; Rose et al., 1995). The majority of work on this issue has been conducted with young adults, but the phenomenon also appears to hold with adolescents. Based on data from the 1994 Continuing Survey of Food Intake for Individuals (CSFII) survey, daily energy intake as well as carbohydrate energy tends to increase among adolescents with an increasing consumption of soft drinks (Harnack et al., 1999).

Intervention studies have yielded comparable results (DiMeglio and Mattes, 2000; Mattes, 1996; Tournier and Louis-Sylvestre, 1991). Interestingly, other studies noted that supplemental noncaloric fluid ingestion is not associated with increased intake or body weight, but the addition of an energy source to a fluid leads to increases in both (Poppitt et al., 1996; Raben et al., 2002; Tordoff and Alleva, 1990). Dietary compensation (energy intake adjustments made during the day to compensate for earlier intake) has been studied with solid, semisolid, and fluid foods. In a meta-analysis including more than 40 studies, the reported mean dietary compensation error for experimental loads of solid foods was 36 percent. This is in contrast to the mean dietary compensation for semisolid foods and for fluids (79 percent and 109 percent, respectively) (Mattes, 1996). This analysis suggests that dietary adjustments are made at other times of the day to offset all but 36 percent of the energy contributed by the experimental solid loads, but there is no compensation, indeed a slight reverse compensation (greater intake of the customary diet), for fluids.

Beverage Consumption and Body Weight

Survey data indicate caloric beverage consumption is associated with higher body weight or body mass index (BMI) (Gillis and Bar-Or, 2003; Ludwig et al., 2001). In a prospective observational study of schoolchildren, increments of soda servings were associated with quarter BMI unit increases (Ludwig et al., 2001). An intervention trial that involved ingestion of 450 kcal daily of sweetened fruit-flavored beverage revealed a significant increase in body weight that was not observed when 450 kcal were consumed in solid form by the same individuals (DiMeglio and Mattes, 2000). Although much of this work has focused on carbonated beverage intake because of its high level of consumption in the population, it is probably incorrect to assume that its effect on body weight is unique. In fact, noncarbonated beverages with energy derived from other macronutrients also elicit weak dietary compensation (de Castro, 1993; Shields et al., 2004), which suggests that they will also affect body weight.

Satiety Properties of Macronutrients

Important features of compensatory responses to beverages have not been adequately characterized. One concern is potential differences across macronutrients. Studies, primarily with solid foods, indicate that when macronutrients are presented as isoenergetic loads (preserving differences in energy density), there is a hierarchy of satiety values wherein protein > carbohydrate > fat (Blundell et al., 1996; Johnson and Vickers, 1993; Stubbs et al., 1997). Although there is some evidence that the hierarchy holds in fluids as well (e.g., Stubbs et al., 1997), the energy-yielding macronutrients have never been directly contrasted in a within-subject design study. Survey data indicate beverages with different macronutrient compositions (e.g., soda, alcohol, milk) are equally ineffective in prompting dietary compensation (de Castro, 1993; Mattes, 1996). A review of the literature reveals that most studies supporting a high satiety value of protein involved manipulations of solid foods (Booth et al., 1970; Hill and Blundell, 1986, 1990; Johnson and Vickers, 1993; Porrini et al., 1995; Stubbs et al., 1996; Vandewater and Vickers, 1996) whereas the high satiety value of protein is not as robust in studies using fluid preloads (de Graaf et al., 1992; Driver, 1988; Geliebter, 1979; Latner and Schwartz, 1999; Stockley et al., 1984; Sunkin and Garrow, 1982).

POSSIBLE MECHANISMS FOR THE WEAK
APPETITIVE EFFECTS OF BEVERAGES

The mechanisms responsible for the weaker appetitive and compensatory dietary responses to fluids than to solids have not been identified. Candidates include cognitive effects, orosensory stimulation, gastrointestinal (GI) tract transit time, osmotic differences, gut hormone activity, absorptive processes, and post-absorptive endocrine or metabolic responses.

Beliefs about the energy content of a food or beverage can have a stronger influence on post-ingestive appetitive responses than the true energy content, at least acutely. When lean and obese individuals were presented with low- or high-energy meals, belief about their energy content was a better predictor of the hunger response than true energy content (Wooley et al., 1972). Beverages may be believed to hold weaker satiation value than isocaloric solid items (DiMeglio and Mattes, 2000). Orosensory cues also modulate the appetitive response to a food or beverage. For example, there is an indirect relationship between the self-reported viscosity of a beverage and hunger (Mattes and Rothacker, 2001). Food that passes through the GI tract more rapidly (a short transit time), such as fluids, may elicit weaker appetitive responses than those with a longer transit time, such as soluble fiber–containing foods. This mechanism might partly explain the recognized satiating effects of fiber (Burton-Freeman, 2000; Delargy et al., 1997; Holt et al., 1992; Howarth et al., 2001). A beverage that holds comparable cognitive and orosensory properties to another beverage, but contains a compound that forms a viscous mass in the gut may be more satiating than the one lacking the compound because of its effects on GI function (Williams et al., 2004; Wolf et al., 2003). Cholecystokinin (CCK) is a gut peptide hormone that enhances satiation, especially in conjunction with gastric distention (Kissileff et al., 2003). A differential effect of ingested solid and fluid foods on CCK may be inferred by contrasting responses across studies. A fluid load (tomato soup) elicits only a modest increment in male adults (Nolan et al., 2003) whereas a more viscous homogenized vegetable load results in a marked CCK elevation in males (Santangelo et al., 1998). Similar, although quantitatively weaker, effects of fluids on CCK release have also been reported in females (Heini et al., 1998).

Several human studies have demonstrated that fluid versus solid forms of the same high-carbohydrate foods lead to comparable early rises of plasma glucose and greater insulin responses (Bolton et al., 1981; Haber et al., 1977). Numerous mechanisms for insulin's satiety effects have been proposed. One is based on evidence that insulin is an independent determinant of the circulating leptin concentration (Mantzoros et al., 1998). Leptin may inhibit food intake (Karhunen et al., 1998; Larsson et al., 1998), in part though a reduction of hunger (Keim et al., 1998; Shimizu et al., 1998). Insulin stimulates both leptin gene expression and glucose oxidation within adipocytes. This leads to increased leptin secretion (Mueller et al., 1998) and higher plasma leptin concentrations in humans (Dirlewanger et al., 2000).

SUMMARY

There is compelling evidence that body weight is increasing in the population. Per capita consumption of energy-yielding beverages has increased in parallel with this trend and energy-yielding beverages evoke a weaker appetitive and compensatory dietary response than do solid foods. Thus, it is reasonable to postulate that the consumption of beverages contributes significantly to positive energy balance. There is also enough evidence suggesting that energy intake in the form of fluid beverages may have less satiating effects and induces more dietary compensation than do solid foods. None of these studies, however, have been conducted under the high-stress situation of combat, which might influence appetite and food intake in diverse ways. Nevertheless, these observations may provide an approach for enhancing the energy intake of individuals, such as soldiers, under emotional and environmental stress. To design diets providing a high proportion of energy in fluid form may be an effective strategy to increase total energy intake, if volume and size constraints are not problematic.

REFERENCES

Blundell JE, Lawton CL, Cotton JR, Macdiarmid JI. 1996. Control of human appetite: Implications for the intake of dietary fat. *Ann Rev Nutr* 16:285–319.

Bolton RP, Heaton KW, Burroughs LF. 1981. The role of dietary fiber in satiety, glucose, and insulin: Studies with fruit and fruit juice. *Am J Clin Nutr* 34(2):211–217.

Booth DA, Chase A, Campbell AT. 1970. Relative effectiveness of protein in the late stages of appetite suppression in man. *Physiol Behav* 5(11):1299–1302.

Burton-Freeman B. 2000. Dietary fiber and energy regulation. *J Nutr* 130(2S Suppl):272S–275S.

Colditz GA, Giovannucci E, Rimm EB, Stampfer MJ, Rosner B, Speizer FE, Gordis E, Willett WC. 1991. Alcohol intake in relation to diet and obesity in women and men. *Am J Clin Nutr* 54(1):49–55.

de Castro JM. 1993. The effects of the spontaneous ingestion of particular foods or beverages on the meal pattern and overall nutrient intake of humans. *Physiol Behav* 53(6):1133–1144.

de Graaf C, Hulshof T, Weststrate JA, Jas P. 1992. Short-term effects of different amounts of protein, fats, and carbohydrates on satiety. *Am J Clin Nutr* 55(1):33–38.

Delargy HJ, O'Sullivan KR, Fletcher RJ, Blundell JE. 1997. Effects of amount and type of dietary fibre (soluble and insoluble) on short-term control of appetite. *Int J Food Sci Nutr* 48(1):67–77.

DiMeglio DP, Mattes RD. 2000. Liquid versus solid carbohydrate: Effects on food intake and body weight. *Int J Obes Relat Metab Disord* 24(6):794–800.

Dirlewanger M, di Vetta V, Guenat E, Battilana P, Seematter G, Schneiter P, Jequier E, Tappy L. 2000. Effects of short-term carbohydrate or fat overfeeding on energy expenditure and plasma leptin concentrations in healthy female subjects. *Int J Obes Relat Metab Disord* 24(11):1413–1418.

Driver CJ. 1988. The effect of meal composition on the degree of satiation following a test meal and possible mechanisms involved. *Br J Nutr* 60(3):441–449.

Geliebter AA. 1979. Effects of equicaloric loads of protein, fat, and carbohydrate on food intake in the rat and man. *Physiol Behav* 22(2):267–273.

Gillis LJ, Bar-Or O. 2003. Food away from home, sugar-sweetened drink consumption and juvenile obesity. *J Am Coll Nutr* 22(6):539–545.

Haber GB, Heaton KW, Murphy D, Burroughs LF. 1977. Depletion and disruption of dietary fibre. Effects on satiety, plasma-glucose, and serum-insulin. *Lancet* 2(8040):679–682.

Harnack L, Stang J, Story M. 1999. Soft drink consumption among US children and adolescents: Nutritional consequences. *J Am Diet Assoc* 99(4):436–441.

Heini AF, Kirk KA, Lara-Castro C, Weinsier RL. 1998. Relationship between hunger-satiety feelings and various metabolic parameters in women with obesity during controlled weight loss. *Obes Res* 6(3):225–230.

Hill AJ, Blundell JE. 1986. Macronutrients and satiety: The effects of a high-protein or high-carbohydrate meal on subjective motivation to eat and food preferences. *Nutr Behav* 3(2):133–144.

Hill AJ, Blundell JE. 1990. Comparison of the action of macronutrients on the expression of appetite in lean and obese human subjects. *Ann NY Acad Sci* 575(575):529–531.

Holt S, Brand J, Soveny C, Hansky J. 1992. Relationship of satiety to postprandial glycaemic, insulin and cholecystokinin responses. *Appetite* 18(2):129–141.

Howarth NC, Saltzman E, Roberts SB. 2001. Dietary fiber and weight regulation. *Nutr Rev* 59(5):129–139.

Hulshof T, De Graaf C, Weststrate JA. 1993. The effects of preloads varying in physical state and fat content on satiety and energy intake. *Appetite* 21(3):273–286.

Johnson J, Vickers Z. 1993. Effects of flavor and macronutrient composition of food servings on liking, hunger and subsequent intake. *Appetite* 21(1):25–39.

Jordan HA, Spiegel TA. 1977. Palatability and oral factors and their role in obesity. In: Kare MR, Maller O, eds. *The Chemical Senses and Nutrition*. New York: Academic Press. Pp. 393–410.

Karhunen LJ, Lappalainen RI, Haffner SM, Valve RH, Tuorila H, Miettinen H, Uusitupa MI. 1998. Serum leptin, food intake and preferences for sugar and fat in obese women. *Int J Obes Relat Metab Disord* 22(8):819–821.

Keim NL, Stern JS, Havel PJ. 1998. Relation between circulating leptin concentrations and appetite during a prolonged, moderate energy deficit in women. *Am J Clin Nutr* 68(4):794–801.

Kissileff HR. 1985. Effects of physical state (liquid-solid) of foods on food intake: Procedural and substantive contributions. *Am J Clin Nutr* 42(5 Suppl):956–965.

Kissileff HR, Carretta JC, Geliebter A, Pi-Sunyer FX. 2003. Cholecystokinin and stomach distension combine to reduce food intake in humans. *Am J Physiol Regul Integr Comp Physiol* 285(5):R992–R998.

Kissileff HR, Klingsberg G, Van Itallie TB. 1980. Universal eating monitor for continuous recording of solid or liquid consumption in man. *Am J Physiol Regul Integr Comp Physiol* 238(1):R14–R22.

Larsson H, Elmstahl S, Berglund G, Ahren B. 1998. Evidence for leptin regulation of food intake in humans. *J Clin Endocrinol Metab* 83(12):4382–4385.

Latner JD, Schwartz M. 1999. The effects of a high-carbohydrate, high-protein or balanced lunch upon later food intake and hunger ratings. *Appetite* 33(1):119–128.

Levitz LS. 1975. The susceptibility of human feeding behavior to external controls. In: Bray GA, ed. *Obesity in Perspective. Proceedings of the Conference.* October 1–3, 1973, Bethesda, MD. DHEW Publication No. 75-708. Washington, DC: US Government Printing Office. Pp. 53–60.

Ludwig DS, Peterson KE, Gortmaker SL. 2001. Relation between consumption of sugar-sweetened drinks and childhood obesity: A prospective, observational analysis. *Lancet* 357(9255):505–508.

Mantzoros CS, Liolios AD, Tritos NA, Kaklamani VG, Doulgerakis DE, Griveas I, Moses AC, Flier JS. 1998. Circulating insulin concentrations, smoking, and alcohol intake are important independent predictors of leptin in young healthy men. *Obes Res* 6(3):179–186.

Mattes RD. 1996. Dietary compensation by humans for supplemental energy provided as ethanol or carbohydrate in fluids. *Physiol Behav* 59(1):179–187.

Mattes RD. 2005. Soup and satiety. *Physiol Behav* 83:739–747.

Mattes RD, Rothacker D. 2001. Beverage viscosity is inversely related to postprandial hunger in humans. *Physiol Behav* 74(4–5):551–557.

Mueller WM, Gregoire FM, Stanhope KL, Mobbs CV, Mizuno TM, Warden CH, Stern JS, Havel PJ. 1998. Evidence that glucose metabolism regulates leptin secretion from cultured rat adipocytes. *Endocrinology* 139(2):551–558.

Nolan LJ, Guss JL, Liddle RA, Pi-Sunyer FX, Kissileff HR. 2003. Elevated plasma cholecystokinin and appetitive ratings after consumption of a liquid meal in humans. *Nutrition* 19(6):553–557.

Poppitt SD, Eckhardt JW, McGonagle J, Murgatroyd PR, Prentice AM. 1996. Short-term effects of alcohol consumption on appetite and energy intake. *Physiol Behav* 60(4):1063–1070.

Porrini M, Crovetti R, Riso P, Santangelo A, Testolin G. 1995. Effects of physical and chemical characteristics of food on specific and general satiety. *Physiol Behav* 57(3):461–468.

Raben A, Tagliabue A, Christensen NJ, Madsen J, Holst JJ, Astrup A. 1994. Resistant starch: The effect on postprandial glycemia, hormonal response, and satiety. *Am J Clin Nutr* 60(4):544–551.

Raben A, Vasilaras TH, Moller AC, Astrup A. 2002. Sucrose compared with artificial sweeteners: Different effects on ad libitum food intake and body weight after 10 wk of supplementation in overweight subjects. *Am J Clin Nutr* 76(4):721–729.

Rolls BJ, Bell EA, Thorwart ML. 1999. Water incorporated into a food but not served with a food decreases energy intake in lean women. *Am J Clin Nutr* 70(5):448–455.

Rolls BJ, Fedoroff IC, Guthrie JF, Laster LJ. 1990. Foods with different satiating effects in humans. *Appetite* 15(2):115–126.

Rose D, Murphy SP, Hudes M, Viteri FE. 1995. Food energy remains constant with increasing alcohol intake. *J Am Diet Assoc* 95(6):698–700.

Santangelo A, Peracchi M, Conte D, Fraquelli M, Porrini M. 1998. Physical state of meal affects gastric emptying, cholecystokinin release and satiety. *Br J Nutr* 80(6):521–527.

Shields DH, Corrales KM, Metallinos-Katsaras E. 2004. Gourmet coffee beverage consumption among college women. *J Am Diet Assoc* 104(4):650–653.

Shimizu H, Tsuchiya T, Sato N, Shimomura Y, Kobayashi I, Mori M. 1998. Troglitazone reduces plasma leptin concentration but increases hunger in NIDDM patients. *Diabetes Care* 21(9):1470–1474.

Stockley L, Jones FA, Broadhurst AJ. 1984. The effects of moderate protein or energy supplements on subsequent nutrient intake in man. *Appetite* 5(3):209–219.

Stubbs RJ, Prentice AM, James WP. 1997. Carbohydrates and energy balance. *Ann NY Acad Sci* 819:44–69.

Stubbs RJ, van Wyk MC, Johnstone AM, Harbron CG. 1996. Breakfasts high in protein, fat or carbohydrate: Effect on within-day appetite and energy balance. *Eur J Clin Nutr* 50(7):409–417.

Sunkin S, Garrow JS. 1982. The satiety value of protein. *Hum Nutr Appl Nutr* 36(3):197–201.

Tordoff MG, Alleva AM. 1990. Effect of drinking soda sweetened with aspartame or high-fructose corn syrup on food intake and body weight. *Am J Clin Nutr* 51(6):963–969.

Tournier A, Louis-Sylvestre J. 1991. Effect of the physical state of a food on subsequent intake in human subjects. *Appetite* 169(1):17–24.

Vandewater K, Vickers Z. 1996. Higher-protein foods produce greater sensory-specific satiety. *Physiol Behav* 59(3):579–583.

Williams JA, Lai CS, Corwin H, Ma Y, Maki KC, Garleb KA, Wolf BW. 2004. Inclusion of guar gum and alginate into a crispy bar improves postprandial glycemia in humans. *J Nutr* 134(4):886–889.

Wolf BW, Wolever TMS, Lai CS, Bolognesi C, Radmard R, Maharry KS, Garleb KA, Hertzler SR, Firkins JL. 2003. Effects of a beverage containing an enzymatically induced-viscosity dietary fiber, with or without fructose, on the postprandial glycemic response to a high glycemic index food in humans. *Eur J Clin Nutr* 57(9):1120–1127.

Wooley OW, Wooley SC, Dunham RB. 1972. Can calories be perceived and do they affect hunger in obese and nonobese humans? *J Comp Physiol Psychol* 80(2):250–258.

A General Model of Intake Regulation: Diurnal and Dietary Composition Components

John M. de Castro, University of Texas at El Paso

INTRODUCTION

A considerable amount of evidence shows that nutrient intakes are affected by a wide range of factors, each of which accounts for only a small portion of the variance in intake. Models that attempt to explain intake control based on any single factor have failed to account for how intake can be controlled in the face of a complex array of influential variables. In addition, the levels and effects of many factors vary from individual to individual, and these individual differences are affected by heredity. These elements have been incorporated into a general model of intake regulation (de Castro and Plunkett, 2002) that is presented in Figure B-49. The model separates sets of uncompensated and compensated factors

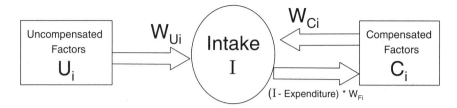

FIGURE B-49 The general intake regulation model wherein intake (I) is controlled by two sets of factors: compensated factors (C_i) that both affect and are affected by intake via negative feedback loops and uncompensated factors (U_i) that affect but are not affected by intake. Inheritance affects the system by (a) determining the preferred level for intake and compensated and uncompensated factors and (b) determining the level of impact of the factors on intake (W). Factors that are affected by heredity are indicated in bold. SOURCE: de Castro and Plunkett (2002), used with permission from Elsevier.

with each factor having preferred levels that are influenced by heredity (e.g., genetic variation). Further, the model specifies that each factor in both sets has an individual impact factor (i.e., weight that specifies the magnitude of the factor's effect on intake). The weights are assumed to be different for each individual, and their values are influenced by heredity. Simulations of the model indicate that although prolonged changes in the level of any factor can result in a prolonged change in intake and body weight, the size of the change depends on the inherited level of responsiveness to that factor. This implies that manipulation of a factor to alter intake will be effective in some individuals but not in others. For this reason, it is important to consider individual differences in responsiveness when developing an intervention designed to alter intake. The responsiveness of the individual to these influences can be measured and used to help construct an individualized intake recommendation.

The Committee on Committee on Optimization of Nutrient Composition of Military Rations for Short-Term, High-Stress Situations was charged with designing the nutrient composition of a ration to be used for short-term, high-stress combat operations. It is a well-known fact that the energy intake of soldiers in these unique situations of high mental and physical stress is lower than the energy expenditure, and this energy deficit status might result in weight losses and other health and perfomance adverse effects. In addition to maintaining health and performance, the ration should be palatable and accepted by soldiers under such unique circumstances. Palatability is only one factor that drives consumption patterns; other factors that might be categorized as psychological factors are also important in defining eating behavior, including level of consumption.

In this paper, the role of diurnal rhythms and dietary energy density on dietary intake behavior is examined; the conclusions are derived with data from reports from 669 free-living normal adult humans who adequately reported intake in a 7-day diet diary. The influence of the time of day and the dietary energy densities on intake were investigated. This model could be applied to soldiers under combat situations. Specifically, this paper attempts to answer the following questions:

- What are the food factors, which regulate food intake, that could maximize the consumption of a food ration given to soldiers under physical, cognitive, and environmental stresses?
- What are the issues to consider when developing a nutritionally enhanced food product in terms of energy density, satiability, behavior and food characteristics to maximize the consumption of the food product in specific relation to soldiers under stress?

DIURNAL FOOD INTAKE PATTERN

There are clear diurnal or circadian influences on intake. Studies using the diet diary technique (de Castro, 1987, 2004c) have demonstrated that substantial changes in intake occur over the course of the day. As the day progresses, the average meal size increases (Figure B-50, left) and the subsequent interval between meals decreases simultaneously (Figure B-50, center). We have found that this pattern is true for both North Americans and Europeans (de Castro et al., 2000) as determined by using the satiety ratio. The satiety ratio is the duration of the interval after the meal divided by the meal size (min/MJ), and it gauges the duration of satiety produced per unit of food energy ingested. This ratio markedly declines over the course of the day and becomes quite low during the late evening (Figure B-50, right) (de Castro, 1987, 2004c). This suggests that the satiating effect of food decreases over the course of the day and that a large proportion of intake in the evening could lead to increased overall intake.

Employing twin data, it was demonstrated that the time of day when people eat is significantly affected by heredity (de Castro, 2001). In particular, people differ in the proportion of daily intake ingested at different times of the day, with some eating a larger proportion of their intake in the morning, some in the afternoon, and some in the evening, and these proportions of intake are heritable. It was also demonstrated that the differences between the morning and afternoon, the morning and evening, and the afternoon and evening were significantly heritable (de Castro, 2001). This suggests that the time-of-day effects on intake vary among individuals and that this difference is, at least, partially caused by heredity. Hence genetic factors appear to affect not only when an individual will tend to eat, but also how big of an effect the selection of that time will have on intake.

Because meal sizes increase during the day, while the after-meal intervals and satiety ratios decrease over the day, it is reasonable to expect that the time of day of nutrient intake would be related to total intake. It was demonstrated that

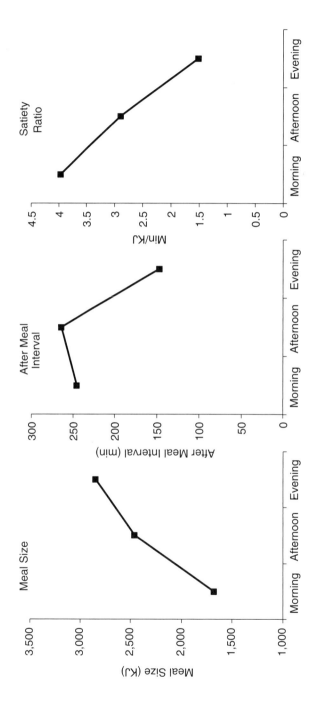

FIGURE B-50 The mean meal sizes (left panel), interval until the following meal (middle panel), and the satiety ratio (right panel) observed during the morning, afternoon, and evening periods.
SOURCE: Adapted from de Castro (2004c).

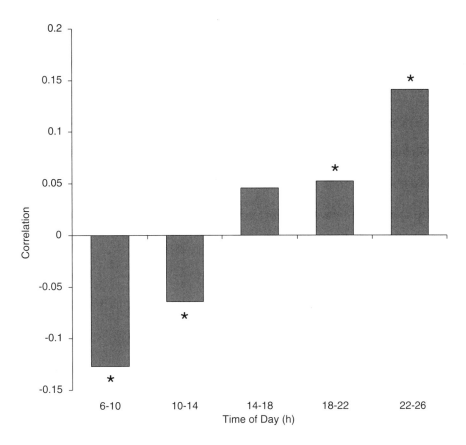

FIGURE B-51 Correlation between proportion of intake during four-hour periods and overall daily intake. The mean correlations between the proportions of food energy ingested and overall daily intake were self-reported in 7 day diet diaries during each of the five time periods and the total amount ingested.
NOTE: *Different from zero ($p < 0.01$).
SOURCE: Adapted from de Castro (2004c).

the proportion of intake ingested in the morning is negatively correlated with overall intake (Figure B-51), while the proportion ingested late in the evening is positively correlated with overall intake (de Castro, 2004c). The energy densities of intake during all periods of the day were positively related to overall intake. The results suggest that a high-density energy intake during any portion of the day could increase overall intake and that an intake in the late night lacks satiating value and can result in greater overall daily intake. Hence the best way to promote higher levels of intake would be to increase the ingestion of high energy dense foods at night.

DENSITY

The energy density of a diet has been shown to markedly affect the total amount of food energy ingested. The greater the food energy content per gram of food consumed, the more total food energy ingested (Bell and Rolls, 2001; de Castro, 2004a; Yao and Roberts, 2001). We have shown that, for study participants consuming diets of varying energy densities during a seven-day period, the dietary energy density (calculated as the food energy content of the foods divided by their total weight) of meals is related to the total energy intakes from the meals; the dietary energy densities over the entire day are related to the total energy intakes over those same days; and the dietary energy densities of the participants' diets are related to their total energy intakes. Dietary energy density is, to a large extent, positively correlated with intake, no matter whethermeals, daily intakes, or overall participant intakes were examined (Figure B-52). These findings resulted in the hypothesis that intake is not controlled on the basis of the energy content of the food, but rather on its volume, that is, the greater the food energy per unit volume of a meal, the more total food energy ingested.

Dietary energy density is calculated as the food energy content of the foods divided by the total weight of those foods. The food energy component comprises the macronutrients, carbohydrate, fat, protein, and alcohol; the weight component comprises the weight of the macronutrients, nonnutritive solids, water contained in the foods, and drinks (water) ingested with the foods. By calculating separately the energy density from carbohydrate, fat, and protein, we investigated whether the components of food energy play different roles in determining the effects of dietary energy density on intake. Each of these densities was positively correlated with intake regardless of whether meals, daily intakes, or weekly intakes were studied (Figure B-53, left). When the carbohydrate, fat, and protein dietary densities were used as independent variables in a multiple regression prediction of energy intake, a variable outcome was produced depending on whether meals, daily intakes, or overall participant intakes were employed (Figure B-53, center). The one consistent outcome was that the dietary energy density of fat always had the strongest positive relationship with energy intake. When the overall dietary energy density was added to the regression, only overall dietary energy density had a strong positive relationship with intake, but all of the macronutrient relationships became negative with respect to intake (Figure B-53, right). This occurred regardless of whether meals, daily intakes, or overall participant intakes were used. The negative relationship suggests that when the overall energy density of a meal is considered, high densities of any macronutrient have a negative influence on intake. Further, this suggested that the overall dietary energy density is more important than the dietary energy density

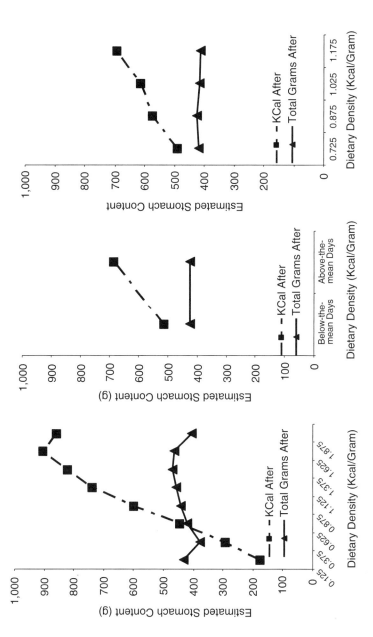

FIGURE B-52 The relationship of dietary density and after meal stomach contents. Participants with a physical activity level of > 1.1. Mean estimated contents of the stomach at the end of meals of food energy (kcal) or volume (total grams) as a function of dietary energy density for meal (left), daily (center), and participant (right) intakes.
SOURCE: Author's unpublished data.

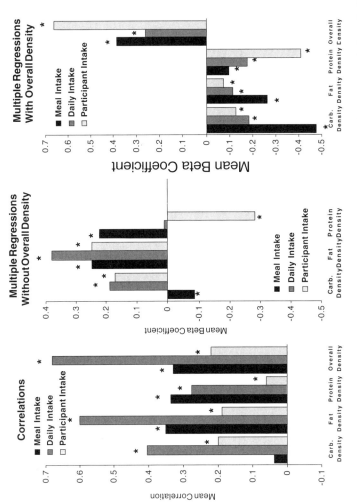

FIGURE B-53 Meal dietary density relationships with meal, daily, and participant intake. Mean univariate correlations (left), multiple regression β coefficients without (center) and with (right) inclusion of overall dietary energy density in the regression for the relationships of carbohydrate dietary energy density, fat dietary energy density, protein dietary energy density, and overall dietary energy density with meal (first bar of each set of three), daily (second bar), and participant (third bar) intakes.
SOURCE: Author's unpublished results.

of any particular macronutrient, implying that it is the meal dietary energy density per se that is the important influence on intake, not the meal's components.

The hypothesis that intake is controlled on the basis of the volume of food ingested infers that the volume of nutrients in the stomach at the end of the meal is the critical factor in determining intake. If the volume in the stomach at the end of the meal is relatively constant, then the food energy ingested would depend on the dietary energy density of the foods. The meal size is not an adequate estimate of the volume in the stomach because it does not include the nutrients from prior intake that still remain in the stomach. We attempted to test these predictions by estimating the contents of the stomach at the end of meals. Because the stomach empties in a very regular and predictable fashion (Hopkins, 1966; Hunt and Knox, 1968; Hunt and Stubbs, 1975), how much of the contents should have emptied over a given interval and how much should therefore be remaining at the time of a second meal is relatively simple to calculate (de Castro, 1987, 1999). Added to this model was an estimate of fluid movement into and out of the stomach according to the model of Toates (1978).

Employing the reported intakes from the seven-day diary records along with these stomach emptying models, both the food energy (kcal) contents and the total gram contents of the stomach at the end of each meal were estimated and expressed as a function of the dietary energy density of the meal (Figure B-52, left). Although the food energy content of the stomach increased significantly with the increase in dietary energy density, the total volume (grams) of contents estimated to be in the stomach was not significantly dissimilar over the nine different dietary energy density levels. An analysis of the mean after-meal stomach contents over the entire day (on days that an individual participant had below- or above-the-mean dietary energy density) revealed a similar picture (Figure B-52, center). Again, food energy content of the stomach was high on the above-the-mean dietary energy density days, but the estimated weight of the contents of the stomach remained unchanged. Finally, the average estimated after-meal stomach contents of participants whose dietary energy densities differed were compared (Figure B-52, right). Exactly as was seen in the meal and daily intake analyses, higher stomach contents of food energy resulted in higher dietary energy densities, but there was no difference in weight of the contents.

Using twin data, it was determined that the level of dietary energy density within the individual diets is affected by heredity (de Castro, 2004b). Additionally, the magnitude of the differences between the members of identical twin pairs in the density of their diet was positively related to the magnitude of the differences in the energy content of their daily intake (de Castro, 2004d). On the other hand, heredity did not seem to influence the relationship between density and intake. There were no significant heritable factors for either the correlation or the slope of the best fitting regression line between density and intake. Hence, it appears that heredity may influence the preferred dietary density that in turn has a marked influence on intake. This infers that heredity does not cause individual differences in responsiveness to dietary density.

SUMMARY

The findings present a relatively clear picture of the roles of diurnal rhythms and dietary energy density in the control of short-term food intake. Intake in the morning appears to reduce overall intake, while intake at night appears to increase it. Dietary energy density, on the other hand, appears to be a major determinant of short-term food energy intake, with higher dietary energy density associated with substantially larger meals, daily intakes, and overall participant intakes. These results support the concept that short-term food intake is controlled on the basis of its weight and volume as opposed to its total food-energy content. This conclusion was supported by the observations that (a) overall dietary energy densities appear to be more important than the energy density of particular nutrients and (b) the estimated after-meal stomach contents appear to be constant regardless of the dietary energy density of the reported diet. These observations further suggest that short-term food regulation may occur on the basis of stomach filling.

Based on these findings, the overall dietary density of assault rations should be maximized, and intake at night should be emphasized. The fact that time-of-day effects on intake appear to be heritable suggests that there may be considerable individual differences in response to manipulating this factor. On the other hand, the effects of dietary energy density on intake do not appear to be influenced by heredity, and this suggests that individual differences in response to dietary energy density manipulation should be minimal. Hence, to maximize intake in the field, maximize energy density and encourage night-time eating.

REFERENCES

Bell EA, Rolls BJ. 2001. Energy density of foods affects energy intake across multiple levels of fat content in lean and obese women. *Am J Clin Nutr* 73(6):1010–1018.

de Castro JM. 1987. Macronutrient relationships with meal patterns and mood in the spontaneous feeding behavior of humans. *Physiol Behav* 39(5):561–569.

de Castro JM. 1999. Inheritance of premeal stomach content influences on food intake in free living humans. *Physiol Behav* 66(2):223–232.

de Castro JM. 2001. Heritability of diurnal changes in food intake in free-living humans. *Nutrition* 17(9):713–720.

de Castro JM. 2004a. Dietary energy density is associated with increased intake in free-living humans. *J Nutr* 134(2):335–341.

de Castro JM. 2004b. The control of eating behavior in free-living humans. In: Stricker EM, Woods, eds. *Handbook of Behavioral Neurobiology.* 2nd ed. Vol 14. *Neurobiology of Food and Fluid Intake.* New York: Plenum Press. Pp. 469–504.

de Castro JM. 2004c. The time of day of food intake influences overall intake in humans. *J Nutr* 134(1):104–111.

de Castro JM. 2004d. When identical twins differ: An analysis of intrapair differences in the spontaneous eating behavior and attitudes of free-living monozygotic twins. *Physiol Behav* 82(4):733–739.

de Castro JM, Plunkett S. 2002. A general model of intake regulation. *Neurosci Biobehav Rev* 26(5):581–595.

de Castro JM, Bellisle F, Dalix AM. 2000. Palatability and intake relationships in free-living humans: Measurement and characterization in the French. *Physiol Behav* 68(3):271–277.

Hopkins A. 1966. The pattern of gastric emptying: A new view of old results. *J Physiol* 182(1):144–149.

Hunt JN, Knox MT. 1968. Regulation of gastric emptying. In: Coyle CF, Heidel W, eds. *Handbook of Physiology*. Vol 4. Alimentary Canal (Motility). Washington, DC: American Physiological Society. Pp. 1917–1935.

Hunt JN, Stubbs DF. 1975. The volume and energy content of meals as determinants of gastric emptying. *J Physiol* 245(1):209–225.

Toates FM. 1978. A physiological control theory of the hunger-thirst interaction. In: Booth DA, ed. *Hunger Models: Computable Theory of Feeding Control.* New York: Academic Press. Pp. 347–373.

Yao M, Roberts SB. 2001. Dietary energy density and weight regulation. *Nutr Rev* 59(8):247–258.

C

Biographical Sketches of Workshop Speakers

Lynn B. Bailey, Ph.D., is a professor at the University of Florida. Her research area of expertise is folate metabolism, estimation of folate requirements, and factors that influence disease and birth defect risk including genetic polymorphisms. Dr. Bailey has conducted human metabolic studies over a period of 25 years generating data that has been instrumental in establishing new dietary intake recommendations for individuals throughout the lifecycle including pregnant women and the elderly. In recognition of Dr. Bailey's established scientific expertise, she has frequently been invited to serve as a scientific advisor for national organizations. For example, she served as a member of the Institute of Medicine's Dietary Reference Intake committee for folate and other vitamins; she was a member of the Food and Drug Administration's Folic Acid Advisory Committee that recommended folic acid fortification of the food supply in the US; and she has served as a scientific advisor to the Centers for Disease Control and the Pan American Health Organization on projects focused on neural tube defect prevention. Dr. Bailey has received very prestigious awards including the USDA Award for Superior Service based on accomplishments in the area of folate nutrition, and the national March of Dimes' Agnes Higgins Award for research related to fetal and maternal health. In addition, she was recently awarded the 2004 American Society of Nutritional Sciences Centrum Center Award for research accomplishments related to human folate requirements. Dr. Bailey received her Ph.D. in nutrition from Purdue University.

Rebecca B. Costello, Ph.D., is the Deputy Director of the Office of Dietary Supplements (ODS) at the National Institutes of Health. Dr. Costello participated in the development of the ODS Strategic Plan in 1998 and more recently in the Strategic Plan for 2004–2009. She is charged with implementing the plan's goals and objectives by organizing workshops and conferences on topics of national interest in dietary supplements, conducting scientific reviews to identify gaps in scientific knowledge, and initiating and coordinating research efforts among NIH Institutes and other federal agencies. Dr. Costello also oversees the development and management of the ODS-USDA National Agricultural Library's IBIDS database of scientific literature on dietary supplements. Prior to her NIH appointment, she was with the Food and Nutrition Board of the National Academy of Sciences, serving as Project Director for the Committee on Military Nutrition Research. From 1987 to 1996, Dr. Costello served as a Research Associate and Program Director for the Risk Factor Reduction Center, a referral center at the Washington Adventist Hospital for the detection, modification, and prevention of cardiovascular disease through dietary and/or drug interventions. She received a B.S. and M.S. in biology from the American University, Washington, D.C., and a Ph.D. in clinical nutrition from the University of Maryland at College Park. Dr. Costello maintains active membership in several nutrition societies and the American Heart Association Council on Epidemiology and Prevention. Her areas of research interest include mineral nutrition, dietary intake methodology, and dietary interventions to reduce cardiovascular disease.

Edward F. Coyle, Ph.D., serves as the director of the Human Performance Laboratory and professor in the Department of Kinesiology and Health Education at the University of Texas at Austin. Dr. Coyle's research has focused upon the metabolic and cardiovascular factors that limit aerobic exercise performance. He is a North American delegate for the sports nutrition working group of the International Olympic Committee. Dr. Coyle has recently received the Distinguished Faculty Award for 2002 at The University of Texas at Austin. He is currently a member of the American Physiological Society, American Institute of Nutrition, American Society for Clinical Nutrition, and the American Academy of Kinesiology and Physical Education. Dr. Coyle received his Ph.D. in animal physiology from The University of Arizona.

John M. de Castro, Ph.D., serves as a professor and chair in the Department of Psychology at the University of Texas at El Paso. He previously served as the chair in the Department of Psychology at Georgia State University in Atlanta. Dr. de Castro's research interests include the control of behavior in free-living humans; psychological, social, nutritional, genetic, and physiological determinants of microregulatory patterns; food and fluid intake regulation; obesity; bulimia nervosa; and behavior genetics. He received his Ph.D. in biopsychology at the University of Massachusetts in Amherst.

Jørn W. Helge, Ph.D., holds the title of Associate Professor at the Department of Medical Physiology, and is on the faculty of Health Sciences. He received his masters and doctorate at the Copenhagen Muscle Research Centre and Department of Human Physiology, August Krogh Institute, University of Copenhagen. His primary research areas are the interaction of diet and training and the effects on endurance performance and muscle substrate utilization and the coupling and importance of physical activity/inactivity for the occurrence and attainment of the metabolic Syndrome.

L. John Hoffer, M.D., is a professor of medicine at McGill University and senior physician in the Divisions of Internal Medicine and Endocrinology at the Lady Davis Institute for Medical Research, Jewish General Hospital in Montreal, Canada, where he serves on the nutrition support service. Dr. Hoffer's research interests include human protein and energy metabolism in response to hypocaloric states and protein restriction. He has served for many years on the Nutrition and Metabolism Committee of the Canadian Institutes for Health Research.

Ronald J. Jandacek, Ph.D., is adjunct professor in the Department of Pathology and Laboratory Medicine at the University of Cincinnati College of Medicine. His undergraduate training was in chemistry at Rice University, and he received a Ph.D. in chemistry from the University of Texas at Austin. After two years in the Army at Walter Reed Army Institute of Research and the Armed Forces Institute of Pathology, he joined Procter & Gamble's Miami Valley Laboratories in Cincinnati, where he worked until 2001. At Procter & Gamble his research centered on the relationship of the chemistry and nutritional properties of lipids, with a focus on intestinal absorption. Since 2001 he has collaborated with Dr. Patrick Tso in studies of nutritional effects on the absorption and metabolism of toxic lipophilic xenobiotics.

Randall J. Kaplan, Ph.D., is the Director, Nutrition and Scientific Affairs at the Canadian Sugar Institute, a nonprofit association representing all Canadian sugar manufacturers on nutrition and international trade issues. The Institute provides a Nutrition Information Service and is guided by a Scientific Advisory Council of nutrition researchers. Dr. Kaplan obtained M.Sc. and Ph.D. degrees in Nutritional Sciences from the Faculty of Medicine at the University of Toronto, and a B.A. in Psychology from the University of Western Ontario. His research involved investigating the effects of macronutrients on cognitive performance, appetite regulation and glucose regulation in healthy elderly individuals and individuals with diabetes, resulting in numerous scientific publications. He received several awards for his research, including those from the Canadian Institutes of Health Research, Natural Sciences and Engineering Research Council of Canada, and Canadian Society for Nutritional Sciences. Dr. Kaplan has also worked as a consultant on research and regulatory issues for the University of Toronto Program in Food Safety Nutrition and Regulatory Affairs, Food and Consumer Product Manufacturers of Canada, and Kellogg Canada Inc. He is currently Chair of the World Sugar Research Organization Scientific and Communications Committee, and a member of the National Institute of Nutrition Scientific Advisory Council, University of Toronto Program in Food Safety Scientific-Technical Committee, and Food and Consumer Products Manufacturers of Canada Scientific and Regulatory Affairs Council. He represents the World Sugar Research Organization as an official Observer at sessions of the Codex Alimentarius Commission of the World Health Organization/Food and Agriculture Organization of the United Nations.

Henry C. Lukaski, Ph.D., is the Assistant Center Director and Research Physiologist at the United States Department of Agriculture, Agricultural Research Service, Human Nutrition Research Center in Grand Forks, North Dakota. He is currently a Clinical Instructor in the Department of Medicine, Adjunct Professor in the Department of Physical Education and Exercise Science and a member of the Sports Medicine Advisory Committee and Research Council at the University of North Dakota. Dr. Lukaski's research focuses on the interaction of physical activity and mineral nutrient intakes in humans with an emphasis on iron, zinc, copper, magnesium, and chromium to promote health and optimal performance throughout the life cycle. He is a Fellow of the American College of Sports Medicine, the Human Biology Council and Mexican Institute of Nutrition. He is a member of the American Physiological Society, American Society for Nutritional Sciences, American Society for Clinical Nutrition, Endocrine Society, New York Academy of Sciences, Sigma Xi, and Phi Kappa Phi. Dr. Lukaski is a Charter Member of the American Heart Association Council on Nutrition, Metabolism and Physical Activity. He serves as a member of the Editorial Boards of Current Nutrition Reviews, International Journal of Applied Sports Science, Nutrition, and CRC Series on Nutrition in Exercise and Sport, and an editorial consultant for a variety of peer-reviewed journals in nutrition, medicine and sport sciences. Dr. Lukaski is a past Associate Editor, Medicine and Science in Sports and Exercise, and a member of the Editorial Boards of the International Journal of Sport Nutrition and Journal of Nutrition. He has served as an advisor and consultant to many national and international health agencies and research organizations, including the National Academy of Sciences, National Institutes of Health, Food and Drug Administration, Department of Defense, Pan American Health Organization, the World Health Organization, and International Olympic Committee. Dr. Lukaski received a master of science and doctoral degrees in physiology and nutrition from the Pennsylvania State University.

Linda K. Massey, Ph.D., serves as a professor and scientist of Human Nutrition in the department of Food Science and Human Nutrition at Washington State University. She obtained her Ph.D. at the University of Oklahoma. Dr. Massey is a national spokesperson for the American Society for Bone and Mineral Research. Her work focuses on how inadequate calcium and magnesium intake and excessive salt intake contribute to chronic diseases associated with aging, such as osteoporosis, hypertension, diabetes, kidney stones and cardiovascular disease. Dr. Massey has received several honors including the Outstanding Dietetics Educator from both the Washington State Dietetic Association and the Western Region Dietetic Educators of Practitioners, Excellence in Clinical Practice and Research from the Washington State Dietetics Association, and the Faculty Excellence award for Washington State University, Spokane.

Richard D. Mattes, Ph.D., is a professor of Foods & Nutrition at Purdue University, an Adjunct Associate professor of Medicine at the Indiana University School of Medicine and an Affiliated Scientist at the Monell Chemical Senses Center. His research focuses on the areas of hunger and satiety, regulation of food intake in humans, food preferences, human cephalic phase responses and taste and smell. At Purdue University, he is presently Chair of the Human Subjects Review Committee, Director of the Analytical Core laboratory for the Botanical Center for Age Related Diseases and is a co-coordinator of the Purdue Resource for Integrative Dietetics and Exercise. He also holds numerous external responsibilities including: editorial board of Ear, Nose and Throat Journal; Chair, adult weight management certificate program at the American Dietetic Association, Chair-elect of the Research Dietetic Practice Group of the American Dietetic Association, Technical Committee member for the Peanut CRSP program in the United States Agency for International Development; and Secretary of the Rose Marie Pangborn Sensory Science Scholarship Fund. Dr. Mattes received his M.P.H. in public health nutrition at the University of Michigan School of Public health and his Ph.D. in Human Nutrition at Cornell University. His professional memberships include the American College of Nutrition, American Dietetic Association, American Society of Clinical Nutrition and Association for Chemoreception Sciences, Society for the Study of Ingestive Behavior, Institute of Food Technologists, just to name a few.

Simin Nikbin Meydani, Ph.D., is Professor of Nutrition and Immunology and the Director of the Cell and Molecular Nutrition Program at the Friedman School of Nutrition Science and Policy and Tufts Sackler Graduate Program in Immunology. She also serves as Director of the Nutritional Immunology Laboratory, at the Jean Mayer USDA Human Nutrition Research Center on Aging at Tufts University. Dr. Meydani's present and past professional activities include FAO/WHO Expert Panel member on Nutritional Requirement of the Elderly; American Aging Association Board of Directors and Fund Raising Committee; Gerontological Society Nutrition Steering Committee; NIA Primate Calorie Restriction Project Advisory Board, External Advisory Committee for the UCLA Claude D. Pepper Older Americans Independence Center; FAO/WHO Joint Expert Committee on Fats and Oils in Human Nutrition; Editorial Board of the Journal of Nutrition, the American Journal of Clinical Nutrition, the Journal of

Nutritional Biochemistry, and the Journal of Experimental Biology and Medicine; NIA, NIH, USDA, and industry grant review Study Sections member. Dr. Meydani received her Ph.D. in nutrition from Iowa State University and her D.V.M. from Tehran University. Her many honors include the American Aging Association Denham Harman Lifetime Research Achievement Award, American Society for Nutritional Sciences Lederle Award in Human Nutrition Research, American College of Nutrition Grace Goldsmith Award, and the Welcome Visiting Professorship at Iowa State University. She also received the HERMES Vitamin Research Award, the Nutritional Immunology Group Award and the Tufts University Outstanding Faculty Award. Dr. Meydani's scientific interests include basic biology of aging as it is related to immune response; nutrition and aging; the impact of nutrition on immune response and resistance to infectious diseases in developed and developing countries; micronutrients, antioxidants, and lipids.

Scott J. Montain, Ph.D., is a Research Physiologist working in the Military Nutrition Division at the US Army Research Institute of Environmental Medicine (USARIEM). He manages the Military Operational Medicine research effort to nutritionally optimize future assault rations and his research has included assessment of the physiological consequences of military sustained operations. Dr. Montain received M.S. from Ball State University and Ph.D. from the University of Texas at Austin, before completing postdoctoral training at USARIEM. He is author or co-author on over 75 peer-reviewed journal articles, book chapters, and reports. Dr. Montain is a member of the American American Physiological Society and a Fellow of the American College of Sports Medicine.

Dennis Passe, Ph.D., is an experimental psychologist specializing in sensory measurement, research design and statistics, and learning and behavior. As former Senior Principal Scientist and head of the Sensory Research & Evaluation Department at the Gatorade Sports Science Institute in Barrington, Illinois, Passe was responsible for the sensory taste panels for Gatorade and all of the other food products made by Quaker Foods and Beverages. He also helped to identify sensory research initiatives to further our understanding of the importance of taste in voluntary fluid intake, and to broaden the use of sensory and psychological measurements during exercise to better understand feelings of well-being, vigor, and energy. He earned his bachelor's degree from Wisconsin State University at LaCrosse, his mater's degree from Western Michigan University in Kalamazoo, and his doctoral degree in psychology from Florida State University (FSU) in Tallahassee. After completing his doctorate, Passe accepted a postdoctoral fellowship at FSU, where he did behavioral psychophysics in taste with dogs. Dr. Passe has published in the human and animal literature in the taste and olfaction areas. He is a member of the American Psychological Association, American College of Sports Medicine, American Society for Testing and Materials (Division E18-Sensory) and the Institute of Food Technologists (Sensory Division).

Ronenn Roubenoff, M.D., received his M.D. from Northwestern University, trained in Internal Medicine and Rheumatology at the Johns Hopkins Hospital, and completed a concurrent fellowship in Clinical Epidemiology at the Johns Hopkins School of Hygiene and Public Health during his Rheumatology fellowship. He then trained in nutrition at Tufts University, and currently focuses his research on the interactions of nutrition, exercise and hormonal and immune regulators of metabolism in chronic disease and aging. He has conducted research on the effects of inflammation, diet and exercise on body composition, strength, and function in rheumatoid arthritis, osteoarthritis, HIV infection, and aging. He was Chief of the Nutrition, Exercise Physiology, and Sarcopenia Laboratory from 1997 to 2002, and Director of Human Studies, at the Jean Mayer USDA Human Nutrition Research Center on Aging at Tufts University from 2001 to 2002. He is an Associate Professor of Medicine and Professor of Nutrition (both Adjunct) at Tufts and continues to practice rheumatology and nutrition at Tufts-New England Medical Center. In September, 2002, Dr. Roubenoff became Senior Director of Molecular Medicine at Millennium Pharmaceuticals, Inc., in Cambridge, Massachusetts.

Susan Shirreffs, Ph.D., completed here first degree in Physiology at Aberdeen University in 1993. Following this she completed a Ph.D. in Exercise Physiology in the area of Post-exercise Rehydration in 1996. After lecturing for 5 years at Aberdeen University, during which time Dr. Shirreffs spent a few months working at the Copenhagen Muscle Research Institute, she moved to Loughborough University to continue her research and teaching interests. Dr. Shirreffs research interests are in sport and exercise physiology and nutrition. Her current research projects focus on exercise in the heat and in particular, recovery from sweat volume and electrolyte losses. Dr. Shirreffs is a member of The Physiological Society, The American College of Sports Medicine, The Nutrition Society, the British Association of Sport and Exercise Sciences and The Medical Research Society.

Joanne L. Slavin, Ph.D., is a professor in the Department of Food Science and Nutrition at the University of Minnesota. Her laboratory is actively involved in research on dietary fiber, phytochemicals in flax, soy, grape extract, and whole grains. She is the author of more than 100 scientific publications and numerous book chapters and review articles and has given hundreds of nutrition seminars for professional and lay audiences. She is a Science Communicator for the Institute of Food Technologists and a member of numerous scientific societies, including the American Dietetic Association, the American Society for Nutritional Sciences, and the American Association for Cancer Research. She is a frequent source for the media on topics ranging from functional foods to sports nutrition. Dr. Slavin received B.S., M.S., and Ph.D. degrees in Nutritional Sciences from the University of Wisconsin-Madison and is a registered dietitian.

Richard J. Stubbs, Ph.D., is the head of the Human Appetite and Energy Balance Program at the Rowett Research Institute in Scotland, United Kingdom. He received his Ph.D. from Cambridge University. Previously Dr. Stubbs had a Glaxo Junior Research Fellowship. He is a Principle Scientific Officer at the Rowett and has over 15 years experience in designing, coordination, and writing up large scale human trials and interventions. Dr. Stubbs has organized numerous scientific meetings and symposia for The Nutrition Society and is well versed in delivering contract research to government agencies and industry alike. He has now conducted over 50 studies at the Rowett on aspects of feeding behavior, appetite control, diet composition and energy balance. Initial work focused on testing models of human intake regulation. More recently he has been concerned with understanding the physiological and psychological responses to induced energy deficits (diet and exercise), detecting and modeling mis-reporting of dietary intakes as a prelude to the accurate modeling of the dietary and phenotypic determinants of energy balance. Currently Dr. Stubbs is working on defining the basis of susceptibility and resistance to diet induced obesity. In research Dr. Stubbs specializes in large multidisciplinary projects involving simultaneous measures of feeding behavior in the context of energy balance. His projects typically involve several human intervention studies conducted in a structured manner. Dr. Stubbs therefore has considerable experience in cocoordinating large-scale, complex human projects as contracts that are bound by time and constrained by budget. Dr. Stubbs has been awarded several times for his achievements in energy balance and obesity research. He is an honorary Senior Research Fellow of Leeds University.

Kevin D. Tipton, Ph.D., is a Senior Lecturer in the School of Sport and Exercise Sciences at The University of Birmingham in Birmingham, England. Prior to that, he was assistant professor at the University of Texas Medical Branch in Galveston. Dr. Tipton's research has focused on the interaction of nutrition and exercise on muscle protein metabolism in humans. He has been Principal Investigator on projects funded by NIH/National Institute of Arthritis and musculoskeletal and Skin Diseases, the Gatorade Sports Science Institute and the National Dairy Council. Dr. Tipton received his undergraduate degree from the University of Kentucky, Lexington, in zoology in 1983. He received his Masters of Science degree from the University of South Florida in 1987 in marine biology and his doctorate in nutrition from Auburn University, Alabama.

Maret G. Traber, Ph.D., is a Principle Investigator at the Linus Pauling Institute in Oregon State University. She is also a professor in the department of Nutrition and Food Management and adjunct professor in the department of Exercise Sports Science at Oregon State University. Recently Dr. Traber became clinical professor in the department of Medicine at the Oregon Health and Science University. She serves as the associate editor of the journal *Lipids*, is on the editorial boards of both the Journal of Nutrition and Free Radical Biology and Medicine. Dr. Traber is a member of the National Institutes of Health, Integrative Nutrition and Metabolic Processes Study Section. She earned her Ph.D. from the University of California in nutrition.

Steven M. Wood, Ph.D., is a Senior Research Scientist at Ross Products Division/Abbott Laboratories, Columbus, Ohio. He conducts and coordinates clinical studies regarding nutritional formulations and their influence on immune function as well as oxidative stress. For the past several years he has worked closely with scientist from the United States Army Research Institute of Environmental Medicine (USARIEM), Natick, Massachusetts, Naval Health Research Center, San Diego, California, and the University of Utah, Salt Lake City, Utah, to conduct studies of soldiers participating in Special Forces Selection and Assessment School, Ranger Training and Marine Mountain Warfare Training. He has also been involved in studies examining the effects of nutritional formulations on immune function in the elderly. He received his Ph.D. in nutritional sciences at the University of Arizona where he studied the relationship of nutrition (b-carotene and selenium) with immune function.

Andrew J. Young, Ph.D., is a research physiologist and Chief of the Military Nutrition Division at the US Army Research Institute of Environmental Medicine (USARIEM) in Natick, Massachusetts. He also is appointed Adjunct Associate Professor in the Sargent College of Allied Health Professions at Boston University. He obtained his B.S. in Biology and Commission in the US Army at the Virginia Military Institute, and his Ph.D. in Physiology at the North Carolina State University. Following graduate school, Dr. Young served in the US Army with assignments at USARIEM and at the Walter Reed Army Institute of Research. After leaving active duty, Dr. Young continued government service as a civilian scientist at USARIEM. Dr. Young's research has concerned the biological basis for, and strategies to mitigate, physical performance degradations in military personnel exposed to physiological stressors such as intense physical exertion coupled with sleep restriction, nutritional deprivation and exposure to extremes of heat, cold and high altitude, all of which could be expected during continuous or sustained military operations. Dr. Young is a graduate of the Command and General Staff Officer's Course, and has been awarded the Army Commendation Medal with Oak Leaf Cluster, the Department of the Army Achievement Medal for Civilian Service, and the Expert Field Medical Badge. He is a member of the American Physiological Society, a Fellow of the American College of Sports Medicine.

D

Biographical Sketches of Committee Members and Staff

John W. Erdman, Jr., Ph.D., (*Chair*) is a professor of nutrition and food science in the Department of Food Science and Human Nutrition and a professor in the Department of Internal Medicine at the University of Illinois at Urbana-Champaign. His research interests include the effects of food processing on nutrient retention, the metabolic roles of lycopene and beta-carotene, and the bioavailability of minerals from foods. His research regarding soy protein has extended into studies on the impact of non-nutrient components of foods such as phytoestrogens on chronic disease. Dr. Erdman has published over 140 peer-reviewed research papers. He chaired the 1988 Gordon Conference on Carotenoids, and has served as a Burroughs Wellcome Visiting Professor in Basic Medical Sciences at the University of Georgia, and the G. Malcolm Trout Visiting Scholar at Michigan State University. His awards include the Borden Award from the American Society for Nutritional Sciences and the Babcock-Hart Award from the Institute of Food Technologists. Dr. Erdman has served on many editorial boards, and he has served as president of the American Society for Nutritional Sciences and on various committees of the Institute of Food Technologists and the National Academy of Sciences. He was elected a fellow of the Institute of Food Technologists and the American Heart Association. Dr Erdman was elected to the Institute of Medicine in 2003. Dr. Erdman received his M.S. and Ph.D. in food science from Rutgers University.

Bruce R. Bistrian, M.D., Ph.D., is Professor of Medicine at Harvard Medical School and Chief of Clinical Nutrition, Beth Israel Deaconess Medical Center. Formerly he was co-director of Hyperalimentation Services, New England Deaconess Hospital, and a lecturer in the Department of Nutrition and Food

Science, Massachusetts Institute of Technology (MIT). He earned his M.D. from Cornell University, his M.P.H. from Johns Hopkins University, and his Ph.D. in nutritional biochemistry and metabolism from MIT. Dr. Bistrian is board certified in Internal Medicine and Critical Care Medicine. Dr. Bistrian's primary research interests include nutritional assessment, metabolic effects of acute infections, nutritional support of hospitalized patients, and the pathophysiology of protein-calorie malnutrition. He is a fellow of the American College of Physicians, and has received an honorary M.A. from Harvard University. Dr. Bistrian is the 2004 recipient of the Goldberger Award of the American Medical Association. Dr. Bistrian has been president of the American Society for Parenteral and Enteral Nutrition, President of the American Society of Clinical Nutrition, and is President-Elect of the Federation of American Societies of Experimental Biology. Dr. Bistrian has served on the editorial boards of numerous nutrition and medical journals, and is the author or co-author of over 400 articles in scientific publications.

Priscilla M. Clarkson, Ph.D., is a professor of exercise science and Associate Dean of the School of Public Health and Health Sciences at the University of Massachusetts, Amherst. She served as President of the New England Regional American College of Sports Medicine (ACSM) Chapter, Vice-president of the National ACSM, President of the National ACSM, and President of the ACSM Foundation. Professor Clarkson has published over 150 scientific articles and has given numerous national and international scientific presentations. The major focus of her research is on how human skeletal muscle responds to environmental challenges such as over-exertion exercise and disuse. She has also published in the area of sport nutrition. Professor Clarkson served as the Editor for the *International Journal of Sport Nutrition and Exercise Metabolism* for 8 years, and is the 2005 Editor-in-Chief of *Exercise and Sport Science Reviews.* Professor Clarkson has served as a scientific advisor to the International Life Sciences Institute (ILSI), as a member of the Science Working Group at NASA to develop laboratories for Space Station, as a scientific advisor to the National Space Biomedical Research Institute, on the Research Review Board of the Gatorade Sports Science Institute, and as a member of the NCAA Competitive and Medical Safeguards Committee.

Johanna T. Dwyer, D.Sc., R.D., is director of the Frances Stern Nutrition Center at New England Medical Center and is a professor in the departments of Medicine and of Community Health at the Tufts Medical School and the School of Nutrition Science and Policy in Boston. She is also a senior scientist at the Jean Mayer USDA Human Nutrition Research Center on Aging at Tufts University. She is currently on part-time assignment to the National Institutes of Health Office of Dietary Supplements. Dr. Dwyer's work centers on life-cycle related concerns such as the prevention of diet-related disease in children and adolescents and maximization of quality of life and health in the elderly. Dr. Dwyer is currently the editor of *Nutrition Today* and on the editorial boards of *Family Economics* and *Nutrition Reviews*. She received her D.Sc. and M.Sc. from the Harvard School of Public Health, her M.S. from the University of Wisconsin, and completed her undergraduate degree with distinction from Cornell University. She is a member of the Institute of Medicine, the Technical Advisory Committee of the Nutrition Screening Initiative, past president of the American Society for Nutritional Sciences, past secretary of the American Society for Clinical Nutrition, and past president of the Society for Nutrition Education.

Barbara P. Klein, Ph.D., is Professor Emeritus of Foods and Nutrition in the Department of Food Science and Human Nutrition, and co-Director, Illinois Center for Soy Foods, University of Illinois. Dr. Klein's research addresses alterations in food quality that occur during storage, processing, and preparing foods for human consumption. Her research is focused on sensory evaluation methodology development and assessment, emphasizing reduced-sodium and low-fat foods; development and evaluation of high soy protein foods such as snacks, cereals, and dairy analogs; and factors affecting phytochemical and nutrient retention in vegetables. Dr. Klein received her B.S. (1957) and M.S. (1959) degrees from Cornell University. She completed her Ph.D. in 1974 at the University of Illinois at Urbana-Champaign and then joined the faculty in the Division of Foods and Nutrition. Dr. Klein is editor of two books, author of seven book chapters, and over 100 journal articles and presentations. She received the Borden Award for Research in Foods and Nutrition in 1988, was elected as a Fellow of the Institute of Food Technologists in 1994, and received the College of Agricultural, Consumer and Environmental Sciences' Paul A. Funk Award for Excellence in 1997.

Helen W. Lane, Ph.D., R.D., is the chief nutritionist for the National Aeronautics and Space Administration, and chief scientist for the Johnson Space Center's Habitability, Environmental Factors, and Bioastronautics Office. She has served as the assistant to the Director for Advanced Program Coordination and Research and branch chief for Biomedical Operations and Countermeasures. Dr. Lane was an associate professor of nutrition at the University of Texas Medical Center from 1977 to 1984, and a professor of nutrition at Auburn University from 1984 to 1989. At present, she serves as an adjunct professor, Department of Preventive Medicine and Community Health, at the University of Texas Medical Branch in Galveston. She has led efforts to define nutritional requirements for healthy crew members during spaceflight. Dr. Lane has completed research on body composition and on nutritional requirements for energy, water, electrolytes, protein, calcium, and iron, as well as clinical and basic research on selenium and breast cancer. As a registered dietitian, she is active in the American Dietetic Association. She is also a member of the American Society for Nutritional Sciences and the American Society for Clinical Nutrition.

Melinda M. Manore, Ph.D., is a professor and chair, Department of Nutrition, Oregon State University, and is a registered dietitian. Her research interests include the interaction of nutrition and exercise in health, exercise performance, disease prevention, and reduction of chronic disease across the life cycle. Dr. Manore's research also focuses on factors regulating energy balance (i.e., energy expenditure, eating behaviors, and body weight and composition), and the role of nutrition, exercise, and energy balance on the reproductive cycle. She is a fellow of the American College of Sports Medicine (ACSM), and a member of American Dietetic Association (ADA), the American Society for Nutritional Sciences, the American Society for Clinical Nutrition, and the North American Association for the Study of Obesity. She is currently chair of the ADA Nutrition Research Practice Group and received the ADA's Sports, Cardiovascular and Wellness Nutritionists Excellence in Practice award in 2001. Dr. Manore currently serves as a member of the USA Gymnastics National Health Advisory Board, the Gatorade Sport Science Institute Nutrition Board, and the Arizona Osteoporosis Coalition Medical Advisory Board. She is associate editor for Medicine and Science in Sports and Exercise and ACSM's Health and Fitness Journal and is on the editorial boards of the Journal of the American Dietetic Association, and the International Journal of Sport Nutrition and Exercise Metabolism. Dr. Manore obtained her M.S. in health education and community health from the University of Oregon and her Ph.D. in human nutrition from Oregon State University.

Patrick M. O'Neil, Ph.D., is professor of psychiatry and behavioral sciences at the Medical University of South Carolina, where he is also Director of the Weight Management Center. Dr. O'Neil has been involved in the study of obesity and its management since 1977, including clinical trials, basic research, teaching and public education. He has been the principal investigator on a number of clinical trials of weight-loss agents. He is the author of over 100 professional publications primarily concerning psychological, behavioral, and other clinical aspects of obesity and its management. Dr. O'Neil has served on the Education Committee of the North American Association for the Study of Obesity (NAASO) since 1994, and was a member of the NAASO Ad Hoc Committee for Development of the Practical Guidelines. He is also immediate Past President of the South Carolina Academy of Professional Psychologists, former member and Chair of the South Carolina Board of Examiners in Psychology, and former Chair of the Obesity and Eating Disorders Special Interest Group of the Association for the Advancement of Behavior Therapy. Dr. O'Neil received his B.S. in economics from Louisiana State University and his M.S. and Ph.D. in clinical psychology from the University of Georgia.

Robert M. Russell, M.D., is a professor of medicine and nutrition at Tufts University and director of the Jean Mayer USDA Human Nutrition Research

Center on Aging at Tufts University in Boston. As a senior scientist at the Jean Mayer USDA Human Nutrition Research Center on Aging, Dr. Russell's primary work involves studying the effects of aging on gastrointestinal absorptive function. He is a noted expert in the area of human metabolism of retinoids and carotenoids. Dr. Russell is a member of numerous professional societies and has served as a councilor and president to the American Society for Clinical Nutrition and a member of the Board of Directors of the American College of Nutrition. Dr. Russell co-authored the standards for parenteral and enteral nutrition to be used in U.S. long-term care facilities. He has served on the editorial boards of five professional journals and is a staff gastroenterologist at the New England Medical Center Hospitals. He has served on national and international advisory boards including the FDA, National Digestive Diseases Advisory Board, USDA Human Investigation Committee (chairman), US Pharmacopoeia Convention, National Dairy Council Scientific Advisory Board, and the American Board of Internal Medicine. He received his B.S. from Harvard University and M.D. from Columbia University.

Beverly J. Tepper, Ph.D., is a professor of food science at Cook College, Rutgers University. Her primary areas of research examine the role of taste genetics on eating behavior and obesity and the effects of disease (especially diabetes) on taste, food ingestion and dietary compliance. She has published more than 50 papers and book chapters in these areas. She currently serves on the editorial boards of the *Journal of Sensory Studies and Food Quality and Preference* and has served as a reviewer for the *American Journal of Clinical Nutrition, Appetite, Brain Research Bulletin, European Journal of Clinical Nutrition, Journal of Food Science, Nutrition Research,* and *Physiology and Behavior*. Dr. Tepper earned her M.S. and Ph.D. degrees in nutrition from Tufts University.

Kevin D. Tipton, Ph.D., is a Senior Lecturer in the School of Sport and Exercise Sciences at The University of Birmingham in Birmingham, England. Dr. Tipton's research has focused on the interaction of nutrition and exercise on muscle protein metabolism in humans. He has been Principal Investigator on projects funded by NIH/National Institute of Arthritis and musculoskeletal and Skin Diseases, the Gatorade Sports Science Institute and the National Dairy Council. Dr. Tipton received his undergraduate degree from the University of Kentucky, Lexington, in zoology in 1983. He received his Masters of Science degree from the University of South Florida in 1987 in marine biology and his doctorate in nutrition from Auburn University, Alabama.

Allison A. Yates, Ph.D., R.D., is the director of nutritional sciences at ENVIRON Health Sciences Institute in Arlington, Virginia. Prior to assuming this position, she served as the Director of the Food and Nutrition Board (FNB) with the

Institute of Medicine of the National Academies from 1994 through September 2003 and as Dean of the College Health and Human Sciences at the University of Southern Mississippi in Hattiesburg from 1988 through 1997. She is a registered dietitian, having completed a masters of science degree in public health at the University of California at Los Angeles and a dietetic internship at the Los Angeles Veteran's Administration Hospital prior to working for the Los Angeles County Department of Health as a public health nutritionist. She earned a doctorate in human nutrition from the University of California at Berkeley, did postdoctoral work there on human sulfur amino acid requirements, and has since served as a faculty member in nutrition and dietetics at the University of Texas Health Science Center in Houston and at Emory University. She has conducted research on essential fatty acid and vitamin E deficiencies in animal models, soy protein utilization and methionine and sulfur requirements in men, and protein and energy requirements in older men and women. Prior to joining the staff of the FNB, she was a member of FNB Committee on Military Nutrition Research.

INSTITUTE OF MEDICINE STAFF

Maria P. Oria, Ph.D., is the study director for the Committee on Military Nutrition Research and its related committees. She is also the director of the Food Forum, an Institute of Medicine activity by which expert members from the various sectors dialogue about issues of concern in food and nutrition areas. She joined the Food and Nutrition Board (FNB) of the Institute of Medicine in February 2002. Her work with the FNB has included serving as program officer for *Scientific Criteria to Ensure Safe Food* and as study director for *Infant Formula: Evaluating the Safety of New Ingredients*, and for *Monitoring Metabolic Status: Predicting Decrements in Physiological and Cognitive Performance*. Prior to joining the National Academies she was a staff scientist for the Institute of Food Technologists, coordinating projects on food safety and human nutrition under a contract with the Food and Drug Administration. She received her B.S. in biology from the University of Navarra (Spain), her M.S. in animal science from the University of Wyoming, and her Ph.D. in food science and nutrition from Purdue University. Her research interests include the cross-cutting areas between food production and food safety/quality and the impact of food production systems in the environment.

Jon Q. Sanders, B.A., is a senior program assistant with the Food and Nutrition Board of the Institute of Medicine. Since joining the National Academies in 2001, Mr. Sanders has worked on a variety of studies ranging from Everglades restoration to review of the WIC food packages. He is currently working on two FNB studies—the first is assessing the progress in childhood obesity prevention efforts at local, state, and national levels based on the recommendations of the IOM report *Preventing Childhood Obesity: Health in the Balance* (2005), and the second is a military nutrition study to asses the mineral requirements for cognitive and physical performance of military personnel. Mr. Sanders received his B.A. degree in anthropology from Trinity University, and is currently working towards his M.S. degree in environmental sciences and policy at Johns Hopkins University. He is a member of the Society for Applied Anthropology and the American Indian Science and Engineering Society. He is coauthor of *Sitting Down at the Table: Mediation and Resolution of Water Conflicts* (2001). Mr. Sanders' research interests include political ecology and environmental decision making.

Leslie J. Sim, B.S., is a research associate at the Food and Nutrition Board (FNB) at the Institute of Medicine (IOM) and also provides Web support for all of the FNB activities. In 2003, she received recognition within the FNB as a recipient of an IOM inspirational staff award. Leslie has previously worked both as a teaching assistant and laboratory assistant for an undergraduate Food Science Laboratory class. She is currently working on two IOM studies—the first is examining the effects of food marketing on the diets and health of children and youth, and the second is a military nutrition study to determine if modifications are needed in the military ration composition to prevent possible adverse health and performance consequences of consuming such rations while in short-term high-stress situations. Previously, she has worked on other military nutrition reports including: *Caffeine for the Sustainment of Mental Task Performance, High-Energy, Nutrient-Dense Emergency Relief Food Product; Weight Management: State of the Science and Opportunities for Military Programs;and Monitoring Metabolic Status: Predicting Decrements in Physiological and Cognitive Performance.* Leslie also provided research support for the IOM reports, *Infant Formula: Evaluating the Safety of New Ingredients* and *Dietary Reference Intakes: Applications in Dietary Planning.* She received her B.S. in biology with an emphasis on food science from Virginia Tech and attended North Carolina State University taking graduate classes in food science.

E

Acronyms and Abbreviations

AAD	Antibiotic associated diarrhea
ACSM	American College of Sports Medicine
ADA	American Dietetic Association
ADP	Adenosine diphosphate
AI	Adequate Intake
ALB	Alpha-lactalbumin
AMDR	Acceptable Macronutrient Distribution Range
AMS	Acute mountain sickness
AO	Antioxidants
AR	Army regulation
ARDS	Acute respiratory distress syndrome
ATO	Army Technology Objective
ATP	Adenosine triphosphate
AVP	Arginine vasopressin
BHA	Butylated hydroxyanisole
BHT	Butylated hydroxytoluene
BMI	Body mass index
BMR	Basal metabolic rate
Bpm	Beats per minute
C	Celsius
cal	Calorie
CS	Casein
CCK	Cholecystokinin

CD4	Cluster of differentiation 4
CDR	Cognitive Drug Research (computerized assessment battery)
CFD	Combat Feeding Directorate
CFU	Colony-forming units
CHD	Coronary heart disease
CHO	Carbohydrate
CK	Creatine kinase
CMNR	Committee on Military Nutrition Research
CoA	Pantothenic acid
CoQ_{10}	Coenzyme Q10
CP	Carbohydrate poor
CR	Carbohydrate rich
CRF	Code of federal regulations
CRP	Combat ration pack
CRH	Corticotrophin-releasing hormone
CRP	C-reactive protein
CSFII	Continuing Survey of Food Intake for Individuals
DBPC	Double-bind placebo controlled
DBRPC-CO	Double-blind randomized placebo-controlled crossover
DEXA	Dual-energy x-ray absorptiometry
DFE	Dietary folate equivalent
DGLA	Dihomo-γ-linoleic acid
DHEA	Dehydroepiandrosterone
dL	Deciliter
DNA	Deoxyribonucleic acid
DoD	Department of Defense
DRI	Dietary Reference Intake
DTH	Delayed type skin hypersensitivity
EAA	Essential amino acid
EAR	Estimated Average Requirement
EEG	Electroencephalogram
EGOT	Erythrocyte glutamate oxaloacetate
EGR	Erythrocyte glutathione reductase
EGRAC	Erythrocyte glutathione activity coefficient
EIEC	Enteroinvasive *E. coli*
EMS	Eosinophilia-Myalgia Syndrome
EPA	Eicosapentaenoid acid
ERGO	Energy rich, glucose-optimized
ESQ	Environmental Symptoms Questionnaire
ETK	Erythrocyte transketolase

F	Fahrenheit
F2-IsoPs	Plasma F2-Isoprostanes
FAO	Food and Agriculture Organization
FAD	Flavin adenine dinucleotide
FDA	Food and Drug Administration
FFM	Fat-free mass
FM	Field manual
fMRI	Functional Magnetic Resonance Imaging
FNB	Food and Nutrition Board
FOS	Fructooligosaccharides
FSR	First Strike Ration
ft	Foot
g	Gram
GABA	γ-aminobutyric acid
GBE	*Ginkgo biloba* extract
GGT	Glutamyl transpeptidase
GH	Growth hormone
GI	Gastrointestinal
GLA	γ-Linolenic acid
GRα	Glucocorticoid-receptor alpha
GRAS	Generally recognized as safe
GTT	γ-Glutamyl transpeptidase
h	Hour
HEX	High exercise
HF	High fat
HMB	β-methyl-hydroxy-β-methybutryrate
HS	High stress
IgA	Immunoglobulin A
IgE	Immunoglobulin E
IGF-1	Insulin-like growth factor 1
IgM	Immunoglobulin M
IL	Interleukin
iNOS	Inducible nitric oxide synthase
IOM	Institute of Medicine
IU	International units
kcal	Kilocalorie
KCl	Potassium chloride
kg	Kilogram
kJ	Kilojoules

km	Kilometer
lb	Pound
LDH	Lactic dehydrogenase
LDL	Low-density lipoprotein
LNAA	Large neutral amino acid
LPS	Lipopolysaccharide
LS	Low stress
MCT	Medium-chain fatty acid triacylglycerol
MCW/LRP	Meal, cold weather/food packet, long range patrol
mEq	Milliequivalent
mg	Milligram
MJ	Megajoule
mM	Millimolar
mmol	Millimole
MDRI	Military dietary reference intake
MMWT	Marine mountain warfare training
MND	Military Nutrition Division
MRDA	Military recommended dietary allowances
MRE	Meal, Ready-to-Eat
NA	Not applicable
NAC	N-acetyl-cysteine
NaCl	Sodium chloride
NAD	Nicotinamide Adenine Dinucleotide
NADP	Nicotinamide Adenine Dinucleotide Phosphate
NADPH	Reduced Nicotinamide Adenine Dinucleotide Phosphate
NAS	National Academy of Sciences
ND	Not determined
NE	Niacin equivalent
Nex	No exercise
NHANES	National Health and Nutrition Examination Survey
NK	Natural killer
nmol	Nanomol
NNIF	Novel nutritional immune formulation
NO	Nitric oxide
NSOR	Nutritional Standards for Operational Rations
NRC	National Research Council
NSC	Natick Soldier Center
OBLA	Onset of blood lactate accumulation
25 (OH) D	25 hydroxy vitamin D

oz	Ounce
PHA	Phytohaemagglutinin
PL	Phospholipid
PLP	Pyridoxal-5'-phosphate
POMC	Pro-opiomelanocortin
POMS	Profile of Mood States
PP	Protein poor
ppm	Parts per million
PR	Protein rich
PUFA	Polyunsaturated fatty acid
RAE	Retinol activity equivalent
RBC	Red blood cell
RC	Randomized control
RDA	Recommended Dietary Allowance
rDNA	Recombinant DNA
RE	Retinol equivalent
RER	Respiratory Exchange Ratio
RDECOM	Research, Development and Engineering Command
RI	Respiratory infections
ROS	Reactive oxygen species
RPE	Rate of perceived exertion
RT	Ranger training
SFAS	Special Forces Selection and Assessment School
SOF	Special Operations Forces
STEC	Shiga toxin producing *E. coli*
STO	Science and Technology Objective
SUSOPS	Sustained operations
TBARS	Thiobarbituric Acid Reactive Substances
TBD	To be determined
TCA	Tricarboxylic acid cycle
TDEE	Total daily energy expenditure
TDP	Thiamin diphosphate
T_{H1}	T helper type 1 cell
T_{H2}	T helper type 2 cell
TLR	Toll-like receptors
TNF	Tumor necrosis factor
TPN	Total parenteral nutrition
TT	Timed trial
TTP	Thiamin diphosphate

μg	Microgram
μM	Micromol
UGR-H&S	Unit Group Ration, Heat & Serve
UL	Tolerable Upper Intake Level
UNU	United Nations University
US	United States
USARIEM	U.S. Army Research Institute of Environmental Medicine
USARMRMC	U.S. Army Medical Research and Materiel Command
UV	Ultraviolet
UVB light	Ultraviolet B light
VO$_2$max or peak	Maximum oxygen consumption
WBGT	Wet Bulb Globe Temperature
WHO	World Health Organization
wk	Week
WP	Whey protein
WPSM	Warfighter Physiological Status Monitoring

F

Glossary

Adequate Intake, AI	The recommended average daily intake level based on observed or experimentally determined approximations or estimates of nutrient intake by a group (or groups) of apparently healthy people that are assumed to be adequate—used when an RDA cannot be determined (IOM, 2004).
Acceptable Macronutrient Distribution Range	A range of intakes (represented as percent of energy intake) for a particular energy source that is associated with reduced risk of chronic disease while providing adequate intakes of essential nutrients.
Antinatriuretic	A substance that decreases urinary excretion of sodium.
acute respiratory distress syndrome	Life-threatening condition in which inflammation of the lungs and accumulation of fluid in the air sacs (alveoli) leads to low blood oxygen levels. While it shares some similarities with infant respiratory distress syndrome, its causes and treatments are different.
body mass index	A key index for relating a person's body weight to their height. The body mass index is a person's weight in kilograms (kg) divided by their height in meters (m) squared and is associated with body fat and health risk.

basal metabolic rate	The rate at which energy is used by the body to maintain basal metabolism when a person is awake but inactive and has fasted for 14 to 18 hours. It typically accounts for 60 to 70 percent of daily energy use, but its value depends on body weight and other factors.
Dietary Reference Intake	Quantitative estimates of nutrient intakes that can be used for planning and assessing diets for apparently healthy people.
Delayed Type Skin Hypersensitivity	Test used as an indicator of the immune system function and that shows skin tissue injury due to phagocytic cell activation and inflammation induced by cell-mediated immunity. In experimental animal models, the injury is characterized by a granulomatous response consisting of macrophages, monocytes, and T lymphocytes.
Estimated Average Requirement	The average daily nutrient intake level estimated to meet the requirement of half the healthy individuals in a particular life stage and gender group (IOM, 2004)
Generally Recognized As Safe	Status of a food ingredient based on common knowledge about the safety of the ingredient through the scientific community that is knowledgeable in food toxicology and related disciplines specific to the safety and intended use of the ingredient under consideration.
Military Dietary Reference Intake	Nutritional standards, based on the Food and Nutrition Board's Dietary Reference Intakes, and intended for use by professional personnel involved in menu development, menu evaluation, nutrition education, nutrition research, and food research and development.
Niacin Equivalent	Because 60 mg of the amino acid tryptophan is equivalent to 1 mg of preformed dietary niacin, niacin equivalents are estimated by adding preformed niacin intake plus one-sixtieth of tryptophan intake.
Profile of Mood States	A 65-item, adjective rating subjective scale that measures moods and was used in the National Hospice Study and The Study to Understand Prognoses and Preferences for Outcomes, and Risks of Treatments.

Recommended Dietary Allowance	The average daily dietary nutrient intake level sufficient to meet the nutrient requirement of nearly all (97 to 98 percent) healthy individuals in a particular life stage and gender group (IOM, 2004).
Retinol Equivalent	The specific biological activity of 1.0 microgram of all-trans retinol, 6.0 micrograms of b-carotene, or 12.0 micrograms of other provitamin A carotenoids; it is equivalent to 3.3 international units of vitamin A activity from retinol (10 from b-carotene).
Tolerable Upper Intake Level	The highest average daily nutrient intake level that is likely to pose no risk of adverse health effects to almost all individuals in the general population. As intake increases above the UL, the potential risk of adverse effects may increase (IOM, 2004).
VO$_2$max	The maximum amount (usually expressed as a volume, liter) of oxygen that an individual can consume in a defined period of time (usually 1 minute). It may be expressed per kilogram of body weight (ml/kg/min). It reflects the upper limit of aerobic metabolism and limited by the amount of oxygen that can be delivered into the working muscle cells. Basically a product of the maximal cardiac output and maximal arterial-venous oxygen difference at the capillary-cell interface.

REFERENCE

IOM (Institute of Medicine). 2004. *Dietary Reference Intakes: Water, Potassium, Sodium, Chloride, and Sulfate.* Washington, DC: The National Academies Press.